DSM-IV Made Easy

DSM-IV Made Easy

THE CLINICIAN'S GUIDE TO DIAGNOSIS

James Morrison, M.D.

THE GUILFORD PRESS

New York   London

© 1995 The Guilford Press
A Division of Guilford Publications, Inc.
72 Spring Street, New York, NY 10012

Printed in the United States of America

This book is printed on acid-free paper.

Last digit is print number: 9 8

Library of Congress Cataloging-in-Publication Data

Morrison, James R., 1940–
    DSM-IV made easy / by James Morrison.
        p.   cm.
    Includes bibliographical references and index.
    ISBN 0-89862-568-8
    1. Mental illness—Diagnosis.   2. Mental illness—Classification.
3. Diagnostic and Statistical Manual of Mental Disorders.
I. Title.
    [DNLM: 1. Mental Disorders—diagnosis.   2. Mental disorders—
classification.   WM   141   1994]
RC469.M676   1994
616.89′075—dc20
DNLM/DLC
for Library of Congress   94-34302
                                                                          CIP

For Mary,
my *sine qua non*

Acknowledgments

Many people helped in the creation of this book. I want especially to thank my wife, Mary, who has provided unfailingly excellent advice and support always.

Others who have read portions of the manuscript in one stage or another include Richard Maddock, M.D., Nicholas Rosenlicht, M.D., James Picano, Ph.D., K. H. Blacker, M.D., Irwin Feinberg, M.D., Lee Robins, Ph.D., and Rita Hargrave, M.D. I am also profoundly indebted to the anonymous reviewers who provided input; you know who you are, even if I don't.

My editor, Kitty Moore, a keen and wonderful critic, helped develop the concept. I also deeply appreciate the many editors and production people at Guilford who, under the careful supervision of Rowena Howells, helped shape and speed this book into print. I would single out Marie Sprayberry, who went the last mile with her thoughtful, meticulous copyediting. And I am indebted to Molly Mullikin, the perfect secretary, who has contributed hours of transcription and years of intelligent service.

To all of these, and to the countless patients who have provided the clinical material for this book, I am profoundly grateful.

Contents

DSM-IV Made Easy

Introduction

Why Did I Write This Book?

Anyone who works with mental health patients needs to know the fourth edition of the *Diagnostic and Statistical Manual of Mental Disorders* (DSM-IV), published by the American Psychiatric Association—it has become the world's standard for evaluation and diagnosis. But the DSM-IV requires a great deal of concentration. Written by a committee with the goal of providing standards for research as well as clinical practice in all the mental health fields, it covers nearly every conceivable contingency. But you'll probably come away from it not knowing how the diagnostic criteria translate to a real live patient.

I wrote *DSM-IV Made Easy* to make DSM-IV accessible to clinicians from all mental health professions. In these pages, you will find descriptions of every mental disorder that occurs in adults. You will learn how to diagnose each one.

What Have I Done to Make DSM-IV Easy?

Whenever possible, I have simplified criteria to make them more understandable. I have emphasized the material a clinician needs to cover when diagnosing an adult mental patient. Some of the explanatory material that DSM-IV includes in the criteria I have moved to the coding notes (see below). It's still there, but I've tried to put it where it won't get in your way unless you really need it. I have also divided certain of the criteria into two or more, in order to limit each criterion to one main principle. Everywhere, I have tried to write simple, declarative sentences that describe what you need to know in diagnosing a patient.

To underscore or augment what you need to know, I have interspersed the text with "Tips." Some of these merely highlight information that will help you make a diagnosis quickly. Some are sidebars that contain historical information and other interesting sidelights about diagnoses. I have also offered editorial asides—my opinions about diagnosis, patients, and clinical matters in general. Throughout, I have tried to give you what you need to know in a form that is clinically relevant and a format that is accessible.

Finally, I have used that reliable device, the clinical vignette. As a student, I found that I often had trouble keeping in mind the points of a diagnosis (such as it was in those days). But once I had evaluated and treated a patient, I always had a mental image to help me remember important points about symptoms and differential diagnosis. I hope that the patients I have described in *DSM-IV Made Easy* will do the same for you.

How to Use This Book

Before you can make any diagnosis, you need information. It will come from three sources: patient records, informants, and interviews with patients themselves. Neither *DSM-IV Made Easy* nor DSM-IV itself will help you much with interview technique. For help, consult texts such as another book of mine, *The First Interview* (New York: Guilford Press, 1995).

Once you have collected your data base of information, select the problem area that seems most likely to include your patient's diagnosis. Problem areas (psychotic disorders, mood disorders, anxiety disorders, etc.) will be covered in one of the various chapters of *DSM-IV Made Easy*. Some patients will have problems in a number of these areas, so you may have to explore several chapters to select just the right diagnosis. Chapter 18 provides some additional pointers on how to construct a differential diagnosis.

Once you have selected a chapter to explore further, turn to the Quick Guide at its beginning. Each of these brief sections outlines the disorders discussed in that chapter; in addition, you will find references to disorders in other chapters that can cause similar symptoms. Based on the Quick Guide description, turn to a disorder that seems a likely candidate. You will find several sorts of information:

Introductory Material. This information is designed to help orient you to the diagnosis. Usually, it will include a brief review of important diagnostic points and demographic information.

The Vignette. You will find well over 100 of them. (I discuss them more fully at the end of this Introduction.)

Diagnostic Criteria. These restate all the requirements printed in DSM-IV, though the wording is somewhat different. I have also substituted bullets (•) and checks (✓) for the numbering system in the DSM-IV criteria. Bulleted criteria are *mandatory* and must be fulfilled. Checked items are part of a list and are *selective*—only a certain number of these must be fulfilled to qualify for the diagnoses. Of course, the changes from the official DSM-IV criteria are only cosmetic. You will draw essentially the same conclusions from both sets of criteria.

Coding Notes. These notes follow many criteria lists and supply additional information about coding, subtypes, and specifiers whenever such information is relevant. As mentioned above, I have also moved some explanatory material that DSM-IV includes in the criteria to these notes.

Evaluation. This is a discussion of the patient presented in the vignette, emphasizing the most likely of the differential diagnoses. I explain how the patient fits the diagnostic criteria and why I think other diagnoses are unlikely. Sometimes I suggest that additional history or medical or psychological testing should be obtained before a final diagnosis is given.

Five-Axis Diagnosis. This embodies all the diagnostic material that seems relevant to the patient, presented in the approved format. It explains how this particular patient should be coded and provides a model for the use of these codes in other patients. (This is an important point: Assigning codes is not always perfectly logical.)

I recommend that you confine your study to relatively short segments. I have done my best to simplify the criteria and to explain the reasoning behind them. But you will probably find that, if you read more than a few diagnoses at a time, they will begin to run together in your mind. I also recommend one other step to help you learn faster. After you have read through a vignette, go back and try to pick out each of the diagnostic criteria before you look at my evaluation. You will retain the material better if you actively match the case history information with the criteria than if you just rely on passively absorbing what I have written.

Important Features of This Book

The first 16 chapters contain descriptions and criteria for the Axis I and II diagnoses. Chapter 17 comprises information concerning other terms that you may find useful. Some of these are V-codes, which are conditions that are not official mental disorders but may require clinical attention anyway. An example would be V65.2 (Malingering). V-codes may be listed on Axis I as the reason why the patient has been referred for evaluation. Also described here are codes that indicate the effects of medication, psychological factors that affect a medical disorder, and the need for more diagnostic information.

Chapter 18 contains a general discussion of diagnostic principles, followed by some additional case vignettes. Generally more complicated than those presented earlier in the book, these histories have been annotated to help you to review the diagnostic principles and criteria covered previously. Of course, I could include only a small fraction of all adult diagnoses in this section.

Using the DSM-IV Multiaxial Classification

DSM-IV offers five axes on which to record the biopsychosocial assessment of your patient. The first three axes are for recording the mental and physical diagnoses; the others enable you to note environmental problems and to provide an assessment of the patient's functioning over the previous year. Here is how you can write up the diagnosis.

Axis I: Mental Disorders

On Axis I, record every mental diagnosis except the personality disorders and Mental Retardation. Nearly every patient will have at least one Axis I diagnosis, and many will have more than one. For example, consider a patient with two Axis I diagnoses: Bipolar I Disorder and Alcohol Dependence. (Note, incidentally, that I capitalize the names of all specific Axis I and II diagnoses, following DSM-IV's style. However, I do not capitalize the names of *groups* of Axis I and II disorders, such as the mood disorders and the personality disorders.) Following the DSM-IV convention, first list the diagnosis most responsible for the current evaluation. In the example just cited, suppose that the patient was a man who had been admitted after a heavy episode of drinking. He had been taking lithium and had had no symptoms of mood disorder for two years. Then his diagnosis should read:

> Axis I   291.8   Alcohol Withdrawal
> 303.90   Alcohol Dependence
> 296.46   Bipolar I Disorder, Most Recent Episode Manic, In Full Remission

In this example, the first diagnosis would have to be Alcohol Withdrawal (that's why the patient sought treatment). But suppose that the patient had taken disulfiram for a year, had not been drinking, and was currently experiencing a severe depression. Then his Axis I diagnosis would read:

> Axis I   296.53   Bipolar I Disorder, Most Recent Episode Depressed, Severe Without Psychotic Features
> 303.90   Alcohol Dependence, Sustained Full Remission

Indicating Certainty of a Diagnosis

When you are uncertain whether a diagnosis is correct, consider using the qualifier (Provisional). This term may be appropriate if you believe that a certain diagnosis is correct, but lack sufficient history to support your impression. Or perhaps it is still early in the course of your patient's illness and you expect that more symptoms will develop shortly. Or perhaps you are waiting for laboratory tests to confirm the presence of a general medical condition that you suspect underlies your patient's illness. Any of these situations could warrant a provisional diagnosis.

TIP What about a patient who comes very close to meeting full criteria, who has been ill for a long time, who has responded to treatment appropriate for the diagnosis, and who has a family history of the same disorder? *I* would probably give that patient a definitive diagnosis, even though the criteria are not quite met. Diagnoses are *not* decided by the criteria; diagnoses are decided by clinicians, who use criteria as guidelines.

Indicating Severity of a Disorder

In the two examples given above, the clinician indicated the severity of the mood disorder. Some diagnostic categories (mood and substance-related disorders, Mental Retardation, Conduct Disorder) specify severity criteria; you will find them described in their appropriate chapters in the text. But if you wish, you can specify severity for *any* Axis I or Axis II diagnosis. Use these generic guidelines:

Mild. The patient has few symptoms other than the minimum criteria needed.

Moderate. Intermediate between Mild and Severe.

Severe. The patient has many more symptoms than the minimum criteria specify, or some symptoms are especially severe, or functioning in society or at work is especially compromised.

In Partial Remission. The patient previously met full criteria for the diagnosis; although some of them now remain, they are too few to fulfill criteria currently.

In Full Remission. The patient has been symptom-free for a period of time that seems clinically relevant to the diagnosis.

Prior History. The patient appears to have recovered from the disorder, but you feel that it is important to mention it.

Axis II: Personality Disorders and Mental Retardation

A separate axis for the personality disorders and Mental Retardation helps to ensure that they will not be ignored when you are dealing with your patient's often more pressing Axis I pathology. Many patients have more than one Axis II diagnosis.

For some patients, an Axis II condition is the most important reason for seeking evaluation. This is especially likely in those with Borderline or Antisocial Personality Disorder. In such a patient, you can indicate that any Axis I disorders are not the focus of clinical attention by adding the words (Principal Diagnosis) after the Axis II diagnosis.

Axis III: Physical Conditions and Disorders

Physical illness may have a direct bearing on the patient's Axis I diagnoses; this is especially true of the cognitive disorders. In other cases, physical illness may affect (or be affected by) the management of an Axis I or Axis II disorder. An example would be hypertension in a psychotic patient who believes that the medication has been poisoned. Of course, you may make multiple diagnoses on Axis III.

Axis IV: Psychosocial and Environmental Problems

Use Axis IV to report any environmental or other psychosocial event or condition that might affect the diagnosis or management of your patient. These may have been caused by the Axis I or Axis II disorder, or they may be independent events. They should have occurred within the year prior to your evaluation. If they occurred earlier, they must have contributed to the development of the mental disorder or must be a focus of treatment. When stating them on Axis IV, be as specific as possible. (Other problems are possible; these are samples.)

Economic Problems. Examples: poverty; debt or credit problems; inadequate welfare or child support.

Housing Problems. Examples: disagreements with landlord or neighbors; homelessness; poor housing; dangerous neighborhood.

Problems with Primary Support Group. Examples: death of a relative; illness in relative; family disruption through divorce or separation; remarriage of parent; physical or sexual abuse, disagreements with relatives.

Occupational Problems. Examples: stressful work conditions or schedule; change of job; dissatisfaction with job; disagreements with supervisor or coworkers; possibility of job loss; unemployment.

Educational Problems. Examples: academic problems; disagreements with classmates or teachers; illiteracy; poor school environment.

Problems Related to the Social Environment. Examples: loss or death of friend; acculturation problems; racial or sexual discrimination; retirement; living alone; social isolation.

Problems Related to Interaction with the Legal System/Crime. Examples: being arrested; being incarcerated; suing or being sued; being a victim of crime.

Other Psychosocial Problems. Examples: disagreements with care giving professionals (counselor, social workers, physician); exposure to war, natural disasters, or other catastrophes; unavailability of social service agencies.

Problems with Access to Health Care Services. Examples: inadequate health care services; no or insufficient health insurance; unavailability of transportation to health care services.

Psychosocial and environmental problems will nearly always be coded on Axis IV. However, occasionally one of these problems may be the focus for evaluation or treatment. Then it should be listed with the appropriate V-code number (see Chapter 17) on Axis I, as in this example:

> Axis I   V62.2   Occupational Problem (disagreement with supervisor)

Axis IV notations will usually relate to distressing conditions, but occasionally there may be a "positive stressor" (a marriage, a promotion at work). Mention only positive stressors that have caused problems for the patient.

Axis V: Global Assessment of Functioning (GAF)

The GAF score reflects the patient's current overall occupational, psychological, and social functioning. It is *not* supposed to reflect physical limitations or environmental problems. It is recorded as a single number on a 100-point scale. The scale specifies symptoms and behavioral guidelines to help you determine your patient's GAF score. Perhaps because of the subjectivity inherent in this scale, its greatest usefulness may be in tracking *changes* in a patient's level of functioning across time. The GAF scale is reproduced in its entirety in Appendix A.

What Is a Mental Disorder?

There are many definitions of *mental disorder*, none of which is both accurate and complete. Perhaps this is because nobody yet has adequately defined the term *abnormal*. (Does it mean that the patient is uncomfortable? Then many patients with Manic Episodes are not abnormal. Is *abnormal* that which is unusual? Then very bright people are abnormal.)

The authors of DSM-IV provide the definition of *mental disorder* that they used to help them to decide whether to include a diagnosis in their book. Paraphrased, here it is:

> A *mental disorder* is a clinically important collection of symptoms (these can be behavioral or psychological) that causes an individual distress, disability, or the increased risk of suffering pain, disability, death, or the loss of freedom.

The symptoms of any disorder must be something more than an expected reaction to an everyday event, such as the death of a relative. Behaviors that primarily reflect a conflict between the individual and society (e.g., over religious or political ideology) are not usually considered mental disorders.

A number of additional points about the criteria for mental disorders bear emphasizing:

1. Mental disorders describe disease processes, not people. This point is made explicit to address the fears of some clinicians that by using the criteria, they are somehow "pigeonholing people." Patients with the same diagnosis may be quite different from one another in many important aspects, including symptoms, personality, and other diagnoses they may have.

2 Don't assume that there are sharp boundaries between disorders or between any disorder and "normality." For example, the criteria for Alcohol Abuse and Alcohol Dependence clearly set these two disorders off from each other (and from people who have neither). In reality, all alcohol users probably fit somewhere along a continuum.

3. There is no essential difference between a physical condition such as pneumonia or diabetes and a mental disorder such as Schizophrenia or Bipolar I Disorder. Either mental disorder could turn out to have a physical basis. In operational terms, the difference between Axis III and Axes I and II is that Axis III diagnoses are not the subject of DSM-IV or of this manual.

4. Basically, DSM-IV follows the *medical model of illness*. By this, I don't mean that it recommends the prescription of medication. I mean that it is a descriptive work derived from scientific studies of groups of patients who appear to have a great deal in common, including symptoms, signs, and life course of their disease.

5. DSM-IV makes no assumptions as to the etiology of most of these disorders. This is the famous "atheoretical approach" that has been much praised and criticized. Of course, most clinicians would agree about the cause of some mental disorders (cognitive disorders such as Dementia Due to Huntington's Disease come to mind). The descriptions of the majority of DSM-IV diagnoses will be well accepted by clinicians whose philosophical perspectives include social and learning theory, psychodynamics, and psychopharmacology.

Warnings

In offering criteria for mental health disorders, DSM-IV posts several warnings that seem worth repeating:

1. The fact that the manual omits a disorder doesn't mean it doesn't exist. With each new edition of the DSM, the number of listed mental disorders has increased. DSM-IV is no exception—it contains some 340 conditions, nearly 120 more than its predecessor, DSM-III-R. The conclusion should be obvious: There are probably still more conditions out there, waiting to be discovered. Prepare to invest in *DSM-V Made Easy*.

2. DSM-IV isn't for amateurs. Owning a list of criteria is no substitute for professional training in interview techniques, diagnosis, and the many other skills that a mental health clinician needs.

3. DSM-IV may not be uniformly applicable to all cultures. Most of the studies on which these criteria are based used patients from the United States and Canada. Although DSM-III-R has been widely used with great success throughout the world, it is not assured that mental disorders largely described by North American and European clinicians will translate to other languages and other cultures. We should be wary of diagnosing pathology in patients who may express unusual beliefs that may be widely held in ethnic or other subcultures. An example would be the belief in witches prevalent among certain Native Americans. Beginning on page 843, DSM-IV lists a number of specific cultural syndromes.

4. DSM-IV isn't meant to have the force of law. Its authors recognize that the definitions used by the judicial system are often at odds with scientific requirements. Thus, having a DSM-IV mental disorder may not exempt a patient from punishment or other legal restrictions on behavior.

The Vignettes

The clinical vignettes in this book are based on real people. Some are composites of several people I have known. In any case, I have altered vital information to protect the identities of all. The vignettes do not present all of the features of the diagnoses they are meant to illustrate (but then hardly any patient does). My intention has been to convey the flavor of each disorder.

Although I have provided vignettes for nearly all of the major DSM-IV conditions, you may notice some omissions. Especially in the mood disorders, I have left out those that elaborate what is obvious or what has already been stated. Some are frankly too numerous; to illustrate every possible substance-related disorder would itself take a book twice the length of this one. And I have included vignettes only for those disorders beginning in early life (Mental Retardation, Attention Deficit/Hyperactivity Disorder, and Tourette's Disorder) that are most likely to be encountered by mental health clinicians who evaluate adults. However, for your convenience you will find in Chapter 16 criteria for all disorders beginning in infancy, childhood, or adolescence. *DSM-IV Made Easy* therefore contains diagnostic criteria for all DSM-IV mental disorders.

CHAPTER 1

Delirium, Dementia, and Amnestic and Other Cognitive Disorders

Quick Guide to the Cognitive Disorders

Although there are many conditions in this diverse category, they are classified logically enough that learning (and remembering) them isn't much of a problem.

Delirium

A delirium is a rapidly developing, fluctuating state of reduced awareness in which the following are true:

- The patient has trouble shifting or focusing attention, *and*
- The patient has at least one defect of memory, orientation, perception, or language, *and*
- The symptoms are not better explained by a dementia.

One of the following causes can be identified (here and throughout, the page number in each case indicates where a more detailed discussion begins):

Delirium Due to a General Medical Condition. Delirium can be caused by trauma to the brain, infections, epilepsy, endocrine disorders, toxicity from medications, poisons, and various other diseases throughout the body (p. 18). I have listed many of these conditions in Appendix B.

Substance-Induced Delirium. Alcohol and other sedative drugs of abuse, as well as nearly every class of street drug, can cause delirium. Medications can also be implicated (p. 21).

Delirium Due to Multiple Etiologies. Occasionally, more than one cause for delirium will be identified in the same patient (p. 25).

Delirium Not Otherwise Specified. Use this category when you don't know the cause of a patient's delirium (p. 27).

Dementia

A dementia differs from a delirium in several ways:

- To diagnose a dementia, there must be memory loss as well as other cognitive deficits (these include amnesia, aphasia, apraxia, agnosia, and loss of executive functioning; see TIP p. 15.
- Any impairment in the ability to focus or shift attention is not prominent.
- The cause of dementia can usually be found within the central nervous system (with delirium, the cause is often elsewhere in the body).
- As compared with delirium, dementia is relatively fixed (unchanging).
- Although patients occasionally recover from a dementia, this is not usual.

One of the following types will be identified:

Dementia of the Alzheimer's Type. This is the most common cause of senility. It begins gradually and usually progresses inexorably. A bit more than half of all dementias are of the Alzheimer's type (p. 30).

Vascular Dementia. Due to vascular brain disease, these patients experience loss of memory and other cognitive abilities. Often this is a stepwise process, with relatively sudden onset and a fluctuating course. Ten to twenty percent of dementias are vascular (p. 35).

Dementia Due to Other General Medical Conditions. A large number of other medical conditions can cause dementia (again, see Appendix B). Some of the most noteworthy include brain tumor, Creutzfeldt–Jakob disease (infection by a slow virus), head trauma, human immunodeficiency virus (HIV) disease, Huntington's disease, Parkinson's disease, and Pick's disease. The most common toxins causing dementia are those resulting from kidney and liver failure (p. 38).

Substance-Induced Persisting Dementia. Five to ten percent of dementias are related to prolonged use of alcohol, inhalants, or sedatives (p. 41).

Dementia Due to Multiple Etiologies. Use this category when evidence for your patient points to more than one of the causes above (p. 44).

Dementia Not Otherwise Specified. This category is useful when you know the patient is demented, but you don't know why (p. 46).

Amnestic Disorders

Amnestic is just a fancy way of saying "amnesia." Here are the main features:

- There is no requirement for reduced ability to focus or shift attention.
- Memory is affected far more than any other function, sometimes to the extent that patients will forget conversations that took place only a few minutes earlier.
- In some cases, especially early in the course of their illness, patients with an amnestic disorder will try to hide a loss of memory by making up (*confabulating*) experiences.

One of the following types will be identified:

Amnestic Disorder Due to a General Medical Condition. These patients have symptoms very much like those of Korsakoff's syndrome (see below), but there is a medical cause (see Appendix B), such as hypoxia, stroke, head trauma, or herpes simplex encephalitis (p. 46).

Substance-Induced Persisting Amnestic Disorder. Popularly known as Korsakoff's syndrome, this is the classical amnestic disorder. It most often occurs in an alcoholic patient who suffers from thiamine (vitamin B1) deficiency (p. 49).

Amnestic Disorder Not Otherwise Specified. Use this category for patients who have severe memory problems and little else in the way of cognitive disability, and you don't know the underlying cause (p. 52).

Other Causes of Cognitive Symptoms

Age-Related Cognitive Decline. Older patients who report trouble remembering names, telephone numbers, or places where they put things may, upon testing, have a memory problem that is consistent with age and not pathological (p. 540).

Dissociative Disorders. Profound, temporary loss of memory may occur in persons who suffer from Dissociative Amnesia (p. 319), Dissociative Fugue (p. 322), or Dissociative Identity Disorder (p. 325).

Pseudodementia. From their apathy and slowed responses, some patients often look as if they have the severe memory loss and other symptoms of dementia. But careful clinical evaluation and psychological testing reveal severe Major Depressive Disorder and cognitive functioning that is relatively intact, though they may have problems with attention and concentration. Pseudodementia accounts for about 5% of patients referred for a dementia workup. Depressive pseudodementia is found only in the elderly.

Malingering. Some patients will intentionally exaggerate or falsify cognitive symptoms to obtain funds (insurance, worker's compensation) or to avoid punishment or military service (p. 539).

Factitious Disorder With Predominantly Psychological Signs and Symptoms. Some patients may feign cognitive symptoms, but not for direct gain. Their motive is to be hospitalized or otherwise cared for (p. 312).

Introduction

Cognition is the mental processing of information. Both memory and thinking are involved in the storage, retrieval, and manipulation of information.

The cognitive disorders are abnormalities of thinking and memory that are associated with temporary or permanent brain dysfunction. Their main symptoms include problems with memory, orientation, language, information processing, and the ability to focus and sustain attention on a task. A clinician obtains information about these symptoms by observing the patient during the interview and by asking the patient to perform certain tasks during the evaluation of mental status. A cognitive disorder is caused by a general medical condition or substance use that leads to defects of brain structure, chemistry, or physiology. However, the underlying causative agent cannot always be defined.

When recognized and properly treated, many cognitive disorders (especially delirium) are reversible; ignored, they can lead to permanent disability. Moreover, although the criteria are relatively simple, their associated symptoms can make the cognitive disorders mimic virtually any other Axis I condition.

For example, delirium can present with symptoms of depression and anxiety; dementia can present with psychosis. Whatever history or symptoms your patient presents, therefore, it is vital to place the cognitive disorders near the top of your differential diagnosis. If you forget about cognitive disorders, emotional symptoms can all too easily obscure an underlying delirium, or you may also diagnose a psychosis such as Schizophrenia when your patient actually has a dementia.

Depending on the underlying cause, cognitive disorders can begin at any age. They are extremely common, especially in a hospital setting. They may constitute as many of one out of five of all mental health admissions.

TIP Although aphasia, amnesia, agnosia, apraxia, and loss of executive functioning play an important role in the diagnosis of cognitive disorders, when they occur in isolation they usually fall under the care of neurologists. The terms may need some explanation.

Amnesia is, of course, a loss of memory. It can be *retrograde* (loss of memory for events that occurred before a certain time) or *anterograde* (loss of ability to form new memories).

Aphasia means a disturbance of language use. Because of brain pathology, the patient becomes unable to use words as symbols.

Apraxia is the inability to perform a motor behavior, even though the muscles and nerves required for the motion are themselves intact.

Agnosia is the inability to recognize familiar objects, even though the senses required for this recognition are intact.

Loss of executive functioning means difficulty in planning, organizing, sequencing, or abstracting information.

Confusion is a term that is often used to describe slowed thinking, loss of memory, or disorientation in patients with cognitive disorders. You should be familiar with it, because other health care providers (neurologists and internists), as well as patients and the general public, may use it. However, the term is inexact and, well, confusing; I've tried to avoid it.

Mental health clinicians often use the term *functional* to describe disorders for which they can find no basis in brain anatomy, chemistry, or physiology. Most mood disorders and psychoses are called functional; we still don't know why or how they have developed. The cognitive disorders are not functional, but are caused by well-defined abnormalities of brain chemistry, anatomy, or physiology.

DELIRIUM

Delirium is a result of a change in the way the brain is working, but the underlying cause is usually a disease process that lies elsewhere in the body, outside the central nervous system (see Appendix B). It is easy to state the basic symptoms of delirium:

- Reduced clarity of awareness of the environment, accompanied by
- Some sort of cognitive deficit.

You can recognize reduced clarity of awareness of the environment by the difficulty patients have in maintaining and shifting attention as you interact with them. Inattention is usually the first symptom; patients may experience it as drowsiness or somnolence. Their thought processes slow down and they may seem vague; they have trouble solving problems and reasoning. You may have to ask questions several times before the patients heed them. On the other hand, inattention may show up instead as a hyperalert distractibility, with rapid shifts from one focus of attention to another.

The cognitive deficit can be a problem with language, memory, orientation, or perception; several of these are often present at the same time. Following are some of the areas in which delirium patients have problems. Those that constitute DSM-IV criteria for delirium I have marked with a bullet.

- **Language.** You will recognize problems with language in speech that is rambling, disjointed, pressured, or incoherent, or speech that leaps from one topic to another. Some patients will have trouble writing or naming things. Speech that is merely slurred, without demonstrating incoherent thoughts, suggests intoxication, not delirium.

- **Memory.** Delirious patients nearly always have trouble remembering things. Recent events are always affected; older memories (especially those from childhood) are usually the last to go.

- **Orientation.** Many patients will be disoriented, sometimes so severely that you cannot examine them adequately. Disorientation is most likely to be for time (date, day, month, year); next comes disorientation for place; last, patients fail to recognize relatives and friends (disorientation for person). Only in very severe cases are patients unsure of their own identities.

- **Perception.** Several sorts of perceptual difficulties can accompany a delirium. Patients with mild or early delirium don't perceive their surroundings as clearly as usual: Boundaries are fuzzy, colors are brighter, images distorted. Some patients misidentify what they see (*illusions*), whereas others experience false perceptions (*hallucinations*; these are especially likely to be visual). If they later experience false beliefs or ideas (*delusions*) grafted onto their hallucinations, these delusions are usually incomplete, changing, or poorly organized. Confronted by visual hallucinations, patients may not be able to tell whether they are dreaming or awake. If they accept their hallucinations as reality, they may become anxious or fearful.

Other areas often revealing disturbance in delirium include the following:

Sleep–Wake Cycle. A change in a patient's normal sleep–wake cycle (insomnia, day–night reversal, vivid dreams or nightmares) almost invariably occurs.

Psychomotor Activity and Behavior. Sometimes physical movements may be slowed down, especially if the delirium is due to metabolic problems; these patients appear retarded and sluggish. Others may have increased motor activity (agitated behavior, picking at bedsheets, etc.). Patients may react to their experiences and emotions by weeping or yelling. A flapping tremor of the hands is common. So are vocalizations, which are sometimes no more than muttering or moans. Patients may strike out if they feel threatened; sometimes they attempt to run away.

Mood. Depression and fear are both common reactions to the experiences mentioned above. (Dysphoria can sometimes be the presenting symptom in delirium; then there is a danger that the patient may be misdiagnosed as having Major Depressive Disorder or Dysthymic Disorder.) Some patients will only react with perplexity; still others will exhibit bland, calm acceptance.

Reasoning. This ability is often impaired.

Delirium usually begins suddenly, and its intensity often fluctuates. Most patients will be more lucid in the morning and worse at night—a transient phenomenon called *sundowning*. When you suspect delirium, interview the patient in separate sessions several hours apart. Because the symptoms of delirium so often fluctuate with time of day, normal or marginal findings at noon may give way to abnormal findings in the evening. If this is not practical, nursing staff (or notes in the patient's chart) may provide the needed information.

Most deliriums last a week or less and then resolve, once the underlying condition has been relieved. Sometimes delirium will evolve into a dementia or an amnestic disorder. After delirium resolves, most patients recall the experiences incompletely; they may have amnesia for certain (or all) aspects. That which is recalled may seem like a dream. Delirium is common on medical wards, where it may be mistaken for other mental disorders, including psychosis, depression, mania, "hysteria," or personality disorder.

Delirium is the most common of the cognitive disorders. In fact, it has the highest incidence of all mental disorders. By some estimates, up to half of hospitalized elderly patients become delirious. It is more common in children and the elderly than in young and middle-aged adults.

Delirium can have many causes, few of which have specific features. The cause of delirium depends on the patient's age group. In children, fever and infection are the most common causes; in young adults, drugs; in middle-aged adults, withdrawal from alcohol and head injury; in the old, metabolic problems, cardiovascular failure, and excessive medications. Often, delirium in an older patient will have multiple causes

Because it may be caused by a disease that can lead to dementia or even kill outright, any delirium is a true emergency. When you suspect one, immediately obtain appropriate medical consultation or testing; often, evaluation by a neurologist will be required. However, formal (neuropsychological) testing can be difficult in patients who cannot adequately sustain attention on a task. Therefore, the diagnosis of delirium may sometimes depend on the clinician's bed-side evaluation.

> **TIP** Delirium has many aliases. Neurologists and internists call it *acute confusional state*. Other terms sometimes used for delirium include *toxic psychosis*, *acute brain syndrome*, and *metabolic encephalopathy*. These terms are useful to know when discussing a delirious patient with professionals who do not specialize in mental health.
>
> Some clinicians regard delirium as a state of agitated mental confusion during which the patient experiences visual hallucinations that are unusually vivid. This would be the case for delirium tremens. However, DSM-IV uses the term *delirium* in a much broader sense, to encompass conditions with the more varied symptoms listed in the criteria.

293.0 Delirium Due to a General Medical Condition

Although the brain itself can be directly involved (as with a brain tumor or seizure disorder), the cause of delirium is usually a disease process that begins outside the central nervous system. These can include endocrine disorders, infections, drug withdrawal or toxicity, vitamin deficiency, fever, liver or kidney disease, poisons, and the effects of surgical operations. A more complete listing is given in Appendix B).

Criteria for Delirium Due to a General Medical Condition

- The patient has a reduced level of consciousness and difficulty focusing, shifting, or sustaining attention.
- There has been a cognitive change (deficit of language, memory, orientation, perception) that a dementia cannot better explain.
- These symptoms develop rapidly (hours to days) and tend to vary during the day.
- History, physical examination, or laboratory data suggest that a general medical condition has directly caused the condition.

Coding Notes

The name of the general medical condition is included as a part of the Axis I code for delirium; that is, the term "General Medical Condition" does not appear in the code.

If the patient has a pre-existing Dementia of the Alzheimer's Type or Vascular Dementia, only one code is needed because "With Delirium" can be coded as a specifier. For example:

Axis I   290.11   Dementia of the Alzheimer's Type, With Early
                    Onset, With Delirium

If the dementia is caused by a general medical condition, it and the delirium must be coded separately. For example:

Axis I   294.1   Dementia Due to Parkinson's Disease
          293.0   Delirium Due to Congestive Heart Failure

Axis III 332.0   Parkinson's disease
          428.9   Congestive heart failure

Note also that all causative agents are coded on Axis III.

Harold Hoyt

After rheumatic heart disease had led to years of gradually worsening short-ness of breath and fatiguability, Harold Hoyt, a 48-year-old bricklayer, finally consented to a mitral valve replacement. Warning him that open heart surgery could cause delirium, his surgeon had recommended mental health consulta-tion as a preventive measure.

"I ain't crazy," said Harold by way of refusal.

The procedure went well, but the recovery room staff noticed right away that Harold seemed withdrawn and uncommunicative. He ignored his wife and grown daughter during their brief hourly visits. When he spoke or wrote notes, it was usually to complain about the tube in his nose or about his inability to sleep in the brightly lighted intensive care unit (ICU).

On the third postoperative day, Harold became increasingly restless. After he pulled out his nasogastric tube, he was quieter for a time, but in the evening he was found crying and trying to get out of bed. He asked a nurse why he was there, and was incredulous when told that he had had open heart surgery. As they spoke, his voice trailed off, and he seemed to forget that anyone was there. When he spoke again, he asked about the outcome of a football game that had been played the week before.

The following morning Harold carried on a normal, though brief, conver-sation with the dietary aide who brought breakfast. But by nightfall he was again talking to himself and had to be restrained from pulling out his IV. He was able to give the date accurately, however.

A mental health consultant diagnosed a "classic postcardiotomy delirium" and recommended that family members sit with Harold to provide stimulation and reality checks. His improving physical condition allowed him to be moved off the ICU. Within 36 hours he was fully oriented and conversing normally with his family. He remembered nothing of his behavior of the past two days and seemed surprised that he had required restraints.

Evaluation of Harold Hoyt

The principal feature differentiating a delirium from a **dementia** is that delirious patients must have an inability to focus and sustain attention. Harold had trouble completing a thought (his voice trailed off in midsentence and he changed the topic to football). It had developed rapidly, which is another criterion for delirium.

Harold's cognitive problem was with short-term memory (among other things, he forgot that he had had surgery). On at least one occasion he was disoriented to time; however, disorientation is not essential to the diagnosis of delirium.

Harold experienced several other symptoms typical of delirium. His symptoms fluctuated with time of day, increasing in the evening and at night—an example of sundowning. He became somewhat agitated and tried to get out of bed; perhaps this was due to anxiety at finding himself in a strange place without knowing why.

When his delirium was first developing, Harold was withdrawn and seemed irritable. These features suggest a **depressive disorder**, which is only one of many Axis I disorders sometimes confused with the cognitive disorders. Because hallucinations are so common, **Schizophrenia** and other psychoic disorders also appear in the differential diagnosis, although the history of an operation and rapid fluctuations in cognition are giveaways. Occasionally a patient (especially one who has a background in health care) will feign the symptoms of delirium to obtain money or for some other gain. This sort of deception can be difficult to detect; when it is found, **Malingering** should be diagnosed. When the motive behind such deception is only to be a patient, **Factitious Disorder With Psychological Symptoms** should be considered.

The variety of **general medical conditions** that can cause delirium is vast. Many of them are included in Appendix B, though even that list is by no means complete. As the consultant noted, cardiotomy is a classical precipitant of delirium (about 25% of open heart surgery patients experience it); somewhat ironically for Harold, the strongest preventative measure against postcardiotomy delirium is a mental health consultation before surgery. When you are coding, be sure to include on Axis III the medical condition(s) responsible for the delirium. In this case, it would not be coded as a health-care-related problem on Axis IV: Harold's problem wasn't that he couldn't get access to health care, but that he had had surgery.

Axis I	293.0	Delirium Due to Chest Surgery
Axis II	V71.09	No diagnosis
Axis III	35.24	Mitral valve replacement (with prosthesis)

```
Axis IV          None
Axis V    GAF = 40   (on admission)
          GAF = 71   (at discharge)
```

Substance-Induced Delirium

People who abuse street drugs or alcohol are at serious risk for developing a delirium. Many drugs can produce intoxication delirium, but abrupt cessation of heavy use of other sedative drugs, such as barbiturates, can produce a withdrawal delirium. The most commonly known is Alcohol Withdrawal Delirium (popularly called *delirium tremens*, or DTs). Its hallmarks are agitation, tremor, disorientation, and vivid hallucinations. In someone who has suddenly stopped after many weeks of heavy drinking, DTs occurs within a few days. DTs can also be precipitated when the patient develops a medical illness (such as liver failure, head trauma, pneumonia, or pancreatitis); alcoholics are at special risk for each of these conditions. Alcohol Withdrawal Delirium isn't especially common, even among the heaviest users of alcohol. But it is so severe that, untreated, as many as 15% die. This makes it an extremely important mental health event.

Delirium—especially intoxication delirium, but also the withdrawal type—can also be caused by a prescribed medication. Medications don't have to be present in high concentrations. In combination with other drugs or illnesses, delirium can occur even at low doses, especially in older people. Drugs with anticholinergic effects (such as antiparkinsonian drugs and antidepressants) are probably the most likely to produce delirium. Although intoxication delirium can occur within minutes of taking cocaine or hallucinogens, for many medications it will occur only after drug levels have built up over several days or longer.

The criteria for Substance Intoxication Delirium and Substance Withdrawal Delirium are quite similar, but not identical:

Criteria for Substance Intoxication Delirium

- The patient has a reduced level of consciousness and difficulty focusing, shifting, or sustaining attention.
- There has been a cognitive change (deficit of language, memory, orientation, perception) that a dementia cannot better explain.
- These symptoms develop rapidly (hours to days) and tend to fluctuate during the day.
- History, physical examination, or laboratory data suggest that *either*:
  ✓ the symptoms developed during a substance intoxication, *or*
  ✓ they are caused by the use of a medication.

Criteria for Substance Withdrawal Delirium

• The patient has a reduced level of consciousness and difficulty focusing, shifting, or sustaining attention.
• There has been a cognitive change (deficit of language, memory, orientation, perception) that a dementia cannot better explain.
• These symptoms develop rapidly (hours to days) and tend to fluctuate during the day.
• History, physical examination, or laboratory data suggest that the symptoms developed during or shortly after substance withdrawal.

Coding Notes

You would not diagnose both a Substance Intoxication (or Withdrawal) Delirium *and* Substance Intoxication (Withdrawal) due to the same substance. Whenever the symptoms are severe enough to warrant, diagnose only the delirium.

Use the exact name of the substance, not the class name (e.g., Toluene Intoxication Delirium, not Inhalant Intoxication Delirium).

Code the Substance Intoxication Delirium according to the specific substance:

| Axis I | 291.0 | Alcohol |
| | 292.81 | All remaining, including Amphetamine [or Amphetamine-Like Substance]; Cannabis; Cocaine; Hallucinogen; Inhalant; Opioid; Phencyclidine [or Phencyclidine-Like Substance]; Sedative, Hypnotic, or Anxiolytic; Other [or Unknown] Substance |

Likewise, code the Substance Withdrawal Delirium according to the specific substance:

| Axis I | 291.0 | Alcohol |
| | 292.81 | All remaining, including Sedative, Hypnotic, or Anxiolytic; Other [or Unknown] Substance |

For multiple substances, list each one separately.

Delirium induced by medications will almost always be due to toxicity. Such medications are categorized as "Other" substances and coded with the exact names of the medications, followed by "-Induced." For example:

Axis I   292.81   Digitalis-Induced Delirium
           292.81   Imipramine-Induced Delirium

Rodney Partridge

A barroom knife fight had left Rodney Partridge with a severed artery in his arm that required several units of whole blood and two hours in the operating room. But apart from a slight tremor, when Rodney awakened from the anesthesia late Sunday morning, he felt almost as good as new. By evening he was eating voraciously and enjoying the attentions of the nursing staff. On Monday, however, when the surgeon came around to make sure the dressing was still dry, the head nurse confided in a worried whisper: "He's been awake most of the night, demanding to be released. The last hour or two, he's been trying to pick things off his sheets."

When the mental health consultant appeared in his doorway, Rodney was propped up in bed; he was restrained by a canvas halter around his chest and by leather cuffs around his ankles and left wrist. His free hand trembled and roamed the bedclothes, pausing occasionally to pinch up a bit of air and fling it to the floor. Then Rodney took a triangle of toast and threw it at the curtain rod over his window.

"Got him! Cheeky bugger."

"Got who?" the consultant wanted to know.

"Oh, my God!" Startled, Rodney lurched against his chest restraints and dropped a second piece of toast onto the sheet. Leaving the toast where it lay, he returned to plucking at his bed clothes.

"Got who?" repeated the consultant.

Rodney's gaze returned to the curtain rod. "It was those guys up there. One of them mooned me."

The guys were about four inches tall and wore short pants, green jackets, and pointed caps. For half an hour they had been parading around on top of the curtain rod, making obscene gestures and throwing multicolored caterpillars onto Rodney's bed. Whenever a caterpillar landed, it would begin crawling toward him, munching a swath across the sheet as it came.

Although he wasn't exactly frightened, Rodney was far from placid. With his gaze constantly darting around the room, he seemed to be watching for other predators. He insisted that the guys and caterpillars were real, but he had no idea why they were there. He was also vague about his orientation. He knew he was in a hospital whose name he had "never been told," thought he had been admitted a week earlier, and missed the date by nearly five months. Tasks such as subtracting serial sevens, which require a patient to focus on a problem, can help identify problems with attention. When Rodney was asked to subtract sevens from 100, he responded: "Ah, 93 . . . 80 . . . um . . . there's a purple one."

With a little urging and a lot of Librium for sedation, Rodney admitted that he had been a heavy drinker most of his adult life. Too many vodka sours had landed him currently between jobs (and wives), and for the last three months he had spent most of his waking hours consuming a quart or more of hard liquor per day. Although his morning shakes often required "a hair of the dog," he had never before had hallucinations. He agreed that he was probably an alcoholic—in fact, he'd started with Alcoholics Anonymous several times, but had never been able to stay the course.

Evaluation of Rodney Partridge

Several points in Rodney's history suggest a cognitive disorder. First, his orientation was poor (he was unclear about the date, and had no idea what hospital he was in). Second, he had rather dramatic hallucinations, which are often encountered in a delirium. The hallucinations of alcohol withdrawal and other deliriums are classically visual, but they may be auditory or tactile. If delusions occur, their content is often related to the hallucinations. The third tipoff to delirium was his reduced attention span (he had difficulty focusing on his conversation with the mental health consultant).

Rodney had several other symptoms typically associated with delirium. He had become so hyperactive (increased startle response, trying to get out of bed) and agitated that he had to be restrained. His tremor was evident. Although Rodney was bemused, many patients are badly frightened by hallucinations, which can be grotesque beyond all belief. His symptoms were clearly more severe than would be encountered in simple Alcohol Withdrawal; by themselves they would warrant clinical attention.

The hallucinations could suggest **Schizophrenia**—a mistake careful clinicians avoid by asking informants how long the patient has been psychotic. As with any delirium, other conditions to rule out include other psychotic disorders, **Malingering**, and **Factitious Disorder**.

The numbering for a Substance-Induced Delirium depends on the substance. They are all specified in the criteria (see above).

Although Rodney Partridge would meet the criteria for Alcohol Withdrawal (p. 73), this diagnosis would be superseded by Alcohol Withdrawal Delirium. Of course, he would also qualify for a diagnosis of Alcohol Dependence (see p. 68)—in addition to the symptoms of withdrawal, he had tried Alcoholics Anonymous without success, and drank in preference to work.

Axis I	291.0	Alcohol Withdrawal Delirium
	303.90	Alcohol Dependence
Axis II	V71.09	No diagnosis
Axis III	39.31	Brachial artery suture
Axis IV		Unemployed
		Divorced

Axis V   GAF = 30   (on admission)
GAF = 60   (at discharge)

Delirium Due to Multiple Etiologies

More patients probably fall into the category of Delirium Due to Multiple Etiologies than are ever diagnosed. Many such diagnoses are undoubtedly missed because the clinician is aware of one cause and fails to identify the others. The signs and symptoms do not differ from those in the foregoing examples.

Delirium Due to Multiple Causes is not really a single diagnosis—it is a collection of two or more diagnoses occurring in a single patient. But this term has been given its own section to remind clinicians of its importance. It is especially common among older people, who are likely to have numerous medical problems.

Criteria for Delirium Due to Multiple Etiologies

- The patient has a reduced level of consciousness and difficulty focusing, shifting, or sustaining attention.
- There has been a cognitive change (deficit of language, memory, orientation, perception) that a dementia cannot better explain.
- These symptoms develop rapidly (hours to days) and tend to fluctuate during the day.
- These symptoms have more than one cause, as judged from history, physical examination, or laboratory data.

Coding Note

Multiple Axis I codes must be used to indicate specific causes of delirium. Also indicate the relevant physical (or substance use) condition on Axis III. For example:

Axis I   293.0   Delirium Due to Cirrhosis
         292.81   Cimetidine-Induced Delirium
Axis III 571.2   Alcoholic cirrhosis

Emil Brion

At age 72, Emil Brion already had such severe emphysema that he required oxygen day and night. "I always warned him about smoking, but he was actually proud of being a three-pack-a-day man," said his wife. "Now, if he takes the oxygen off to smoke, he gets goofy and scared."

She meant that Emil would see things: A light cord would become a snake; a pile of clothes on the chair looked for an instant like a lion ready to spring. He might wake up whimpering from a nightmare. Sometimes he seemed so distracted that she could hardly persuade him to put the oxygen back on. But all things considered, he was doing pretty well. He could even drive a little, as long as he used his oxygen.

That lasted until the Fourth of July, when Emil strolled barefoot into the back yard and sliced the outer sole of his heel on a broken piece of glass. The cut didn't hurt much, so he forgot to clean it up when he got back inside. It was several days before either he or his wife noticed how red and swollen the injured area had become. By that time, according to the specialist in infectious diseases who admitted him to the hospital, he had developed a severe septicemia.

Even with continuous IV antibiotics, for three days Emil's temperature hovered above 102 degrees. Even with nasal oxygen, his arterial oxygen saturation was low. During much of the day he slept; at night he was awake, mumbling to himself and groaning. When he spoke clearly enough to be understood, he complained that he was a miserable old man and wished that he were dead.

On Emil's seventh hospital day, his fever finally broke. He removed the oxygen tube and told the nurse, "Wheel me outside so I can have a smoke."

Evaluation of Emil Brion

Emil's wife noted that when he went without his oxygen, he was sometimes so distracted that he couldn't even focus on restarting his oxygen. When a second disorder (systemic infection) was added to the anoxia, he rapidly became somnolent. His cognitive difficulties included illusions (the light-cord snake) and nightmares, and he began to mumble (language difficulties).

Several other symptoms typically associated with delirium were also apparent. He had a change in his sleep–wake pattern (drowsy during the day, awake at night). He became depressed and even wished himself dead; perhaps at times he recognized how desperately ill he was.

Emil's mental condition had more than one cause, as shown by the fact that he became sicker, even when nasal oxygen was running. Once the infection in his bloodstream was resolved and his fever broke, his cognition suddenly improved. However, a complete evaluation of his mental status would be needed to be sure there were no residual symptoms of **dementia** or a **depressive disorder**. His perceptual problems would not be confused with **Schizophrenia** because they developed so rapidly.

Note that in the coding of Emil's delirium, each specific cause is indicated by a separate line on Axis I. The code numbers themselves are identical.

Axis I	293.0	Delirium Due to Anoxia
	293.0	Delirium Due to Septicemia
Axis II	V71.09	No diagnosis
Axis III	492.8	Emphysema
	038.9	Septicemia
Axis IV		None
Axis V	GAF = 25	(on admission)
	GAF = 80	(at discharge)

780.09 Delirium Not Otherwise Specified

The catch-all category of Delirium Not Otherwise Specified is for any disorder that does not meet the criteria for one of the previously described types of delirium. DSM-IV specifically mentions the following:

Delirium with cause not proven. A delirium for which a causal link to a specific etiology cannot be established.

Delirium due to sensory deprivation. A type of delirium experienced by people whose sensory input is markedly reduced (e.g., volunteer subjects of a psychological experiment).

DEMENTIAS

All patients with dementia have a number of features in common. Again, the DSM-IV criteria in the following list are marked with a bullet.

- **Decline.** *Dementia* means "loss," so there must be a decline from a previous level of functioning. Patients who have always functioned at a low level (individuals with Mental Retardation) are not considered demented. (Like anyone else, a mentally retarded person can *become* demented. In fact, many patients with Down syndrome eventually develop Dementia of the Alzheimer's Type.)
- **Memory Loss.** All dementias involve amnesia. In mild cases this may only involve recent memory; as a dementia worsens, more remote memories are also affected. Although a sense of self is generally preserved until late in the disease, severely demented patients may fail to recognize their relatives or long-time friends, or even answer to their own names.

- **Other Cognitive Deficits**. In addition to memory loss, dementia patients must show at least one other cognitive deficit listed below. (It should be noted that most demented patients will have some loss in their ability to sustain attention; this inattention neither necessitates the diagnosis of delirium nor rules out a dementia.)

    Agnosia. Patients cannot recognize or identify familiar objects (such as the parts of a ballpoint pen), even though sensory functioning is intact.

    Aphasia. Patients may use circumlocutions to get around words they can't remember. Increasingly, they may come to depend on clichés; they may become vague, circumstantial or even mute. Use of language is usually spared until late in the disease.

    Apraxia. Patients cannot perform certain motor acts, even though they are physically capable of doing so, their senses are intact, and they understand what they are being asked to do. These deficits may be shown by inability to build with blocks or copy designs and figures. Overlearned motor behaviors such as the use of a fork and knife are usually preserved until late in the course of the dementia.

    Loss of Executive Functioning. This is the mechanism people use to organize simple ideas and bits of behavior into complex behaviors, such as dressing and other functions of self-care. When executive functioning is affected, patients have trouble interpreting new information and adapting to new situations.

Every dementia patient will have at least one of these cognitive deficits, but most won't have them all. The "three A's"—agnosia, aphasia, and apraxia—are somewhat more common in Dementia of the Alzheimer's Type and other degenerative disorders than in Vascular Dementia or Dementia Due to Other General Medical Conditions. The three A's are also more likely to occur late in the course of any dementia.

- **Impairment**. The loss of ability to think and to remember must be severe enough to interfere with the patient's work or social life. For any dementia, the criteria require that *each* of the symptoms must be severe enough to cause such interference. That is, if the patient has memory loss, aphasia, and loss of executive functioning, each of these three symptoms must affect the patient's life in an important way. This requirement helps set off dementias, which *must* have a cognitive problem other than memory decline, from amnestic disorders, which *may* have another cognitive problem, provided that it is mild as compared to the memory loss.

- **No Delirium**. Dementia cannot be diagnosed if the symptoms occur only when the patient is delirious. If there was a delirium in the past, it must now have become a dementia. However, these two conditions can (and often do) coexist, as when a patient with Dementia of the Alzheimer's Type is given medication that produces a Substance Intoxication Delirium.

The onset of dementia is often gradual (of course, this depends a great deal on the cause). The first indication may be loss of interest in work or leisure activities. Family or friends may note a change in long-standing personality traits. When executive functioning is affected, judgment and impulse control suffer. Loss of the social graces ensues, as shown when the patient makes crude jokes or doesn't attend to personal hygiene and appearance. Stripped of the ability to analyze, to understand, to remember, and to apply old knowledge to new situations, the patient may be left to rely upon the skeleton of habits.

Demented patients become increasingly vulnerable to psychosocial stresses: What would have been a minor problem a few years earlier now assumes monumental proportions. Some become paranoid or irritable; others may even shoplift. Still others try to compensate for failing memory by compulsively making lists. The misperceptions (hallucinations or illusions) so common in delirium are often absent, especially early in the process. As the dementia worsens, paranoid ideas and delusions of infidelity can lead to assaultive behavior.

Some patients are placid, especially early in the illness as apathy leads to gradually reduced activity. Patients who retain some insight may become depressed or anxious. Later, especially if patients become frustrated or frightened, there may be outbursts of anger. They may become restless and pace. Often these people will wander from home, sometimes remaining lost for hours or days. In the final stage of dementia, patients may lose all useful speech and self-care. Then they lie in bed, unaware of attendants or family.

Although dementia is usually found in older patients, it can be diagnosed any time after the age of three or four, which is when a person's intelligence becomes reliably measurable. The course depends on the underlying cause. Most often it is one of chronic deterioration; however, the dementia can be static or can even remit. Remission is especially likely in hypothyroidism, subdural hematoma, and normal-pressure hydrocephalus. When one of these causes is diagnosed early and successfully treated, a full recovery can occur.

The diagnosis of any dementia demands medical and neurological evaluation, to confirm causation and to intervene with treatment whenever either is possible. In many cases, a biological cause can be identified. These include primary diseases of the central nervous system, such as Huntington's disease, multiple sclerosis, and Parkinson's disease; infectious diseases, such as neurosyphilis and acquired immune deficiency syndrome (AIDS); vitamin deficiencies; tumors; trauma; a variety of diseases of the liver, lung, and cardiovascular system; and endocrine disorders. (A more complete listing is given in Appendix B.) However, some dementias must be diagnosed not on the basis of demonstrated pathology, but by inference from clinical features (and by ruling out other nonorganic causes). This is the case with Alzheimer's and Pick's diseases.

Dementia of the Alzheimer's Type

The most common cause of senility, Dementia of the Alzheimer's Type has been recognized throughout the 20th century. It affects about 3% of people over the age of 65 and increases steadily with advancing age. (Each year, about 2% of people over the age of 65 become demented; Dementia of the Alzheimer's Type accounts for about twice as many of these as does Vascular Dementia.) Alzheimer's disease accounts for over half of all dementias; the majority of elderly patients in nursing homes have been stricken with this degenerative disorder. It is especially common among patients over 40 who have Down syndrome, but any clinician who treats older patients is bound to encounter this disorder frequently. Patients with early-onset Alzheimer's disease are especially likely to have relatives with the same disorder.

Alzheimer's is also important because so many other disorders, both cognitive and otherwise, can be mistaken for it. Therefore, it is a diagnosis of exclusion that should only be made once all other causes (especially those that can be treated) have been ruled out.

The first sign of Dementia of the Alzheimer's Type may be an apparent change in personality. Commonly, existing personality traits are accentuated: The patient may become more obsessional, secretive, or sexually active. Other early indications of dementia may be apathy, emotional lability (sudden weeping or temper outbursts), or the loss of a previously acute sense of humor.

Memory loss is the first symptom experienced by about half of Alzheimer's patients, but eventually, as in other dementias, all patients will become forgetful. Recent memory (the ability to remember information that was learned within the previous few minutes) is the first aspect to be affected. Patients may forget familiar names or re-ask questions that have just been answered. To compensate, some write themselves notes or compile lists. Immediate memory (the ability to recall information that has just been presented) and remote memory (information learned years ago) are relatively well preserved.

Loss of *executive functioning* (usually attributed to frontal lobe damage) can be tested directly by asking the patient to tell similarities and differences or to carry out a sequence of steps, as on the Mini-Mental State Exam (see Appendix B). But executive functioning is often best evaluated from the history or from observation of some of these behaviors: closely trailing the clinician or a companion (imitation behavior), frozen expression until prompted (lack of spontaneity), putting on more than one pair of trousers (perseveration), or repeatedly getting lost on the ward though oriented at home (environmental dependency). The picture that will emerge is of a person who can navigate and function reasonably well in a fixed, familiar environment, but who has difficulty adapting to changing circumstances. Many patients are referred for evaluation only when they cannot cope with the unfamiliar surroundings of a new house. As is true of most intellectual tasks, patients may do better when they are rested.

Aphasia may be manifested at first by trouble finding words. The vocabulary contracts as clichés and stereotyped phrases are substituted for real communication, and the patient no longer uses complex sentences. Reading and writing may deteriorate; conversation rambles. Agnosia may appear first as trouble recognizing a new acquaintance; later, even family members may not be recognized. In advanced cases, apraxia may appear at first as clumsiness or trouble dressing.

Many patients with Alzheimer's disease will also have perceptual defects such as illusions or hallucinations. They may become inordinately suspicious and develop paranoia. About 20% have depression; even those who are not depressed often experience insomnia or anorexia. Therefore, it is important to consider dementia in the differential diagnosis of any older patient who presents with symptoms suggestive of a depressive disorder.

The typical Alzheimer's patient lives six to eight years after the disease begins. The clinical course, though variable, is typically a steady decline through three stages:

1. One to three years of growing forgetfulness.

2. Two to three years of increasing disorientation, loss of language skills, and inappropriate behavior. Although physical exam reveals typical "frontal release signs" (such as the *palmomental reflex*, which is a pursing of lips when the palm is stroked), until advanced stages most patients look grossly normal. (Also, some elderly people develop frontal release signs without having evidence of dementia.) Hallucinations and delusions may appear during this stage.

3. A final period of severe dementia, during which there is disorientation for person and complete loss of self-care.

There is almost always a complete loss of insight; sooner or later, judgment becomes impaired. At the end, complete muteness and unresponsiveness may ensue. Alzheimer's patients tolerate physical illness poorly; infection or malnutrition that would not severely affect a nondemented person may trigger a superimposed delirium.

Although Alzheimer's disease is quite common, the diagnosis of Dementia of the Alzheimer's Type must usually be inferred from the absence of other causes. Because some other causes of dementia are treatable, and because Alzheimer's disease has a dismal prognosis, it is vitally important to rule out all other possible causes. (DSM-IV lists Dementia of the Alzheimer's Type *first*; don't let this lead you astray.)

Criteria for Dementia of the Alzheimer's Type

- The patient has developed problems with thinking, as shown by both of these:
  - Impaired memory (can't learn new information or can't recall information previously learned), *plus*

- At least one of these:
  - ✓ Aphasia
  - ✓ Apraxia
  - ✓ Agnosia
  - ✓ Impaired executive functioning
- Each of these symptoms materially impairs work or social functioning, and each indicates a decline in the patient's level of functioning.
- The decline in mental functioning begins gradually and worsens steadily.
- These impairments aren't due to any other disorder that causes dementia, such as:
  - Central nervous system disease (brain tumor, cerebrovascular disease, Huntington's disease, normal-pressure hydrocephalus, Parkinson's disease, subdural hematoma)
  - Systemic disease (hypothyroidism, vitamin deficiency, HIV infection, neurosyphilis)
  - Substance-related disorders
- These impairments don't occur *solely* during a delirium.
- They aren't better explained by another Axis I disorder, such as a depressive disorder or Schizophrenia.

Coding Notes

There are several ways to code Dementia of the Alzheimer's Type, depending on the age of onset and accompanying symptoms. If more than one of these symptoms is present, code according to the most prominent symptom. The exact diagnosis may even change during the course of a patient's illness.

Prominent symptom	With Late Onset (over 65)	With Early Onset (65 or less)
Uncomplicated	290.0	290.10
With Delusions	290.20	290.12
With Depressed Mood*	290.21	290.13
With Delirium	290.3	290.11

* With Depressed Mood is only coded when depression meets the full symptomatic criteria for Major Depressive Episode (see p. 191). In such a case, you would not also code mood disorder.

Specify if: With Behavioral Disturbance. This specifier is added to the end of the diagnosis whenever the patient wanders a great deal or is markedly combative.

On Axis III, also code 331.0 (Alzheimer's disease).

Sarah Neal

After her husband died, Sarah Neal had made the rounds of her three children and had finally settled in with Jason (who provided the details of her history). She had now lived with him for four years. Even when she was 74, she had managed the gardening, the marketing, and most of the cooking. The arrangement had worked out well for both of them—Jason had remained single after a stormy divorce decades before. But for nearly a year, problems had been evident.

Around Christmas, Sarah had spent two days searching the house for the presents she had hidden. She and Jason finally found them in the storage shed, but this was only the beginning of her forgetfulness. She had always prided herself on her ability to remember telephone numbers, but in February, when Jason was assigned a new extension number at work, she could never seem to recall what it was or where she had written it down. After several days of frustration, he finally pasted the new number to both of their telephones. She began to avoid her circle of friends from the mobile home park where they lived.

Late that spring, they suffered the first of several kitchen fires. These all started because Sarah had forgotten about food left bubbling on the stove. Although the last one caused $1,500 worth of damage to their kitchen, Sarah had seemed strangely unaffected. "She's always been so careful about money," Jason mused, "but when I got home to find the fire department there and water soaking everything, she didn't turn a hair. It's as if a stranger had moved inside my mother's head." A physical examination by her internist had revealed no evidence of medical illness.

Sarah looked a good 10 years younger than her stated age. She was clean and neatly dressed, though her silk blouse was missing a button from one sleeve and she wore two sweaters. Throughout the 45 minutes, she gave good eye contact and seemed to pay attention to the conversation. She smiled continually while asserting (several times) that she had been "just fine." When the interviewer pointed out that her son said she had almost burned down the house, she replied, "Stuff and nonsense. He's a rotten little poop!"

"It sounds like you're upset," remarked the interviewer.

"Stuff and nonsense. I couldn't feel happier."

The interviewer asked how an apple and an orange were alike, and learned that she "had them in my 'fridge." A child and a dwarf were different because "that's just the way they are."

When asked to elaborate, she said, "A child's a child and a dwarf's a dwarf."

When asked to name the president of the United States, she said, "That's what you should know for yourself. I don't feel like helping you any more."

Later in the interview she was asked to identify a ballpoint pen. "It's a whatsis for writing, of course! Stuff and nonsense."

Evaluation of Sarah Neal

Aside from her memory deficit (telephone numbers, hiding places), did Sarah's symptoms fulfill the criteria for dementia? Because she was alert and focused well during the interview, she could not have a delirium. For real communication, she frequently substituted stereotypic phrases ("Stuff and nonsense")—evidence of impaired language ability. She also had an agnosia: She couldn't name so commonplace an object as a pen. Loss of executive functioning was shown by such problems as starting fires in the kitchen and an inability to abstract similarities and differences; she also wore two sweaters, which suggested perseveration. (Although she had lost a button from her sleeve, which might also indicate loss of executive functioning, this could happen to nearly anyone.) These behaviors had evidently begun gradually, were progressive, and severely disrupted her life and her son's.

Further evaluation of Sarah would properly include a complete mental status exam, which might include use of a scale such as the Mini-Mental State Exam (see Appendix C). Reportedly in good health, she would still need a complete neurological exam and enough laboratory (especially radiological) testing to rule out other causes of dementia.

In the elderly, a dementia that begins gradually is most likely due to Alzheimer's disease, but a number of treatable causes *must* be ruled out. Sarah had had no history of blows to the head, so was unlikely to have **subdural hematoma**. Her son was positive that she had never used drugs or alcohol, eliminating **Substance Intoxication** as a cause. Physical exam revealed no evidence of **Parkinson's disease.** Her affect was good and there was no history of depression, so **pseudodementia due to a depressive disorder** seemed unlikely. Skull X-rays and magnetic resonance imaging (MRI) would rule out **brain tumors** and **normal-pressure hydrocephalus**; blood tests would rule out **hypothyroidism** and **vitamin B12 deficiency** as possible causes. With no history of stepwise progression in her disease, **Vascular Dementia**, the second most common cause of dementia in the elderly, seemed unlikely. Other than memory loss, patients with an **amnestic disorder** do not have cognitive symptoms (such as Sarah's aphasia and agnosia).

All this would leave Dementia of the Alzheimer's Type as the disorder of exclusion. Most often it occurs in the very old, but a form of it can develop in younger people. In such a case, concern may first come from coworkers or supervisors, who report the patient's inability to respond to workplace pressures. This early-onset form, though uncommon, should be considered as a diagnosis of last resort in younger patients presenting with dementia.

Axis I	290.0	Alzheimer's Dementia, With Late Onset, Uncomplicated
Axis II	V71.09	No diagnosis
Axis III	331.0	Alzheimer's disease

Axis IV   None
Axis V   GAF = 35 (current)

290.4X Vascular Dementia

Approximately 20% of dementias have a vascular origin. This condition has also been called *multi-infarct dementia* because its presumed cause is a series of strokes. Whereas patients with Dementia of the Alzheimer's Type deteriorate gradually, many patients with Vascular Dementia become worse through a series of small steps as the strokes occur. Vascular dementia is especially likely to develop in a patient who has diabetes or hypertension.

Besides memory loss, patients experience the loss of executive functioning, which (as noted above) can show up as the inability to deal with novel tasks. Apathy, slowed thinking, and deterioration of hygiene are also often noted. Relatively mild stresses may precipitate pathological laughing or crying. These patients are less likely than Alzheimer's patients to have aphasia, apraxia, or agnosia, though loss of any aspect of mental functioning is possible.

TIP Some authorities advocate a division of dementias into *cortical* (or *degenerative*, such as Dementia of the Alzheimer's Type), and *subcortical* (dementia due to most other causes). The subcortical dementias (some texts also call these *secondary dementias*) are allegedly less likely to produce agnosia, apraxia, and aphasia. Other authorities object, pointing out that the pathology of disease is never that neat and that all dementias have some degree of both cortical and subcortical pathology. Because there is so much overlap in symptoms, DSM-IV's seems the safer classification. It categorizes the dementias much more simply, on the basis of presumed underlying cause.

Criteria for Vascular Dementia

- The patient has developed deficits of thinking, as shown by *both* of these:
  - Impaired memory (can't learn new information or can't recall information previously learned), *plus*
  - At least one of these:
    - ✓ Aphasia
    - ✓ Apraxia

✓ Agnosia
✓ Impaired executive functioning
- Cerebral vascular disease has probably caused the deficits above, as judged by laboratory data (radiographic evidence of multiple infarctions that involve cortex and white matter) or by focal neurologic signs and symptoms (increased deep tendon reflexes, weakness in limbs, abnormal gait, extensor Babinski reflex).
- Each of these symptoms materially impairs work or social functioning, and each indicates a decline in the patient's level of functioning.
- These impairments don't occur *solely* during a delirium.

Coding Notes

If more than one of the following symptoms is present, code according to the most prominent symptom:

290.40	Uncomplicated
290.41	With Delirium
290.42	With Delusions
290.43	With Depressed Mood*

* Only code With Depressed Mood when depression meets the full symptomatic criteria for Major Depressive Episode (see p. 191). In such a case, you would not also code mood disorder.

Specify if: With Behavioral Disturbance. This specifier is added to the end of the diagnosis whenever the patient wanders a great deal or is markedly combative.

On Axis III, also code the specific cerebrovascular condition. For example:

434.9 Cerebral artery occlusion

Minnie Bell Leach

At her family physician's request, her daughter and son-in-law had brought Minnie Bell Leach for consultation. She had lived with them for the past year, since her second stroke. Nearly five years earlier, her first stroke had left her with a partly paralyzed left leg, but she had been able to care for herself and even do her marketing until the second stroke a year ago. Since then, she had been largely wheelchair-bound. Her daughter provided an increasing share of her personal care.

Bit by bit over the last few months, she had begun to slip. Her daughter remembered that at first Minnie Bell often forgot to take her medicine for high blood pressure. Despite the fact that she kept them in their container (which had three compartments for each day of the week), she had at first needed reminding to take the pills at breakfast, lunch, and bedtime. After a week or two, this had improved, and for a time she had seemed almost back to her former self.

But upon her awakening the previous Sunday morning, it was clear that Minnie Bell had slipped some more. She had neglected to zip her skirt and had gotten the buttons of her blouse into the wrong holes. None of these mistakes did she seem to notice. She also had trouble expressing herself—at breakfast she asked for "red stuff" for her toast (it was strawberry jam that she and her daughter had made together last summer). Since Sunday she had reverted to taking her medicine only when reminded.

Minnie Bell looked a bit older than her 68 years. She sat quietly in her wheelchair, cradling her left wrist in her right hand. Over her cotton house dress she wore a cloth overcoat that had fallen off one shoulder; she did not appear to notice. Although she maintained good eye contact throughout the consultation, she spoke only when spoken to. Her speech was clear and coherent. She denied having hallucinations, delusions, or depression, but she spontaneously complained of a cough, shortness of breath, and numerous aches and pains. She did not mention the fact that she couldn't walk.

On the Mini-Mental State Exam (see Appendix C) Minnie Bell scored 20 out of 30. She knew the year but missed the month and date by over two months; she could name the city and state, a watch and a pencil. Although she could repeat the names of three objects (ball, chair, telephone) immediately after she heard them, five minutes later she could recall only the ball. She became confused when asked to follow the three-part instruction, and she persistently forgot to place the folded paper on the floor. There were no apraxias: She could use a pencil to copy a simple figure.

On neurological exam, her left hand was weak; there was an abnormal Babinski sign (upgoing great toe when the sole of her foot was scratched) on that side.

Evaluation of Minnie Bell Leach

The evidence for Minnie Bell's having a cognitive disorder was as follows: She had had increasing difficulty with her memory, as shown by the history of forgetting to take her medication and by the obvious problem with short-term memory. From the Mini-Mental State Exam, she appeared to have no agnosias or apraxias. However, her daughter noted the aphasia for "jam." She also had increasing problems with executive functioning, as shown by her neglected appearance and her inability to follow a three-step instruction. These problems represented a major decline from her previous level of functioning, and they did interfere with her everyday life.

From the fact that Minnie Bell retained eye contact during her evaluation, we may infer that her attention was not impaired, as would be the case with a

delirium. (The prolonged course of her disease also points away from a delirium.) The presence of several cognitive deficits besides memory loss pointed away from an **amnestic disorder**. She denied depression, delusions, or hallucinations, rendering unlikely the diagnosis of a noncognitive disorder such as a **pseudodementia**.

A vascular etiology for her disease was suggested by her history of hypertension and by the stepwise progression of her disability following several strokes. The fact that she had neurological signs (weakness of her hand, upgoing toe) from the start of her decline provided further evidence that **Dementia of the Alzheimer's Type** was not involved.

Because Minnie Bell's principal symptom seemed to be trouble with her memory, she would be scored as follows:

Axis I	290.40	Vascular Dementia, Uncomplicated
Axis II	V71.09	No diagnosis
Axis III	434.9	Cerebral Artery Occlusion
Axis IV		None
Axis V	GAF = 31	(current)

Dementia Due to Other General Medical Conditions

Dementias Due to Other General Medical Conditions is likely to begin more abruptly than Dementia of the Alzheimer's Type. The symptoms and course of illness depend heavily on the underlying medical cause. So does treatment and prognosis.

An impressive list of underlying disease processes can lead to dementia. It includes infections, metabolic disorders, trauma, toxins, and tumors. Neurological disorders can also be responsible, including Huntington's and Parkinson's diseases, multiple sclerosis, and normal-pressure hydrocephalus. A more complete list can be found in Appendix B.

Although HIV disease is not one of the more common causes of dementia, it has rapidly become one of the most important, occurring in young people and laying waste otherwise vigorous lives.

Criteria for Dementia Due to Other General Medical Conditions

- The patient has developed deficits of thinking, as shown by *both* of these:
  - Impaired memory (can't learn new information or can't recall information previously learned), *plus*

- At least one of these:
  - ✓ Aphasia
  - ✓ Apraxia
  - ✓ Agnosia
  - ✓ Impaired executive functioning
- Each of these symptoms materially impairs work or social functioning, and each indicates a decline in the patient's level of functioning.
- These symptoms don't occur *solely* during a delirium.
- A general medical condition has probably directly caused the deficits above, as judged by history, laboratory data, or physical examination.

Coding Notes

As distinct from Dementia of the Alzheimer's Type and Vascular Dementia, none of these dementias has a codable subtype. Besides coding the specific dementia on Axis I, you should also code the underlying disease on Axis III. Some of the more common responsible general medical conditions are listed in the table below.

Type of dementia	Axis I	Axis III
Dementia Due to HIV Disease	294.9	043.1
Dementia Due to Head Trauma	294.1	854.00
Dementia Due to Parkinson's Disease	294.1	332.0
Dementia Due to Huntington's Disease	294.1	333.4
Dementia Due to Pick's Disease	290.10	331.1
Dementia Due to Creutzfeldt–Jakob Disease	290.10	046.1
Dementia Due to [Other General Medical Condition]	294.1	*

* Specify these numbers on Axis III. They might include normal-pressure hydrocephalus, hypothyroidism, brain tumor, Vitamin B12 deficiency, and many others. See Appendix B for more.

If one of these disorders is superimposed onto Dementia of the Alzheimer's Type or Vascular Dementia, code both diagnoses on Axis I and the specific general medical conditions on Axis III.

Arlen Wing

When he was admitted to the hospital for the third time in four months, Arlen Wing had lost 30 pounds, which was nearly 20% of his body weight. He also seemed to have lost much of his will to live: He had often neglected to take his zidovudine and the other medications prescribed to shore up his failing immune system. That, plus the apathy that was so obvious on admission, prompted the request for mental health consultation. Arlen's physician noted that a computed tomography (CT) brain scan showed diffuse cortical atrophy; an electroencephalogram (EEG) had been read as indicating "nonfocal slowing."

Arlen had trained to be a dancer. After he just missed landing a job with the Joffrey Ballet, he had joined his long-time companion, Alex, in the business of buying and selling antique dolls. The two had made a good living traveling around the country to auctions and doll shows, until Alex rather suddenly died of pneumocystis pneumonia. Arlen soon discovered he was HIV-positive; at once he began taking prophylactic zidovudine. He had continued to operate his business until the last few months, when his CD4 cell count dropped below 200, triggering his recent series of hospitalizations.

Arlen made eye contact and listened politely while the consultant explained the purpose of the visit. His speech was slow and labored, but there were no other abnormalities in the flow of his speech. He had no delusions, hallucinations, or other abnormal content of thought. He denied feeling especially sad or anxious—"just tired."

Arlen knew his own name, the name of the hospital, and the month, but he gave the date and year incorrectly. He thought that he had been admitted only the day before, whereas it had actually been a week earlier. He could not recall the name of the physician who had attended him for the past three years. He scored only 14 out of 30 on the Mini-Mental State Exam. When asked to pick up a sheet of paper, fold it, and put it on the floor, he twice dropped the paper unfolded onto the floor. When asked to tell how an apple and an orange were similar, he could offer no response. Although he acknowledged being seriously ill, he admitted that recently he had often neglected to take his medication. "I was feeling terrible," he said, "and I thought it might be making me sick."

Evaluation of Arlen Wing

Arlen's history and obvious intellectual deficits pointed clearly to the cognitive disorders. He was alert and he adequately focused his attention on the exam; these two factors made a delirium unlikely. (However, trouble continuing with a task or shifting attention from one task to another can occur later in the course of Dementia Due to HIV Disease.) His loss of recent memory was obvious; this is especially common in an HIV-related dementia. Also typical were his apathy and slowed speech (retarded motor movements in general are typical of this disorder). His impairments represented a significant decline from his previous level of functioning. There were no obvious agnosias, apraxias, or aphasias, which is what would be expected from a non-Alzheimer's type of dementia.

Informants who knew him well would be the most satisfactory source of information about Arlen's executive functioning (had he been having trouble dressing himself, shopping, or taking care of other routine daily tasks?). However, his inability to follow a sequence of events in the Mini-Mental State Exam also provided evidence. Discontinuing his zidovudine and other medications suggested a lapse in judgment, typical of the later stages of an HIV-related dementia. He denied feeling depressed—evidence against a mood disorder with pseudodementia.

Axis I	294.9	Dementia Due to HIV Disease
Axis II	V71.09	No diagnosis
Axis III	043.1	HIV infection affecting central nervous system functioning
Axis IV		None
Axis V	GAF = 21 (current)	

Substance-Induced Persisting Dementia

Dementia can result from prolonged use of alcohol, sedatives, and inhalants, though the vast majority of cases of Substance-Induced Persisting Dementia are due to alcohol use. Patients will have difficulty with constructional tasks (e.g., drawing), behavioral problems, and memory defects. These patients are often described as having delusional jealousy or hallucinations.

This condition is called "Persisting" to underscore the fact that, unlike many other substance-related cognitive disorders, it is not transitory. However, the criteria for Substance-Induced Persisting Dementia are little different from those for any other dementia. Although the onset is typically gradual, nothing may be noted amiss until the patient has dried out for several days or weeks.

TIP A fine line may divide patients with Substance-Induced Persisting Dementia from those who have Substance-Induced Persisting Amnestic Disorder, also known as Korsakoff's psychosis (see p. 49). Some autopsy studies show that patients diagnosed as having alcoholic dementia have typical Wernicke–Korsakoff pathology. It is a convention to diagnose demented patients who have a long history of heavy drinking as having Alcohol-Induced Persisting Dementia.

Criteria for Substance-Induced Persisting Dementia

- The patient has developed deficits of thinking, as shown by *both* of these:
  - Impaired memory (can't learn new information or can't recall information previously learned), *plus*
  - One or more of these:
    - ✓ Aphasia
    - ✓ Apraxia
    - ✓ Agnosia
    - ✓ Impaired executive functioning
- Each of these symptoms materially impairs work or social functioning, and each indicates a decline in the patient's level of functioning.
- These symptoms don't occur *solely* during a delirium.
- They last longer than the typical effects of Substance Intoxication or Withdrawal.
- Substance use is evident from history, physical examination, or laboratory data, and the clinician believes that this use has directly caused the impaired memory.

Coding Notes

The following code numbers can be utilized:

291.2	Alcohol
292.82	All remaining, including Inhalant; Sedative, Hypnotic, or Anxiolytic; Other [or Unknown] Substance

Also code Substance Dependence as appropriate on Axis I.

Mark Culpepper

Despite drinking nearly a fifth of hard liquor every day until he was 56, Mark Culpepper had successfully avoided hospitalization. He had taught developmental biology for 30 years, but six months earlier the university had offered him early retirement. Soon afterwards, his daughter, Amarette, had moved in with him as housekeeper and companion. She provided most of the history of his illness.

Amarette never understood how her father had managed to retain his position while drinking nearly a fifth of hard liquor each day. Of course, in later years his teaching assignments had always been lower-division, and he had published no research for over a decade. He was "COT," as the students put it— "coasting on tenure." Tenure was a powerful influence at the university; it forgave him the occasional missed class he was too hung over to attend and the fact that he hardly ever graded a paper at all.

By the time his daughter moved in, Mark was fully retired and devoting all of his time to drinking. Amarette quickly took care of that. She confiscated the contents of his bar and, by combining shame with threats, obtained such control over his finances that he was forced to stop drinking altogether. She remained steadfast through a week during which he vomited and had the shakes. At a stroke, she had rid her father of a 30-year habit.

The results were both more and less than Amarette had expected. In the next four months Mark didn't touch a drop, but neither did he accomplish much of anything else. Even sober, he neglected his appearance, often going for days without shaving. He spent much of his time "working on a paper" that was, as far as she could tell, recycled material from decades-old notebooks. He had simply copied it out unaltered. "Anything there that made any sense at all, you could read in an old freshman biology text. A very old text," she said while he was being admitted.

An event the day before had precipitated the admission. When she returned from a brief errand, she found him in the living room trying to mop up water from the bathtub that he had turned on and apparently forgotten about. The taps were still running.

Mark was a pleasant enough man whose red nose and cheeks gave him a somewhat boyish appearance. He carried a sheaf of papers and a dog-eared manila folder; the title page read, "Limb Regeneration in the Newt." His speech was normal and he denied delusions, hallucinations, depression, and suicidal ideas. Although he seemed to pay attention during the Mini-Mental State Exam, he scored only 19 out of 30. He was unable to recall two of three objects after five minutes. With difficulty, he correctly spelled "world" backward. When asked to follow the three-part instruction (to pick up a piece of paper, fold it, and place it on the floor), he persistently neglected to fold the paper. When asked about this, he brushed it off, saying, "Well, I was thinking about my research."

Evaluation of Mark Culpepper

The core feature of any dementia is memory impairment. In Mark's case, this was not apparent on casual observation. He was pleasant, carried on a conversation in a natural manner, and even appeared to be working on a scientific paper. However, after five minutes he could recall only one of the three objects given to him on the Mini-Mental State Exam.

Mark had no evidence of aphasia, apraxia, or agnosia, but from the history his daughter gave, he had been having difficulty caring for himself (he neglected his appearance and flooded the house with bathwater). This loss of executive functioning was reflected in formal testing by his inability to follow a three-part instruction.

Judging from the history, Mark's overall functioning had declined significantly, interfering with his life. He focused attention well and it did not appear to wander during the interview, suggesting that a **delirium** was not responsible. Other Axis I pathology was not evident: He denied symptoms of **depression** and **psychosis**, which are the two major conditions that might present with neglect and memory loss. Of course, a physical exam would be needed to rule out other **general medical conditions**. Considering his history of heavy alcohol abuse, however, an alcohol-induced persisting dementia would seem highly probable.

The matter of Mark's alcohol use would require some thought. At the time he stopped drinking, when he developed shakiness and vomiting, he would have been diagnosed as having Alcohol Withdrawal. Alcohol had clearly interfered with his work and with his relationship with Amarette. Although he had probably not increased his intake of alcohol in the past year, the effects of his drinking were still being felt. (This last statement may represent a somewhat liberal interpretation of the criterion for Substance Dependence, new in DSM-IV, that there be at least three symptoms within a given 12-month period.) Applying the criteria strictly, we should diagnose him as having Alcohol Abuse, but this would seem to trivialize his problem with alcohol.

Mark had recently retired and had time on his hands. He might profit from occupational or recreational therapy, or even from referral to day care. These interventions might be facilitated by mentioning retirement on Axis IV.

Axis I	291.2	Alcohol-Induced Persisting Dementia
	303.90	Alcohol Dependence, With Physiological Dependence, Early Full Remission
Axis II	V71.09	No diagnosis
Axis III		None
Axis IV		Retirement
Axis V	GAF = 41	(current)

Dementia Due to Multiple Etiologies

Whether it has one cause or many, the basic symptoms of a dementia remain the same. Because so many medical and neurological disorders can cause dementia, the combinations are nearly endless. Any patient's symptoms should be consistent with the underlying pathology, but it may be hard to discriminate the contributing factors on purely clinical grounds.

Dementia Due to Multiple Etiologies is especially common in older people, who are most likely to have multiple illnesses. Also likely to fall into this category are substance abusers, whose drinking or drug use puts them at risk for a variety of medical disorders. For example, a patient with Alcohol-Induced Persisting Dementia may also have head trauma, infection, or a degenerative condition such as Marchiafava–Bignami disease (in which the corpus callosum of the brain is affected by chronic alcohol intake).

Because the symptoms are likely to be similar to those for many other dementias, I have not provided a case vignette for this category.

Criteria for Dementia Due to Multiple Etiologies

- The patient has developed deficits of thinking, as shown by *both* of these:
  - Impaired memory (can't learn new information or can't recall information previously learned), *plus*
  - At least one of these:
    - ✓ Aphasia
    - ✓ Apraxia
    - ✓ Agnosia
    - ✓ Impaired executive functioning
- Each of these symptoms materially impairs work or social functioning, and each indicates a decline in the patient's level of functioning.
- These symptoms don't occur *solely* during a delirium.
- These impairments have more than one cause, as judged by history, physical examination, or laboratory data.

Coding Notes

Multiple codes are used to record the multiple causes of this dementia. In addition, multiple Axis III codes may be required for the physical causes themselves. For example, a demented patient with Huntington's disease who has also suffered a blow to the head may be recorded as follows:

Axis I	294.1	Dementia Due to Head Trauma
	294.1	Dementia Due to Huntington's Disease
Axis III	854.00	Head trauma
	333.4	Huntington's disease

Here is another example:

Axis I	290.10	Dementia of the Alzheimer's Type, Uncomplicated, With Behavioral Disturbance
	292.82	Barbiturate-Induced Persisting Dementia
Axis III	331.0	Alzheimer's disease

294.8 Dementia Not Otherwise Specified

The category of Dementia Not Otherwise Specified can be used for demented patients for whom no cause can be clearly defined.

AMNESTIC DISORDERS

In the uncommon conditions known as *amnestic disorders*, loss of short-term memory is sometimes so severe that the patient cannot even recall events that took place only a few minutes earlier. As in other cognitive disorders, remote memories are better retained than more recent ones. Immediate recall (the ability to repeat a few seconds later what has just been heard) is not affected. Reduced attention span is not a prominent feature of the amnestic disorders, though it is often minimally present. When other cognitive symptoms are present (aphasia, apraxia, agnosia, loss of executive functioning), as they sometimes are, they are not nearly as important (for work or social life) as the failure of memory. Although these patients tend to be friendly enough, their *affect* (i.e., their behavioral indication of emotional state) is likely to be shallow.

As in any amnesia, patients generally have some disorientation for time, and often for place. A patient may successfully navigate a familiar house but may quickly become lost once hospitalized. Some are apathetic to the memory problem; others try to hide it by *confabulating* (i.e., they make up events to fill the information void). Confabulation may be spontaneous or may occur in response to prompting (Q: "Did I see you in the bar last night?" A: "Sure, I was there with my girlfriend"). If present at all, confabulation tends to be present early in the course of the disorder, then diminish.

The most frequent cause of amnestic syndromes is chronic alcohol use with accompanying vitamin B1 (thiamine) deficiency. Often, there are other symptoms of the underlying disorder. If the cause is alcohol, these may include peripheral neuropathy and cerebellar ataxia. The onset is usually rather sudden, although there are some reports of more gradual onset. Recovery can occur, though chronicity is more often the rule.

294.0 Amnestic Disorder Due to a General Medical Condition

All amnestic disorders are due to brain damage. Head trauma is probably the most common cause; other causes include surgery of the temporal lobe, hypoxia, stroke, and some forms of encephalitis (e.g., those resulting from tuberculosis, herpes simplex). When recovery occurs, it may take an extended period of time.

Criteria for Amnestic Disorder Due to a General Medical Condition

- The patient develops impaired memory (can't learn new information or can't recall information previously learned).
- These symptoms materially impair work or social functioning, and they indicate a decline in the patient's level of functioning.
- These symptoms don't occur *solely* during a delirium or dementia.
- A general medical condition has probably directly caused this memory impairment, as judged by history, physical exam, or laboratory data.

Coding Notes

Specify whether:
>   Transient: Duration is one month or less, *or*
>   Chronic: Duration is longer than one month.

In the wording for the name of the amnestic disorder, indicate the *exact* name of the cause, not the *class* name—for example, Amnestic Disorder Due to Herpes Simplex Encephalitis.

Code the general medical condition on Axis III.

Gerald Pratt

The symptoms of Gerald Pratt's depression had included insomnia and weight loss, and he had complained endlessly that he could not concentrate on his studies. He had never had a previous episode of depression or mania; he had been in good health and had never abused alcohol or drugs. After two months of misery, he had been found in a garage with the engine of his car still running.

This had happened six months ago. Although Gerald had survived the attempt, he had "not been right since," according to his mother (the main informant). He had tried to return to his forestry studies in junior college, but had soon dropped out. Since then, Gerald had remained at home. Although he was not depressed, he was extremely forgetful. His mother was afraid that the carbon monoxide had "affected his brain."

Gerald was a pleasant-appearing young man who was neatly dressed and showed no behavioral abnormalities. He paid careful attention during the examination and seemed eager to do well. His affect was about medium, and he said that he felt "normal"; he denied having any hallucinations, delusions, or suicidal ideas. His speech was clear, coherent, relevant, and spontaneous; he used no *neologisms* (i.e., invented words or peculiar meanings for established words).

Gerald's memory for material learned prior to the suicide attempt was very good, and he talked knowledgeably about the forestry courses he had once taken. He had no memory at all for the suicide attempt and could not imagine why he would have done anything so foolish. He could repeat up to five numbers that had just been recited to him; two minutes later, he remembered none of them. His memory for three objects at five minutes was nil. Although he could not state the month and date correctly, he knew the year and knew that it was winter. He scored 17 out of 30 on the Mini-Mental State Exam, failing after one subtraction of serial sevens. He quickly and accurately followed the three-part instruction. He named a watch and a pencil and repeated a simple phrase without errors. He copied a design and wrote a sentence flawlessly. He denied that his memory was impaired; when repeatedly questioned about this, he became rather angry.

Evaluation of Gerald Pratt

As in any other amnestic disorder, Gerald's most striking finding was the loss of short-term memory. Although his immediate recall (for a series of numbers) was unimpaired, he clearly had an anterograde amnesia (he could recall nothing he had been told only a few minutes earlier). His occupational functioning (in this case, going to school) had suffered a disastrous decline. His indignation and utter lack of insight are not unusual for this condition.

Gerald performed well on much of the Mental Status Exam. He focused his attention on the tasks he was given and demonstrated no aphasia, apraxia or agnosia. His executive functioning was intact, as judged by his neat appearance and his ability to follow a three-part command. From this information, we can rule out **delirium** and **dementia**. There was no evidence to suggest that he had manufactured his symptoms for financial gain or for other motives (**Malingering** or **Factitious Disorder**). Although Gerald had had a **mood disorder** at the time he made the suicide attempt, he now had no remnants of depressed mood or suicidal ideas. **Dissociative Amnesia** and **Dissociative Identity Disorder** could be eliminated on the basis of the previous history and his recall of much of his life before the suicide attempt.

Gerald's symptoms would suggest a diagnosis of Amnestic Disorder Due to Cerebral Anoxia. Because it had lasted far longer than one month, the specifier of "Chronic" would be added. The causative general medical condition would be specified on Axis III.

Even though it was not a current complaint, his mood disorder would also be specified (this would help alert clinicians and family members to a possible recurrence). He had had no manias and only a single episode of depression that met the full criteria for Major Depressive Episode (see p. 193). He had had no symptoms of depression since the suicide attempt, giving him the fifth digit severity score for In Full Remission (see p. 195). His complete diagnosis would be as follows:

Axis I	294.0	Amnestic Disorder Due to Cerebral Anoxia, Chronic	
	296.26	Major Depressive Disorder, Single Episode, In Full Remission	
Axis II	V71.09	No diagnosis	
Axis III	348.1	Cerebral anoxia	
Axis IV		None	
Axis V	GAF = 41 (current)		

Substance-Induced Persisting Amnestic Disorder

In theory, numerous substances can cause an amnestic disorder; in practice, clinicians have by far the most experience with alcoholism in this regard. This is the prototype of all amnestic disorders, one that has been known for years by the terms *Korsakoff's syndrome* and *Korsakoff's psychosis*. It is probably caused by a combination of prolonged thiamine deficiency and the direct effects of alcohol on the brain. This disorder may have become less common in the past few decades, since it has become routine to give thiamine to patients being detoxified from alcohol.

Although these patients may be apathetic and have other changes in personality, they are often attentive, alert, and capable of solving simple problems. Immediate memory is preserved (they can repeat words or digits just after hearing them), yet they have essentially no ability to form new, permanent memories. Many of their old memories have also been obliterated, though very old memories (those dating from childhood) are relatively unaffected. Of course, the word "Persisting" appears in the title to point out that the effects of the substance last far longer than would symptoms of intoxication or withdrawal.

Korsakoff's psychosis may begin as *Wernicke's encephalopathy*, a usually quiet delirium accompanied by paralysis of eye movements and trouble walking. If it is quickly treated with thiamine, it usually resolves within a few weeks. If this does not happen, it may evolve into the permanent memory deficit of Korsakoff's psychosis.

Criteria for Substance-Induced Persisting Amnestic Disorder

- The patient develops impaired memory (can't learn new information or can't recall information previously learned).

- These symptoms materially impair work or social functioning, and they indicate a decline in the patient's level of functioning.
- These symptoms don't occur *solely* during a delirium or dementia.
- Enduring effects of substance use have probably caused these deficits, as judged by history, physical exam, or laboratory data.

Coding Notes

The following code numbers can be utilized:

291.1	Alcohol
292.83	All remaining, including Sedative, Hypnotic, or Anxiolytic; Other [or Unknown] Substance

Also code Substance Dependence as appropriate on Axis I.

Patients who abuse sedatives, hypnotics, or anxiolytics can have intoxication and withdrawal syndromes identical to those seen in users of alcohol. On occasion, these can cause an amnestic disorder. When this is the case, the disorder should be coded as 292.83 with the exact substance specified, if known—for example, 292.83 Phenobarbital-Induced Persisting Amnestic Disorder. Of course, multiple diagnoses can be made when multiple substances are responsible.

If you can't identify the substance responsible, use this code: 292.83 Unknown Substance-Induced Persisting Amnestic Disorder.

Charles Jackson

A powerfully built six-footer, Charles Jackson still showed traces of a military bearing. Before he left the Army a year before, he had been demoted to buck private; this was the culmination of a string of disciplinary actions for drunkenness. Fortunately, he had served 21 years and did not forfeit his retirement pay.

For over a year he had had monthly consultations with the current interviewer. On his last Mini-Mental State Exam, Charles had scored 17: the full nine points for language, three for spelling "world" backwards as *drolw*, three for registration (immediately repeating three items), and two for knowing the city and state.

On this occasion, the interviewer asked when they had last met. Charles replied, "Well, I just don't know. What do you think?" To the follow-up question, he said that he guessed he had seen the interviewer before. "Maybe it was last week."

Asking him to remain seated, the interviewer went into the waiting room to ask Mrs. Jackson how she thought her husband was doing. She said, "Oh, he's about the same as before. He sketches some. He can still draw a pretty good caricature of you, as long as you're sitting right in front of him. But mostly, he just sits around the house and watches TV. I come home and ask him what he's been watching, but he can't even tell me."

At any rate, Charles was no longer drinking, not since they had moved to the country. It was at least two miles to the nearest convenience store, and he didn't walk very well any more. "But he still talks about drinking. Sometimes he seems to think he's still in the Army. He orders me to go buy him a quart of gin."

Charles remembered quite a few things, if they had happened long enough ago—the gin, for example, and getting drunk with his father when he was a boy. But he couldn't remember the name of his daughter, who was two and a half. Most of the time, he just called her "the girl."

The interviewer walked back into the inner office. Charles looked up and smiled.

"Have I seen you before?" asked the interviewer.

"Well, I'm pretty sure."

"When was it?"

"It might have been last week."

Evaluation of Charles Jackson

Charles had not only an especially severe anterograde memory loss (he could form no new memories), but also a considerable degree of retrograde amnesia (he couldn't even recall his daughter's name). He showed no evidence of shifting attention or reduced awareness, which ruled out a **delirium**. There was no evidence of agnosia, apraxia, aphasia, or loss of executive functioning, one of which would be needed to diagnose a **dementia**. In **Alcohol-Induced Persisting Dementia**, other impairments of thinking (such as judgment or ability to form abstractions) will be found, whereas in **Alcohol-Induced Persisting Amnestic Disorder**, memory is nominally the only faculty affected. His wife described no evidence of lapses in judgment unrelated to his desire to drink. With only a little prompting, Charles appeared to confabulate a previous meeting with the examiner. Although confabulation is not a criterion for diagnosis, it is one of the classic symptoms.

The main items of differential diagnosis include other causes of amnestic disorder and other complications of alcoholism. Either of these sources of confusion should be clear from the history. Of course, there is little danger that his condition would be mistaken for the **memory blackouts** associated with **Alcohol Intoxication**.

Although the history is not given completely in the case vignette, Charles would probably also receive an Axis I diagnosis of Alcohol Dependence. He had not met the criteria during the past year, so he would be given the added qualifier of Sustained Full Remission (see p. 76). The vignette does not contain information on which to judge whether or not the dependence was physiological. Any associated physical conditions, such as cirrhosis of the liver, would be scored on Axis III.

Axis I	291.1	Alcohol-Induced Persisting Amnestic Disorder
	303.90	Alcohol Dependence, Sustained Full Remission
Axis II	V71.09	No diagnosis
Axis III		None
Axis IV		None
Axis V	GAF = 41	(highest level past year)

294.8 Amnestic Disorder Not Otherwise Specified

The category of Amnestic Disorder Not Otherwise Specified can be used for patients who have an amnestic disorder but no established cause.

294.9 Cognitive Disorder Not Otherwise Specified

The category of Cognitive Disorder Not Otherwise Specified includes patients whose cognitive deficit does not clearly suggest delirium, dementia, or amnestic disorder. For example:

Mild Neurocognitive Disorder. DSM-IV specifically mentions that some patients may show deficits on psychological testing that are not severe enough to cause significant impairment. You will find suggested criteria for this diagnosis on page 706 of DSM-IV.

Postconcussional Disorder. Suggested research criteria for this rather self-explanatory condition are provided on page 704 of DSM-IV.

Mental Disorders Due to a General Medical Condition

Quick Guide to Mental Disorders Due to a General Medical Condition

Amnestic Disorder. A medical illness can cause a profound loss of memory (including the inability to form new memories), but such patients can focus attention and otherwise perform well cognitively (p. 46).

Anxiety Disorder. Panic attacks or generalized anxiety can be caused by various medical illnesses (p. 280).

Catatonic Disorder. A variety of medical and neurological conditions can produce catatonia and other psychotic symptoms that may not meet criteria for any of the psychotic disorders (p. 54).

Delirium. Medical conditions that can cause delirium include trauma to the brain, infections, epilepsy, endocrine disorders, and various other diseases throughout the body (p. 18).

Dementia. A large number of diseases can cause dementia. Some of the most noteworthy include brain tumor, Creutzfeldt–Jakob disease (infection with a slow virus), head trauma, HIV disease, Huntington's disease, Parkinson's disease and Pick's disease. The most common endogenous toxins causing dementia are those resulting from uremia and hepatic failure (p. 38).

Mood Disorder. Either highs or lows of mood can be caused by various physical illnesses (p. 229).

Personality Change. Medical illnesses can affect a patient's personality for the worse. As noted above, this does not qualify as a Personality Disorder, because it may be less pervasive and not present from an early age (p. 57).

Psychotic Disorder. A variety of medical and neurological conditions can produce psychotic symptoms that may not meet criteria for any of the other psychotic disorders (p. 178).

Sexual Dysfunction. Sexual problems are often the result of physical illnesses (p. 357).

Sleep Disorder. Many patients who have medical problems complain that they sleep too much or not enough; numerous parasomnias can also occur under these circumstances (p. 396).

Introduction

This chapter covers a DSM-IV section that is new to the manual. The criteria for most disorders caused by a general medical condition (they are listed in the Quick Guide, above) have been given in their appropriate DSM-IV sections; for the sake of uniformity, the same practice is followed in the chapters of this book.

However, two conditions are treated here in their entirety, because they really don't belong anywhere else. Catatonic Disorder Due to a General Medical Condition does not belong with Schizophrenia, and because it doesn't necessarily involve hallucinations or delusions, it doesn't fit the more general criteria for a Psychotic Disorder Due to a General Medical Condition. (It could have been included as a Psychotic Disorder Not Otherwise Specified, but it wasn't.)

Personality Change Due to a General Medical Condition has not been included with the personality disorders for several reasons:

- It isn't necessarily present from the patient's teen years (or earlier).
- The behavior doesn't necessarily affect many aspects of the patient's life (in DSM-IV lingo, it may be less pervasive than a personality disorder).
- A medical disorder *can* be identified that could account for the change in personality.

293.89 Catatonic Disorder
Due to a General Medical Condition

Although the criteria listed for Catatonic Disorder Due to a General Medical Condition include excited as well as retarded behavior, a patient with a general medical condition is most likely to have the characteristic symptoms of re-tarded catatonia. These symptoms include *posturing* (assuming an odd position voluntarily); *catalepsy* (holding a pose when told that it is not necessary); and *waxy flexibility* (the contraction of flexor and extensor muscles at the same time; for example, when you bend the patient's arm at the elbow, it feels as if you were bending a rod made of wax). Patients may also drool, stop eating, or become mute. Some of these behaviors are further described and discussed in the section on Schizophrenia, Catatonic Type (see p. 152).

Catatonia of any cause was once encountered fairly frequently; now it is uncommon. Most descriptions of Catatonic Disorder Due to a General Medical Condition only mention one, sometimes two, patients. The medical conditions responsible include viral encephalitis, postpartum psychosis, subarachnoid hemorrhage, ruptured berry aneurysm in the brain, subdural hematoma, hyperparathyroidism, arteriovenous malformation, temporal lobe tumor, akinetic mutism, and penetrating head wounds. There has even been a description of one patient who had a reaction to fluorides. A busy neurologist or mental health clinician who does a lot of consulting in a large medical center may occasionally encounter a case.

Criteria for Catatonic Disorder
Due to a General Medical Condition

- The patient has catatonic symptoms, as shown by immobility, extreme and apparently aimless physical activity, pronounced negativism, muteness, echolalia, echopraxia, or peculiarities of voluntary movement (such as posturing or waxy flexibility).
- History, physical exam, or laboratory findings suggest that these symptoms are caused directly by a general medical condition.
- The symptoms don't occur solely during a delirium.
- No other mental disorder better explains these symptoms.

Coding Note

Use the name of the general medical condition on Axis I. On Axis III, record the general medical condition diagnosis responsible for the catatonia.

Marion Wright

Since graduating from high school 12 years earlier, Marion Wright had worked as a sign painter. In school he had shown some aptitude for art, though not enough that he saw himself as the next Pablo Picasso. Nor did he like school enough to study for a career in commercial art. But painting signs on buildings and billboards was undemanding, well-paying, immediately available, and largely open-air. Within a few years he was married, had two kids and a small house in a subdivision, and was still painting signs. He thought he was set for life.

One afternoon not long after his 30th birthday, his foreman drove by to inspect the billboard Marion had just finished. "You've painted the logo in script. The blueprint calls for block letters," the foreman pointed out. Marion said that he thought the script looked better, but without much grumbling he changed it. A week later he completed an ad for a local premium beer; the female model holding the bottle was naked from the waist up. The following day he was out of work.

Marion made a few efforts to find a new job, but within a week he was staying at home and watching daytime TV. His wife noted that he seemed to be talking less and less, but he ignored her suggestion to seek clinical evaluation. Although he continued to eat and sleep normally, his interest in sex vanished. By the fourth week after losing his job, he had no spontaneous speech at all and would only answer a question if it was directly put to him. With the added persuasion of Marion's brother, his wife finally got him to the clinic. He was immediately hospitalized.

On admission Marion would answer questions appropriately, if briefly. Fully oriented, he denied feeling depressed or suicidal. He had no delusions, hallucinations, obsessions or compulsions. He earned a perfect score on the Mini-Mental State Exam, though the examiner noted that he was slow to carry out instructions.

The following morning he deliberately turned away from the nurse who approached his bedside. Although he willingly accompanied the nurse to a table in the dining room, he refused to eat and was completely mute. In fact, the clinician who examined him later that morning found that Marion would readily move in any direction at the slightest touch of an examiner's hand. In the evening he seemed improved and even spoke a few words.

But the following morning, he again silently refused to cooperate. When his pillow was removed, his head remained elevated about two inches above the mattress. This position appeared to cause him no discomfort; he seemed ready to maintain it all day. Later, an examiner noted that when Marion's arm was twisted into an awkward position (elevated at an angle over the bed), he maintained that position even when he was told that he could relax.

Marion's clinicians considered the diagnosis of Schizophrenia, but they noted that he had been only briefly ill and had no family history of psychosis. His wife assured them that he had never abused drugs or alcohol. Despite the fact that his neurological exam remained normal, an MRI of his head was obtained. It revealed a tumor the size of a golf ball sitting on the convexity of his right frontal lobe. Once this was surgically removed, he quickly regained full consciousness. Two months later he was back on his ladder painting billboards, following instructions to the letter.

Evaluation of Marion Wright

Marion had several symptoms that are classical for catatonia. These included negativism (turning away from the nurse when she approached his bedside), muteness (this can be complete, as in Marion's case, or relative), exaggerated compliance (moving at the slightest touch by an examiner), a "psychological pillow" (holding his head unsupported above the mattress), and catalepsy (maintaining an uncomfortable posture even when told that he could relax). He did not show the additional symptoms of *echolalia* (parroting back what has just been said) or *echopraxia* (repeatedly imitating someone's actions).

Marion did not have the wandering attention found in **delirium**. Catatonic behavior can be found in **Schizophrenia**, which his clinicians correctly rejected because he had been ill too briefly. Too few symptoms ruled out **Schizophreniform Disorder**. Muteness and marked retardation, even to the point of immobility, can be encountered in **Major Depressive Episode**, but he specifically denied mood symptoms. Muteness may occasionally be encountered in **Somatization Disorder** and in **Malingering** or **Factitious Disorder**, but it would be unusual to encounter a full, persisting catatonic syndrome in one of these conditions.

Note that catatonic behavior can include excessive or even frenzied motor activity. Then the differential diagnosis would include **Manic Episode** and **Substance Intoxication**. Of course, neither of these applied to Marion's case.

On laboratory and surgical examination, Marion was found to have a (benign) brain tumor, the direct physiological result of which can be catatonic symptoms. This fulfilled the criteria for his Axis I diagnosis:

Axis I	293.89	Catatonic Disorder Due to Meningioma
Axis II	V71.09	No diagnosis
Axis III	225.2	Cerebral meningioma, benign
Axis IV		None
Axis V	GAF = 21	(on admission)
	GAF = 90	(at discharge)

310.1 Personality Change Due to a General Medical Condition

Some medical conditions can cause a personality change, which is defined as some alteration (usually a worsening) of the patient's previous personality traits. If the medical condition occurs early enough in childhood, the change can last throughout the person's life. Most personality changes are caused by an injury to the brain or by some other central nervous system disorder, such as epilepsy or Huntington's disease, but systemic diseases (e.g., systemic lupus erythematosis) that affect the brain are also sometimes implicated.

Several sorts of personality changes commonly occur. Mood may become unstable, perhaps with outbursts of rage or suspiciousness. Other patients may become apathetic and passive; paranoid ideas are also common. Changes in mood are especially common with damage to the frontal lobes of the brain. Patients with temporal lobe epilepsy may be overly religious, verbose, and lacking in a sense of humor; some become markedly aggressive. Belligerence can accompany these outbursts of temper, to the extent that some patients can have markedly impaired social judgment. The type specifiers listed in the Coding Notes are used to categorize the nature of the personality change.

If there is a major alteration in the structure of the brain, these personality changes can persist. If the problem stems from a correctable chemical problem, the changes may resolve. When severe, they can ultimately lead to dementia, as is sometimes the case in patients with multiple sclerosis.

Criteria for Personality Change
Due to a General Medical Condition

- There has been a lasting change from the patient's established personality.
- History, physical exam, or laboratory findings suggest that a general medical condition has directly caused the personality change.
- No other mental disorder (including those caused by a general medical condition) better accounts for these symptoms.
- The symptoms don't occur solely during a delirium and don't fulfill criteria for dementia.
- This problem causes important clinical distress or impairs work, social, or personal functioning.

Coding Notes

Specify type (depending on the main feature):

Aggressive Type: Aggressive behavior

Apathetic Type: Indifference

Disinhibited Type: Loss of impulse control, as shown by such behavior as sexual indiscretions

Labile Type: Unstable affect

Paranoid Type: Paranoid ideas or suspiciousness

Other Type: DSM-IV gives the example of personality change that occurs with a seizure disorder

Combined Type: More than one feature of the clinical picture stands out

Unspecified Type

Use the name of the general medical condition on Axis I. On Axis III, record the general medical condition diagnosis responsible for the personality change.

To make this diagnosis in children, there must be at least a year-long, pronounced deviation from normal development or a material change in the child's usual patterns of behavior.

Eddie Ortway

The potential for rehabilitation of 28-year-old Eddie Ortway was evaluated following a gunshot wound. Born in central Los Angeles, Eddie was reared by his mother whenever she was neither in jail for prostitution nor in the hospital for drug and alcohol use. His parents, he always suspected, had been only briefly acquainted.

Eddie avoided school whenever possible, and grew up with no role model in sight. His principal accomplishment was learning to use his fists. By the time he was 15, he and his gang had participated in several turf wars. He was making a name for himself as an aggressive enemy.

But Eddie was not a criminal, and the necessity for earning a living soon sent him to work. With little education and no training, he found his opportunities pretty much limited to fast food and hard labor. Sometimes he held several jobs at a time. But, as an old probation report noted, he still had "a raging sense of injustice." Although he gradually stopped associating with his gang, through his middle 20s he continued to deal aggressively with any situation that seemed to require direct action.

His 27th birthday was one of these. Eddie was delivering a pizza to an apartment building in his old neighborhood when he encountered a teenager forcing an old woman into an alley at gunpoint. Eddie stepped forward and for his pains received a bullet that entered his head through the left eye socket and exited at the hairline.

He was admitted to the hospital by way of the operating room, where surgeons debrided his wound. He never even lost consciousness and was released in less than a week. But he did not return to work. The social worker's report noted that Eddie's physical condition had rebounded within a month, but that he "lacked drive." He appeared for every scheduled job interview, but his prospective employers uniformly reported that he "just didn't seem very interested in working."

"I needed time to recuperate," Eddie told the interviewer. He was a good-looking young man whose hair had begun receding from his forehead. An incisional scar ran up onto his scalp. "I still don't think I'm quite ready."

He had been recuperating for two years. Now he was being tested to try to learn why. Other than a slight droop of his left eyelid, his neurological examination was completely normal. An EEG showed some slow waves over the frontal lobes; the MRI showed a localized absence of brain tissue.

Eddie never failed to cooperate with testing procedures, and all of the clinicians who examined him noted that he was polite and pleasant. However, as one of them put it, "There seems something slightly mechanical about his cooperation. He complies but never anticipates, and he shows little interest in the proceedings."

His affect was about medium and showed almost no lability. His speech was clear, coherent, and relevant. He denied delusions, hallucinations, obsessions, compulsions, or phobias. When asked what he was interested in, he thought for a few seconds and then answered that he guessed he was interested in going back home. He made a perfect score on the Mini-Mental State Exam.

In the time since his injury, Eddie admitted, he had lived on workers' compensation and spent most of his time watching television. He didn't argue with any one anymore. When one examiner asked him what he would do if he again saw someone being mugged, he shrugged and said that he thought people should "just live and let live."

Evaluation of Eddie Ortway

Eddie's history and examinations presented an obvious general medical cause for his personality change. (Note that it was the *physiology* of trauma to the brain that produced Eddie's personality change. This is an explicit requirement for this diagnosis, which cannot be made when personality change accompanies a nonspecific medical condition such as severe pain.)

A normal attention span and lack of memory deficit ruled out **delirium** and **dementia**. An Axis II disorder such as **Dependent Personality Disorder** could not explain Eddie's condition, because his behavior represented a marked change from his *premorbid personality* (i.e., the way he was until his injury). And the features of Eddie's personality change were not better explained by a different Mental Disorder Due to a General Medical Condition. A Mood Disorder Due to Brain Trauma would be one of several possible examples.

Besides head trauma, a variety of neurological conditions can cause personality change. These include multiple sclerosis, cerebrovascular accidents, brain tumors, and temporal lobe epilepsy. Other causes of behavioral change that can *look* like a change in personality include such Axis I disorders as **Delusional Disorder**, **Impulse Control Disorder**, **Mood Disorders**, and **Schizophrenia**. But Eddie's problems began abruptly after he was shot, and he had no prior history that was consistent with any other Axis I disorder. However, many other patients experience personality change associated with Axis I disorders, including Substance Dependence.

The fact that Eddie's condition impaired him socially and occupationally completed the criteria for this diagnosis. In his clinical picture, apathy (and passivity) clearly stood out as the main feature. This determined the specific subtype.

Axis I	310.1	Personality Change Due to a General Medical Disorder, Apathetic Type
Axis II	V71.09	No diagnosis
Axis III	851.31	Open gunshot wound of cerebral cortex, without loss of consciousness
Axis IV		None
Axis V	GAF = 55	(highest level past year)

293.9 Mental Disorder Not Otherwise Specified Due to a General Medical Condition

The Not Otherwise Specified category can be used to code a patient whose symptoms appear to be caused by a medical disorder but do not qualify for any of the 10 disorders listed in the Quick Guide. DSM-IV specifically mentions the following:

Dissociation. This can occur with partial complex seizures.

Substance-Related Disorders

Quick Guide to the Substance-Related Disorders

Mind-altering substances all yield four basic types of disorder: Substance Dependence, Abuse, Intoxication, and Withdrawal. Most of these DSM-IV terms apply to nearly all of the substances discussed; exceptions are noted below.

Substance Use Disorders

Substance Dependence. This means that the user has taken a substance frequently enough to produce clinically important distress or impaired functioning, as well as certain behavioral characteristics. Found in connection with all classes of drugs but caffeine, Substance Dependence doesn't have to be intentional; it can develop from medicinal use, such as the treatment of chronic pain. A discussion of Substance Dependence, in which Alcohol Dependence is used as a model, begins on page 67.

Substance Abuse. This is a *residual category* (i.e., a diagnosis of last resort) for patients whose substance use produces problems but does not fulfill the more rigorous criteria for Substance Dependence. This diagnosis applies to all substances but caffeine and nicotine. It conveys less information than Substance Dependence; as of this writing, it is still unclear whether the diagnosis has much predictive value. It is discussed beginning on page 79. (Alcohol Abuse is used as an illustration.)

Substance-Induced Disorders

Substance Intoxication. This acute clinical condition results from recent overuse of a substance. Anyone can become intoxicated; this is the only substance-related diagnosis that can apply to a person who uses a substance only once. All drugs but nicotine have a specific syndrome of intoxication. The definitions of these syndromes can be found in the text at the positions indicated in the first column of Table 3.1 (page 64). Using Alcohol Intoxication as the model, a general discussion of Substance Intoxication begins on page 81.

Substance Withdrawal. This collection of symptoms, specific for the class of substance, develops when a person who has frequently used a substance discontinues or markedly reduces the amount used. All substances except caffeine, cannabis, PCP, the hallucinogens, and the inhalants have an officially recognized withdrawal syndrome. Again with Alcohol Withdrawal as the model, a discussion of Substance Withdrawal begins on page 72.

Various other substance-induced disorders (described in detail elsewhere in this book) have been described for each of the substances except nicotine. These include Substance-Induced Delirium, Persisting Dementia, Persisting Amnestic Disorder, Psychotic Disorder, Mood Disorder, Anxiety Disorder, Sexual Dysfunction, and Sleep Disorder. They can be experienced during intoxication, during withdrawal, or as consequences of the substance use that endure long after misuse and withdrawal symptoms have ended. You will find discussions of these disorders located in their respective chapters, on the pages indicated in the column heads of Table 3.1.

As a concise reference to all of the substance-related disorders, it is hard to improve upon the table given in DSM-IV (which I have adapted here as Table 3.1). Unhappily, there is little to go on in the way of indicating the prevalence of these disorders.

Introduction

Citizens of the late 20th century have an ever-widening variety of mind-altering substances to use, but doing so still leads to a few basic sorts of problems with behavior, cognition, and physiological symptoms. These behaviors and substances are discussed in this chapter. The substances, all of which affect the central nervous system, include medications, toxic chemicals, and illegal drugs. Several substances, however, can be obtained legally without a prescription: alcohol, caffeine, and nicotine, as well as some of the inhalants.

DSM-IV lists 120 numbered substance-related disorders. When all the subcodes

Table 3.1 Substances and Their Mental Effects

	Substance - related disorder					
Substance	Delirium[a] (p. 21)	Persisting Dementia (p. 41)	Persisting Amnestic Disorder (p. 49)	Psychotic Disorder[b] (p. 180)	Mood Disorder (p. 233)	Anxiety Disorder (p. 282)
Alcohol (p. 67)	291.0 I/W	291.2	291.1	291.5/.3 I/W	291.8 I/W	291.8 I/W
Amphetamines (p. 86)	292.81 I			292.11/.12 I	292.84 I/W	292.89 I
Caffeine (p. 92)						292.89 I
Cannabis (p. 94)	292.81 I			292.11/.12 I		292.89 I
Cocaine (p. 99)	292.81 I			292.11/.12 I	292.84 I/W	292.89 I/W
Hallucinogens (p. 104)	292.81 I			292.11/.12[c] I	292.84 I	292.89 I
Inhalants (p. 110)	292.81 I	292.82		292.11/.12 I	292.84 I	292.89 I
Nicotine (p. 114)						
Opioids (p. 116)	292.81 I			292.11/.12 I	292.84 I	
PCP (p. 122)	292.81 I			292.11/.12 I	292.84 I	292.89 I
Sedatives, hypnotics, anxiolytics (p. 126)	292.81 I/W	292.82	292.83	292.11/.12 I/W	292.84 I/W	292.89 W
Other (or unknown) (p. 132)	292.81 I/W	292.82	292.83	292.11/.12 I/W	292.84 I/W	292.89 I/W

Adapted with permission from the *Diagnostic and Statistical Manual of Mental Disorders* (4th ed., p. 177) by the American Psychiatric Association, 1994, Washington, DC: Author. Copyright 1994 by the American Psychiatric Association.

The page number given for each substance and each type of disorder indicates the point in text at which a discussion of that substance or disorder begins. Abbreviations in table body: I, with intoxication; W, on withdrawal; PD, perceptual disturbances.

[a] Any delirium is called Substance Intoxication Delirium or Substance Withdrawal Delirium, according to whether it occurs during intoxication or withdrawal. The code numbers are the same regardless.

[b] For the psychotic disorders, the first set of numbers after the decimal point indicates the code for "With Delusions;" the second set of numbers indicates the code for "With Hallucinations."

[c] Also 292.89 Hallucinogen Persisting Perception Disorder (Flashbacks).

Table 3.1 Substances and Their Mental Effects 65

Table 3.1 Substances and Their Mental Effects *(cont'd)*

Substance - related disorder

Sexual Dysfunction (p. 541)	Sleep Disorder (p. 652)	Disorder NOS	Dependence (p. 105)	Abuse (p. 122)	Intoxication (p. 126)	Withdrawal (p. 112)
291.8 I	291.8 I/W	291.9	303.90	305.00	303.00	291.8 PD
292.89 I	292.89 I/W	292.9	304.40	305.70	292.89 PD	292.0
	292.89 I	292.9			305.90	
		292.9	304.30	305.20	292.89 PD	
292.89 I	292.89 I/W	292.9	304.20	305.60	292.89 PD	292.0
		292.9	304.50	305.30	292.89	
		292.9	304.60	305.90	292.89	
		292.9	305.10			292.0
292.89 I	292.89 I/W	292.9	304.00	305.50	292.89 PD	292.0
		292.9	304.90	305.90	292.89 PD	
292.89 I	292.89 I/W	292.9	304.10	305.40	292.89	292.0 PD
292.89 I	292.89 I/W	292.9	304.90	305.90	292.89 PD	292.0 PD

and qualifiers are taken into account, there are hundreds of ways to code a patient with a substance-related disorder. For any substance-related disorder, the diagnostician must specify the substance(s) responsible, the type of problem, and in some cases the time relationship of substance use to the onset of the problem behavior.

DSM-IV uses 11 groupings, plus the usual Not Otherwise Specified, to categorize substances. All of these groupings, however, are artificial, and among these 11 we can identify certain similarities:

- Central nervous system depressants (alcohol and the sedatives, hypnotics, and anxiolytics)
- Central nervous system stimulants (cocaine, amphetamines, and caffeine)
- Perception-distorting drugs (inhalants, cannabis, hallucinogens, and phencyclidine [PCP])
- Narcotics (opioids)
- Nicotine
- Other (corticosteroids and other medications)

In addition, Polysubstance Dependence is diagnosed when, over a period of six months, a patient has used at least three mind-altering substances and none of them predominates.

TIP The terminology keeps changing, but the basic disorders are the same: alcoholism and drug abuse. One of the problems with substance use has been that because it has been so variously defined (by different writers, for different substances, in different eras), there is substantial disagreement as to exactly what it is and who engages in it. The genius of DSM-IV is to define the disorders related to all the substances more or less uniformly. These definitions replace older terms such as *alcoholism*, *problem drinking*, *loss of control*, *physiological dependence*, *addiction*, *habituation*, and other (often pejorative) terms applied over the years to people who use mind-altering substances.

Most adults use some substances; most do not use them pathologically. But what is *pathological use*? It is use beyond which any positive effects are outweighed by negative effects. Often, this point comes very early—for some patients and substances, with their first exposure. Usually, the use is frequent; it always involves symptoms and maladaptive changes in behavior.

Finally, the term *drug abuse* is variously defined. The National Institute on Drug Abuse defines it as using a substance because of its psychic effect, because of dependence, because of a wish to commit suicide, or for any other reason that is not consistent with accepted medical practice. The DSM-IV definition is different: By Substance Abuse, it refers to problem behavior that is less than addictive (see Quick Guide).

The terms *denial* and *craving* are nowhere to be found in the DSM-IV criteria, yet they are clearly important in the development of substance-related disorders. (Perhaps the authors found them too hard to quantify. This is a problem that needs further consideration.)

Note also that none of the symptoms for Substance Dependence or Abuse explain why users like their chosen substances. In an effort to be objective and consistent, the DSM-IV criteria ignore many of the nuances of dependence on specific substances. Gone, for example, is the descriptive richness of the stages of alcoholism. You should consult mental health textbooks, scientific articles, and literary works to supplement these criteria.

THE BASIC SUBSTANCE-RELATED CATEGORIES, ILLUSTRATED BY ALCOHOL-RELATED DISORDERS

My approach in this part of the chapter differs somewhat from the DSM-IV format for discussing Substance Dependence, Abuse, Intoxication, and Withdrawal. First, instead of discussing these basic disorder types by themselves, I use the alcohol-related disorders in these categories as illustrations. Second, instead of pairing the substance use disorders (in this case, Alcohol Dependence and Abuse) and the substance-induced disorders (Alcohol Intoxication and Withdrawal), I pair Alcohol Dependence with Withdrawal and Alcohol Abuse with Intoxication, in order to illustrate the first two in one patient and the second two in another (the first patient's wife). Later in the chapter, I discuss whatever intoxication and/or withdrawal syndromes apply to each of the other 10 substance groupings listed in Table 3.1. (Note that the criteria for Substance Dependence and Abuse, given below in connection with Alcohol Dependence and Abuse, are applicable to all substance groupings.) I also briefly mention other disorders related to each substance, as well as other substances.

Substance Dependence

For years, clinicians and researchers have argued about the definitions of substance abuse. The DSM-IV approach is to define Substance Dependence as the core behavior of those who misuse substances. These criteria specify a type of dependence that includes behavioral, physiological, and cognitive symptoms. As an exercise, let us dissect some of the language regarding Substance Dependence (see the criteria set on page 69). It is described in the following terms:

- **The use is maladaptive**. Its use (perhaps to cope with other problems) only makes things worse for the user, as well as the user's relatives and associates.
- **There is a pattern to the use**. The repetition of this use forms a predictable habit pattern.
- **The effects are clinically important**. This usage pattern either has come to the attention of professionals or warrants such attention. (Actually, the original DSM-IV language reads "clinically significant." However, the word *significant* has statistical implications that cannot be sustained in clinical practice. I think *important* is better here. In this text I have also substituted the word *material* for significant.)
- **The use causes distress or impairment**. This says that the substance use must be serious enough to interfere in some way with the patient's life. Substance Dependence is thereby defined in exactly the same terms as are used for many other non-substance-related Axis I disorders. To support this analysis of Substance Dependence, you must be able to identify at least three of the seven symptoms noted in the criteria set.

Finally, in diagnosing not only Substance Dependence but Substance Abuse, Intoxication, and Withdrawal, remember that rapidity of onset and excretion affect the likelihood that a patient will develop problems with a given substance. Rapidly absorbing a substance (by smoking, snorting, or injection) favors quicker onset of action, shorter duration of action, and greater likelihood of Substance Dependence or Abuse. A longer *half-life* (the time it takes the body to eliminate half the remaining substance) extends the period during which the user will experience Substance Withdrawal, but reduces the likelihood of withdrawal symptoms.

303.90 Alcohol Dependence

Although nearly half of all adult Americans have had some sort of problem with alcohol (driving drunk, hangover that kept them from work) at least once in their lives, far fewer (about 10%) have had so many problems that they qualify for a diagnosis of Alcohol Dependence. Note that the criteria are the same as for any other type of Substance Dependence; they are given below as generic Substance Dependence criteria.

Generic Criteria for Substance Dependence

- The patient's maladaptive pattern of substance use leads to clinically important distress or impairment, as shown in a single 12-month period by three or more of the following:
  - ✓ Tolerance, shown by *either* of these:
    - ✓ markedly increased intake of the substance is needed to achieve the same effect, *or*
    - ✓ with continued use, the same amount of the substance has markedly less effect.
  - ✓ Withdrawal, shown by *either* of these:
    - ✓ the substance's characteristic withdrawal syndrome is experienced *or*
    - ✓ the substance (or one closely related) is used to avoid or relieve withdrawal symptoms.
  - ✓ The amount or duration of use is often greater than intended.
  - ✓ The patient repeatedly tries without success to control or reduce substance use.
  - ✓ The patient spends much time using the substance, recovering from its effects, or trying to obtain it.
  - ✓ The patient reduces or abandons important work, social, or leisure activities because of substance use.
  - ✓ The patient continues to use the substance, despite knowing that it has probably caused ongoing physical or psychological problems.

Coding Notes

Specify whether:

With Physiological Dependence. There is evidence of tolerance or withdrawal (see above).

Without Physiological Dependence.

Choose one or none of the following to specify course (see p. 76):

Early Full Remission (months 2 through 12)

Early Partial Remission (months 2 through 12)

Sustained Full Remission (months 13+)

Sustained Partial Remission (months 13+)

Specify neither, either, or both of these:

On Agonist Therapy (does not apply to cannabis, hallucinogens, inhalants, PCP)

In a Controlled Environment (does not apply to nicotine)

Quentin McCarthy

"I can get off it, but I can't stay off it." Quentin McCarthy was 43, and he was talking about alcohol. He liked to say that throughout his adult life he had been successful at two things—drinking and selling insurance. Now he was having trouble with both.

Quentin was the second of three sons born to parents who were both attorneys. Both of his brothers had been excellent students. Quentin was bright, but he had been hyperactive and the class clown. In school, he had never been able to focus his attention well enough to excel at anything but physical education.

To please his parents, after high school Quentin tried a semester of junior college. It was worse than high school—the only thing that kept him going was guilt. Whereas his older brother was admitted to law school (with honors at entrance) and his younger brother mopped up the prizes at the state science fair, Quentin felt almost joyful when his birthday was that year's number four pick in the national draft lottery. The following day he enlisted in the Army.

Somewhere in his schooling Quentin had learned to type, so he was assigned to his battalion's administrative section. Throughout four years in the military, he never fired his weapon in anger. By comparison with some of the older men, his drinking was moderate. Although he had about the usual number of fights, he managed to avoid serious trouble. When he left the service at age 22, he had held onto his sergeant's stripes through two tours of duty in Vietnam.

After that, life suddenly became serious. Working part-time after hours in the post exchange, Quentin had discovered that he was a natural salesman. So it seemed a logical move to take a job selling life insurance. It also seemed sensible to marry the boss's daughter. When his father-in-law died suddenly two years later, Quentin became sole proprietor of the agency.

"The business made me and it ruined me," he said. "I made a lot of money having lunch with people and selling them large policies. I told myself that I had to drink with them in order to make a sale, but I suppose that was just rationalization."

As time went on, Quentin's two-martini lunches turned into four-martini lunches. By the time he was 31, he was skipping lunch completely and nipping throughout the afternoon to "keep a glow on." At the end of the day, he was sometimes surprised to see how much had disappeared from the bottle he kept in his desk drawer.

The past year had brought Quentin two unpleasant surprises. The first came when his doctor informed him that the nagging pain just above his navel was an ulcer; for the sake of his health, he would have to stop drinking. The second, which in a way seemed worse because it injured his pride, occurred one afternoon over lunch. A long-time client of the agency apologetically said that he would be taking his substantial business elsewhere; his wife didn't feel comfortable that he was "doing business with a lush." Thinking back, Quentin realized that there had been several other, less blatant instances of customers departing the fold.

The result had been his resolve to quit, or at least to reduce the amount of his drinking. ("Quitting is easy," he remarked ruefully. "I did it twice in one month.") At first he promised himself he would not drink before 5 p.m.; that proved impractical, and he later amended it to "around lunchtime." With the level in his desk drawer bottle receding as fast as ever, Quentin decided he would try Alcoholics Anonymous. "That was worse than useless," he explained. "The stories I heard from some of those people made me feel like a teetotaler."

A comment made by his wife, herself no stranger to alcohol, eventually brought him in for evaluation. "You used to drink to have a good time," she told him. "Now you drink because you need it."

Evaluation of Quentin McCarthy

The criteria for Substance Dependence are not especially complicated, just long. Quentin's history of alcohol use illustrates most of the major features of Substance Dependence. At least three of these characteristics are needed to qualify for the diagnosis, and they must have all occurred within a one-year period. This is not to say that they must have begun within the year prior to evaluation, only that the problems must have been present within a relatively compact time frame. (Incidentally, not all experts in chemical dependence would agree with DSM-IV's somewhat restrictive insistence on the one-year time frame for symptoms of Substance Dependence. Some patients may deteriorate very slowly, presenting new symptoms and abandoning old ones sporadically. Many experienced clinicians would argue that such patients shouldn't be excluded from the Substance Dependence diagnosis.)

- **Tolerance.** *Tolerance* means that a substance has been taken long enough for the user's body to grow accustomed to the chemical effects. Therefore, a greater quantity of the substance is needed to produce the same effect. This is especially apparent in regard to alcohol, opioids, and sedatives, but it can be found in all other substance groups, with the possible exception of PCP. As a result of tolerance, the patient either requires more of the substance to obtain the same effect or feels less effect from the same dose. Quentin experienced some of this when he began drinking throughout the afternoon to keep his "glow" on.
- **Withdrawal.** The symptoms of withdrawal are discussed below.
- **Using more.** Many patients start out to consume a relatively small amount (e.g., "just a nip before dinner"), but end up skipping dinner and just nipping. As a result, they use more of their substance of choice than they intend.
- **Attempts at control.** Quentin tried to quit by setting rules and attend-

ing Alcoholics Anonymous. For others, quitting completely may seem too drastic and frightening. They may instead try to reduce the amount they use.

- **Time investment**. This symptom is especially characteristic of those who use substances other than alcohol. (Alcoholics often carry on with other activities, drunk or sober.) And alcohol, like nicotine, is legal and hence easy to obtain. Quentin spent a good deal of time drinking, which probably qualified him on this criterion, even though he was also working during much of that time. Other patients, especially those who use drugs other than alcohol, may spend a great deal of time ensuring their supplies. For example, see the case of Kirk Aufderheide (page 127).
- **Reduction in other activities**. Substance-dependent patients commonly ignore work and social activities. This was not the case with Quentin, who devoted the necessary time to work (though some clients objected to his drinking).
- **Warnings ignored**. Quentin drank despite the dangers from ulcers. Other patients may ignore warnings about liver disease (cirrhosis or hepatitis) or esophageal varicose veins, which can rupture after prolonged retching. IV drug users often continue to share needles, despite the well-known risk of AIDS. Suicidal ideas, mood disorders, and psychoses can be exacerbated by the use of nearly any drug in common use.

In this vignette, Quentin showed at least five of the seven criteria for Alcohol Dependence. The next vignette will reveal whether he would also meet the criteria for Alcohol Withdrawal.

Substance Withdrawal

The symptoms of Substance Withdrawal develop as the concentration of a substance decreases in the user's brain. The generic criteria for Substance Withdrawal are simple: They require only that the patient develop specific symptoms after ceasing to take a substance that has been used heavily for a long time. Stress or impairment must result, and no general medical condition or other mental disorder must better explain the symptoms.

Generic Criteria for Substance Withdrawal

- A syndrome specific to a substance develops when someone who has used it frequently and for a long time suddenly stops or markedly reduces its intake.
- This syndrome causes clinically important distress or impairs work, social, or other functioning.

• This syndrome is neither the result of a general medical condition nor better explained by a different mental disorder.

The symptoms that develop during Substance Withdrawal are specific to the substance used and are described in the relevant sections of this chapter. However, certain symptoms are found in withdrawal from many substances:

- Alteration in mood (anxiety, irritability, depression)
- Abnormal motor activity (restlessness, immobility)
- Sleep disturbance (insomnia or hypersomnia)
- Other physical problems (fatigue, changes in appetite)

For a substance to cause withdrawal symptoms, patients must first become tolerant to it. This requires frequent use for a period of time that depends on the specific substance. For heroin, this may be only a few injections. For alcohol, weeks of heavy drinking are usually needed to produce clinically important tolerance. Most patients who are dependent on a substance will experience withdrawal if it is taken away from them suddenly.

Several substances do not produce Substance Withdrawal. Hallucinogens, for example, can induce dependence, yet a withdrawal syndrome has not been reported. (Although DSM-IV lists no official Caffeine Withdrawal syndrome, any coffee drinker who suddenly switches to decaf knows it exists.)

The time course of withdrawal depends on the *half-life* of the drug in the body. (As noted earlier, this is the time it takes for the body to eliminate one-half of the substance.) Usually, withdrawal symptoms begin within 12 to 24 hours after the last dose is consumed and last no longer than a few days. A powerful urge to continue using the substance often accompanies the withdrawal symptoms.

Analysis of blood, breath, or urine can prove that the patient has used alcohol or another substance, but more often evidence is obtained from history. Denial often biases self-report, so histories are more reliable if someone other than the patient (a relative or friend) provides the information. As a rule of thumb, many clinicians mentally double the amount of a substance the patient claims to have used.

291.8 Alcohol Withdrawal

Heavy drinking of several days or more is required to produce Alcohol Withdrawal. (Drinkers can tolerate greatly varying amounts of alcohol, so it is difficult to be more precise.) Symptoms begin a few hours after drinking stops and coincide with a rapidly declining blood alcohol level. Nearly all patients will show evidence of central nervous system overactivity, such as sweating, racing pulse, or increased reflexes. The most common symptom is tremor; nausea and vomiting may also occur. (The number 100 serves as a good reminder when looking for physiological signs of Alcohol Withdrawal: pulse over 100 beats per minute; temperature over 100°; diastolic blood pressure approaching 100 mm Hg. Rapid respirations may constitute another sign.) Some patients may have brief hallucinations that last 12 to 24 hours. After two or three days, a few may even have seizures.

Sometimes this common syndrome is called "uncomplicated withdrawal." It is usually brief, peaks on the second day, and lasts only a few days. However, the accompanying anxiety, irritability, and sleeplessness may last a good deal longer.

The heavier the drinking has been, the more likely symptoms are to be severe, and so "uncomplicated withdrawal" shades into other, more serious syndromes. The best-known of these is delirium, which affects only about 5% of those hospitalized for withdrawal. When delirium occurs during the course of severe alcohol withdrawal, it is commonly called delirium tremens (DTs). When a patient has both seizures and delirium, the seizures almost invariably come first. Rodney Partridge, a patient with Alcohol Withdrawal Delirium, has been described in Chapter 1 (see p. 23).

Another alcohol withdrawal syndrome is Alcohol-Induced Psychotic Disorder with Hallucinations. Formerly known as alcoholic auditory hallucinosis, it is an uncommon (though not rare) disorder whose symptoms can almost exactly mimic Schizophrenia. Danny Finch, a patient with this disorder, is described in Chapter 4 (see p. 182).

Criteria for Alcohol Withdrawal

- A patient who has been drinking heavily and for a long time suddenly stops or markedly reduces alcohol intake.
- Within a few hours to several days of reducing intake, two or more of the following develop:
  ✓ Autonomic overactivity (sweating or rapid heartbeat)
  ✓ Worsened tremor of hands
  ✓ Sleeplessness
  ✓ Nausea or vomiting
  ✓ Short-lived hallucinations or illusions (visual, tactile, or auditory)
  ✓ Speeded-up psychomotor activity
  ✓ Anxiety
  ✓ Grand mal seizures
- These symptoms cause clinically important distress or impair work, social, or other functioning.
- These symptoms are neither the result of a general medical condition nor better explained by a different mental disorder.

Coding Notes

Specify if: With Perceptual Disturbances. The patient has altered perceptions: auditory, tactile, or visual illusions or hallucinations with intact insight. (*Intact insight* implies that the patient recognizes that the symptoms are unreal, caused by the substance use. Hallucinations without this insight suggest a diagnosis of Alcohol-Induced Psychotic Disorder.)

If the patient meets criteria for Alcohol Withdrawal Delirium, do *not* also code 291.8 (Alcohol Withdrawal).

Quentin McCarthy Again

By the time Quentin sought help, he was drinking the equivalent of nearly a pint of hard liquor per day. He declined the offer of a brief hospitalization to detoxify, and instead began an outpatient withdrawal regimen of decreasing doses of a benzodiazepine. He was asked to return in three days.

On Quentin's next visit, he looked gray and unhappy. He signed in at the registration desk with a wobbly scrawl, and his hand shook as he reached out an arm to have his blood pressure and pulse taken. Both of these measures were elevated.

For three days Quentin had drunk no alcohol. Beginning the second morning, he had felt increasingly anxious. It was a sensation that he could only compare to the feelings he had had his first night in Vietnam, when he had awakened to the booming of howitzers. His anxiety grew throughout the day. Although he was exhausted by bedtime, he hardly slept at all. When he arrived four hours early for his clinic appointment, he admitted that he had taken none of the medicine he had been given. "I wanted to do it myself," he explained.

Over the next several days, Quentin's withdrawal symptoms abated. Within two weeks, he no longer needed the medication. However, because he felt strongly tempted to drink when he was having lunch with clients, he requested disulfiram (Antabuse) therapy.

Three months later, Quentin was still taking disulfiram and still hadn't touched alcohol. He attended at least one Alcoholics Anonymous meeting each day. He had rescued his insurance business from the doldrums and had even persuaded two of his old clients to return with their business. However, he admitted that he occasionally felt acute episodes of anger when he wanted a drink.

Further Evaluation of Quentin McCarthy

Can someone go into Substance Withdrawal without having Substance Dependence? It is theoretically possible. The criteria don't say it couldn't happen, but, outside of a patient who is medically addicted, it must be a rare event. Quentin's is one of those cases where common sense would tell you to diagnose Alcohol Dependence, as well as Alcohol Withdrawal.

When he stopped using alcohol, Quentin developed typical Alcohol Withdrawal symptoms. They included rapid pulse, insomnia, anxiety, and tremor, and they made him uncomfortable enough that he returned early to the mental health clinic. Going longer without medication might have put him at serious risk for withdrawal seizures or perceptual disturbances such as auditory or visual hallucinations. Then he might qualify for other diagnoses—for example, **Alcohol-Induced Delirium** or **Alcohol-Induced Psychotic Disorder with Hallucinations**. Of course, Quentin's withdrawal symptoms would only further underscore his primary diagnosis of **Alcohol Dependence**.

Could any other **general medical conditions** or Axis I disorders have caused these symptoms? The differential diagnosis for withdrawal symptoms is long and substance-specific. For opioid withdrawal it includes **flu-like** syndromes. Patients withdrawing from cocaine and amphetamines typically have symptoms of **depression**. But both Quentin's history and symptoms were so typical for Alcohol Withdrawal that other diagnoses would seem highly unlikely.

Before coding Quentin's diagnosis, however, we must consider the matter of course modifiers for Substance Dependence.

Course Modifiers for Substance Dependence

New in DSM-IV, the course modifiers for Substance Dependence state that a patient cannot be considered in any sort of remission until there have been no substance-related symptoms (other than craving) for at least 30 days. This means that the patient must not have had symptoms of either Substance Dependence or Substance Abuse for that substance. (It is possible that a patient might continue to use a substance, but no longer experience symptoms; it also seems highly improbable.) Until a patient has experienced at least one month of partial or full remission, no course modifier (including *On Agonist Therapy* and *In A Controlled Environment*) can be added to the diagnosis of Substance Dependence.

Criteria for Substance Dependence Course Modifiers

Course modifiers only refer to the criteria for Substance Dependence. This is because there is still not enough information to feel confident about the typical course for patients who *abuse* a given substance but are not *dependent* on it.

Remission

No patient can be said to be in any sort of remission until the full criteria for Substance Dependence are no longer met for one month or more. (Note that the criteria for remission include all the symptoms of both Dependence and Abuse.) In particular, for at least one month, the patient must have no problems from the use of the substance.

All remissions can be divided in two ways: into *full* versus *partial* and *early* versus *sustained*.

Early Remission. Early remission comprises months 2–12 after the patient last experienced problems with the substance. This period of time was singled out because most patients are especially vulnerable to relapse during the first year of sobriety.

Sustained Remission. After the first year, the patient is said to be in sustained remission.

During both of these time periods, a patient will be in partial or full remission:

Full Remission. There have been no symptoms of dependence or of abuse. A person who has stopped using a substance but is still trying to get it, for example, would not qualify for this type of remission. During months 2–12 this would be called Early Full Remission; after the first year it is termed Sustained Full Remission.

Partial Remission. The patient has met at least one criterion for either Substance Dependence or Abuse, but does not fully qualify for Dependence on this substance. The terms Early Partial and Sustained Partial Remission apply, as above.

On Agonist Therapy

This term describes patients who (1) have previously met criteria for Substance Dependence, (2) have not met criteria for Substance Dependence or Abuse for at least one month, and (3) are currently taking medication to block the effects of the substance in question. Example: A heroin-dependent patient takes methadone.

In a Controlled Environment

Patients who are in full remission but live in an environment where it would be very difficult to obtain the substance may merit the modifier In a Controlled

Environment. Such an environment would include a therapeutic community or a jail or locked hospital ward with good control of contraband. This term would not be applied during the first month.

Coding Note

Some patients may qualify for both "On Agonist Therapy" and "In a Controlled Environment." An example of the full coding for such a heroin-dependent patient might read: "Opioid Dependence, Early Full Remission, On Agonist Therapy, In a Controlled Environment."

Evaluation of Course Modifiers for Quentin McCarthy

When he first came to the clinic, Quentin had been alcohol-free for only a few hours; at this point, his diagnosis of Alcohol Dependence would have qualified for no course modifier. On his return after three days, moreover, he would have qualified for a diagnosis of Alcohol Withdrawal. But at his re-evaluation, three months into recovery, he had symptoms of neither Alcohol Dependence nor Abuse; his withdrawal symptoms had abated; and he was still taking disulfiram. (The occasional episodes of anger, when a patient would like a drink, are pretty typical for alcoholism recovery; alcoholics themselves sometimes refer to them as "a dry drunk.") His diagnosis (finally!) at three months would thus read:

Axis I	303.90	Alcohol Dependence, Early Full Remission
Axis II	V71.09	No diagnosis
Axis III		None
Axis IV		None
Axis V	GAF = 40	(on admission)
	GAF = 75	(current)

TIP DSM-IV mentions the term *recovered* as it applies to Substance Dependence. It defines *recovery* as the absence of a current substance use disorder, but it does not say when you can consider a patient recovered. Rather, this is something you must judge on clinical grounds. This is not entirely satisfactory. For one thing, a large number of experts (including several million people with substance-related problems) believe, "Once an addict, always an addict." A considerable body of experience supports this impression. It includes patients who have been clean and sober for years who, for one reason or another, begin to use again and quickly become dependent. It is significant, and a bit sobering, that nowhere in DSM-IV is there a code number for recovered *anything*, including all substance-related disorders, mood disorders, and Schizophrenia.

Substance Abuse

Substance Abuse is a residual category for patients who do not fulfill the criteria for Substance Dependence, but who use a substance in ways that harm or distress the patients and/or others in their environments. Note that these patients do not have symptoms of tolerance or withdrawal. The four sorts of problems that do qualify for Substance Abuse, according to DSM-IV, are as follows:

- **Failure to fulfill important roles.** Despite the expectations of others, a substance abuser may be repeatedly late to work or school, show neglect in the care of small children, or repeatedly fail to cook dinner.
- **Repeated use when it is physically dangerous to do so.** The abuser may repeatedly drive or operate machinery when intoxicated. Here, it is the physical *safety* of the action (driving when drunk) that is at issue, rather than a medical condition that could be worsened by drinking.
- **Use despite recurrent legal problems.** These include arrests for driving under the influence and other legal problems.
- **Use despite social or interpersonal problems.** These would include loss of friends, verbal or physical fights.

Substance Abuse is a relatively new category, and there are not as yet enough data to enable us to define its course clearly. To what degree does a patient with Alcohol Abuse correspond to what used to be called a "problem drinker"? Is Substance Abuse only a way station on the road to Substance Dependence? How long may Abuse continue before it becomes Dependence? What percentage of abusers never become dependent? DSM-IV makes one thing perfectly clear: A patient who qualifies for Substance Dependence can *never* return to be "only" an abuser of substances within that class.

Nonetheless, the differences between Substance Dependence and Abuse are sometimes hard to tease out. Substance Dependence implies physiological changes and loss of control; Substance Abuse refers to social and legal problems. In Dependence, the preoccupation with the substance of choice reduces the time available for social, occupational, or recreational activities. In Abuse, the emphasis is not on time available, but on failure to follow through with responsibilities. Substance-dependent patients continue to use despite knowledge that the behavior is causing physical or emotional problems, whereas substance abusers continue to use despite social or interpersonal problems. Clearly, this is a somewhat artificial classification—but what classification isn't?

305.00 Alcohol Abuse

Many abusive drinkers would be called "alcoholics" by clinicians and by themselves. These people probably drink less heavily than those who are dependent on alcohol. They are certainly less likely to experience symptoms of Alcohol Withdrawal, though theoretically an abuser could drink enough to experience physiological symptoms upon stopping. Note that the criteria for Alcohol Abuse are the same as for any other type of Substance Abuse; they are given below as generic Substance Abuse criteria.

Generic Criteria for Substance Abuse

- The patient's maladaptive substance use pattern causes clinically important distress or impairment, as shown in a single 12-month period by one or more of the following:
  ✓ Because of repeated use, the patient fails to carry out major obligations at work, home, or school.
  ✓ The patient repeatedly uses substances even when it is physically dangerous to do so.
  ✓ The patient repeatedly has legal problems resulting from substance use.
  ✓ Despite knowing that it has caused or worsened social or interpersonal problems, the patient continues to use the substance.
- For this class of substance, the patient has never fulfilled criteria for Substance Dependence.

Dolores McCarthy

One of Dolores McCarthy's earliest memories was of when she was four years old, sitting on her grandfather's lap. She would rest her head against his soft old cotton sweater. He would wrap his arms securely around her, and she would cling to his neck. Also clinging to him was a particular smell that she always associated with her grandfather. It wasn't until she was a teenager that she realized what it was: beer.

By the time Dolores was 10, she had watched in horror as by degrees the old man died of cirrhosis. When she was a teenager, she saw her father's drinking wreck her parents' marriage. In college, when she discovered that two glasses of wine would ease her chronic sense of tension, she promised herself that she would use alcohol and never let it use her.

Accordingly, she had evolved a set of rules to limit her consumption. She allowed herself only one drink before dinner, and never more than three in a day (except on weekends and vacations, when she could have four). From her father's unfortunate example, she had learned: Regardless of the occasion, never drink during work and never allow "extras." Even the day of her 22nd birthday, when she married Quentin, the young salesman in her father's office, she had only four glasses of champagne—just enough to maintain her customary comfortable glow.

Despite her control, Dolores had had two lapses. The first had occurred 12 months earlier, when she became pregnant for the first and only time. Although she wanted a child, she took the precaution of having an amniocentesis. When it revealed that she was carrying a Down's syndrome baby, she gulped several extra drinks and drove around while deciding what to do. A Breathalyzer-measured blood alcohol level of 1.2 landed her in traffic court just one week after the abortion.

Her second arrest for driving while intoxicated had occurred six months later, when she lost her self-control once again after her mother died of Alzheimer's disease. The day Quentin entered treatment was therefore only the third time he had ever known his wife to be drunk.

Evaluation of Dolores McCarthy

Although Dolores drank far more than the average American, she had had few problems from her alcohol use, because of her vigilance and the unfortunate examples of her father and husband. She had never drunk enough to develop tolerance or withdrawal symptoms, and her control had been almost unwaveringly iron-fisted. When it slipped, however, she had legal problems: two arrests for driving under the influence of alcohol within a 12-month period. Driving while drunk would qualify as an illustration of her maladaptive use of alcohol. (Stipulating "in a single 12-month period" might at first seem a bit odd, when only one of the criteria needs to be met. What it means is that Dolores's two arrests for driving under the influence of alcohol would not have counted had they occurred farther apart.)

There are no modifiers for Substance Abuse, so Dolores's Axis I diagnosis would be 305.00 (Alcohol Abuse). Her full diagnosis is given later.

Substance Intoxication

Anyone can get drunk. Anyone can be exposed to toxic fumes. Although most people who become intoxicated do so voluntarily, people can also be affected accidentally (e.g., through exposure to industrial chemicals or drinking a "spiked" lemonade). Regardless of intent, for a diagnosis of Substance Intoxication to be appropriate, the central nervous system effects of the substance must cause maladaptive psychological changes or behaviors. Note that all Substance Intoxication is by definition reversible. When there are permanent effects of substance use, another disorder (e.g., Substance-Induced Persisting Dementia) will be diagnosed instead.

When people are intoxicated, their behavior changes in ways that work to their disadvantage; that is, the changes are *maladaptive*. These include work or social problems, abnormally *labile* (i.e., unstable) mood, impaired thinking, defective judgment, and belligerence. This is an important criterion, because it helps to discriminate patients who are only intoxicated in the physiological sense (excessive digitalis, for example) from those who also have maladaptive behavior. For a patient to be diagnosed as having Substance Intoxication, behavioral changes and physiological signs must both be present.

> **TIP** Clearly, in some cases we must interpret somewhat liberally what we mean by *maladaptive*. If a person drinks a six-pack of beer, then goes quietly to bed without disturbing anyone, are we to say that intoxication did not occur? Because of the phenomenon of tolerance, a person's symptoms are often independent of the amount of an agent consumed. Probably this person will have some impairment of attention or feel some depression (or euphoria), and that will be enough to qualify. Or perhaps just going to bed represents behavioral change. In any event, remember that the DSM-IV criteria are only guidelines; don't let rigid interpretation of the criteria contravene your common sense.

In addition, signs of intoxication will be noted. Although these tend to be substance-specific, there are certain common themes:

- Motor incoordination or agitation
- Loss of ability to sustain attention
- Impaired memory
- Reduced alertness (drowsiness, stupor, or even coma)
- Effects on the autonomic nervous system (dry mouth, heart palpitations, gastrointestinal symptoms, changes in blood pressure)
- Mood changes (depression, euphoria, anxiety, and others)

Of course, there is also the ubiquitous requirement that all general medical conditions and other mental disorders must be ruled out as more likely causes of the symptoms. As a general rule, symptoms of intoxication (or withdrawal) that last longer than about four weeks may point to another mental or physical disorder. For example, a drinker who still has depressive symptoms a month after drying out should be evaluated for Major Depressive Episode.

Generic Criteria for Substance Intoxication

- The patient develops a reversible syndrome due to recent use of or exposure to a substance that affects the central nervous system.
- During or shortly after using the substance, the patient develops clinically important behavioral or psychological changes that are maladaptive.
- This condition is neither the result of a general medical condition nor better explained by a different mental disorder.

Coding Note

Although DSM-IV specifies that the symptoms and behavioral and psychological changes of intoxication are "substance-specific," it notes that various substances can produce syndromes of intoxication that are similar, or even identical.

303.00 Alcohol Intoxication

The picture of acute alcohol intoxication is so familiar that it seems almost unnecessary to describe it again here. However, a number of observations should be made.

There is a great deal of variability in the blood levels people can tolerate without appearing drunk. The range may be as great as from 0.3 to 1.5 mg/ml, despite the fact that many states now set the sobriety level for driving at 0.8 mg/ml. Furthermore, the symptoms of Alcohol Intoxication are usually more prominent when the blood level is rising (during the early part of the period of drinking) than when it is falling (when the person is sobering up). Levels of alcohol in the body can be measured in urine, blood, breath, or even saliva.

Alcohol Intoxication should only be diagnosed when there is evidence (usually historical) that the patient has drunk enough, rapidly enough, to intoxicate most people. In borderline cases, this may mean factoring in the drinker's weight, age, and general state of health.

Some people develop marked behavioral changes after drinking small amounts of alcohol. This condition, called Alcohol Idiosyncratic Intoxication, is coded as an Alcohol-Related Disorder Not Otherwise Specified (see p. 86).

Criteria for Alcohol Intoxication

- The patient has recently drunk alcohol.
- During or shortly after drinking, the patient develops clinically important behavioral or psychological changes that are maladaptive. These may include inappropriate sexuality or aggression, lability of mood, impaired judgment, and impaired work or social functioning.
- Shortly after drinking, one or more of these occurs:
  - ✓ Slurring of speech
  - ✓ Poor coordination
  - ✓ Unsteady walking
  - ✓ Nystagmus (involuntary rhythmic eye movements)
  - ✓ Impaired attention or memory
  - ✓ Stupor or coma
- These symptoms are neither the result of a general medical condition nor better explained by a different mental disorder.

Dolores McCarthy Again

Dolores accompanied her husband to his second clinic appointment. She had been worried about Quentin for several months, and when his agitation kept them both awake most of that night, she had gone down to the kitchen and poured them each a drink. When he refused his, she drank it for him. Then she lost count and had a couple more.

"Anything was besher—was *better* than what he was going through," Dolores told the clinician that morning. After correcting herself, she spoke slowly and deliberately.

On the spur of the moment Dolores had decided that she should accompany Quentin to his appointment, to be sure he didn't get into trouble. They had taken her car, and she had insisted on driving. Quentin hadn't dared remind her what had happened on the other occasions she had driven after drinking. Fortunately, traffic was light, and her only difficulty was that she needed two extra tries when parking in an unusually long space at the curb.

As Dolores entered the clinic building, however, she stumbled and might have fallen had someone not grabbed her elbow and steadied her as she wobbled into the waiting room. She fumbled with the large buttons of her coat until her husband undid them for her. She then slumped into a chair where, with her coat thrown over her, she appeared to doze until they were called into the clinician's office.

Further Evaluation of Dolores McCarthy

Especially in light of her prior experience, Dolores's insistence on driving when she had been drinking suggests that her judgment was badly askew. In other patients, evidence of maladaptive behavior might include fights or arguments with family or friends, lapses in business judgment, or embarrassing behavior (e.g., making sexually inappropriate remarks).

Dolores showed several symptoms specific for Alcohol Intoxication. She slurred her words, walked unsteadily, and had difficulty unbuttoning her coat (motor incoordination). When she finally got into the office, she appeared to doze. Any one of these symptoms would qualify for the diagnosis of Alcohol Intoxication.

A clinician attending Dolores would have to consider whether a history, physical exam, or laboratory data would be needed to be sure her symptoms were not due to a **general medical condition**. (They might instead be accounted for by another Axis I disorder, such as a **Substance Intoxication Delirium** caused by some other substance.) However, her typical symptoms and history of recent alcohol use would make that seem nearly unnecessary.

A diagnosis of **Alcohol Intoxication Delirium** would not be warranted in Dolores's case. Although her reduced attention span and lowered state of consciousness had come on quickly, the vignette contains no evidence of cognitive changes such as disorientation, memory loss, language problems, or perceptual disturbance. (Her speech was slurred, but her thought processes seemed to be intact.)

The generic criteria for Substance Intoxication specify, as noted earlier, that the syndrome must be reversible. Of course, the question of reversibility could not be answered for several hours, until the symptoms had had a chance to wear off. Until then, the diagnosis could be made only on a presumptive basis. The full diagnosis for Dolores would be as follows:

Axis I	305.00	Alcohol Abuse
	303.00	Alcohol Intoxication
Axis II	V71.09	No diagnosis
Axis III		None
Axis IV		Abortion
		Death of mother
Axis V	GAF = 75	(current)

Other Alcohol-Related Disorders

Other possible alcohol-related disorders are listed (with code numbers) in Table 3.1. Additional alcohol-related vignettes are provided elsewhere: Mark Culpepper had Alcohol-Induced Persisting Dementia (see p. 41), and Charles Jackson had Alcohol-Induced Persisting Amnestic Disorder (see p. 49). One alcohol-related disorder that is no longer a DSM diagnosis in its own right (and thus is not included in Table 3.1) is nonetheless worth mentioning here:

Alcohol Idiosyncratic Intoxication. This interesting disorder refers to the tendency in a few people to react strongly to a very small amount of alcohol (too little to cause intoxication in most people). For example, a person who is usually withdrawn and unassuming may become hostile and belligerent after a single glass of wine. This condition occurs within minutes of the drinking, and lasts a few hours at most. Predisposing factors may be advancing age, fatigue, and brain injury (such as that resulting from trauma or infection). In DSM-III-R, it had a code number of its own; it has also been called *pathological intoxication*. In DSM-IV, it would be coded as 291.9 (Alcohol-Related Disorder Not Otherwise Specified).

AMPHETAMINE (OR AMPHETAMINE-LIKE)-RELATED DISORDERS

Amphetamines are valued for the euphoria, appetite suppression, and increase in energy they provide. Although many people begin amphetamine use by snorting, blood vessel constriction in the nose makes absorption unpredictable, so other routes are sought. Smoking or injection produces a more rapid effect. Binge users take the drug repeatedly for half a day to two or three days. Tolerance develops rapidly, so the effects of the drug fall off. It is almost inevitable that a period of nonuse will occur, but users remember how "wonderful" the drug was (euphoria) and want more. This institutes a cycle of use–withdrawal that usually lasts about 10 days.

When they were first synthesized in 1887, there were no regulations on the amphetamines. Through the middle years of the 20th century, it was commonplace to use them for weight control, depression, and nasal stuffiness; they were widely abused in the 1960s and into the 1970s. Since then, however, rigid controls and changing prescribing practices have greatly reduced their availability. Virtually their only legitimate uses now are for the diagnosis and treatment of obesity, Narcolepsy, depressive disorders, and childhood Attention-Deficit/Hyperactivity Disorder.

Amphetamines may be taken intermittently at relatively modest doses by truckers, students, and others who want something beyond caffeine to keep them awake. Some users take these drugs to produce euphoria, often leading to "speed runs" that may last for weeks. There may be episodes of delirium during these runs and "crashes" when the supply runs out. Others use stimulants to counterbalance the effects of sedatives and other drugs of abuse.

Cocaine has largely filled the niche once occupied by amphetamines. (The effects of amphetamines are nearly identical to those of cocaine, but their half-life in the body is much longer. This may explain cocaine's greater addicting powers—and appeal). Now, only about 2% of emergency room drug-related visits are due to amphetamines and their related substances. Some data suggest that those dependent on amphetamines may stop using them after a decade or so.

The substances related to amphetamine that are available by prescription include methamphetamine (Desoxyn), dextroamphetamine (Dexedrine), diethylopropion (Tenuate), methylphenidate (Ritalin), and pemoline (Cylert).

292.89 Amphetamine Intoxication

If amphetamine is injected, feelings of euphoria, confidence, and well-being begin quickly. Users experience a "rush." Their thoughts may seem profound, and their sexual interest may appear to be heightened, but they pay the price of anorexia and agitation. When the intoxication is severe, they become confused and their speech rambles.

With longer use, the person may begin to withdraw from other people and focus more or less exclusively on obtaining and using drugs. Hallucinations (such as bugs crawling on the skin) or paranoid ideas can develop. Delirium may be accompanied by violence. Some people adopt stereotyped behaviors: ritualistic reenactments of things they normally like to do (e.g., assembling and disassembling electronic equipment). Any of these syndromes can resemble Schizophrenia, but the alert clinician will focus on the longitudinal history as obtained from informants. Laboratory studies help confirm the toxic origins of the behavior.

Criteria for Amphetamine Intoxication

- The patient has recently used amphetamine or a related substance.
- During or shortly after its use, the patient develops clinically important behavioral or psychological changes that are maladaptive. These may include blunted affect, hypervigilance, interpersonal sensitivity, anger, anxiety or tension, changes in sociability, stereotyped behaviors, impaired judgment, and impaired work or social functioning.
- Shortly after use, two or more of these occur:
  - ✓ Slowed or rapid heart rate
  - ✓ Dilated pupils
  - ✓ Raised or lowered blood pressure
  - ✓ Chills or sweating

✓ Nausea or vomiting
✓ Weight loss
✓ Speeded-up or slowed psychomotor activity
✓ Muscle weakness, shallow or slowed breathing, chest pain, or heart arrhythmias
✓ Coma, confusion, dyskinesias (involuntary muscular activity), dystonias (disordered muscle tone), or seizures
• These symptoms are neither the result of a general medical condition nor better explained by a different mental disorder.

Coding Note

Specify if: With Perceptual Disturbances. The patient has altered perceptions: auditory, tactile, or visual illusions or hallucinations with intact insight. (*Intact insight* implies that the patient recognizes that the symptoms are unreal, caused by the substance use. Hallucinations without this insight suggest a diagnosis of Amphetamine-Induced Psychotic Disorder.)

Freeman Cooke

"I was hyperactive when I was a child," said Freeman Cooke to the interviewer. "My mother used to give me coffee to slow me down."

Moving restlessly around the office, he looked as if he'd just had several cups too many. He had already twice excused himself to the bathroom, where he nearly threw up. The nurse who checked him noted that his blood pressure was up, and his pulse was racing along at 132 beats per minute. He admitted that he had snorted half a gram of "crystal meth" not long before coming to the office.

Freeman had been the oldest of four children. His mother was an unhappy, nervous woman who always seemed unwell. His father made good money as a finish carpenter, but his appetite for vodka grew as his family increased. When still a child, Freeman had promised himself that he would avoid alcohol and treat his wife, if he ever had one, with more respect than his father had done. He managed to keep half his promise.

After completing high school, Freeman got married and obtained a job as a helper with a long-distance moving company. The pay was good but the hours were awful. When he and his boss were on the road, they sometimes worked 18 hours straight. Like most of the other truckers, he used dextroamphetamine to pep him up and keep him awake. At first, he took them only when he was working. When he came home from a 10-day trip, he would "crash and burn," sometimes sleeping as long as 20 hours at a stretch. But by the time he had enough seniority and experience to buy his own truck, he was using amphetamines recreationally, too.

Freeman had started to snort powdered methamphetamine—"meth"—but he rapidly switched to smoking because it gave him a better "flash." When he was high he felt insanely happy, tireless, and powerful. "Like I could lift a grand piano, all by myself," he explained. He also developed the tendency to argue, and would sometimes keep his wife up late at night with a tirade about matters that the next day seemed inconsequential even to him. After a few hours, as the effect of the high began to wear off and only the memory of the flash remained, he felt driven to smoke up again and again. But with each use during a run, it took more of the drug to produce the flash. Eventually, either his supply or his constitution would give out, and he would once again crash and burn. When he struggled back to consciousness, he was often astonished at how much of the stuff he had consumed.

When Freeman awakened after an unusually memorable two-day run, he found a note saying that his wife was leaving him. For the first time, he realized how exactly like his father he had become.

Evaluation of Freeman Cooke

Like any other type of Substance Intoxication, Amphetamine Intoxication must be documented with marked, detrimental behavioral or psychological changes. In Freeman's case, that requirement presented no problem: His drug use had led to arguments with his wife, which culminated in her leaving him. Of the physical signs and symptoms required, he had elevated pulse and blood pressure, as well as agitation and nausea. At the time he was evaluated, he had no hallucinations or illusions that would constitute the specifier of perceptual disturbances.

Freeman also qualified for a diagnosis of Amphetamine Dependence. He clearly reported tolerance: He required more drug to achieve a high on successive occasions of use. He sometimes used more methamphetamine than he intended, and he spent a great deal of time and energy in using it and recovering from the effects. (Evidence of Amphetamine Withdrawal is discussed below.)

Axis I	292.89	Amphetamine Intoxication, With Physiological Dependence
	304.40	Amphetamine Dependence
Axis II	V71.09	No diagnosis
Axis III		None
Axis IV		Separated from wife
Axis V	GAF = 55	(current)

292.0 Amphetamine Withdrawal

Finally, a few hours after the last use of amphetamines, there comes the crash: agitation, anxiety, depression, and exhaustion. The user experiences an intense craving that may later wane in the face of ensuing depression, fatigue, and insomnia (which is paradoxically accompanied by a marked need for sleep). Still later, voracious appetite may develop. The fatigue and apathy worsen in the half day to four days following the crash. Suicide attempts may result. In short, the user becomes a patient.

Criteria for Amphetamine Withdrawal

- A patient who has been using an amphetamine or a similar substance heavily and for a long time suddenly stops or markedly reduces its intake.
- Within a few hours to several days of reducing intake, the patient develops dysphoric mood *and* two or more of the following:
  ✓ Fatigue
  ✓ Unpleasant, vivid dreams
  ✓ Excessive sleepiness or sleeplessness
  ✓ Increase in appetite
  ✓ Speeded-up or slowed psychomotor activity
- These symptoms cause clinically important distress or impaired work, social, or other functioning.
- These symptoms are neither the result of a general medical condition nor better explained by a different mental disorder.

Freeman Cooke Again

When he checked into Detox, Freeman was still wired from the last half gram of meth he had smoked that morning. Coming off a two-day binge, he knew from past experience that if he was going to do something about his habit, he had to take the plunge when he was still intoxicated. If he waited until he crashed, he wouldn't do anything except sleep. Then he'd go out looking for drugs.

Freeman had declined lunch and was playing cards with three other patients at a table in the corner of the day room when he felt himself begin to slip. He noted almost with amusement how exactly like a wind-up turntable he felt, running more slowly every moment. With each hand it seemed harder to play the cards; they might have been made of lead. Suddenly, he was overwhelmed with depression so profound that, tired as he was, he had to try to escape. His body ached for some speed.

Back in his room, he started to pack the few things he had brought in.

When the gym bag was half full, he put it aside and collapsed onto the bed. He knew that he utterly lacked the energy to go out and hustle. The drug craving was gradually giving way to the need for sleep, but his eyes remained resolutely open. He knew he was doomed to lie there for hours, paralyzed by fatigue but unable to sleep. It was going to be a long night.

Further Evaluation of Freeman Cooke

After he stopped using amphetamines, Freeman rapidly became depressed. He also suffered from fatigue, psychomotor slowing, and insomnia (even though he badly wanted to sleep). His profound craving for speed is not a criterion of withdrawal, but it is typical. The misery these symptoms caused him, together with the lack of any other disorder that could better explain them, would qualify him for the diagnosis of Amphetamine Withdrawal.

The differential diagnosis of Freeman's condition would include either **Bipolar I Disorder** (because of his fluctuating moods) and other substance-induced disorders, such as **Cocaine Withdrawal** and **Phencyclidine Intoxication**. Patients who develop psychosis during intoxication may be mistakenly diagnosed as having **Schizophreniform Disorder** or other psychotic disorders.

Even after most of the acute effects of withdrawal have dissipated, mood symptoms may last for weeks or months. If this is the case, consider a diagnosis of Amphetamine-Induced Mood Disorder.

An Axis I diagnosis of 292.0 (Amphetamine Withdrawal) would be added to Freeman's five-axis diagnosis as given earlier.

Other Amphetamine-Related Disorders

You will find a complete listing of amphetamine-related disorders in Table 3.1. Some are described more fully at other points in this book. Two others are briefly mentioned here:

292.11 Amphetamine-Induced Psychotic Disorder, With Delusions. These patients often, though not always, develop paranoia with ideas of reference and well-formed delusions. Their awareness of the environment is accentuated. They may watch other people very carefully, and later become "aware" that others are watching them. They may also overreact to any perception of movement; they may actually hallucinate. The delusions can last a week or longer. When this disorder is well developed, it may resemble Schizophrenia, Paranoid Type in all but the time course.

292.12 Amphetamine-Induced Psychotic Disorder, With Hallucinations. Patients with this type of psychotic disorder may scratch excessively if they think they see bugs crawling on their skin.

CAFFEINE-RELATED DISORDERS

Caffeine, the most widely used psychoactive substance in the world, is present in coffee, cola beverages, tea, chocolate, and a variety of prescription and over-the-counter drugs. Perhaps two-thirds to three-quarters of adults frequently consume at least one of these. Although tolerance and some degree of withdrawal are undeniably associated with caffeine, few people ever experience enough social problems to qualify for dependence; in any case, DSM-IV includes no diagnosis for dependence on caffeine.

Caffeine withdrawal (this is not an *official* DSM-IV diagnosis, either, but it has been included in an appendix of DSM-IV for further study) may be especially likely during changes in the person's social schedule—as when on vacations, over weekends, and the like. The symptoms most likely to occur include fatigue, headache, and sleepiness. Somewhat less frequent symptoms include impairment of concentration and motor performance. Research criteria for this proposed diagnosis are provided on page 708 of DSM-IV.

Black coffee has long been used as a folk remedy to sober up people who have drunk too much alcohol. However, caffeine does nothing to relieve their symptoms. Instead, the persons who were "only" inebriated become agitated as well.

305.90 Caffeine Intoxication

The symptoms caused by "Mr. Coffee Nerves" (once the star of advertisements for a popular hot drink) may seem too familiar to rate much space. However, it has been estimated that as many as 10% of adults may sometime have symptoms of Caffeine Intoxication, which is also known as caffeinism. The symptoms are much like those of Generalized Anxiety Disorder (see p. 276). The patient feels "wired," excessively energetic, excitable, and driven. Loud speech, irritability, and jitteriness are also commonly associated with Caffeine Intoxication.

The effects are determined by several factors. Of course, the patient's degree of tolerance is important, but so is the amount ingested. A naïve user might experience symptoms from as little as 250 mg of caffeine. Even chronic coffee drinkers risk symptoms when they take in more than 500 mg per day. Other individual characteristics, such as age, fatigue, medical condition, and expectations, can also play a role. A diagnosis of Caffeine Intoxication is usually not made in people who are younger than 35; perhaps it takes years to develop awareness that there is even a problem.

Although I have not included a separate vignette for Caffeine Intoxication in this section, a patient described in Chapter 12, Dave Kincaid, illustrates this diagnosis. (For Dave's full case vignette, see the description of Substance-Induced Sleep Disorder, p. 436.)

Criteria for Caffeine Intoxication

- The patient has recently consumed caffeine (usually more than 250 mg, or two to three cups of coffee).
- Beginning during or shortly after ingestion, five or more of these occur:
   ✓ Restlessness
   ✓ Nervousness
   ✓ Excitement
   ✓ Sleeplessness
   ✓ Red face
   ✓ Increased urination
   ✓ Gastrointestinal upset
   ✓ Muscle twitching
   ✓ Rambling speech
   ✓ Rapid or irregular heartbeat
   ✓ Periods of tirelessness
   ✓ Speeded-up psychomotor activity
- These symptoms cause clinically important distress or impair work, social, or other functioning.
- These symptoms are neither the result of a general medical condition nor better explained by a different mental disorder.

Evaluation of Dave Kincaid

Dave Kincaid worked in a coffee roastery while he was writing his novel. He had free access to the rich, thick coffee they served there. He also consumed quite a few chocolate-covered coffee beans. He probably consumed over 1000 mg of caffeine per day, so he had reason to feel nervous ("up"). He couldn't sit still when he was trying to type, and at night he lay awake with insomnia. Rapid heartbeat and abdominal upset are also fairly typical symptoms that can be encountered even with relatively mild caffeinism.

In the criteria listed above, most of the symptoms may be found after as little as two cups of coffee. Muscle twitching ("live flesh," as Dave Kincaid called it), agitation, and periods of tirelessness require caffeine intake substantially greater (a gram of caffeine or more per day).

Because its symptoms are sometimes confused with other Axis I disorders, it is important to keep Caffeine Intoxication in mind. If we assume that Dave included his mental health when he said that his health had been excellent, he probably would not have had a past history of Axis I disorders such as anxiety disorders (especially **Generalized Anxiety Disorder** and **Panic Disorder**), mood disorders (especially **Manic** or **Hypomanic Episode**), and various **sleep disorders**. He had once smoked a little marijuana, but he had never used **other substances** whose effects might be confused with caffeinism. These would especially include the central nervous system stimulants (**cocaine, amphetamines** and related substances).

Ruling out **Caffeine-Induced Anxiety Disorder** and **Caffeine-Induced Sleep Disorder** would require some clinical judgment: for these disorders, the symptoms must be more severe than are usually found in Caffeine Intoxication, and they must be serious enough to need independent clinical attention.

Dave's complete five-axis diagnosis is given on page 438.

Other Caffeine-Related Disorders

You will find a complete listing of caffeine-related disorders in Table 3.1.

> **292.9 Caffeine-Related Disorder Not Otherwise Specified**. This is how Caffeine Withdrawal would have to be coded, if you ever found a patient with enough symptoms.

CANNABIS-RELATED DISORDERS

Cannabis is the generic name of the hemp plant, *Cannabis sativa*, whose active ingredient is tetrahydrocannabinol (THC). Depending on the variety of hemp and where it is grown, the leaves and tops may contain anywhere from 1% to about 10% THC. (In some California locales, careful nurturing of selected cultivars has produced the latter figure and higher—a dubious triumph of U.S.

agriculture.) Hashish, which is a resin produced from the leaves of the hemp plant, contains about 10% THC. Cannabis is the most widely used illicit substance in the United States. As many as 4% of all American adults may at some time qualify for a diagnosis of Cannabis Abuse or Dependence. Its popularity may be once again on the rise among teenagers.

The serious behavioral and psychological consequences seen in those withdrawing from other substances (cocaine, opioids, alcohol, and the like) are not generally a problem with cannabis. Therefore, DSM-IV does not include criteria for Cannabis Withdrawal. However, people who suddenly quit after heavy cannabis use can experience mild physiological symptoms that can last several weeks; these include anxiety, sleeplessness, and other symptoms similar to sedative withdrawal. Symptoms of tolerance have also been noted in heavy users. Its use can thus lead to Cannabis Dependence, though this takes a long time (relative to other types of Substance Dependence) to develop.

Flashbacks are rare. So is acute depression, which, when present, is usually mild and temporary. Some patients experience paranoia, which can last as long as several days. Using cannabis may worsen the psychosis of someone who already has Schizophrenia.

Cannabis may be one of the most difficult of substances for some patients to discontinue using, simply because it causes relatively few medical complications. Some complications are powerful motivating factors for discontinuing the use of other, more dangerous substances. Many heavy cannabis users do not realize that they have become tolerant. Although cannabis is usually smoked, THC can be absorbed from the gastrointestinal tract (hence the stories you hear about marijuana brownies). Because of erratic absorption from the gastrointestinal tract, THC that has been swallowed is especially dangerous.

292.89 Cannabis Intoxication

The devotees of cannabis value it for the relaxation and elevation of mood it brings them. It causes their perceptions to seem more acute; they may notice that colors seem brighter. Adults see the world afresh, much as children do. Their appreciation for music and art is enhanced. Their ideas flow rapidly; they may find their own conversation especially witty.

The effects of cannabis are many and varied. These reactions (both negative and positive) are strongly influenced by setting and mind set. Time sense often changes—a few minutes may seem like an hour. Usually, cannabis also produces red eyes and a rapid heartbeat. Users may become passive and drowsy; mood often becomes apathetic. Motor performance suffers (e.g., cannabis impairs driving performance).

Although there may be illusions, hallucinations rarely occur, and users generally retain insight. They are not convinced by their own misperceptions; they may even laugh at them. Often a user will appear more or less normal, even when highly intoxicated.

Especially in first-time users, intoxication often begins with anxiety, which can progress to panic. In fact, the most common untoward reaction to cannabis is an anxiety disorder. Some patients fear that body distortions mean impending death.

Some clinicians believe that there is also a syndrome of chronic cannabis use. Though variable, the symptoms are said to include mild depression, reduced drive, and decreased interest.

Criteria for Cannabis Intoxication

- The patient has recently used cannabis.
- During or shortly after its use, the patient develops clinically important behavioral or psychological changes that are maladaptive. These may include motor performance deficits, anxiety, euphoria, impaired judgment, social withdrawal, and the sensation that time has slowed down.
- Within two hours of use, two or more of these occur:
  ✓ Red eyes
  ✓ Increase in appetite
  ✓ Dry mouth
  ✓ Rapid heart rate
- These symptoms are neither the result of a general medical condition nor better explained by a different mental disorder.

Coding Note

Specify if: With Perceptual Disturbances. The patient has altered perceptions: auditory, tactile, or visual illusions or hallucinations with intact insight. (*Intact insight* implies that the patient recognizes that the symptoms are unreal, caused by the substance use. Hallucinations without this insight suggest a diagnosis of Cannabis-Induced Psychotic Disorder.)

TIP As for any Substance Intoxication, the criteria for Cannabis Intoxication require that recent substance use produce *maladaptive* behavioral or psychological manifestations. It would be hard to argue that social withdrawal and defective judgment are anything but maladaptive, but euphoria? Suppose the patient is euphoric, but nothing comes of it? Is the patient then not intoxicated? Some DSM-IV criteria work better than others. Some still leave too much to the interpretation of the individual clinician.

Russell Zahn

"You got a candy bar on you?" Russell Zahn shambled into the interviewer's office and slumped onto the sofa. He flicked a lock of hair back across one shoulder of his torn denim jacket. "I know it's only an hour since breakfast, but I'm really hungry."

At age 27, Russell lived on general relief and was often homeless. In the hills of northern California where he grew up, the principal cash crop was marijuana. For the first several years since leaving high school, he had worked at its cultivation and marketing; more recently, he had been more or less exclusively a consumer. Now he had been referred to the mental health clinic by a judge who had grown weary of his repeated courtroom appearances for possession of small amounts of marijuana. Russell volunteered that he had finished a joint in the alley outside, just before coming in to his appointment.

Russell wasn't especially unhappy about being evaluated; he just didn't see much need for it. He required very little to live on. Whatever his relief check didn't cover, he earned by begging. He had his own corner in the business section of town, where for six hours a day he lounged behind a sign requesting contributions. Every couple of hours he would walk back to the alley and sneak a toke. "I don't smoke on duty," he said. "It's bad for business."

All in all, life seemed a lot better now than when he was a kid. Russell's parents had both died in an automobile accident when he was six. For two years after that, he had been passed around among grandparents, aunts and uncles, and a cousin. No one really wanted him, and he interrupted a six-year tour of various foster homes by running away when he was 14.

The alternative life style of the northern California marijuana industry had suited Russell just fine, until he discovered that no industry at all suited him even better. It had been years since he had worked at anything, and he supposed he never would again. His mood was always good. He had never had to see a doctor. He had tried all the other drugs ("except smack"), but he didn't really care for any of them.

Russell stood and stretched. He rubbed his already brick-red eyes. "Well, thanks for listening."

The interviewer asked where he was going and pointed out that his appointment wasn't over. "You've only been here about 20 minutes."

"Really!" Russell said, and slouched back into his chair. "It seemed more like an hour. I've always had a lousy sense of time."

Evaluation of Russell Zahn

According to DSM-IV, Russell's time distortion (typically, time seems to pass slowly) would fulfill the requirement for a maladaptive behavior due to Cannabis Intoxication. It is not clear how clinically important this was for Russell, but it was certainly noticeable. Red eyes and increased appetite (suggested by his desire for a midmorning candy bar) provided the physical indicators necessary to make the diagnosis. For coding purposes, note that he had no evidence of disturbed perception (such as illusions or hallucinations).

Of course, possible use of other substances (notably **alcohol** and **hallucinogens**, if perceptual problems are noted) should be considered in the differential diagnosis of Cannabis Intoxication. History and the odor of alcohol can be important to this differentiation and to ruling out mental disorders such as **anxiety** and **mood disorders**.

Was Russell dependent? He had used cannabis for a number of years. Although he might have greater tolerance to the drug than the average user, there was no evidence that he used more than he intended or that he had ever tried to cut down. Of course, by DSM-IV criteria, there is no withdrawal syndrome for cannabis. Russell did spend considerable time procuring and using marijuana, and it could be argued that his homeless, aimless life was partly due to the use of the drug. (It could also be argued that a personality disorder caused these problems and the use of cannabis.) The vignette does not suggest any physical or psychological problem caused by the cannabis. Still, considering the overall deterioration of Russell's work ethic, the time he spent using cannabis, and his probable tolerance to the drug, a diagnosis of Cannabis Dependence would seem warranted.

You can see that it is a bit of a stretch to force cannabis into the DSM-IV generic Substance Dependence criteria. Anyone who believes in strict adherence to the criteria for Substance Dependence could, on the basis of Russell's repeated court appearances, diagnose him as having Cannabis Abuse.

Russell's complete diagnosis would be as follows:

Axis I	292.89	Cannabis Intoxication
	304.30	Cannabis Dependence
Axis II	799.9	Diagnosis Deferred
Axis III		None
Axis IV		Homeless
		Unemployed
		Repeated arrests
Axis V	GAF = 50	(highest level past year)

Other Cannabis-Related Disorders

You will find a complete listing of cannabis-related disorders in Table 3.1. Two of these are mentioned here:

292.11 Cannabis-Induced Psychotic Disorder, With Delusions. This disorder involves delusions that are usually persecutory. It lasts only a day, or several days at the most. In the United States, it is rare and most often seen in juveniles. But in other countries and cultures (e.g., Gambia), it may be more common. Most U.S. patients who have delusions associated with cannabis probably have other diagnoses as well (e.g., Schizophrenia or drug–drug interactions).

292.89 Cannabis-Induced Anxiety Disorder. The case of Bonita Ramirez, a college student who had Cannabis-Induced Anxiety Disorder, is given in Chapter 6 (see p. 284).

COCAINE-RELATED DISORDERS

Cocaine is a central nervous system stimulant with symptoms of intoxication and withdrawal identical to those for the amphetamines. Long out of fashion after a brief spurt of popularity in the early 1900s, cocaine use enjoyed a resurgence when the U.S. government clamped down on the manufacture and distribution of amphetamines during the 1970s. Since then, plummeting cost and skyrocketing availability have made it one of the most widely used illegal drugs in the United States. In recent years, about a quarter of drug-related visits to emergency rooms were due to cocaine. Men and women are almost equally affected by this scourge.

Cocaine that has been heated with bicarbonate yields a white lump that is not destroyed by heating. It produces a popping sound when smoked; hence the name *crack*. The availability of crack cocaine has accounted for much of the recent rise in cocaine use.

Most users of cocaine begin by taking it intermittently, but rapidly progress to "runs" similar to those of amphetamine users. Dependence on crack cocaine usually occurs after only a few weeks of use. Although runs usually last a day or less, there is almost no tolerance to cocaine, so they can continue for several days.

The cross-sectional evaluation may not adequately discriminate patients who use cocaine from those who use amphetamines or related drugs. History can also be unreliable: What is sold on the streets doesn't always conform to what is advertised. Even the more reliable purveyors have no control over impurities or contaminants. The only sure way to determine what substance a patient is using is to obtain a urine or blood specimen for toxicology.

292.89 Cocaine Intoxication

Cocaine is probably the strongest pharmacological reinforcer ever produced. Laboratory animals will choose it in preference to food, water, and sex; given free access, they will use it again and again until they die. Humans use it by snorting, injecting, or smoking. Smoking crack can produce a rush of euphoria and a feeling of well-being that ensues within a few seconds. The user feels alert and self-confident, and has increased sex desire. These positive feelings last for a few minutes, then give way to dysphoria and an intense craving for more of the drug. With continued acute use, the euphoric effects lessen and the dysphoric effects (anxiety, depression, fatigue) increase. Motivation diminishes to the point that the user is interested in only one thing: obtaining more cocaine.

Behavioral changes associated with Cocaine Intoxication include aggression and agitation, often leading to fighting and hypervigilance. Cocaine postpones fatigue, and the resulting increase in energy breeds impaired judgment and an increased willingness to take risks. Violence and crime are frequent products of the cocaine-intoxicated state.

Cognitive symptoms range from feelings of omnipotence to ideas of reference, (beliefs that external events have a special meaning unique to oneself), delusions, and *haptic* (tactile) hallucinations. Other symptoms include irritability, increased sensory awareness, anorexia, insomnia, and spontaneous ejaculation. If the intoxication is severe, there may be rambling speech, confusion, anxiety, headache, and palpitations of the heart.

Criteria for Cocaine Intoxication

- The patient has recently used cocaine.
- During or shortly after its use, the patient develops clinically important behavioral or psychological changes that are maladaptive. These may include blunted affect, hypervigilance, interpersonal sensitivity, anger, anxiety or tension, changes in sociability, stereotyped behaviors, impaired judgment, and impaired work or social functioning.
- Shortly after use, two or more of these occur:
  - ✓ Slowed or rapid heart rate
  - ✓ Dilated pupils
  - ✓ Raised or lowered blood pressure
  - ✓ Chills or sweating
  - ✓ Nausea or vomiting
  - ✓ Weight loss
  - ✓ Speeded-up or slowed down psychomotor activity
  - ✓ Muscle weakness, shallow or slowed breathing, chest pain, or heart arrhythmias

✓ Coma, confusion, dyskinesias (involuntary muscular activity), dystonias (disordered muscle tone) or seizures

• These symptoms are neither the result of a general medical condition nor better explained by a different mental disorder.

Coding Note

Specify if: With Perceptual Disturbances. The patient has altered perceptions: auditory, tactile, or visual illusions or hallucinations with intact insight. (*Intact insight* implies that the patient recognizes that the symptoms are unreal, caused by the substance use. Hallucinations without this insight suggest a diagnosis of Cocaine-Induced Psychotic Disorder.)

Amanda Brandt

Since her graduation from college at age 22, Amanda Brandt had worked as a futures trader on the Chicago Stock Exchange. It was a fast-paced, high-pressured life, and she loved it. "I was an economics major in college," she explained, "and what can you do with that? Teach?"

Futures trading exactly suited Amanda's temperament. Since early high school she had been energetic and outgoing. Her job introduced her to a lot of young people who were as bright and well paid as she.

Amanda's father was a Baptist minister; he and her mother were both teetotalers. Though both of her grandfathers were long dead, she thought that they had been alcoholics. She supposed that this might have had something to do with her parents' attitude toward alcohol. "I'm sure they never dreamed I smoked pot in college," Amanda said. "But it never seemed to bother me, and it was the social thing to do."

What was social in her corner of the Exchange, she soon discovered, was cocaine. She and her fellow traders made more than enough money to afford quantities of the powdery stuff, though not as much as they actually used. With the advent of crack in the mid-1980s, the price decreased and Amanda's use soared. She had always hated the pain of needles, so instead of snorting, she learned to smoke it.

"Within a few seconds of lighting up, you felt wonderful. It was like a total body climax," she said. "I felt like even my lungs were coming."

The rush of the intense high blasted her with a pleasure that obliterated any concern she might have had about the pounding heartbeat and the feelings of agitation. For 15 minutes or so she felt incalculably witty; she loved and controlled the world. While she orbited, she didn't need sex, people, food, water, or even air. For a quarter of an hour, she felt that she could live forever.

Evaluation of Amanda Brandt

Amanda's use of cocaine produced profound behavioral and psychological changes, including alterations in her judgment and social life. She noted that the pleasure produced by the drug was worth the side effects it caused—in her case, rapid heartbeat and a sense of agitation. Someone observing while she was acutely intoxicated would probably have noticed some of the other symptoms listed in the criteria. Her subjective feelings give some idea of why people become addicted to cocaine.

Besides **Amphetamine Intoxication** (the symptoms are exactly the same), some of the other Axis I disorders that feature hyperactivity or mood instability should be considered. These would include either **Bipolar Disorders** and **general medical conditions** such as hyperthyroidism. **Phencyclidine Intoxication** can have perceptual distortions similar to Cocaine Intoxication. Patients who become psychotic or delirious when intoxicated must be discriminated from those with **Schizophrenia** and other psychotic disorders, or with **Delirium Due to a General Medical Condition**.

From the information given in this vignette, Amanda's Axis I diagnosis at this point would be 292.89 (Cocaine Intoxication). A fuller diagnosis is provided below.

292.0 Cocaine Withdrawal

After the acute intoxication phase, blood cocaine levels drop rapidly. Unless more of the drug is immediately consumed, the patient rapidly crashes into depression. The patient may also experience irritability, suicidal ideas, fatigue, loss of interest, and a decreased ability to experience pleasure. Panic attacks are common, and the craving for cocaine is intense. Although most of these symptoms tend to abate after increasing for two to four days, depression can linger for months. Suicide attempts are fairly common and sometimes successful.

About half of all those who have problems with cocaine use also have a mood disorder. Many are bipolar or cyclothymic; this sets them quite apart from individuals with opioid-related disorders.

Criteria for Cocaine Withdrawal

- A patient who has been using cocaine heavily and for a long time suddenly stops or markedly reduces its intake.
- Within a few hours to several days of reducing intake, the patient develops dysphoric mood *and* two or more of the following:
  ✓ Fatigue
  ✓ Unpleasant, vivid dreams
  ✓ Excessive sleepiness or sleeplessness

✓ Increase in appetite
✓ Speeded-up or slowed psychomotor activity
- These symptoms cause clinically important distress or impair work, social, or other functioning.
- These symptoms are neither the result of a general medical condition nor better explained by a different mental disorder.

Amanda Brandt Again

In the aftermath of her intoxication, Amanda died, or so it seemed. She would feel suddenly, incurably depressed. The supreme self-confidence of only a few moments before would be replaced by an anxious uncertainty that gradually overwhelmed her over the next day or two. The only remedy was to smoke another lump of crack, and then another and another, until her supply ran out. Then she would be left sleepless and exhausted, while every cell in her body remembered exactly how exhilarating it felt to be high and craved to experience it again.

By the summer of Amanda's fourth year on the Exchange, her life had begun to unravel. Compared to the importance of using cocaine, work now seemed irrelevant. For days in a row, she would call in sick; when she did go in, her mind was focused on when and how she would score her next vial of crack. When she was finally fired, she responded by moving to a smaller apartment and selling her BMW. Now that she could devote all of her time to acquiring and using crack, it took her exactly two months to smoke up her life savings and the proceeds from selling her car.

It was her final binge of using that brought Amanda in for treatment. After smoking her last pipeful, she roamed the hallway in her apartment building, weeping and knocking on doors. When anyone answered, she tried to get inside. Someone called the police, who took her to the emergency room. There she became enraged and lashed out with her fists. Ultimately, she had to be restrained and admitted to a mental health inpatient unit.

Further Evaluation of Amanda Brandt

Amanda's history made it painfully clear that cocaine was the source of her disorder. When she ran out of it, she showed (by weeping) the requisite dysphoria and several of the physical symptoms listed in the criteria: insomnia, fatigue, and speeded-up psychomotor activity. For any withdrawal syndrome to be diagnosed by DSM-IV criteria, it must cause marked distress or greatly affect the patient's life; Amanda conformed to this rule. Not included in the criteria, but typical nonetheless, was her perfect memory of the experience of using crack and her desire for more.

At this point, there is enough information to give Amanda another substance-related diagnosis: Cocaine Dependence. She spent nearly all of her time using crack cocaine, which cost her her job and her car. Finally, she developed withdrawal symptoms.

A number of other cocaine-related disorders are listed in DSM-IV, some of which are more frequently encountered than others. If Amanda's depression persisted substantially longer than the period of withdrawal, **Cocaine-Induced Mood Disorder** might be added to her list.

Other patients may have associated mental disorders, such as **Pathological Gambling**, **Antisocial Personality Disorder**, and **Posttraumatic Stress Disorder**.

Axis I	292.0	Cocaine Withdrawal
	304.20	Cocaine Dependence
Axis II	V71.09	No Diagnosis
Axis III		None
Axis IV		Unemployment
Axis V	GAF = 35	(current)

Other Cocaine-Related Disorders

You will find a complete listing of cocaine-related disorders in Table 3.1 One of these is mentioned here:

292.81 Cocaine Intoxication Delirium. Some patients experience an agitated delirium associated with intoxication. They may perform remarkable feats of strength, and their wild, irrational behavior occasionally results in death.

HALLUCINOGEN-RELATED DISORDERS

Also called *psychedelic* and *psychotomimetic* drugs, hallucinogens as a rule produce illusions, not hallucinations. Two such drugs that occur naturally are psilocybin (obtained from certain mushrooms) and peyote (obtained from cactus).

The prototype of the manufactured hallucinogens is lysergic acid diethylamide (LSD), which in the 1960s was embraced as the first new mind-altering substance to be developed in generations. In the United States, legal manufacture of LSD has long since disappeared; all supplies currently come from illicit (street) labs. Morning glory seeds contain lysergic acid amide, a substance similar to LSD.

Newer synthetics, such as MDA, MDMA, and others, continue to turn up. These are sometimes called "designer drugs" because they resemble the pharmacological properties of known hallucinogens while escaping (temporarily) their illegal status. PCP is also a hallucinogen, but is classified separately (see p. 122) because it has somewhat different toxic effects.

During the past 20 years or so, the popularity of LSD appears to have plummeted. It is now used by under 5% of college students, mostly young men. However, the use of designer drugs (especially MDMA) may have increased. It is unusual for a hallucinogen to be the sole substance used.

In many cases, as noted earlier in connection with cocaine, drugs sold on the street are quite different from what is promised. Lacking a quality control ethic, vendors freely substitute cheap for dear, available for rare. Thus, for example, "psilocybin" may in fact be ordinary mushrooms onto which some entrepreneur has sprayed LSD or PCP.

Tolerance to LSD occurs so rapidly that it is rarely used more than once a week. More frequent use simply doesn't produce effects worth the trouble. No withdrawal syndrome from LSD or other hallucinogens is defined, though some people reportedly crave them after stopping.

TIP Because one hallmark of DSM-IV has been renaming disorders in the interests of greater descriptive accuracy, it is astonishing that the hallucinogens have not been renamed. Typically, they do not produce hallucinations at all, but illusions. In fact, in Canada these drugs are sometimes referred to as *illusionogens*. There is still work for DSM-V.

292.89 Hallucinogen Intoxication

The first symptoms of Hallucinogen Intoxication are usually somatic. Patients may mention dizziness, tremor, weakness, or numbness and tingling of extremities. Perceptual changes (usually illusions) include the apparent amplification of sounds and visual distortions (e.g., body image), as well as synesthesias (in which one type of sensory experience produces the sensation of another—e.g., a color results in the sensation of a sound). Hallucinations, if they occur at all, may be of vivid geometric forms or colors. Auditory hallucinations can also occur. Many people experience intense euphoria, depersonalization (i.e., a sense of detachment from oneself), derealization (i.e., a sense of unreality in one's perceptions), dream-like states, or an altered sense of time (it speeds up or slows down). Attention may be impaired, though most users retain insight.

The specific features are greatly influenced by setting and by a person's expectations. Some users find the experience pleasant; others become extraordinarily anxious. A "bad trip" usually includes feelings of anxiety and depression; panic attacks may occur. These reactions will occasionally be prolonged, characterized by fears of becoming psychotic. Usually, acutely negative reactions subside within 24 hours (the time it takes to excrete all of the drug).

LSD is an extremely potent agent; a dose of a few micrograms (an amount that can be soaked into a postage stamp) can produce significant symptoms. It is absorbed from the gut, and action usually begins within an hour. The effects tend to peak at two to four hours, and may last half a day.

Like users of PCP, users of the hallucinogens can injure or even kill themselves if they act on their illusions. For example, they may judge that they can leap safely to the ground from atop a tall building.

Criteria for Hallucinogen Intoxication

- The patient has recently used a hallucinogen.
- During or shortly after its use, the patient develops clinically important behavioral or psychological changes that are maladaptive. These may include severe depression or anxiety, ideas of reference, fear of becoming insane, persecutory ideas, impaired judgment, and impaired work or social functioning.
- During or shortly after use, while fully alert the patient has perceptual changes (depersonalization, derealization, illusions, hallucinations, synesthesias, or subjective intensification of experience).
- Shortly after use, two or more of these occur:
  ✓ Dilated pupils
  ✓ Rapid heart rate
  ✓ Sweating
  ✓ Irregular heartbeat
  ✓ Blurred vision
  ✓ Tremors
  ✓ Poor coordination
- These symptoms are neither the result of a general medical condition nor better explained by a different mental disorder.

Wanda Pittsinger

At age 26, Wanda still worked at the cinema. She had started this job on a part-time basis when she was a high school senior; after graduation, she moved to full-time and had stayed on ever since. It didn't pay especially well, but it was comfortable. The work (making change and popcorn) was undemanding, and she got to see a lot of first-run movies, though not necessarily in start-to-finish order.

Wanda's job had lasted longer than her marriage. When she was 22, she had been married to Randy for almost 10 months. Other than a pregnancy (which she also terminated), the main thing she got out of the relationship was an introduction to LSD. She still saw Randy occasionally, but by this time they were not much more than friends—about the only activity they pursued together was tripping, which almost invariably wiped out their sex drive.

Wanda had tried other drugs. Marijuana gave her headaches; cocaine made her nervous. She had snorted heroin once, and it made her throw up. But acid was just about right. It always raised her spirits and made her feel giddy. Sometimes, if she was looking into a mirror, she seemed to see herself melting. This didn't bother her; you expected weird things to happen when you dropped acid. Besides the usual colored diamonds, triangles, and squares, she thought that LSD sometimes revealed new meanings or insights. She valued the sensation of thinking deeply. The experience was almost always worth the palpitations and blurred vision that were her only side effects.

Acid even gave Wanda a better feeling about Randy. She still sometimes tripped with him on a day off, and he continued to supply her with the little squares of blotting paper impregnated with LSD. As a present, he had once given her two movie tickets that had been soaked in LSD. She'd kept them tucked into the corner of her dresser mirror.

Evaluation of Wanda Pittsinger

Wanda's psychological and behavioral changes while taking LSD were minor, and the pluses and minuses were pretty much a wash. They helped her tolerate Randy, but she lost interest in sex. One could argue whether these were clinically important—they weren't enough to get her into treatment, as a "bad trip" might. But she did have other symptoms of Hallucinogen Intoxication: She noted the typical side effects of blurred vision and palpitations of her heart. She also had the typical marked perceptual changes: illusions of lights, patterns, and shapes, and the sensation of having special insight. Moreover, she felt euphoric—another common experience with this drug.

The differential diagnosis of Hallucinogen Intoxication includes **delirium**, **dementia**, **epilepsy**, and **Schizophrenia**. Beyond her illusions, Wanda had symptoms suggestive of none of these disorders. However, her clinician would have to do a complete workup, including a mental status evaluation, to rule out these possibilities completely. **Hypnopompic hallucinations** (i.e., hallucinations experienced between the sleeping and waking states) can take on the aspect of a flashback, but Wanda's illusory experiences occurred at times other than when she was waking up.

DSM-IV allows a diagnosis of Hallucinogen Dependence, but it is probably rare. Like Wanda, most users take it infrequently; rapid tolerance (loss of effect) results from use more often than once or twice a week. There was no evidence presented that she had lost control over the use of this substance or that its use altered the way she approached her job or social life.

Any time Wanda used LSD, she could qualify for an Axis I diagnosis of 292.89 (Hallucinogen Intoxication). A fuller diagnosis is given below.

292.89 Hallucinogen Persisting Perception Disorder (Flashbacks)

Flashbacks may be triggered by stress, by entering a dark room, or by using marijuana or phenothiazines. Symptoms can include seeing faces, geometric forms, flashes of color, trails, afterimages, or halos; micropsia (in which things look small); and macropsia (in which things look huge). Diminished sex interest may be a feature. The patient usually has insight into what is happening.

Although brief flashbacks (lasting perhaps a few seconds) are common, only a small percentage of users have enough of these symptoms to be distressing or to interfere with their activities. They usually decrease with time; however, they can occur weeks or months after use and can persist for years.

Criteria for Hallucinogen Persisting Perception Disorder (Flashbacks)

- After stopping the use of a hallucinogen, the patient re-experiences at least one of the symptoms of perception that occurred during intoxication. These may include flashes of color, trails of images, afterimages, halos, macropsia, micropsia, geometric hallucinations, and false peripheral perception of movement.
- These symptoms cause clinically important distress or impair work, social, or other functioning.
- These symptoms are neither the result of a general medical condition nor better explained by hypnopompic (while awakening) hallucinations or by a different mental disorder, such as Schizophrenia or a dementia.

Wanda Pittsinger Again

Wanda came for help when she found herself tripping at times when she had not dropped acid for several days.

"I noticed it one night at work when I walked into the auditorium just before the main feature. I saw myself on the screen, first all in green, and then sort of sparkly. Then my image seemed to sort of dissolve, and I saw that it was only a trailer for a Woody Allen film that would be playing in two weeks."

When Wanda told Randy about this the next day, he called it a flashback and said that it was "cool." Despite Randy's reassurance, these experiences worried her. She stayed home from work for a day or two, because she felt she couldn't cope with the flashbacks at work. She had never used drugs of any sort since.

In the nearly two months since she had last used LSD, Wanda had experienced a number of flashbacks. Most of them amounted to seeing "trails"—ghostly afterimages of people or objects that had traversed her field of vision. A couple of times she had seen Randy's face on the ceiling of her bedroom. Once the kitchen table seemed to grow in size to the point that she thought that she would never be able to reach it to eat her breakfast. But she never again experienced her own image on the silver screen.

Further Evaluation of Wanda Pittsinger

When Wanda walked into the darkened theater, she basically experienced a recurrence of the illusions she had had during LSD intoxication, although the details had changed. Flashbacks of some degree or other are common; perhaps one-quarter of LSD users have them. They would probably not qualify for a diagnosis at all, if they hadn't so upset her.

As in Hallucinogen Intoxication, Wanda's clinician would have to rule out **delirium, dementia, Schizophrenia, epilepsy,** and **space-occupying lesions in the brain.** She would not qualify for a diagnosis of **Hallucinogen-Induced Psychotic Disorder, With Hallucinations,** because she had insight that her perceptions were caused by substance use. The past history of LSD use and the typical presentation would make her current diagnosis secure:

Axis I	292.89	Hallucinogen Persisting Perception Disorder
Axis II	V71.09	No diagnosis
Axis III	None	
Axis IV	None	
Axis V	GAF = 70	(current)

Other Hallucinogen-Related Disorders

You will find a complete listing of Hallucinogen-Related Disorders in Table 3.1. Here are several that merit special mention:

292.84 Hallucinogen-Induced Mood Disorder. Depression or anxiety is relatively common; euphoria is rare. Sleep is often decreased. Patients may be restless and experience feelings of guilt. They may express fear that they have destroyed their brains or gone crazy. Hallucinogen-Induced Mood Disorder may last relatively briefly, or it may endure for months.

292.9 Hallucinogen-Related Disorder Not Otherwise Specified. Here there are at least two possible diagnoses worth mentioning. Both of these must be catalogued as Not Otherwise Specified, because they are not officially sanctioned by DSM-IV. They may be experienced with hallucinogens other than LSD.

Hallucinogen-induced personality change. Chronic use may lead to character change, such as the development of magical thinking or basic change in attitude.

Hallucinogen-induced persisting psychosis. Occasionally, a hallucinogen seems to trigger a psychosis that may last a long time, perhaps forever. There has been a good deal of controversy as to whether this is "only" an underlying psychosis that might eventually have developed, whether or not the patient used drugs.

INHALANT-RELATED DISORDERS

Inhalant users will breathe almost anything that evaporates or can be sprayed from a container. Used on purpose to produce intoxication, a volatile substance is called an *inhalant*; if it is accidentally inhaled, it is called a *toxin*. The inhalants include glue and gasoline (which are perhaps the most popular), solvents, thinners, various aerosols, correction fluid, and refrigerants. Preference may be guided more by availability than by effect.

Users value inhalants for a number of reasons. They relieve boredom and alleviate concern. They alter perceptions (producing changes of color, size, or shape of objects, or frank hallucinations), ideas, moods, and the sense of time. Users also like inhalants because they are cheap and, like everything that is absorbed from the lungs, quick to take effect.

Neurological damage from prolonged use of inhalants can be quite varied. Encephalopathy and peripheral neuropathy are widely experienced. Also, there can be ataxia, symptoms of parkinsonism, loss of vision, and involvement of the fifth and seventh cranial nerves (producing numbness and paralysis of the face). With chronic use there may be weight loss, weakness, disorientation, inattentiveness, and loss of coordination. Death is rare; it usually results from a patient's using a bag or mask that does not allow oxygen to be mixed with the substance being breathed.

Three groups of patients use inhalants. Youngsters (males or females) experiment with them, often as a group activity. Adults (mostly males) can become dependent on them. Finally, they are used by individuals who are also chronic users of other drugs. Many inhalant users come from underprivileged minorities. Personality disorders, especially Antisocial Personality Disorder, are quite common among inhalant users.

292.89 Inhalant Intoxication

Patients with Inhalant Intoxication are rarely encountered in emergency rooms or medical offices. Many of their symptoms are similar to those of Alcohol Intoxication. Early symptoms include drowsiness, agitation, lightheadedness, and disinhibition. Later symptoms include ataxia, disorientation, and dizziness. More severe intoxication produces insomnia, weakness, trouble speaking, disruptive behavior, and occasionally hallucinations. After a period of sleep, the patient will often be lethargic and feel hung over.

Toluene, a widely used solvent, is a principal component of many of the substances abused. It is associated with headache, euphoria, giddiness, and cerebellar ataxia. With smaller doses there may be fatigue, headache, inhibited reflexes, and tingling sensations.

Inhalants are usually absorbed by bagging or by huffing. When bagging, people spray, squeeze, or pour the contents into a plastic bag and then inhale from the bag. They huff by placing substance-soaked rags into their mouths and inhaling. Either of these methods can enable the users to maintain a high that lasts for hours.

When evaluating patients whom you suspect of using inhalants, be sure to ask carefully about all other substance classes. Polysubstance use is common in these patients, and some symptoms may be due to the use of alcohol, cannabis, hallucinogens, nicotine, or PCP. The only sure way to determine what a patient has been using is chemical analysis of the substance(s) in the patient's blood or urine.

Criteria for Inhalant Intoxication

- Recently the patient has intentionally used volatile inhalants or has had brief, high-dose exposure to them.
- During or shortly after this experience, the patient develops clinically important behavioral or psychological changes that are maladaptive. These may include apathy, assaultiveness or belligerence, impaired judgment, and impaired work or social functioning.
- During or shortly after this experience, two or more of these occur:
  ✓ Dizziness
  ✓ Nystagmus
  ✓ Poor coordination
  ✓ Slurring of speech
  ✓ Unsteady walking
  ✓ Lethargy
  ✓ Diminished reflexes
  ✓ Slowed psychomotor activity
  ✓ Tremors
  ✓ General muscular weakness

✓ Blurred or double vision
✓ Stupor or coma
✓ Euphoria
• These symptoms are neither the result of a general medical condition nor better explained by a different mental disorder.

Coding Notes

Do not include anesthetic gases or short-acting vasodilators in this category. Intentional use of these substances is coded under Other (or Unknown) Substance-Related Disorders (see p. 132). The "other" category is also used for accidental exposure to inhalants (e.g., exposure resulting from an industrial accident).

Because most commercial products contain a number of different gases and other volatile substances, it is often impossible to determine which have produced the effects observed. That is why, in coding, it is often necessary to use the generic term Inhalant Intoxication.

Dudley Langenegger

The sea was calm when Dudley Langenegger was taken to the brig, but he stumbled, swayed, and almost fell onto the bunk. He rubbed his eyes, which were already brick-red, and seemed to be trying to determine where he was. "It couldn't be the barracks," he said with a giggle, "there's no Playmate posters on the wall."

Dudley had been in the Army for six months, just long enough to finish his basic training. Since he was 12 he had been in trouble for running away, breaking and entering, and something called "incorrigibility." Days before his 18th birthday, the judge had given him a choice: "Jail or the Army."

Even when he was clean and sober, which wasn't often, Dudley hadn't been an especially good soldier. Often insolent, he was only compliant enough to spend most of his weekends confined to base rather than the stockade. When his unit boarded a ship for its joint operation with the Navy, Dudley went along.

So, apparently, did several tubes of model airplane cement. At least, those were what Dudley said he had been huffing in the galley at midnight. As he told his story, he required several sharp commands and at least one good shaking from the first sergeant to keep him from wandering off the subject or falling asleep. His breath smelled like a paint shop.

Dudley had been inhaling various vapors, mainly organic solvents, for about three years. Where he grew up, a lot of the guys did this—the stuff was easy to get, cheap, even legal. He admitted that the issue of legality didn't weigh upon him, but cheapness and ease were important.

Airplane glue produced a quick, reliable high. Dudley liked it because it raised his mood and made long hours seem to flash by. Tonight he had had his own private party. Everyone else had gone to bed, and he wanted to boost himself out of the low mood he had been in. It had worked so well that he had thought that it might be a good idea to throw pots and pans around in the galley, which was how he had been discovered by the military police.

"I never use it more than once or twice a week," he said with another giggle. "Too musha stays vits s'posed, uh, bad for your brain."

Evaluation of Dudley Langenegger

As a result of sniffing glue, Dudley had the bad judgment to throw things in the galley; by giggling, he also demonstrated maladaptive emotional changes. In addition to the obvious ill timing of his drug use, he had a number of the physical symptoms of Inhalant Intoxication. These included slurred speech, lethargy (his first sergeant had to keep him awake during the interview), and poor coordination. The giggling would suggest euphoria, but a direct question about his mood would be needed to be sure. His eyes were irritated, and he had the odor of solvents on his breath. (A physical examination might well have revealed nystagmus and depressed reflexes as well.)

Dudley would come close to fulfilling criteria for Inhalant Intoxication Delirium. When apprehended and interviewed, he was obviously less than fully alert and could not sustain attention without a lot of direction from his first sergeant. He was also disoriented (he didn't know where he was), and he couldn't speak clearly. However, delirium would only be diagnosed if Dudley's impairment lasted longer than expected for an intoxication *and* independently required clinical attention.

This vignette does not provide enough information to allow a diagnosis of **Inhalant Dependence**. Huffing had certainly interfered with Dudley's work, but there is no evidence that other criteria had been met. Dudley's problems with fights, poor work performance, and the legal system might all be related to his use of inhalants, but they could also be attributed to a personality disorder. (There isn't enough information for a definitive diagnosis on Axis II, either. This would have to be explored later.) However, any of these behaviors would qualify him for a diagnosis of **Inhalant Abuse**. Until more extensive knowledge about his usage patterns could be obtained, this diagnosis, rather than Inhalant Dependence, would have to be used.

Differential diagnosis would include use of other drugs such as **alcohol**; the history is usually sufficient to discriminate these causes, and the odor of airplane glue on the patient's breath can be a dead giveaway. Various neurological conditions (such as **multiple sclerosis**) must also be ruled out.

Dudley's five-axis diagnosis would be as follows:

Axis I	292.89	Inhalant Intoxication
	305.90	Inhalant Abuse

Axis II   V71.09   No diagnosis; antisocial personality traits
Axis III   None
Axis IV   Arrested by MPs
Axis V   GAF = 40   (current)

Other Inhalant-Related Disorders

You will find a complete listing of Inhalant-Related Disorders in Table 3.1.

NICOTINE-RELATED DISORDERS

Because tens of millions of adults are dependent on nicotine, the potential for withdrawal problems is enormous. In part because of the intense craving nicotine induces, it has been called the most widely used addictive drug in the United States. In terms of lethality, it is responsible for at least 60 times as many deaths each year as heroin.

It is hard to find clear evidence of primary reinforcers in nicotine. That is, its chemical effects do not include the direct production of euphoria, elevated self-esteem, or the enhancement of energy—the effects so valued by those who use drugs such as cocaine or opioids. Rather, nicotine produces nausea, vomiting, and anxiety, especially in the novice smoker. (Although it has been reported to reduce anxiety, this is probably the effect of "curing" the person's Nicotine Withdrawal.) So why do people smoke? In a nutshell, social factors get them started; then they are hooked.

There is a strong positive correlation between Nicotine Dependence and Alcohol Dependence, Schizophrenia, and other mental disorders. When interviewing alcoholics and schizophrenics, ask about tobacco use.

292.0 Nicotine Withdrawal

A patient who is withdrawing from nicotine often complains most, not of the specific symptoms listed in these criteria, but of craving a cigarette. This incessant desire can overwhelm the ability to focus on other, more substantive (but less pressing) issues. The result is a moody, anxious patient who sleeps poorly and eats too much, knowing that everything could be fixed by one dose of a perfectly legal substance that is being used every day by millions worldwide. No wonder these people are irritable. Onset of withdrawal symptoms occurs within a day of last use, and is often detectable within just a few hours.

No separate case vignette is provided for Nicotine Withdrawal. However, Hoyle Garner had a Sleep Disorder Due to Chronic Obstructive Pulmonary Disease that was caused by smoking; his story is given in Chapter 12 (see p. 433). He was also diagnosed as having Nicotine Dependence, and at one time had Nicotine Withdrawal.

Criteria for Nicotine Withdrawal

- The patient has used nicotine daily for several weeks or more.
- Within 24 hours of abruptly reducing nicotine intake, the patient develops four or more of these:
  ✓ Dysphoria or depression
  ✓ Insomnia
  ✓ Anger, frustration, or irritability
  ✓ Anxiety
  ✓ Trouble concentrating
  ✓ Restlessness
  ✓ Slowed heart rate
  ✓ Increase in appetite or weight
- These symptoms cause clinically important distress or impair work, social, or other functioning.
- These symptoms are neither the result of a general medical condition nor better explained by a different mental disorder.

Other Nicotine-Related Disorders

The other nicotine-related disorders are listed in Table 3.1. A special word on Nicotine Dependence is in order here:

305.10 Nicotine Dependence. Like caffeine, nicotine is legal, easy to obtain, and cheap (relative to heroin). Most people can use it without interfering in any material way with their other, non-substance-related pursuits. But in the course of a single year, they may repeatedly try to stop, suffer from withdrawal symptoms, and eventually return to smoking despite the knowledge that they are making a pulmonary or cardiovascular disorder worse.

OPIOID-RELATED DISORDERS

Not long ago, opioids were the most feared of the mind-altering substances. (That distinction has now been claimed by cocaine.) In terms of human wastage and criminal activity, opioids are still among the most costly of illegal drugs. Typically, users will spend over $200 a day on their habits, mostly obtained through criminal activities. In terms of problematic use, heroin remains the most devastating of the opioid drugs.

Opioid users value their drugs because of the high, which they experience as euphoria and diminished concern for the present. Heroin has several times the power of morphine to produce euphoria and blunt the perception of pain, to the point that users become indifferent to pain. However, first-time opioid users often experience vomiting and dysphoria.

Some users (especially those who are middle-class and middle-aged) may start to abuse opioids during the course of medical treatment. Being a health care professional places people at special risk for opioid use. However, most users begin in their teens or 20s as a result of peer pressure. Opioid use is generally preceded by the use of other drugs, such as alcohol or marijuana. In this group, risk factors for opioid use include low socioeconomic status, residence in an urban area, divorced parents, and relatives who abuse alcohol.

Some writers interpret the fact that users of "hard" drugs often begin with alcohol and marijuana as meaning that the use of alcohol or marijuana leads to opioid addiction. That conclusion could be correct, but no one really knows whether it is. It is entirely possible that a common precursor (hereditary or environmental) leads to a variety of drug use behaviors, including the use of alcohol, marijuana, and opioids.

Some degree of tolerance to any opioid drug develops within the first few doses; the lives of users quickly become dominated by the pursuit and use of the drug. However, nobody knows why some people exposed to narcotics become addicted and others do not. Once hooked, users will go to nearly any length to obtain drugs. They will plead, steal, lie, and promise just about anything in the world.

Overall, there is a 0.7% lifetime prevalence of severe opioid use in the adult population. Males outnumber females by about three to one. Even after detoxification, once opioid users return to familiar environments, many begin to use again; usually this occurs within three months. But of those who live long enough, a good number eventually shake off their addiction.

Most users of heroin use the drug intravenously, and up to half of IV drug users are positive for HIV. Always check for HIV when you encounter a heroin user. Needle marks indicate the injection of heroin or *speedballs* (mixed heroin and cocaine).

292.89 Opioid Intoxication

When an opioid drug is injected, its effects are felt almost immediately. This "rush" has been described as similar to an orgasm, and is rapidly followed (depending on the individual) by euphoria, drowsiness, the perception of warmth, dry mouth, and heaviness in the extremities. Some users experience a flushed face and itching nose. As opposed to Cocaine Intoxication, violent behavior is rare during Opioid Intoxication.

Although opioid users can become tolerant to enormous doses, overdose with opioids remains a medical emergency. It can produce clouding of consciousness (including coma), severe respiratory depression, shock, and ultimately death from anoxia. It is often recognized by extremely constricted (pinpoint) pupils, or by dilated pupils if the overdose is severe. Opioid overdose is treated intravenously with naloxone, a potent opioid antagonist.

Sedative or Alcohol Intoxication can sometimes be confused with Opioid Intoxication. The presence of pinpoint pupils can help make the distinction. Once again, a urine or blood test may be necessary to differentiate among the various possible causes of a patient's symptoms.

Patients who use opioid drugs often wear dark glasses. Sometimes this is the fashion of their culture; sometimes they do this to hide their pupils. When you are interviewing opioid users, ask them to remove dark glasses. Other physical stigmata of opioid use include scarring of the arms, other places where veins are prominent, and just about any other location where drugs can be injected. The subcutaneous route of administration, called *skin-popping,* is a last resort for those who have already destroyed their veins by years of using dirty needles.

Criteria for Opioid Intoxication

- The patient has recently used an opioid.
- During or shortly after its use, the patient develops clinically important behavioral or psychological changes that are maladaptive. These may include euphoria leading to apathy, depression or anxiety, speeded up or slowed psychomotor activity, impaired judgment, and impaired work or social functioning.
- During or shortly after use, the patient develops constricted pupils (or dilation due to brain damage following a severe overdose) *and* one or more of these:
  ✓ Sleepiness or coma

✓ Slurring of speech
✓ Impaired memory or attention
• These symptoms are neither the result of a general medical condition nor better explained by a different mental disorder.

Coding Note

Specify if: With Perceptual Disturbances. The patient has altered perceptions: auditory, tactile, or visual illusions or hallucinations with intact insight. (*Intact insight* implies that the patient recognizes that the symptoms are unreal, caused by the substance use. Hallucinations without this insight suggest a diagnosis of Opioid-Induced Psychotic Disorder.)

Herm Cry

Herm Cry was admitted to the detox unit exactly 24 hours after he last shot up. The junk had been good-quality—he knew, because he had slept for nearly eight hours afterwards. But then he awakened to the all-too-familiar aching muscles and runny nose that told him it was time to go out and earn his next fix. He had had no regular job for at least a year, but he knew some ways of getting money that didn't involve waiting for a paycheck.

At a young age, Herm had become familiar with the symptoms of withdrawal. His father's drinking was well known in their working-class neighborhood in St. Louis. By the time he was 10, Herm had watched his father suffer through at least two episodes of DTs. Alcohol had never done much for Herm. He didn't much care for the taste, and he certainly didn't need the hangover. His mother, a public health nurse, had her own problems with Demerol.

Off and on since he was 12, Herm had smoked marijuana. But it wasn't until a neighborhood block party the night he turned 16 that he first snorted heroin. "All of a sudden," he told the clinician who admitted him, "I knew I'd found the way."

Within a few minutes, he felt happier than he had ever been in his life. It was as if a warm bath had leached out all the anger, depression, and anxiety he had ever contained. For a few hours, he even forgot how much he hated his old man. All he had left was an overwhelming sense of tranquility that gradually gave way to drowsy apathy.

The following day, using a sterile syringe he stole from his mother, Herm injected heroin for the first time. Almost immediately, he vomited; this was followed at once by a sense of pleasure that seemed to race outward to the tips of his fingers and toes. Rubbing his itching nose, he fell asleep. When he aroused himself, several hours had passed. He injected again, using a smaller quantity of the drug (all he had left). When he awakened this time, he briefly considered stopping. His next thought was the realization that, more than anything else he could remember, he wanted to use heroin again.

Evaluation of Herm Cry

The sense of tranquility and peace that Herm experienced after injecting heroin is what causes people to return to the drug after the first time, even if it makes them sick at first. Of course, after they have used it for a few days, they no longer need a positive reason—simply avoiding the curse of withdrawal is enough to make them go out and steal so they can continue.

Herm's most notable behavioral symptom was the impairment in his social functioning (for a year or more he had forsaken work for criminal activities). He also had at least one typical symptom of Opioid Intoxication: profound drowsiness that lasted for several hours after injecting. (The runny nose and aching muscles are symptoms of the impending withdrawal. See the next vignette, which continues Herm's story.)

The criteria for Opioid Intoxication also require that the patient have pinpoint pupils. This is sometimes so pronounced that the user cannot see clearly. Patients are unlikely to complain about this feature; to make a diagnosis of Opioid Intoxication, a clinician must make this observation.

Most opioid users meet criteria for another mental disorder. These include **mood disorders** (up to 75%), **alcohol-related disorders** (about 30%), **Antisocial Personality Disorder** (25%), and the **anxiety disorders** (12%). Up to 13% of opioid users make suicide attempts. Considering the situation they are in, it is small wonder.

Herm had no perceptual disturbances, such as illusions or hallucinations. Assuming that he had constricted pupils and that no other **mental disorder** or **general medical condition** better explained his symptoms, criteria for the diagnosis of Opioid Intoxication would be fulfilled.

Because there is very little material in this first vignette pertaining to the issue of personality disorder, Herm's Axis II diagnosis would have to be deferred. This would keep future clinicians alert to the possibility, without prejudicing them as to its nature. He would also seem a likely candidate for problems with the legal system, thereby earning an entry on Axis IV, but the first vignette produces no such evidence.

Much of the material that would qualify Herm for a diagnosis of Opioid Dependence is contained in the next vignette. His diagnosis at this point would be as follows:

Axis I	292.89	Opioid Intoxication
Axis II	799.9	Diagnosis Deferred
Axis III		None
Axis IV		None
Axis V	GAF = 55	(highest level past year)

292.0 Opioid Withdrawal

Although some symptoms of Opioid Withdrawal may appear after a very few doses, it takes a week or two of continuous use to produce the typical withdrawal syndrome. Opioid Withdrawal strongly resembles a flu-like viral illness: It comprises symptoms such as nausea and vomiting, dysphoria, muscle aches and pains, tearing and runny nose, fever, and diarrhea. Another symptom of autonomic nervous system activation that occurs during withdrawal is piloerection—small hairs stand up, producing "goose flesh." (This is the derivation of the term "going cold turkey.") How rapidly symptoms of withdrawal appear depends principally on which drug is used; consult a reference on opioids for information about specific drugs' half-lives. Even after most of the symptoms have abated, some patients may suffer a protracted abstinence syndrome characterized by anxiety and low self-esteem, which can last as long as five or six months.

Criteria for Opioid Withdrawal

- The patient has either:
  - ✓ Recently stopped or reduced use of opioids after heavy, prolonged use (at least several weeks) or
  - ✓ Been given an opioid antagonist after using opioids for some time.
- Within minutes to several days after this experience, the patient develops three or more of these:
  - ✓ Dysphoria
  - ✓ Nausea or vomiting
  - ✓ Aching muscles
  - ✓ Tearing or runny nose
  - ✓ Dilated pupils, piloerection, or sweating
  - ✓ Diarrhea
  - ✓ Yawning
  - ✓ Fever
  - ✓ Sleeplessness
- These symptoms cause clinically important distress or impair work, social, or other functioning.
- These symptoms are neither the result of a general medical condition nor better explained by a different mental disorder.

Herm Cry Again

Sixteen hours after his last fix, Herm still had not scored. His usual suppliers had refused to extend his credit. He had tried to borrow money from his mother, but she had refused, and the earrings he had stolen from her dresser top had proven worthless. Although the abdominal cramps were worsening and he felt nauseated, he managed to make it to the apartment of a former girlfriend for whom he had briefly pimped. But she had just injected the last of her own heroin supply and was asleep. He appropriated her used syringe for his own use later, in case he scored.

Ducking into the restroom in the bus station, Herm narrowly averted disastrous consequences from a bout of explosive diarrhea. As he was about to emerge from the stall, he suddenly retched into the grimy toilet bowl. He sat down on the cool tile floor and tried to rub away the goose flesh on his arm. He dabbed his runny nose with a bit of toilet paper. He was too weak, he realized, to go out and hustle. He would have to go to detox for a few days and get his strength back. Then he could go out and get what he needed to really make him well.

Further evaluation of Herm Cry

Earlier, Herm had awakened to muscle cramps and a runny nose—typical early symptoms of Opioid Withdrawal. As the day went on and he could not obtain more heroin, he developed gastrointestinal symptoms of nausea, vomiting, and diarrhea. He had goose flesh, and by the time he was admitted, a clinician would also probably find dilated pupils. Although it does not constitute one of the criteria for Opioid Withdrawal, craving for the drug is almost universal in addicts who, like Herm, suddenly stop using opioids.

On the basis of the symptoms related in the two vignettes, Herm should also be given a diagnosis of Opioid Dependence. Of course, he suffered from withdrawal. He spent a great deal of time trying to obtain heroin, and he had had no job for a year or more, presumably because his drug habit fully occupied his time. He probably met other criteria for Opioid Dependence as well, such as tolerance and attempts to quit, but these are not addressed in the vignette. Because it was the main reason for Herm's entering treatment, Opioid Withdrawal is listed below as the first diagnosis.

Herm's Axis II diagnosis would not change. He showed several symptoms of **Antisocial Personality Disorder** (such as thievery and pimping), but as far as we know, these occurred only in the context of his substance use. This personality disorder is certainly well represented among other users of opioids, however.

Axis I	292.0	Opioid Withdrawal
	304.00	Opioid Dependence, With Physiological Dependence
Axis II	799.9	Diagnosis Deferred
Axis III		None
Axis IV		None
Axis V	GAF = 55	(current)

Other Opioid-Related Disorders

You will find a complete listing of opioid-related disorders in Table 3.1.

PHENCYCLIDINE (OR PHENCYCLIDINE-LIKE)-RELATED DISORDERS

Phencyclidine (PCP) was originally developed as an anesthetic agent; its only legitimate use now is in veterinary medicine. However, because it is cheap and easy to produce (it can be mixed up almost literally in a bathtub), it continues to be popular with young men in their 20s who value it for the euphoria it produces.

Called *angel dust* on the street, PCP is a hallucinogen. But it also has stimulant and depressant qualities that cause it to be classified separately. It is a highly potent drug that, in its typical street dose of 5 mg, can produce psychotic symptoms so convincing that they sometimes cannot be distinguished from Schizophrenia. Schizophrenia patients who take it run a risk of activating severe pathology.

Although whether it produces either tolerance or withdrawal is not known with any certainty, PCP's addictive potential is pronounced—as high as that of "hard" drugs, some say. If it is swallowed, its symptoms begin within an hour of use; if it is smoked, they begin within a few minutes. A high lasts from four to six hours and can be repeated in runs lasting several days. PCP can be taken just about any way the user wants it—by snorting, by swallowing, or by injection. It has even been absorbed vaginally. Now it is usually smoked in cigarettes, which are preferred because smoking produces its effects so quickly that it allows the user to titrate them with some precision (and thus to avoid emergency room visits for overdoses).

292.89 Phencyclidine Intoxication

With much variability, the effects of PCP are related to the dose. Besides euphoria, PCP can produce lethargy, anxiety, depression, delirium and behavioral problems that include agitation, impulsivity, and assault. Even catatonic symptoms and suicide have been reported. Some users experience violent, exaggerated, unpredictable responses to light or sound; this is the reason why sensory restriction is recommended for intoxicated patients. Physical symptoms include high fever, muscle rigidity, muteness, and hypertension. Heavy doses can result in coma, convulsions, and death from respiratory arrest.

Criteria for Phencyclidine Intoxication

- The patient has recently used PCP or a related substance.
- During or shortly after its use, the patient develops clinically important behavioral or psychological changes that are maladaptive. These may include assault, belligerence, impulsivity, agitation, unpredictability, impaired judgment, and impaired work or social functioning.
- Within an hour of use (less, if PCP is snorted, smoked, or injected), the patient develops two or more of these:
  - ✓ Nystagmus
  - ✓ Rapid heartbeat or high blood pressure
  - ✓ Numbness or decreased response to pain
  - ✓ Trouble walking
  - ✓ Trouble speaking
  - ✓ Rigid muscles
  - ✓ Coma or seizures
  - ✓ Abnormally acute hearing
- These symptoms are neither the result of a general medical condition nor better explained by a different mental disorder.

Coding Note

Specify if: With Perceptual Disturbances. The patient has altered perceptions: auditory, tactile, or visual illusions or hallucinations with intact insight. (*Intact insight* implies that the patient recognizes that the symptoms are unreal, caused by the substance use. Hallucinations without this insight suggest a diagnosis of Phencyclidine-Induced Psychotic Disorder.)

Jennie Meyerson

At age 24 Jennie Meyerson had been troubled half her life. When she was 12, her father had walked out on the family in the midst of the worst argument she could remember between her two warring parents. The divorce had preoccupied her mother and chased her older sister out of the house, and Jennie had been left pretty much on her own.

By the time Jennie was 14, she had begun smoking marijuana after school and sometimes between classes. Within a year she was smoking instead of going to classes. On her 18th birthday, her mother kicked her out of the house. She lived with a succession of boyfriends, each of whom introduced her to a new recreational drug. She had been in and out of mental hospitals and was a double alumna of the Betty Ford Clinic.

Jennie's last interviewer was Patrolman Reggie Polansky, a young police officer. One Saturday afternoon, he was called to the sixth floor of a run-down apartment building, where a young woman was sitting on a ledge high above the street. The sweetish smell of marijuana smoke enveloped Polansky as he walked through the room to the window.

The ledge just outside the window was perhaps 10 inches wide. About a yard to his left sat Jennie, barefoot and bare-legged, wearing a cotton blouse and a thin dress. She sat quietly, her face tilted up to the late summer sunshine. On the pavement 80 feet below, a crowd had gathered.

Gripping the window sill, Polansky poked his head out. "What are you doing out there?"

"Just ress—jes' res-*ting*." With an effort, she finally pronounced the word. She didn't open her eyes or turn her head. "I'm gonna fly."

"You don't want to do that. Come on back in here."

"You c'mon out—*here*. I'm Amelia Earhart. We can both fly." Jennie giggled and told him that she was Amelia Earhart, and that she was a flyer. They talked for several minutes. She admitted that she was joking about being Amelia Earhart, but thought that she could learn to fly. It had come to her in a flash this morning, after she "got dusted." She had used angel dust off and on for the past several months.

Patrolman Polansky pointed to her hand. The webbed space between her thumb and finger was bleeding. "You've cut yourself."

Jennie said she must have done it on the jagged window cornice as she was climbing out. Perhaps it was a message from God. That must be it, she said, because she hadn't felt it at all. It was "like God's wounds." Instead, she felt happy, strong, and light. She felt like practicing for the Labor Day air show on Monday.

"Look how close the ground is," she said. "It seems like I can just step down there."

She slowly stretched out both arms until they extended straight out from her shoulders, and stepped lightly forward onto the wind.

Evaluation of Jennie Meyerson

Jennie experienced several behavioral and psychological changes before her death that would qualify her for a diagnosis of Phencyclidine Intoxication. Her judgment was also badly affected, as she ultimately demonstrated. Of the physical symptoms that must be present to make the diagnosis, two are documented in the vignette: trouble speaking (her speech was slurred) and reduced pain perception (she hadn't noticed that she had torn the skin of her hand while climbing out the window).

Jennie also had an illusion (the ground looked close to her, rather than six stories down), which would meet the requirement for the qualifier of With Perceptual Disturbance. Other drugs can produce perceptual distortions during intoxication, including **cocaine, amphetamines, opioids**, and **cannabis**. The odor in the room suggested to Patrolman Polansky that marijuana was used, but PCP users often spray their drug onto something they can smoke (usually marijuana or tobacco). When reliable information is lacking, a definitive diagnosis often depends on a toxicology report.

The vignette gives no information as to the extent of Jennie's problem with PCP, so a diagnosis of either Phencyclidine Dependence or Abuse would not be possible. The vignette clearly indicates that Jennie had had, at a minimum, previous occupational (school) problems from the use of a variety of substances. However, DSM-IV does not allow a diagnosis of Polysubstance Abuse (only Polysubstance Dependence). Further diagnosis would depend on additional information about her usage patterns.

Jennie's statements that she could fly and that she had stigmata ("God's wounds") were not firmly held, and therefore not delusional. This would rule out **Schizophrenia** and any other psychosis. There was no evidence that her disorder was due to a **general medical condition**. In other patients, rapid resolution (often without treatment) may help differentiate Phencyclidine Intoxication from other mental disorders such as **mood** and **anxiety disorders**. PCP users should also be evaluated for personality disorders and the use of other mind-altering substances.

The posthumous five-axis diagnosis for Jennie Meyerson would be as follows:

Axis I	292.89	Phencyclidine Intoxication, With Perceptual Disturbance (Provisional)
	305.90	Phencyclidine Abuse (Provisional)
Axis II	799.9	Diagnosis Deferred
Axis III		None
Axis IV		None
Axis V	GAF = 0	(expired)

Other Phencyclidine-Related Disorders

You will find a complete listing of Phencyclidine-Related Disorders in Table 3.1.

SEDATIVE-, HYPNOTIC-, OR ANXIOLYTIC-RELATED DISORDERS

Sedatives, hypnotics, and anxiolytics are used for different purposes but share many features. Most specifically, they have in common symptoms of intoxication and withdrawal.

The terms applied to these substances are somewhat confusing, and not always precisely used. A *sedative* is anything that reduces excitement and induces quiet without producing drowsiness. A *hypnotic* helps the patient get to sleep and stay there. And an *anxiolytic* is one that reduces anxiety. However, most of the drugs discussed in this section can have any of these actions, depending on the dose.

The major drug classes covered in this section are the benzodiazepines, such as diazepam (Valium) and alprazolam (Xanax), and the barbituates, such as pentobarbital (Nembutal); other classes include the carbamates and the barbituate-like hypnotics. Users value the barbiturates and benzodiazepines for the disinhibition they produce, which means that they induce euphoria, reduce anxiety and guilt, and boost self-confidence and energy. There are two main patterns of abuse, which can be summarized roughly as follows.

Some people get started with a prescription, usually obtained to combat the effects of insomnia or anxiety. Then they increase the dose to varying degrees. Although they would probably have withdrawal symptoms if they abruptly stopped using the drug, many of these patients would never meet the behavioral criteria for Substance Dependence given earlier in this chapter. That is, these people don't use more of the drug than they intend, try to cut down, devote inordinate time to drug use, give up important social activities, or use the drug despite knowledge that they are being harmed.

More frequently, some young people use these drugs to produce euphoria. This is the history we classically associate with the misuse of most of the substances described in DSM-IV. In the past, this has especially been true of the use of barbiturates and specialty drugs such as methaqualone and glutethimide. In recent years, however, the legitimate manufacture of these drugs has been either greatly curtailed (barbiturates) or banned altogether (methaqualone). Also, physicians' prescribing practices have changed. Government regulation has been an important catalyst for all these changes.

Benzodiazepines are only infrequently the primary substance used, but they are often used to mitigate the undesired effects of other drugs. For example, they can help calm the jitters induced by central nervous system stimulants. Benzodiazepines are also sometimes used to boost the high of methadone or to ease the symptoms of heroin withdrawal. In 1979, 3.5% of those who responded to a household survey had taken nonprescribed benzodiazepines at least once in the previous year. The benzodiazepines preferred by users are diazepam and alprazolam, and users will pay premium prices to be sure they are getting the real thing. The street value of a Valium tablet in the mid-1990s was about $1.

292.89 Sedative, Hypnotic, or Anxiolytic Intoxication

As with the use of most drugs, the effects achieved through the use of sedatives, hypnotics, or anxiolytics depend strongly on the setting where they are consumed and the expectations of those who use them. Mood is often labile, with case reports ranging from euphoria to hostility and depression. Loss of memory similar to that occurring in heavy alcohol consumption has also been reported. Other common effects include unsteady gait, slurred speech, nystagmus, poor judgment, and drowsiness. In very high doses, these drugs produce respiratory depression, coma, and death; this outcome is far less likely with the benzodiazepines than with the barbiturates. The DSM-IV criteria for this category are exactly the same as those for Alcohol Intoxication.

Criteria for Sedative, Hypnotic, or Anxiolytic Intoxication

- The patient has recently used a sedative, hypnotic, or anxiolytic drug.
- During or shortly after use, the patient develops clinically important behavioral or psychological changes that are maladaptive. These may include inappropriate sexuality or aggression, lability of mood, impaired judgment, and impaired work or social functioning.
- Shortly after use, one or more of these occur:
  ✓ Slurring of speech
  ✓ Poor coordination
  ✓ Unsteady walking
  ✓ Nystagmus
  ✓ Impaired attention or memory
  ✓ Stupor or coma
- These symptoms are neither the result of a general medical condition nor better explained by a different mental disorder.

Kirk Aufderheide

When the forklift load of galvanized iron pipe crushed his pelvis at work, Kirk Aufderheide promised himself that he would never complain about anything else again, if only he could regain the use of his legs. Four months later, on the day he hobbled out of the hospital using an aluminum walker, he began trying to fulfill that promise. What he hadn't reckoned on were the muscle spasms.

Kirk was 35 when the warehouse accident happened. Even though he had had insulin-dependent diabetes for the past 15 years, he considered himself healthy. His only previous hospitalization had been for febrile convulsions as a child. The combination of his diabetes and a strict religious upbringing had caused him to avoid street drugs, alcohol, and tobacco. Until his accident, he had prided himself on never taking so much as an aspirin tablet.

But the muscle spasms changed all that. They had probably been there ever since the accident, though Kirk didn't notice them until the first day he was allowed out of bed. Thereafter, any time he was up and about, he was likely to be seized with excruciating cramps in the muscles of his lower back. Reluctantly, he accepted a prescription for diazepam. A 5-mg tablet four times a day, his doctor assured him, would help relax his muscles.

Miraculously, it worked. For nearly two weeks Kirk was able to move around comfortably, if not pain-free. When the spasms returned and his doctor told him that 20 mg a day was the maximum dose he should take, he sought the advice of another doctor.

Within a few months, Kirk was seeing four physicians and taking between 60 and 80 mg of diazepam every day. He saw one of them under an assumed name (the prescription of benzodiazepines is tightly controlled in the state where Kirk lives). The other two physicians he consulted worked across the state line, which was only a few miles from where he lived. A fifth doctor had noticed his low mood and warned him not to take too much of the drug; he had never returned to see that physician again.

What with waiting for his appointments and driving to pharmacies remote from his neighborhood, Kirk needed several hours each week to obtain his supply. Much of the rest of his time—he hadn't yet been able to return to work, so he stayed home and kept house for his wife and two daughters—he spent dozing in front of the television set. His wife complained that he had changed; he had become moody and he seemed to have trouble following the thread of a conversation.

Evaluation of Kirk Aufderheide

Kirk's wife described him as moody, which is the sort of psychological change that would be expected from diazepam intoxication. He had at least two of the specific symptoms from the list above: drowsiness and unsteady gait.

Although the present criteria are exactly the same as for Alcohol Intoxication, historical information and the smell of alcohol on the breath should allow easy discrimination. In Kirk's case, there was no history to implicate alcohol. However, a blood test may be needed to determine that a patient has used both.

Would Kirk qualify for a diagnosis of Diazepam Dependence? He had developed a degree of tolerance that caused him to take four times the maximum dose recommended—far more than any one of his physicians would prescribe. He spent considerable time going to four different doctors and pharmacies to obtain his supply. He also continued to use diazepam even though one physician told him that high doses could harm him.

Kirk's five-axis diagnosis at this point would be as follows:

Axis I	292.89	Diazepam Intoxication
	304.10	Diazepam Dependence, With Physiological Dependence
Axis II	V71.09	No diagnosis
Axis III	809.0	Fracture (crush) of pelvis
	250.01	Insulin-dependent diabetes mellitus
Axis IV		Unemployed
Axis V	GAF = 60	(current)

292.0 Sedative, Hypnotic, or Anxiolytic Withdrawal

When a patient stops using (or markedly reduces a high dose of) a sedative, hypnotic, or anxiolytic drug, the result is much like the abrupt cessation of alcohol use; the criteria for withdrawal are identical. (In this context, a high dose means several times the therapeutic dose—for example, 60 mg or more of diazepam.) However, the time course varies with the half-life of the drug. As in the case of the opioids, consult a reference on these drugs for information about specific drugs' half lives.

One diagnostic challenge is to distinguish withdrawal symptoms from the re-emergence of those symptoms that led to treatment in the first place (anxiety, agitation, and insomnia play a prominent role in both). The time course can help: Any symptoms that remain (or that appear) two to three weeks after the drug has been discontinued are probably old symptoms re-emerging.

Criteria for Sedative, Hypnotic, or Anxiolytic Withdrawal

- A patient who has been using a sedative, hypnotic, or anxiolytic drug heavily and for a long time suddenly stops or markedly reduces its intake.
- Within a few hours to several days, two or more of the following develop:
  - ✓ Autonomic overactivity (sweating, rapid heartbeat)
  - ✓ Worsened tremor of hands
  - ✓ Sleeplessness
  - ✓ Nausea or vomiting
  - ✓ Short-lived hallucinations or illusions (visual, tactile, or auditory)
  - ✓ Speeded-up psychomotor activity
  - ✓ Anxiety
  - ✓ Grand mal seizures

- These symptoms cause clinically important distress or impair work, social, or other functioning.
- These symptoms are neither the result of a general medical condition nor better explained by a different mental disorder.

Coding Note

Specify if: With Perceptual Disturbances. The patient has altered perceptions: auditory, tactile, or visual illusions or hallucinations with intact insight. (*Intact insight* implies that the patient recognizes that the symptoms are unreal, caused by the substance use. Hallucinations without this insight suggest a diagnosis of Sedative-, Hypnotic-, or Anxiolytic-Induced Psychotic Disorder.)

Kirk Aufderheide Again

Four days short of the first anniversary of his accident, Kirk's wife received notice that she was being transferred to a branch office in the interior of the state. The transfer forced the family to move. At the new location, Kirk found that there were tighter controls on the prescription of benzodiazepines, and far fewer physicians and pharmacies. Once they had settled into their new house, he realized that he had no choice but to reduce his dose of diazepam.

Although Kirk intended to taper his usage, he put off doing so until he was nearly out of medication. So on a warm summer morning he found himself suddenly facing the prospect of taking only four tablets, whereas the day before he had had 16. At first, he was surprised at how little it bothered him. For several days he experienced insomnia, but he had expected that. (With no work to go to, he had had time to read some magazine articles about the effects of substance use.)

But at 4 A.M. of the third day, Kirk awakened to a sense of anxiety that bordered on panic. He felt nauseated and noticed that his pulse was racing. For two days his agitation mounted, to such an extent that he had difficulty sitting still long enough to eat the supper he had prepared. On the fifth day, his wife arrived home after work to find him having a grand mal seizure.

Further evaluation of Kirk Aufderheide

When he drastically decreased his intake of diazepam, Kirk noted some of the classic symptoms of withdrawal: racing pulse, insomnia, and nausea. He had had no illusions or hallucinations to qualify for the specifier of With Perceptual Disturbances.

Anxiety and panic attacks commonly occur as rebound phenomena; therefore, **anxiety disorders** form an important part of the differential diagnosis. When hallucinations occur during withdrawal, they can be mistaken for a **Manic Episode** or various **psychotic disorders**. **Delirium** is also a relatively common complication. **Antisocial Personality Disorder** is often found among patients who obtain these medications illegally.

Kirk's seizure occurred after several days of withdrawal. (Childhood febrile seizures might have made him more susceptible to withdrawal seizures.) Because the seizure was the focus of treatment on admission, it is listed first on Axis I. (The rest of the five-axis diagnosis remains as it was before.)

Axis I	292.0	Diazepam Withdrawal
	304.1	Diazepam Dependence, With Physiological Dependence
Axis III	780.3	Withdrawal Seizure

Other Sedative-, Hypnotic-, or Anxiolytic-Related Disorders

You will find a complete listing of these disorders in Table 3.1. One of these is mentioned briefly here:

292.81 Sedative, Hypnotic, or Anxiolytic Withdrawal Delirium. When delirium occurs, it is almost always within a week of the patient's discontinuing a drug. Like delirium due to other causes, it features reduced attention span and problems with orientation, memory, perception (visual, auditory, or tactile hallucinations or illusions) or language disturbance. It is usually preceded by insomnia.

POLYSUBSTANCE-RELATED DISORDER

304.80 Polysubstance Dependence

The category of Polysubstance Dependence denotes use for at least six months of three or more substances at once, none of which predominates. Criteria must be met for Substance Dependence for these substances as a group, but not for any single one of these. Presumably, if the dependence criteria are met for one substance, "*Dependence*" should be diagnosed for that substance, with Substance-Related Disorder Not Otherwise Specified diagnosed for the others.

Nicotine and caffeine are excluded from the substances that can play a role in Polysubstance Dependence. The reasons for this are obvious: They are legal and they are used by substantial portions, if not by an outright majority, of the general population.

OTHER (OR UNKNOWN) SUBSTANCE-RELATED DISORDERS

The category of Other (or Unknown) Substance-Related Disorders covers disorders linked to substances not included in the 11 categories listed in Table 3.1 and described above; the category is also used when the specific substance a patient has used is unknown. The generic criteria for Substance Dependence, Abuse, Intoxication, and Withdrawal given earlier in this chapter, or the criteria for substance-induced disorders described in other chapters (e.g., Substance-Induced Delirium, Substance-Induced Persisting Dementia, etc.), are applied here as appropriate. Some examples of the substances included in this category are as follows:

> **Anabolic steroids.** The value to users of the anabolic steroids derives from enhanced physical attractiveness and athletic ability. For body builders and other athletes, this desire can be a powerful motivator to use drugs. Besides the obvious effects on the physique, users report euphoria, increased libido, and at times aggression (so-called *'roid rage*). Anabolic steroids differ in some respects from other substances that are misused: They are often used in a social context, and this use continues unabated for months or years. However, they are similar to other misused substances in that patients use them longer than initially desired, cannot stop using them, spend excessive time using or trying to get them, and use them even though they know they cause harm. Cessation of their use can also cause withdrawal symptoms, which include depression, fatigue, restlessness, insomnia, loss of appetite, and reduced interest in sex. Some users develop an intense drug craving.

> **Nitrous oxide.** Nitrous oxide is an anesthetic inhalant that produces lightheadedness and mild euphoria; hence its nickname, *laughing gas*. It can be obtained from cans of whipped cream or from dentists.

Over-the-counter/prescription drugs. Over-the-counter and prescription drugs that can induce dependence include antiparkinson drugs, cortisone and its derivatives, antihistamines, and others.

Betel nut. People in many cultures chew betel nut to achieve a mild high or sensation of floating.

Kava. Made from a pepper plant that grows in the South Pacific, kava causes sedation and loss of coordination and weight.

CHAPTER 4

Schizophrenia and Other Psychotic Disorders

Quick Guide to the Psychotic Disorders

When psychosis is a prominent reason for a mental health evaluation, the diagnosis will be one of the disorders or categories listed below. The page number following each item indicates where a more detailed discussion begins. (Note that the order in which the psychotic disorders other than Schizophrenia are presented here differs slightly from the order in which they are discussed both in DSM-IV and later in this chapter.)

Schizophrenia

Schizophrenia patients have been ill for at least six months with at least two of these five symptom types, discussed on page 137 ff: delusions, hallucinations, disorganized behavior, disorganized speech, and negative symptoms. They do not have significant manic or depressive symptoms, and both substance use and general medical conditions have been ruled out (p. 143).

Five subtypes of Schizophrenia are defined:

Paranoid Type. These patients have persecutory delusions and auditory hallucinations, but no negative symptoms, disorganized speech, or catatonic behavior (p. 148).

Disorganized Type. In this subtype, delusions and hallucinations are less prominent than negative symptoms and disorganized speech and behavior (p. 149).

Catatonic Type. The cardinal symptoms of this subtype are excessively retarded or excited activity and bizarre behavior (p. 152).

Undifferentiated Type. These patients will have some or all of the five basic types of psychotic symptoms. None of these symptoms dominates the clinical picture (p. 155).

Residual Type. After an acute psychosis has markedly improved, these patients still seem somewhat unusual, odd, or peculiar (p. 158).

Schizophrenia-Like Disorders

Schizophreniform Disorder. This category is for patients who have all the symptoms of schizophrenia, but who have been ill for only one to six months—less than the time specified for Schizophrenia (p. 160).

Schizoaffective Disorder. For at least one month, these patients have had symptoms of Schizophrenia; at the same time, they have prominent symptoms of mania or depression (p. 164).

Brief Psychotic Disorder. These patients will have had at least one of the basic psychotic symptoms for less than one month (p. 172).

Disorders with Delusions

Delusional Disorder. Although these patients have delusions (which are not bizarre), they have none of the other symptoms of Schizophrenia (p. 169).

Shared Psychotic Disorder. This condition may be diagnosed when a patient develops delusions similar to those held by a relative or other close associate (p. 175).

Other Psychotic Disorders

Psychotic Disorder Due to a General Medical Condition. A variety of medical and neurological conditions can produce psychotic symptoms that may not meet criteria for any of the conditions above (p. 178).

Substance-Induced Psychotic Disorder. Alcohol or other substances (intoxication or withdrawal) can cause psychotic symptoms that may not meet criteria for any of the conditions above (p. 180).

Psychotic Disorder Not Otherwise Specified. This category is for patients with postpartum psychosis or other symptoms that do not seem to fit any of the categories above (p. 184).

Disorders with Psychosis as a Symptom

Some patients have psychosis as a symptom of mental disorders discussed in other chapters. These disorders include the following:

Mood disorder with psychosis. Patients with severe Major Depressive Episode (p. 194) or Manic Episode (p. 198) can have hallucinations and mood-congruent delusions.

Cognitive disorder with psychosis. Many demented patients have hallucinations or delusions (p. 27).

Personality disorders. Patients with Borderline Personality Disorder may have transient periods (minutes or hours) when they appear delusional (p. 478).

Disorders That Masquerade as Psychosis

The symptoms of some disorders *appear* to be psychotic, but are not. These disorders include the following:

Specific Phobia. Some phobic avoidance behaviors can appear quite strange without being psychotic (p. 259).

Mental Retardation. These patients may at times speak or act bizarrely (p. 501).

Somatization Disorder. Sometimes these patients will report pseudohallucinations or pseudodelusions (p. 294).

Factitious Disorder. These patients may feign delusions or hallucinations in order to obtain hospital or other medical care (p. 312).

Malingering. These patients may feign delusions or hallucinations in order to obtain money (insurance or disability payments), avoid work (such as in the military), or avoid punishment (p. 439).

Introduction

During the second half of the 20th century, one of the great leaps forward in mental health has been to recognize that psychosis can have many causes. At least a part of this progress can be credited to DSM-III and its successors, which have established and popularized criteria for many forms of psychosis.

The existence of psychosis is usually not hard to determine. Delusions, hallucinations, and disorganized speech or behavior are generally obvious; they often represent a dramatic change from a person's normal behavior. But differentiating the various causes of psychosis can be difficult. Experienced clinicians cannot definitively diagnose some patients, even after several interviews.

Symptoms of Psychosis

A psychotic patient is out of touch with reality. Psychosis can be manifested by one or more of five basic types of symptoms; some of these have been defined briefly in earlier chapters, but a more detailed discussion is provided here.

Delusions

A *delusion* is a false belief that cannot be explained by the patient's culture or education; the patient cannot be persuaded that the belief is incorrect, despite evidence to the contrary or the weight of opinion. Delusions can be of several types:

Grandeur. Patients believe they are persons of exalted station, such as God or a movie star.

Guilt. Patients feel they have committed an unpardonable sin or grave error.

Ill Health. Patients believe they have a terrible disease.

Jealousy. Patients are convinced that their spouses or partners have been unfaithful.

Passivity. Patients believe they are being controlled or manipulated by some outside influence, such as radio waves).

Persecution. Patients feel they are being interfered with.

Poverty. Patients fear they are facing destitution, contrary to such evidence as a job and ample money in the bank.

Reference. Patients feel they are being talked about, perhaps in the press or on TV.

Thought Control. Patients believe ideas are being put into their minds by others.

Delusions must be distinguished from *overvalued ideas*, which are beliefs that are not clearly false but continue to be held despite lack of proof that they are correct. Examples include belief in the superiority of one's own race or political party.

Hallucinations

A *hallucination* is a false sensory perception that occurs in the absence of a related sensory stimulus. Hallucinations are nearly always abnormal and can affect any of the five senses, but auditory and visual hallucinations are the most common.

To count as psychotic symptoms, hallucinations must occur when the person is fully conscious. This means that hallucinations that occur during delirium cannot be taken as evidence of one of the psychotic disorders discussed in this chapter. The same can be said for hallucinations that occur when someone is going to sleep or waking up; these are regarded as normal experiences.

Illusions are experiences that must be discriminated from hallucinations. Illusions are simply misinterpretations of actual sensory stimuli. They usually occur in conditions of decreased sensory input, such as at night. (For example, a person awakens to the belief that a burglar is bending over the bed; when the light comes on, it is only a pile of clothes on a chair.) Illusions are common and usually normal.

Disorganized Speech

Even without delusions or hallucinations, a psychotic patient may have *disorganized speech* (sometimes also called *loose associations*), in which mental associations are governed not by logic but by rhymes, puns, and other rules not apparent to the observer, or by no clear rules at all.

Some disorganization of speech is quite common (try reading an exact transcript of some politicians' off-the-cuff remarks, for example!). But by and large, when those words were spoken, members of the audience understood perfectly what was intended. To be regarded as psychotically disorganized, the speech must be so badly impaired that it materially interferes with communication.

Disorganized Behavior

Disorganized behavior, or physical actions that do not appear to be goal-directed (e.g., taking off one's clothes in public, repeatedly making the sign of the cross, assuming and maintaining postures), may indicate psychosis. Again, note the importance of understandability in deciding that a given behavior is bizarre.

Negative Symptoms

Negative symptoms include reduced range of expression of emotion (flat or blunted *affect*), markedly reduced amount or fluency of speech, and loss of the will to do things (*avolition*). They are called negative because they give the impression that something has been taken away from the patient, not added, as is the case with hallucinations and delusions. Negative symptoms reduce the apparent textural richness of a patient's personality.

> **TIP** In evaluating patients who have delusions or hallucinations, be sure to consider the Cognitive Disorders. This is especially true in instances where the psychosis has developed quite rapidly.
>
> Schizophrenia patients who have active hallucinations or delusions should be asked about symptoms of dysphoria. They are likely to have either depression or anxiety, or both.

Distinguishing Schizophrenia from Other Disorders

DSM-IV uses four types of information to distinguish among the various types of psychosis: psychotic symptoms, course of illness, consequences of illness, and exclusions. Each of these categories of information (plus a few other features) can help you distinguish Schizophrenia, the most common psychotic disorder, from other psychotic disorders or other disorders involving psychosis. The reason for this emphasis on Schizophrenia is that the differential diagnosis of psychosis very often boils down to Schizophrenia versus non-Schizophrenia. In terms of the numbers of patients affected for long periods of time, as well as the seriousness of its implications for treatment and prognosis, it is the single most important cause of psychotic symptoms.

Psychotic Symptoms

The five ways in which a patient can be identified as psychotic—delusions, hallucinations, disorganized behavior, disorganized speech, and negative symptoms—are described at the beginning of this chapter. Any psychotic patient must have at least one of these symptoms, but to be diagnosed as having Schizophrenia, a patient must have at least two. Therefore, the first task in diagnosing any psychosis is to determine the extent of the psychotic symptoms.

When two or more of these symptoms of psychosis have been present for at least one month, the "A" criteria for Schizophrenia are said to be satisfied (see the basic criteria list, p. 144). DSM-IV (p. 285) specifies that these two or more psychotic symptoms must be present during a "significant portion of time" during that month. But what does *significant* mean in this context? There are probably several ways it can be interpreted: (1) These symptoms have been present on more than half the days in the month; (2) several persons independently may have observed on several days that the patient is having symptoms; and/or (3) the symptoms may have occurred at times when they are especially likely to have an effect on the patient and the environment—for example, if a patient has repeatedly interrupted a social gathering by screaming. Finally, note that a duration of less than one month is allowed if treatment has caused the symptoms to remit.

Delusions and hallucinations are the most commonplace symptoms of psychosis. As noted earlier, delusions must be discriminated from overvalued ideas, and hallucinations from illusions. Note that DSM-IV requires only one symptom if it is:

- A delusion that is bizarre (e.g., spending the night in a space capsule making love with Martians).
- The hallucination of a voice that keeps commenting on the patient's behavior or thoughts.
- The hallucination of at least two voices that talk with each other.

For behavior to be psychotic, it must be grossly disorganized and must not merely appear bizarre, and the patient must lack insight into its nature. For example, a patient with Obsessive–Compulsive Disorder may perform rituals (which can seem pretty bizarre), but the patient will agree that they are excessive or unreasonable. This is *not* psychotic.

Disorganized speech means speech that is not merely circumstantial, but shows marked loosening of associations. Examples: "He tells me something in one morning and out the other," "Half a loaf is better than the whole enchilada." Or, in response to the question, "How long did you live in Wichita?": "Even anteaters like to French-kiss."

Negative symptoms can be hard to pinpoint, unless you ask an informant about changes in affective lability, volition, or amount of speech. Negative symptoms can also be mistaken for stiffening of a patient's affect due to use of a neuroleptic medication.

TIP What exactly does *bizarre* mean? Unhappily, the definition isn't exact. The problem of deciding what is bizarre and what isn't becomes especially acute when a clinician is trying to assess behavior in a person from another culture. In general, however, *bizarre* refers to something that is so far from the usual experiences of life that most people would not understand it and would regard it as unlikely to occur. Examples of bizarre delusions include falling down a rabbit hole to Wonderland, being controlled (thoughts or actions) by aliens from Halley's Comet, or having one's brain replaced by a computer. Examples of nonbizarre delusions include being spied upon by neighbors or being betrayed by one's spouse.

Course of Illness

In DSM-IV, the cross-sectional symptoms are less important to the differential diagnosis of psychosis than is the course of illness. That is, the type of psychosis is largely determined by the longitudinal patterns and associated features of the disorder. Several of these factors are noted here:

Duration. How long has the patient been ill? A duration of at least six months is required for a diagnosis of Schizophrenia. This rule was formulated in response to the observation that psychotic patients who have been ill a long time (longer than six months) tend at follow-up to have Schizophrenia. Patients with a briefer history of psychosis often turn out to have some other condition.

Precipitating factors. Severe emotional stress sometimes precipitates a brief period of psychosis. For example, the stress of childbirth may be specifically associated with a postpartum psychosis. A chronic course is less likely if there are precipitating factors.

Previous Course of Illness. A prior history of complete recovery (no residual symptoms) from a psychosis suggests a disorder other than Schizophrenia.

Premorbid Personality. Good social and job-related functioning in an adult patient *before* psychotic symptoms develop directs the diagnostic focus away from Schizophrenia and toward another psychotic disorder or disorder involving psychosis, such as a mood disorder.

Consequences of Illness

Psychosis almost always seriously affects the functioning of both patient and family. How severe this is and whom it affects are other features that can help discriminate Schizophrenia from other causes of psychosis. For a patient to be diagnosed as having Schizophrenia requires that the patient's social or occupational functioning be materially impaired. For example, most people who have Schizophrenia never marry, and either do not work at all or hold jobs that require a lower level of functioning than is consistent with their education and capabilities. None of the non-Schizophrenia psychotic disorders require this criterion for diagnosis, and the criteria for Delusional Disorder specify that functioning is not impaired in any important way except as it relates specifically to the delusions.

Exclusions

Once the fact of psychosis is established, can it be attributed to any Axis I disorder other than Schizophrenia? At least three sets of possibilities must be considered.

First, is there a general medical condition? The top place in any differential diagnosis belongs to disorders caused by general medical factors (see Appendix B for a listing of some of these factors). History, physical examination and laboratory testing must be scrutinized for evidence.

Next, rule out substance-related disorders. Has the patient a history of abusing alcohol or street drugs? Some of these (cocaine, alcohol, psychostimulants, and the psychotomimetics) can cause psychotic symptoms that almost exactly mimic Schizophrenia. The use of prescription medications (e.g., adrenocorticosteroids) can also produce symptoms of psychosis.

Finally, consider mood disorders. Are there prominent symptoms of either mania or depression? The history of mental health treatment is awash with patients whose mood disorders have for years been diagnosed as Schizophrenia. Mood disorders should be included early in the differential diagnosis of any patient with psychosis.

Other features

You should also know about some features of psychosis that are not included in the DSM-IV criteria sets. Some of these have been found to help predict outcome. They include the following:

Family History of Illness. A close relative with Schizophrenia increases your patient's chances of having Schizophrenia. Bipolar I Disorder With Psychotic Features also runs in families. Always learn as much as you can about the family history.

Response to Medication. Regardless of how psychotic the patient appears, previous recovery with lithium treatment suggests a diagnosis of mood disorder.

Age at Onset. Schizophrenia usually begins by a person's mid-20s. Onset of illness after the age of 40 suggests something other than Schizophrenia. It could be Delusional Disorder, but you should consider a mood disorder. However, late onset does not completely rule out the diagnosis of Schizophrenia.

Schizophrenia

In an effort to achieve precision, the DSM criteria for Schizophrenia have been made more complicated over the years. But the basic pattern of a Schizophrenia diagnosis is relatively straightforward. It can be outlined briefly:

1. Before becoming ill, the patient may have a withdrawn or otherwise peculiar personality.

2. The illness begins gradually, often imperceptibly. At least six months before the diagnosis is made, behavior begins to change. Right from the start this may involve delusions or hallucinations, or it may begin with milder symptoms, such as beliefs that are peculiar but not psychotic.

3. During at least one month of those six, the patient has been frankly psychotic. There have been two or more of the five basic symptom types described earlier.

4. The illness causes important problems with work and social functioning.

5. The clinician can exclude mood disorders, substance use, and general medical factors as probable causes.

6. Although most patients improve with treatment, relatively few recover to such an extent that they are completely back to normal.

There are several reasons why it is important to diagnose Schizophrenia accurately:

Frequency. Approximately 1% of the general adult population will contract this disorder; it is a common disease.

Chronicity. Most patients who develop Schizophrenia continue to have symptoms throughout their lives.

Severity. Although most patients do not require months or years of hospitalization, as used to be the case, incapacity for social and work functioning can be profound.

Management. Adequate treatment almost always means using neuroleptic medications, which carry a risk of tardive dyskinesia and often must be taken on a lifelong basis.

Although nearly everyone does so, it is probably incorrect to speak of Schizophrenia as if it were one disease. It is almost certainly a collection of several different diseases for which the same basic set of diagnostic criteria is used, with variations. The DSM-IV basic criteria refer simply to Schizophrenia, but patients cannot be coded until they also receive a subtype diagnosis. I first present the basic criteria, and then discuss each subtype in turn.

Finally, it is important to note that many other symptoms are often found in patients with Schizophrenia, even though they do not constitute formal criteria for the basic diagnosis. Here are a few:

Cognitive Dysfunction. Distractibility, disorientation, or other cognitive problems are often noted, though Schizophrenia is classically described as occurring in a clear sensorium.

Dysphoria. Anger, anxiety, and depression are all common emotional reactions to ensuing psychosis.

Absence of Insight. The belief that they are not ill often leads patients to refuse to take medicine.

Sleep disturbance. Many patients stay up late and arise late when they are attempting to deal with the onset of hallucinations or delusions.

Suicide. About 10% of these patients (especially newly diagnosed young men) die by suicide.

Basic Criteria for Schizophrenia

- Symptoms (the "A" symptoms of DSM-IV). For a substantial part of at least one month (or less, if effectively treated), the patient has had two or more of:
  - ✓ Delusions (only one symptom is required if a delusion is bizarre, such as being abducted in a space ship from the sun)
  - ✓ Hallucinations (only one symptom is required if hallucinations are of at least two voices talking to each other or of a voice that keeps up a running commentary on the patient's thoughts or actions)
  - ✓ Speech that shows incoherence, derailment, or other disorganization
  - ✓ Severely disorganized or catatonic behavior
  - ✓ Any negative symptom, such as flat affect, reduced speech, or lack of volition
- Duration. For at least six continuous months, the patient has shown some evidence of the disorder. At least one month must include the symptoms of frank psychosis mentioned above. During the balance of this time (as either prodromal or residual indications of the illness), the patient must show *either or both* of these:
  - ✓ Negative symptoms as mentioned above
  - ✓ In attenuated form, at least two of the other symptoms mentioned above (example: deteriorating personal hygiene, *plus* an increasing suspicion that people are talking behind one's back)
- Dysfunction. For much of this time, the disorder has materially impaired the patient's ability to work, study, socialize, or provide self-care. (If the illness

begins in childhood or adolescence, the criteria for dysfunction require only that the patient fail to achieve the expected occupational, scholastic, or social level.)
- Mood exclusions. Mood disorders with psychotic features and Schizoaffective Disorder have been ruled out, because the duration of any depressive or manic episodes that have occurred during the psychotic phase has been brief.
- Other exclusions. This disorder is not directly caused by a general medical condition or the use of substances, including prescription medications.
- Developmental Disorder exclusion. If the patient has a history of any pervasive developmental disorder (such as Autistic Disorder), Schizophrenia is diagnosed only if prominent hallucinations or delusions are also present for a month or more (less, if treated).

Coding Notes

After at least one year has passed since onset, classify the course of psychosis. Until a year has passed, you cannot assign any of these course specifiers.

Continuous. There has been no remission of "A" symptoms. If negative symptoms stand out, you can also add With Prominent Negative Symptoms.

Episodic With Interepisode Residual Symptoms. During episodes, "A" criteria are met. Between episodes, the patient has clinically important residual symptoms. If negative symptoms stand out, you can also add With Prominent Negative Symptoms.

Episodic With No Interepisode Residual Symptoms. During episodes, "A" criteria are met. Between episodes, the patient has remissions with no clinically important symptoms.

Single Episode In Partial Remission. There has been one episode during which "A" criteria are met. Now there are some clinically important residual symptoms. If negative symptoms stand out, you can also add With Prominent Negative Symptoms.

Single Episode In Full Remission. No clinically important symptoms remain.

Other or Unspecified Pattern.

Lyonel Childs

When he was young, Lyonel Childs had always been somewhat isolated, even from his two brothers and his sister. During the first few grades in school, he seemed almost suspicious if other children talked to him. He seldom seemed to feel at ease, even with those he had known since kindergarten. He never smiled or showed much emotion, so that by the time he was 10, even his siblings thought he was peculiar. Adults said he was "nervous." For a few months during his early teens, he was interested in magic and the occult; he read extensively about witchcraft and casting spells. Later he decided he would like to become a minister. He spent long hours in his room learning Bible passages by heart.

Lyonel had never been much interested in sex, but at age 24, still attending college, he was attracted to a girl in his poetry class. Mary had blonde hair and dark blue eyes, and he noticed that his heart skipped a beat when he first saw her. She always said "Hello" and smiled when they met. He didn't want to betray too great an interest, so he waited until an evening several weeks later to ask her to a New Year's Eve party. She refused him, politely but firmly.

As Lyonel mentioned to an interviewer months later, he thought that this seemed strange. During the day Mary was friendly and open with him, but when he ran into her at night, she was reserved. He knew there was a message in this that eluded him, and it made him feel shy and indecisive. He also noticed that his thoughts had speeded up so that he couldn't sort them out.

"I noticed that my mental energy had lessened," he told the interviewer, "so I went to see the doctor. I told him I had gas forming on my intestines, and I thought it was giving me erections. And my muscles seemed all flabby. He asked me if I used drugs or was feeling depressed. I told him neither one. He gave me a prescription for some tranquilizers, but I just threw it away."

Lyonel's skin was pasty white and he was abnormally thin, even for someone so slightly built. He sat quietly without fidgeting during the interview, and his casual clothing seemed quite ordinary. His speech was entirely ordinary; one thought flowed normally into the next, and there were no made-up words.

By summer, he had become convinced that Mary was thinking about him. He decided that something must be keeping them apart. Whenever he had this feeling, his thoughts became so "loud" that he felt sure other people must know what he was thinking. He neglected to look for a summer job that year and moved back into his parents' house, where he kept to his room, brooding. He wrote long letters to Mary, most of which he destroyed.

In the fall, Lyonel realized that his relatives were trying to help him. Although they would wink an eye or tap a finger to let him know when she was near, it did no good. She continued to elude him, sometimes only by minutes. Sometimes there was a ringing in his right ear, which caused him to wonder whether he was becoming deaf. His suspicion seemed confirmed by what he privately called "a clear sign." One day while driving he noticed, as if for the first time, the control button for his rear window defroster. It was labeled REAR DEF, which to him meant "right-ear deafness."

When winter deepened and the holidays approached, Lyonel knew that he would have to take action. He drove off to Mary's house to have it out with her.

As he crossed town, people he passed nodded and winked at him to signal that they understood and approved. A woman's voice, speaking clearly to him from just behind him in the back seat, said, "Turn right" and "Atta boy!"

Evaluation of Lyonel Childs

Lyonel was psychotic. Two of the five symptoms listed above (the "A" symptoms) must be present for a diagnosis of Schizophrenia, and two was the number Lyonel had. His symptoms (hallucinations and delusions) were those that are most often encountered in Schizophrenia.

The hallucinations of Schizophrenia are usually auditory. Visual hallucinations often indicate a **Substance-Induced Psychotic Disorder** or **Psychotic Disorder Due to a General Medical Condition**; they can also occur in **dementia** or **delirium**. Hallucinations of sense or smell are more commonly experienced by a person whose psychosis is due to a medical factor, but they would not rule out Schizophrenia.

Like Lyonel's, auditory hallucinations are typically clear and loud; often patients will agree with the examiner who asks, "Is it as loud as my voice is right now?" Although the voices may seem to come from within a patient's head, often they are reported as coming from the hallway, an appliance, or a family pet.

The special messages that Lyonel received (finger tapping, eye winking) are called **delusions of reference**. Patients with Schizophrenia may also experience other sorts of delusions; these have been listed beginning on page 137. Many of these are to some extent **persecutory** (i.e., the patient feels in some way pursued or interfered with). None of Lyonel's delusional ideas were so far from normal human experience as to deserve the term **bizarre**. (If they were, he would need only that one psychotic symptom for the diagnosis of Schizophrenia.)

Lyonel did not have disorganized speech, disorganized behavior, or negative symptoms, but other Schizophrenia patients often have these psychotic symptoms. His illness significantly interfered with his work (he didn't get a summer job) and relationships with others (he stayed in his room and brooded). In each of these areas, he functioned much less well than before he became ill.

Although Lyonel had heard voices for only a short time, he had been delusional for several months. The prodromal symptoms (his beliefs about intestinal gas and reduced mental energy) had begun a year or more earlier. He easily fulfilled the requirement of a total duration (prodrome, active symptoms, and residual period) of at least six months. (Many relapses of psychosis occur without appreciable prodromal symptoms. When they do occur, high levels of prodromal symptoms predict high levels of subsequent psychotic symptoms.)

The doctor Lyonel consulted found no evidence of a **general medical condition**. Auditory hallucinations that may exactly mimic the Paranoid Type of

Schizophrenia (see below) can occur in **Alcohol-Induced Psychotic Disorder**. People who are withdrawing from **amphetamines** may even harm themselves as they attempt to escape terrifying persecutory delusions. Either of these disorders would be suspected if Lyonel had recently used substances.

Lyonel also denied feeling depressed. **Major Depressive Disorder With Psychotic Features** can produce delusions or hallucinations, but often these are mood-congruent (they center about feelings of guilt or deserved punishment). **Schizoaffective Disorder** could be excluded because he had no prominent mood symptoms (depressive or manic). From the duration of his symptoms, we know that Lyonel could not have **Schizophreniform Disorder**.

The next section presents Lyonel's subtype diagnosis and the course criteria for this diagnosis.

295.30 Schizophrenia, Paranoid Type

Patients with Schizophrenia, Paranoid Type, often appear the most "normal" among Schizophrenia patients—despite their obviously psychotic ideas, their behavior and physical appearance remain relatively unaffected. They are usually also better able to take care of their own day-to-day needs, even when they are at their sickest. This relative preservation of social (and, at times, school or work) functioning also sets them quite apart from those with other forms of Schizophrenia. These patients have a relatively late age of onset (some studies report an average of 35 years), whereas most other Schizophrenia patients become ill in their 20s.

Criteria for Schizophrenia, Paranoid Type

- The patient meets the basic criteria for Schizophrenia.
- The patient is preoccupied with delusions or frequent auditory hallucinations.
- *None* of these symptoms is prominent:
  - Disorganized speech
  - Disorganized behavior
  - Inappropriate or flat affect
  - Catatonic behavior

Further Evaluation of Lyonel Childs

In addition to the basic Schizophrenia criteria, a diagnosis of Schizophrenia, Paranoid Type, requires the absence of features typical of the Disorganized and Catatonic Types (see below). Paranoid patients do not have speech that is incoherent or affect that is blunted or inappropriate. Lyonel's speech and affect were both typically well preserved. He also had no abnormal or disorganized motor behaviors, which would be typical of the Catatonic Type. As is generally true in the Paranoid Type, Lyonel's hallucinations were related to the topics of his delusions.

It is worth noting here that Schizophrenia patients do not necessarily remain true to one subtype or another. A patient may appear Paranoid during one acute episode and subsequently show Disorganized features.

Many patients with Schizophrenia also have an abnormal premorbid personality. Often, this takes the form of Schizoid or Schizotypal Personality Disorder. When he was a child, Lyonel had at least five features of Schizotypal Personality Disorder (see p. 470). These included constricted affect, no close friends, odd beliefs (interest in the occult), peculiar appearance (as judged by peers), and suspiciousness of other children.

Throughout his current episode, Lyonel had had no change of symptoms that might suggest anything other than a continuous course. (Of course, he had no negative symptoms.) He had been ill for just about one year, so his overall diagnosis was as follows:

Axis I	295.30	Schizophrenia, Paranoid Type, Continuous
Axis II	301.22	Schizotypal Personality Disorder (Premorbid)
Axis III		None
Axis IV		Unemployed
Axis V	GAF = 30	(current)

295.10 Schizophrenia, Disorganized Type

The Disorganized Type of Schizophrenia was first recognized nearly 150 years ago. It was originally termed hebephrenia because it began early in life (hebe is Greek for *youth*). Patients with the Disorganized Type are frequently the most obviously psychotic of all Schizophrenia patients. They often deteriorate rapidly, talk gibberish, and neglect hygiene and appearance.

Criteria for Schizophrenia, Disorganized Type

- The patient meets the basic criteria for Schizophrenia.
- *All* of these symptoms are prominent:
  - Disorganized behavior
  - Disorganized speech
  - Affect that is flat or inappropriate

- The patient does not fulfill criteria for Schizophrenia, Catatonic Type (see below).

Bob Naples

As his sister told it, Bob Naples was always quiet when he was a kid, but not what you'd call peculiar or strange. Nothing like this had ever happened in their family before.

Bob sat in a tiny consulting room down the hall. His lips moved soundlessly, and one bare leg dangled across the arm of his chair. His sole article of clothing was a red-and-white-striped pajama top. An attendant tried to drape a green sheet across his lap, but he giggled and flung it to the floor.

It was hard for his sister, Sharon, to say when Bob first began to change. He was never very sociable, even a loner. He hardly ever laughed and always seemed rather distant, almost cold; he never appeared to enjoy anything he did very much. In the five years since he'd finished high school, he had lived at their house while he worked in her husband's machine shop, but he never really lived *with* them. He had never had a girlfriend—or a boyfriend, for that matter, though he sometimes used to talk with a couple of high school classmates if they dropped around. About a year and a half ago, Bob had completely stopped going out and wouldn't even return phone calls. When Sharon asked him why, he said he had better things to do. But all he did when he wasn't working was stay in his room.

Sharon's husband had told her that at work, Bob stayed at his lathe during breaks and talked even less than before. "Sometimes Dave would hear Bob giggling to himself. When he'd ask what was funny, Bob would kind of shrug and just turn away, back to his work."

For over a year, things didn't change much. Then, about two months earlier, Bob had started staying up at night. The family would hear him thumping around in his room, banging drawers, occasionally throwing things. Sometimes it sounded like he was talking to someone, but his bedroom was on the second floor and he had no phone.

He stopped going in to work. "Of course, Dave'd never fire him," Sharon continued. "But he was sleepy from being up all night, and he kept nodding off at the lathe. Sometimes he'd just leave it spinning and wander over to stare out the window. Dave was relieved when he stopped coming in."

In the last several weeks, all Bob would say was "Gilgamesh." Once Sharon asked him what it meant and he answered, "It's no red shoe on the backspace." This astonished her so much that she wrote it down. After that, she gave up trying to ask him for explanations.

Sharon wasn't sure how Bob got to the hospital. When she'd come home from the grocery store a few hours earlier, he was gone. Then the phone rang and it was the police, saying that they were bringing him in. A security guard down at the mall had taken him into custody. He was babbling something about Gilgamesh and wearing nothing but a pajama top. Sharon blotted the corner of her eye with the cuff of her sleeve. "They aren't even his pajamas—they belong to my daughter."

Evaluation of Bob Naples

Bob fully met the basic criteria for Schizophrenia. He had several psychotic symptoms. Besides his badly disorganized speech and behavior, he had the negative symptoms of inappropriate affect and lack of volition (he just stopped going to work). However, even with these typical features it is difficult to rule *in* the Disorganized Type of Schizophrenia during a first interview, because of the several exclusions that must first be met.

Bob would say only one word when he was admitted, so it could not be determined whether he had a cognitive deficit, as would be the case in a **Delirium Due to a General Medical Condition** or in a **Substance-Induced Psychotic Disorder** caused by amphetamines or PCP. Only after treatment was begun might this be known for sure. Other evidence of gross brain disease could be sought with skull X-rays, MRI, and blood tests as appropriate.

Bipolar I patients can show gross defect of judgment by refusing to remain clothed, but Bob did not have any of the other typical features of mania, such as euphoric mood, hyperactivity, or pressured speech. The absence of prominent mood symptoms would rule out **Major Depressive Episode** and **Schizoaffective Disorder**. Over a year earlier, Bob had been found giggling to himself at his lathe, so the early manifestations of Bob's illness had been present for far longer than the six-month minimum for Schizophrenia. This would rule out **Schizophreniform Disorder**.

What about other forms of Schizophrenia? Bob had none of the disorders of motion characteristic of **Schizophrenia, Catatonic Type**. He did have each of the three symptoms required for a diagnosis of **Schizophrenia, Disorganized Type**. His affect was inappropriate (he laughed without apparent cause), though reduced lability (termed flat or blunted) would also qualify. By the time of his evaluation, his speech had been reduced to a single word, but earlier it had been incoherent (and peculiar enough that his sister even wrote some of it down). Finally, there was loss of volition (the will to do things): He had stopped going to work and spent most of his time in his room, apparently accomplishing nothing. Of course, his symptoms had been continuous for longer than a year and included prominent negative symptoms; hence the Continuous specifier would be appropriate.

From Sharon's information, a premorbid diagnosis of Schizoid Personality Disorder (p. 466) also seemed warranted. Bob's specific symptoms included the following: no close friends, not desiring relationships, choosing solitary activities, lack of pleasure in activities, and no sexual experiences. As noted earlier, premorbid Schizoid Personality Disorder is often found in patients later diagnosed as having Schizophrenia.

Although Bob's eventual diagnosis would seem evident, the results of lab testing to rule out non-schizophrenia causes of psychosis should be awaited. Therefore, a qualifier of (Provisional) should be added to the Axis I diagnosis.

Axis I	295.10	Schizophrenia, Disorganized Type, Continuous With Prominent Negative Symptoms (Provisional)
Axis II	301.20	Schizoid Personality Disorder (Premorbid)
Axis III		None
Axis IV		None
Axis V	GAF = 15	(current)

295.20 Schizophrenia, Catatonic Type

The Catatonic Type is one of the classic Schizophrenia subtypes. It was first described in 1874; in 1896, Emil Kraepelin included it with the Disorganized and Paranoid Types as a major subgroup of *dementia praecox*. During the early part of the 20th century, each of these subtypes constituted about a third of all U.S. hospital admissions for Schizophrenia. Since that time, the prevalence of the Catatonic Type has declined markedly, until now it is unusual to encounter such a patient on an acute care inpatient service. The case of Edward Clapham was abstracted from admission and discharge summaries dating to the early 1970s.

Catatonic Type patients may have any of the basic symptoms of Schizophrenia, but their abnormal physical movements set them apart. Although motor activity may be speeded up, catatonic behavior is more typically slow or retarded, sometimes to the point of stupor. Most of the classic behaviors of this subtype are illustrated in the vignette.

Criteria for Schizophrenia, Catatonic Type

- The patient meets the basic criteria for Schizophrenia.
- At least two catatonic symptoms predominate:
  - ✓ Stupor or motor immobility (catalepsy or waxy flexibility)
  - ✓ Hyperactivity that has no apparent purpose and is not influenced by external stimuli
  - ✓ Mutism or marked negativism
  - ✓ Peculiar behavior such as posturing, stereotypies, mannerisms, or grimacing

✓ Echolalia or echopraxia

Coding Notes

Some of the terms used above require definition:

Negativism is demonstrated when the patient (1) refuses to follow all instructions without apparent motive, *or* (2) maintains a rigid posture despite the examiner's physical attempts to move the patient.

Mannerisms are unnecessary movements that are part of goal-directed behavior, such as a flourish of the pen when signing a document.

Stereotypies are behaviors that do not appear to be goal-directed, such as flashing a "Victory" sign with two upraised fingers every few seconds.

Posturing means that the patient spontaneously poses or assumes a posture that is bizarre or inappropriate.

Echolalia and *echopraxia* are involuntary and apparently meaningless repetitions of another person's words and actions, respectively.

Edward Clapham

Edward Clapham, a 43-year-old, single man, was admitted to the university hospital's mental health service. He gave no chief complaint; he was entirely mute. He had been transferred from the state psychiatric hospital, where his diagnosis had been Schizophrenia, Catatonic Type. For the past eight years, he had not communicated by speech or writing.

According to the transfer note, Edward had been intensively treated with neuroleptics during his entire hospitalization, though none of these medications had helped him. He reportedly spent the entire day every day lying on his back, toes pointing towards the foot of his bed, fists clenched and turned inward. From years of maintaining this position, he had developed severe muscle contractures at both ankles and both wrists. Most of the time he could be spoon-fed, but occasionally he refused to swallow and had to be fed by nasogastric tube. This had often been the case during the past six months; despite the tube feedings, he had lost about 30 pounds.

Ten days earlier Edward had developed a high fever (104.6° F) and had been transferred to the medical service, where the staff treated a Klebsiella pneumonia with tetracycline. Subsequently he was moved to the mental health service, where this evaluation took place.

Very little was known about Edward's background. He had been reared in the Midwest, the second child of a farm family. He may have attended some college, and he had worked for approximately 10 years as a tractor salesman.

On admission, his mental status examination read as follows:

> Mr. Clapham lies flat on his back in bed. He is totally mute, so nothing can be learned of his thought content or flow of thought. Similarly, his cognitive processes, insight, and judgment cannot be assessed. His toes point down and his fists are rotated inward. There is a noticeable tremor of his feet and his hands; he contracts the muscles of his arms and legs so strongly that they actually shake.
>
> Besides being mute, he shows other signs of catatonia. *Negativism*: When he is approached from one side, he gradually turns his head so that he gazes in the opposite direction. *Catalepsy*: When a limb is placed in any position (for instance, raised high above his head), he will maintain that position for several minutes, even if told that he can drop his hand. *Waxy flexibility*: Any attempt to bend his arm at the elbow, where there are no contractures, is met with resistance. It is evident that the biceps and triceps muscles are contracting together, causing motion at the joint to feel as if one were bending a rod made of wax or some other stiff substance. *Facial grimacing*: Every four or five minutes, he wrinkles his nose and purses his lips. This expression lasts for 10 or 15 seconds, then relaxes. There is no apparent purpose to these motions, and they are not accompanied by any motions of the tongue or other indications of tardive dyskinesia.

Evaluation of Edward Clapham:

Edward fulfilled the generic criteria for Schizophrenia. His illness had lasted far longer than the minimum six months; it is hard to imagine how it could have had a greater effect on every aspect of his life. Nonetheless, on admission to the mental health unit, he was given an Axis I diagnosis of 298.9 (Psychotic Disorder Not Otherwise Specified). This provisional diagnosis was given because the clinician could not be sure from the initial presentation whether the symptoms were due to the effects of his dehydration and loss of weight (a general medical condition), Schizophrenia, or another cause such as a mood disorder, which is perhaps the most frequent cause of a catatonic syndrome.

The list of general medical conditions that can produce catatonic behavior includes liver disease, strokes, epilepsy, and uncommon disorders such as Wilson's disease (a defect of copper metabolism). These possibilities should be vigorously pursued with neurological and medical consultation and with the appropriate laboratory and X-ray studies. Urine or blood screens for toxic substances or drugs of abuse should be considered a part of every such patient's workup. Any patient who presents with a first episode of catatonia should probably have an MRI.

For patients who have catatonic excitement, mania should be carefully considered. Many patients who have been diagnosed as having Schizophrenia, Catatonic Type, really have a manic phase of Axis I **Bipolar Disorder**. On the other hand, a patient with severe psychomotor retardation should be considered for a diagnosis of **Major Depressive Disorder With Melancholic Features.** Although patients with **Somatization Disorder** are occasionally mute or have abnormal motor activity, such episodes are usually short-lived, lasting only a few hours or days, not years.

Edward's symptoms were classic for Schizophrenia, Catatonic Type. He demonstrated grimacing, muteness, waxy flexibility, and catalepsy. He could not be called stuporous because he was alert enough to turn away from an approaching stimulus (negativism). His behavior did not include enough range to show other typical catatonic behaviors.

After a careful review of the options, Edward was given a course of electroconvulsive therapy (ECT). Although the first three bilateral ECT sessions produced no noticeable effect, after the fourth he asked for a glass of water. After a total of 10 sessions, he was conversing with others on the ward, feeding himself, and walking—always on tiptoe because of the severe contractures at his ankles. Although he continued to show residual symptoms of his disease, he lost all of his catatonic symptoms and eventually left the hospital, whereupon he was lost to follow-up.

Edward's eight-year course of illness had been continuous. After appropriate medical investigations and additional history ruled out other possible causes of his abnormal behavior, his revised diagnosis was as follows:

Axis I	295.20	Schizophrenia, Catatonic Type, Continuous
Axis II	V71.09	No diagnosis
Axis III	718.47	Contractures of ankles
	718.43	Contractures of wrists
Axis IV		None
Axis V	GAF = 60	(at discharge)

295.90 Schizophrenia, Undifferentiated Type

The Undifferentiated Type of Schizophrenia is a diagnosis of exclusion. If the actively psychotic Schizophrenia patient meets criteria for none of the previously described subtypes, Undifferentiated is what is left. The criteria for this diagnosis are essentially identical to the basic criteria for Schizophrenia.

Criteria for Schizophrenia, Undifferentiated Type

- The patient meets the basic criteria for Schizophrenia.
- The patient does *not* meet the criteria for the Paranoid, Disorganized, or Catatonic Types.

Natasha Oblamov

"She's nowhere near as bad as Ivan." Mr. Oblamov was talking about his two grown children. At 30 years of age, Ivan had such severe Schizophrenia of the Disorganized Type that, despite neuroleptics and a trial of ECT, he could not put 10 words together so they made sense. Now Natasha, three years younger than her brother, had been brought to the clinic with similar complaints.

Natasha was an artist. She specialized in oil-on-canvas copies of the photographs she took of the countryside near her home. Although she had had a one-woman exhibition in a local art gallery two years earlier, she still had never earned a dollar from her art work. She had a room in her father's apartment, where the two lived on his retirement income. Her brother lived on a back ward of the state mental hospital.

"I suppose it's been going on for quite a while now," said Mr. Oblamov. "I should have done something earlier, but I didn't want to believe it was happening to her, too."

The signs had first been there about 10 months ago, when Natasha stopped attending class at the art institute and gave up her two or three drawing pupils. Mostly she stayed in her room, even at mealtimes; she spent much of her time sketching.

Her father finally brought Natasha for evaluation because she kept opening the door. Perhaps six weeks earlier she had begun emerging from her room several times each evening, standing uncertainly in the hallway for several moments, then opening the front door. After peering up and down the hallway, she would retreat to her own room. In the past week, she had reenacted this ritual a dozen times each evening. Once or twice, her father thought he heard her mutter something about "Jason." When he asked her who Jason was, she only looked blank, and turned away.

Natasha was a slender woman with a round face and watery blue eyes that never seemed to focus. Although she volunteered almost nothing, she answered every question clearly and logically, if briefly. She was fully oriented and had no suicidal ideas or other problems with impulse control. Her affect was as flat as one of her canvases. She would describe her most frightening experiences with no more emotion than if she was making a bed.

Jason was an instructor at the art institute. Some months earlier, one afternoon when her father was out, he had come to the apartment to help her with "some special stroking techniques," as she put it (referring to her brush). Although they had ended up naked together on the kitchen floor, she had spent most of that time explaining why she felt she should put her clothes back on. He left unrequited, and she never returned to the art institute.

Not long afterward, Natasha "realized" that Jason was hanging about, trying to see her again. She would sense his presence just outside her door, but each time she opened it, he vanished. This puzzled her, but she couldn't say that she felt depressed, angry, or anxious. Within a few weeks she started to hear a voice quite a bit like Jason's, which seemed to be speaking to her from the photographic enlarger she had set up in the tiny second bathroom.

"It usually just said the 'C' word," she explained in response to a question. "The 'C' word?"

"You know, the place on a woman's body where you do the 'F' word." Unblinking and calm, Natasha sat with her hands folded in her lap.

Several times in the past several weeks, Jason had slipped through her window at night and climbed into her bed while she slept. She had awakened to feel the pressure of his body on hers; it was especially intense in her groin area. By the time she had fully awakened, he would be gone. The previous week when she went in to use the bathroom, the head of an eel—or perhaps it was a large snake—emerged from the toilet bowl and lunged at her. She lowered the lid on the animal's neck and it disappeared. Since then, she had only used the toilet in the hall bathroom.

Evaluation of Natasha Oblamov

Natasha had a variety of psychotic symptoms. They included hallucinations (visual in this case—the eel in the toilet) and a nonbizarre delusion about Jason. She also had the negative symptom of flat affect (she talked about eels in her toilet without showing any emotion at all). Although her active symptoms had been evident for only a few months, the prodromal symptom of staying in her room had been present for about 10 months. Her disorder obviously interfered with her ability to complete a canvas, though she did not suffer from lack of volition.

Nothing in Natasha's history would suggest a **general medical condition**. However, a certain amount of routine lab testing might be ordered initially: complete blood count, routine blood chemistries, urinalysis. No evidence is given in the vignette to suggest that she had a **Substance-Induced Psychotic Disorder**, and her affect, though flat, was pleasant and nothing like the severely depressed mood of a **Major Depressive Disorder With Psychotic Features**. Furthermore, she had never had suicidal ideas. There was nothing to suggest that she had ever had a **Manic Episode**. The gradual onset of illness that persisted for longer than six months would rule out **Schizophreniform Disorder** and **Brief Psychotic Disorder**. Finally, her brother had Schizophrenia. About 10% of the first-degree relatives (parents, siblings, and children) of patients with Schizophrenia also develop this condition.

The subtype of Natasha's disease is easily settled. She had no motor symptoms that would qualify her for a diagnosis of **Catatonic Type**; her flat affect would rule out **Paranoid Type**. Her affect suggested **Disorganized Type**, but she did not have the other symptoms (disorganization of speech and behavior) required for this diagnosis. By the process of elimination, then, she had Undifferentiated Type, Continuous. Although she did not fulfill the criteria for Disorganized Type, she did have fairly prominent flat affect; the clinician who interviewed Natasha added a specifier to her diagnosis to reflect this symptom. Others might not.

Axis I	295.90	Schizophrenia, Undifferentiated Type, Continuous, With Prominent Negative Symptoms
Axis II	799.9	Diagnosis Deferred
Axis III		None
Axis IV		None
Axis V	GAF = 30	(current)

TIP As a postscript, it should be noted that this picture of nonspecific symptoms is often found in Schizophrenia patients after they have been treated with neuroleptic medications. When this is the case, these patients are better classified according to the symptoms observed during the most recent untreated psychotic episode.

295.60 Schizophrenia, Residual Type

The Residual Type of Schizophrenia is essentially a place filler—a diagnosis that ought to exist but is probably seldom used in clinical practice. It may be used for a patient whose diagnosis of Schizophrenia is already established, and who has either been treated or improved spontaneously to the point of no longer having enough symptoms for a diagnosis of active disease. Why would such a patient come for an evaluation? Perhaps the patient comes for an insurance-related or forensic evaluation; perhaps a colleague refers a partly treated patient for consultation. When possible, it is better to use the diagnosis originally given the patient, with Episodic With Interepisode Residual Symptoms or Single Episode In Partial Remission as a qualifier. There is no information about prevalence and other demographic data concerning the Residual Type diagnosis.

Criteria for Schizophrenia, Residual Type

• The patient at one time met criteria for Schizophrenia, Catatonic, Disorganized, Paranoid, or Undifferentiated Type.

- The patient no longer has pronounced catatonic behavior, delusions, hallucinations, or disorganized speech or behavior.
- The patient is still ill, as indicated by *either* of the following:
  - ✓ Negative symptoms such as flattened affect, reduced speech output, or lack of volition, *or*
  - ✓ An *attenuated* form of *at least* two characteristic symptoms of Schizophrenia, such as odd beliefs (related to delusions), distorted perceptions or illusions (hallucinations), odd speech (disorganized speech), or peculiarities of behavior (disorganized behavior).

Ramona Kelt

When she was 20 and had been married only a few months, Ramona Kelt was hospitalized for the first time with what was called "hebephrenic schizophrenia." According to records, her mood had been silly and inappropriate, her speech disjointed and hard to follow. She had been admitted after putting coffee grounds and orange peels on her head. She talked about television cameras in her closet that spied upon her whenever she had sex.

Since then she had had several additional episodes, widely scattered across 25 years. Whenever she fell ill, her symptoms were the same. Each time she recovered enough to return home to her husband.

Every morning Ramona's husband had to prepare a list that spelled out her day's activities, even including meal planning and cooking. Without it, he might arrive home to find that she had accomplished nothing that day. The couple had no children and few friends.

Ramona's most recent evaluation was prompted by a change in medical care plans. Her new clinician noted that she was still taking neuroleptics; each morning her husband carefully counted them out onto her plate and watched her swallow them. During the interview she winked and smiled when it did not seem appropriate. She said that it had been several years since television cameras had bothered her, but she wondered whether her closet "might be haunted."

TIP As you read through the criteria for the various forms of Schizophrenia, a pattern emerges for assigning subtype diagnosis. Catatonic symptoms take precedence over all others, even if there are prominent negative or paranoid symptoms. If there are no catatonic symptoms, Disorganized Type is diagnosed, if the patient has the required negative symptoms. If the patient qualifies for neither the Catatonic nor the Disorganized Type, and has prominent delusions or hallucinations, Paranoid Type will be the diagnosis. Finally, if all else fails, diagnose Undifferentiated Type.

Evaluation of Ramona Kelt

Although the information contained in the vignette is sketchy, there is enough to support a strong presumption of Schizophrenia. Ramona had been ill for many years with symptoms that included disorganized behavior and a delusion about television cameras. The early diagnosis of Disorganized Type (hebephrenic) would seem warranted from her inappropriate affect and bizarre speech and behavior. However, she did not now meet the basic criteria for Schizophrenia. Between episodes (e.g., during the most recent interview), she continued to show peculiarities of affect (winking) and ideation (the closet might be haunted) that suggested attenuated psychotic symptoms. She also had a serious negative symptom, avolition: If her husband didn't plan her day for her, she would accomplish nothing.

Of course, to have any type of Schizophrenia, Ramona would have to have none of the exclusions (general medical conditions, Substance-Induced Psychotic Disorder, mood disorders, Schizoaffective Disorder). If we assume that this was still the case, her current diagnosis would be as follows:

Axis I	295.60	Schizophrenia, Residual Type, Episodic With Interepisode Residual Symptoms, With Prominent Negative Symptoms
Axis II	V71.09	No diagnosis
Axis III		None
Axis IV		None
Axis V	GAF = 51	(current)

Ramona Kelt could also be diagnosed as follows:

Axis I	295.10	Schizophrenia, Disorganized Type, Episodic With Interepisode Residual Symptoms, With Prominent Negative Symptoms

This would convey somewhat more information about the nature and course of her illness.

295.40 Schizophreniform Disorder

Although its name sounds as if it must be related to Schizophrenia, the diagnosis of Schizophreniform Disorder was devised in the 1950s specifically to deal with the problem of patients who may have something different. These patients look as if they have Schizophrenia, but may later recover completely with no residual effects. The Schizophreniform diagnosis is valuable because it prevents closure: It alerts all clinicians that the underlying cause of the patient's psychosis has not yet been proven. (The -form suffix means this: The symptoms look like Schizophrenia and may turn out to be Schizophrenia. But with limited information, the conservative clinician feels uncomfortable making a diagnosis that implies lifelong treatment.)

The *symptoms* and *exclusions* required for Schizophreniform Disorder are identical to those of basic Schizophrenia. The two diagnoses differ in terms of *duration* and *dysfunction*. DSM-IV doesn't require evidence that Schizophreniform Disorder has interfered with the patient's life. However, when you think about it, most people who have had delusions and hallucinations for a month have probably suffered some inconvenience in work or social life.

The real distinguishing point is the length of time the patient has been symptomatic: From one to six months is the period required. This interval is of practical importance, because numerous studies have shown that psychotic patients who have been ill briefly have a much better chance of full recovery than do those who have been ill for six months or longer. Still, over half of those who are initially diagnosed as having Schizophreniform Disorder are eventually found to have Schizophrenia or Schizoaffective Disorder.

Criteria for Schizophreniform Disorder

- For a substantial part of at least one month (or less, if effectively treated), the patient has had two or more of these (the "A" criteria for Schizophrenia):
  - ✓ Delusions (only one symptom is required if a delusion is bizarre, such as being abducted in a space ship from the sun)
  - ✓ Hallucinations (only one symptom is required if hallucinations are of at least two voices talking to each other or of a voice that keeps up a running commentary on the patient's thoughts or actions)
  - ✓ Speech that shows incoherence, derailment, or other disorganization
  - ✓ Severely disorganized or catatonic behavior
  - ✓ Any negative symptom such as flat affect, reduced speech, or lack of volition
- Including prodromal, active, and residual phases, an episode of the illness has lasted at least one month but not longer than six months.
- Mood disorders with psychotic features and Schizoaffective Disorder have been ruled out, because the duration of any depressive or manic episodes that have occurred during the psychotic phase has been brief.
- This disorder is not the direct physiological result of a general medical condition or the use of substances, including prescription medications.

Coding Notes

A statement of prognosis should be added to the diagnosis:

With Good Prognostic Features (two or more of the following):

✓ Actual psychotic features begin within four weeks of the first noticeable change in the patient's functioning or behavior.
✓ The patient is confused or perplexed when most psychotic.
✓ Premorbid social and job functioning are good.
✓ Affect is neither blunt nor flattened.

Without Good Prognostic Features (zero or one of the foregoing)

If the diagnosis is made without waiting for recovery, which will often be the case, the term (Provisional) should be appended.

Jonathan Capp

Jonathan Capp was the second of three children born to a barber and his wife, who lived in a small town in northern California. Jonathan had attended a small Catholic school, where he had only really cared for math and science. Throughout his childhood, his physical health had been good. Although he had experimented once with marijuana when he was 13, he had neither enjoyed the experience nor repeated it. He scrupulously avoided other drugs.

After high school he had attended junior college for one year, then started work in the construction trade and moved into a small studio apartment. He spent most of his free time hanging out with other young people he had known in high school. He dated several women and had "about the usual amount" of sexual experience, but no steady girl friend.

On a warm July afternoon, Jonathan had just picked up his mail and unlocked his front door when, immediately behind his left shoulder, he heard a woman's voice say, "I think he understands." He spun around to see who could have approached him so stealthily, but no one was there. He was so astonished that he dropped the utility bill and advertising circular he was holding. As he stooped to pick them up, a man's voice, also located behind him and just as clear, said, "He's got better things to do than that."

"Man, it was brutal! I'd never been so scared in my life," he told the interviewer at the mental health center six weeks later. "I was just plain positive I couldn't have imagined it. Still am. Those voices were real!"

At age 20, Jonathan was tall, muscular, and tan, with a wispy beard and hair pulled back into a ponytail. He wore faded denims and a turtleneck shirt. His gaze was solemn and unwavering, almost unblinking. He went on to tell about the events of the following day.

"We'd been putting up that new subdivision north of town. I was framing out units on the second floor. I was just raising my nail gun when I heard that same woman's voice behind me. She said, 'He's doing that perfectly!' And then the man said, 'You mean, as well as . . . ' And then his voice kinda trailed off." Initially, he had no idea what they meant. But as they continued to comment on his behavior, he finally figured out that they were comparing him favorably with Jesus.

Jonathan had never had experiences like this before; neither had anyone in his family. His mood was good, neither depressed nor high, though he certainly wondered what was happening to him. His sleep and appetite were normal, and his substance use was limited to an occasional beer.

During the intervening time, Jonathan heard these same voices many times. Occasionally it happened only once or twice a day, but sometimes they seemed to keep up a steady stream of chatter for hours on end. Usually it was when he was alone, after work or on a weekend, but one other time he heard them on the job. Then they seemed so loud that he looked around, astonished that no other worker appeared to overhear. They always said the same sort of thing, although with time they became more explicit. Last week he had distinctly heard the woman say, "He's the Second Coming!" Then the man's voice replied, "Any day now."

Jonathan's statements were calm but emphatic. His demeanor was earnest. He made excellent eye contact and leaned forward slightly, one forearm resting on a corner of the interview table. His speech was clear and goal-directed. His cognitive processes seemed intact: He was fully oriented, had a good memory for recent and remote events, could retain and recall information, and could perform mental arithmetic. He scored a perfect 30 on the Mini-Mental State Exam.

Asked whether he had any ideas that would account for his experiences, he replied, "I wish I did! Of course, I *am* a carpenter. My parents used to send me to Sunday school when I was a kid, but I've never been especially religious, so that shouldn't have anything to do with it. It seems almost like a trick of the mind, but I've always been healthy. So I can't believe that I'm crazy, either."

Evaluation of Jonathan Capp

Jonathan had a single psychotic symptom: auditory hallucinations. (He was not convinced that he was Jesus; therefore, he was not delusional.) However, his hallucinations were so striking (two voices talking to each other) that DSM-IV does not require the usual two psychotic symptoms for diagnosis. This would also be the case if Jonathan had heard a single voice continually commenting on his thoughts or actions. Note that these diagnostic criteria do not require that the patient have any interference with social or job functioning.

The clinical features of Jonathan's psychosis were not much different from those of Schizophrenia, Paranoid Type. Of course, that's the whole point of

Schizophreniform Disorder: At the time the diagnosis is first made, the clinician doesn't know whether the outcome will be full recovery or long-term illness. Jonathan didn't use alcohol to excess, or use drugs at all; this would rule out a **Substance-Induced Psychotic Disorder**. The usual **general medical** causes of psychosis would have to be investigated. **Bipolar Disorder** would be improbable: Jonathan didn't have any symptoms of mania or depression. His psychosis had been present too long for **Brief Psychotic Disorder**, which lasts less than one month, and too briefly for **Schizophrenia**.

The criteria require that a qualifier of (Provisional) be appended if the diagnosis of **Schizophreniform Disorder** is made before the patient recovers, which is usually the case. Once the patient has recovered completely (within the six-month limit), this qualifier can be removed. Eventually, the diagnosis may be changed to Schizophrenia, if the illness lasts longer than six months and it interferes with the patient's work or social life.

With Schizophreniform Disorder patients, a statement of prognosis should be made whenever possible. In Jonathan's case, the treating clinician noted the following evidence of good prognosis: (1) As far as anyone could tell, his illness had begun abruptly with prominent psychotic symptoms (auditory hallucinations). (2) His premorbid functioning (both work and social life) had been good. (3) Lacking flattening or inappropriateness, his affect was intact throughout his illness. Thus, he had three of the features that favor a good prognosis; only two are needed. (He did not have the fourth good-prognosis feature specified by DSM-IV: perplexity or confusion during the worst of the psychotic symptoms.)

Jonathan refused admission to the hospital on the grounds that he was not ill; he did agree to take small amounts of trifluoperazine, a medium-dose neuroleptic. Within four weeks the voices had remitted completely, and he stopped the medicine. At a two-year follow-up, they had not returned. Therefore, Jonathan Capp's complete diagnosis should read:

Axis I	295.40	Schizophreniform Disorder, with Good Prognostic Features
Axis II	V71.09	None
Axis III	None	
Axis IV	None	
Axis V	GAF = 65	(on admission)
	GAF = 90	(at follow-up)

295.70 Schizoaffective Disorder

Schizoaffective Disorder is just plain confusing. Over the years, it has meant many things to many clinicians. Because there were so many interpretations in use for this confusing category, DSM-III included no criteria for it at all in 1980. DSM-III-R first attempted to specify criteria in 1987. These endured for seven years and have been substantially rewritten for DSM-IV.

Most interpretations suggest that Schizoaffective Disorder is some sort of cross between a mood disorder and Schizophrenia. Some writers regard it as a form of Bipolar Disorder, because some patients seem to respond well to lithium. Other commentators believe it is closer to Schizophrenia. Still others hold that it is an entirely separate type of psychosis, or simply a collection of confusing, sometimes contradictory symptoms.

DSM-IV criteria specify that the patient must have all of the following during a single, continuous period of mental illness:

- The "A" criteria for Schizophrenia for at least a month.
- Delusions or hallucinations without major mood symptoms for two weeks or more.
- Mood symptoms that meet criteria for Major Depressive, Manic, or Mixed Episode for a "substantial" period of the total illness.

There are the usual exclusions for substance use and general medical conditions. Obviously, the entire illness must last at least one month, though many patients will be ill much longer.

No one knows much about the demographic features of Schizoaffective Disorder. It is probably less common than Schizophrenia; its prognosis lies between that of Schizophrenia and the mood disorders. Recent studies indicate that Schizoaffective Disorder patients who have predominant manic symptoms (the Bipolar Type) may have a better prognosis than those with the Depressive Type of this condition (see below).

Criteria for Schizoaffective Disorder

- During a continuous period of illness, for a substantial part of at least one month (or less, if effectively treated) the patient has had two or more of the following symptoms:
  - ✓ Delusions (only one symptom is required if a delusion is bizarre, such as being abducted in a space ship from the sun)
  - ✓ Hallucinations (only one symptom is required if hallucinations are of at least two voices talking to each other or of a voice that keeps up a running commentary on the patient's thoughts or actions)
  - ✓ Speech that shows incoherence, derailment, or other disorganization
  - ✓ Severely disorganized or catatonic behavior
  - ✓ Any negative symptom such as flat affect, reduced speech, or lack of volition
- During this same continuous period of illness the patient has had:
  - ✓ A Major Depressive Episode (see p. 191) that includes depressed mood,

or

✓ A Manic Episode (see p. 195), *or*
✓ A Mixed Episode (see p. 199).

- For at least two weeks of this period, there have been delusions or hallucinations and *no* prominent mood symptoms.
- The mood episode symptoms have been present during a substantial part of the active and residual portions of the illness.
- This disorder is not caused directly by a general medical condition or the use of substances, including prescription medications.

Coding Notes

Specify whether:

Bipolar Type. The episode either is Manic or Mixed, or is now Major Depressive with a history of either Manic or Mixed.

Depressive Type. The history includes only Major Depressive Episodes.

Velma Dean

Velma Dean's lips curled upwards, but the smile didn't reach her eyes. "I'm really sorry about this," she told her therapist, "but I guess—well, I don't know what." She reached into the large shopping bag she had carried into the office and pulled out a six-inch kitchen knife. First she grasped it in her hand, with her thumb along the blade. Then she tried clutching it in her fist. The therapist reached for the alarm button under the desk top, ruefully aware of yet another change of course in this patient's multifaceted history.

A month before her 18th birthday, Velma Dean had joined the Army. Her father, a colonel of artillery, had wanted a son, but Velma was his only child. Over the feeble protests of her mother, Velma's upbringing had been strict and semimilitary. After working three years in the motor pool, Velma herself had just been promoted to sergeant when she became ill.

Her illness started with two days in the infirmary for what seemed like bronchitis, but as the penicillin took effect and her fever came down, the voices began. At first they seemed to be located toward the back of her head. Within a few days they had moved to her bedside water glass. As nearly as she could tell, their pitch depended on the contents of her glass: If the glass was nearly empty, the voices were female; if it was full to the top, they spoke in a rich baritone. They were always quiet and mannerly. Often they gave her advice on how to behave, but at times she said they "nearly drove me crazy" by constantly commenting on what she was doing.

A psychiatrist diagnosed Velma's condition as Schizophrenia and prescribed neuroleptics. The voices improved, but never quite disappeared. She concealed the fact that she had "figured out" that her illness had been caused by her first sergeant, who for months had tried unsuccessfully to get her into bed. She also hid the fact that for several weeks she had been drinking nearly a pint of Southern Comfort each evening. The Army retired her as medically unfit, 100% disabled. When she was well enough to travel, her father drove her the 600 miles back home.

For her treatment, Velma enrolled at her local Department of Veterans Affairs (VA) outpatient clinic. There, her new therapist verified (1) the continuing presence (now for nearly eight months) of her barely audible hallucinations, and (2) her increasingly profound symptoms of depression. These included low self-esteem and hopelessness (much worse in the morning than in the evening); loss of appetite; a 10-pound weight loss over the past eight weeks; insomnia that caused her to awaken early most mornings; and the guilty conviction that she had disappointed her father by "deserting" the Army before her hitch was up. She denied thoughts of injuring herself or other people.

Velma's VA clinician gave her an Axis I working diagnosis of 799.9 (Diagnosis Deferred), noting that she had been ill too long for Schizophreniform Disorder and that her mood symptoms seemed to rule out Schizophrenia. Physical exam and laboratory testing ruled out general medical conditions. Although Alcoholics Anonymous helped her stop drinking, her depressive and psychotic symptoms continued.

Because Velma's depressive symptoms might be secondary to a partly treated psychosis, her neuroleptic dose was increased. This completely eliminated the hallucinations and delusions, but the depressive symptoms continued virtually unabated. The antidepressant imipramine at 200 mg a day only produced side effects; after four weeks, lithium was added. Once a therapeutic blood level was reached, her depressive symptoms melted completely away. For six months she remained in a good mood and free of psychosis, though she never obtained a job or did very much with her time.

Now it seemed that Velma might actually be suffering from a Major Depressive Disorder With Psychotic Features. At this point, her clinician became uneasy that the neuroleptic could produce side effects such as tardive dyskinesia. With Velma's consent, the neuroleptic was gradually reduced by about 20% per week. After three weeks she began once again to hear voices commanding her to run away from home. During this time her mood remained good; with the exception of some difficulty getting to sleep at night, she developed none of the vegetative symptoms she had formerly had with depression. She was rapidly restarted on her full former dose of neuroleptic medication.

After several months of renewed stability, Velma and her therapist decided to try again. This time they began cautiously to reduce the imipramine, by 25 mg each week. Each week they met to evaluate her mood and check for symptoms of psychosis. By December she had been free of the antidepressant for two months, and had remained symptom-free (except for habitual bland, smiling affect). Now her therapist took a deep breath and decreased her lithium by one tablet per day. The following week Velma returned to the office, hallucinating and wondering whether to hold her kitchen knife in her hand or in her fist.

Evaluation of Velma Dean

This patient illustrates current thinking about Schizoaffective Disorder. Velma's condition really seemed to be a mixture of mood and psychotic symptoms. She had what appeared to be a single period of illness (her only "well" periods were when she was taking medication; even then, she had residual lack of initiative). During this period she had mood symptoms both with and without psychotic symptoms. Although she abused alcohol at one time during her illness, both her mood and psychotic symptoms continued long after she quit drinking.

Although these criteria can be stated relatively simply, Velma's history illustrates how difficult it can be to apply them. The therapist, whose thinking has already been described in the vignette, was correct to code her initially as **Diagnosis Deferred on Axis I**. This category reminded her clinicians to keep thinking about her diagnosis and to reject any label that might close their minds to further attempts at therapy. She could not be diagnosed as having **Schizophrenia**, because of the exclusion of prominent mood symptoms. A **mood disorder with psychosis** could be eliminated because she had psychotic symptoms even when not depressed. After many months of care, she still showed no evidence of a **general medical condition**.

The relative duration of psychosis and mood symptoms is very important in Schizoaffective Disorder. DSM-IV states that the mood symptoms must be present for a period of time that is "substantial" relative to the overall duration of the entire episode of illness. Velma's depressive symptoms lasted for at least two months, which her clinician regarded as "substantial" in comparison with the overall duration of her illness. If her overall illness had lasted 10 years, her clinician might have judged that eight weeks of depression was not substantial enough.

Many patients with both mood and psychotic symptoms will eventually comfortably fit the criteria for Schizophrenia or a mood disorder. If they are followed long enough, perhaps the majority of patients with Schizoaffective Disorder will be rediagnosed. Given the highly restrictive nature of the current definition, it seems likely that this diagnosis will rarely be used. If you ever make the diagnosis, ask yourself, "Have I overlooked another diagnosis that is more reasonable?" Schizoaffective Disorder is a diagnosis best used for patients who have a long-standing history of both sets of symptoms. **Psychotic Disorder Not Otherwise Specified** may prove to be much more useful to most clinicians.

Velma's mood symptoms were depressive, which defined her subtype diagnosis:

Axis I	295.70	Schizoaffective Disorder, Depressive Type
Axis II		None
Axis III		None
Axis IV		Unemployment
Axis V	GAF = 20	(current)

297.1 Delusional Disorder

As the name indicates, the chief characteristics of Delusional Disorder are persistent delusions that at face value often seem entirely believable (they are nonbizarre). In fact, the patients themselves can appear quite normal, as long as you don't touch on any of their delusional themes. There are half a dozen possible themes, which are outlined in the Coding Notes.

Although the symptoms can seem very similar to those of Schizophrenia, there are several reasons to list Delusional Disorder separately:

The age of onset is often late.

Family histories of the two illnesses are dissimilar.

At follow-up, these patients are rarely rediagnosed as having Schizophrenia.

The infrequent hallucinations take a back seat to the delusions.

Compared to that of Schizophrenia, the course of Delusional Disorder is less fraught with intellectual and work-related deterioration. Nonetheless, domestic problems are frequent, and, depending on subtype, these patients are often swept up in litigation or endless medical tests.

Delusional Disorder usually starts late in life, as noted above. It is quite rare (Schizophrenia is perhaps 30 times more common). Chronically reduced sensory input (being deaf or blind) may contribute to its development, as may social isolation (e.g., being an immigrant in a strange country). Delusional Disorder may also be associated with family traits that include suspiciousness, jealousy, and secretiveness. Persecutory Type is the most common of the subtypes (see below).

Criteria for Delusional Disorder

• For at least one month the patient has had delusions that are nonbizarre (the content is something that could reasonably happen).

- The patient has never met the "A" criteria for Schizophrenia (p. 144), except that hallucinations of touch or smell may be present if they are related to the theme of the delusions.
- Functioning and behavior are not markedly affected, apart from direct consequences of the delusions.
- The duration of any mood symptoms accompanying delusions has been brief as compared to the duration of delusions.
- This disorder is not directly caused by a general medical condition or the use of substances, including prescription medications.

Coding Notes

Specify type, based on theme of delusions:

Erotomanic Type. Someone (often of higher social station) is in love with the patient.

Grandiose Type. The patient has a special identity, knowledge, power, self-worth, talent, or relationship to God or someone famous.

Jealous Type. The patient's spouse or lover has been unfaithful.

Persecutory Type. The patient (or a close associate) is in some way being intentionally cheated, drugged, followed, slandered, or otherwise mistreated.

Somatic Type. The patient notes physical sensations or bodily dysfunctions (foul odors, insects crawling on or under skin) that imply a general medical condition or physical defect.

Mixed Type. The patient has two or more of the themes above in about equal portions.

Unspecified Type.

Molly McConegal

Molly McConegal, a tiny sparrow of a woman, sat perched on the front of her waiting room chair. On her lap she tightly clutched her scuffed black handbag; her gray hair was caught up in a fierce little bun at the back of her head. Through spectacles as thick as highball glasses, she darted myopic, suspicious glances about the room. She had already spent 45 minutes with the consultant behind closed doors. Now she was waiting while her husband, Michael, had a turn.

Michael confirmed much of what Molly had already said. The couple had been married for over 40 years, had two children, and had lived in the same neighborhood (the same house, in fact) nearly all of their married life. Both were retired from the telephone company, and they shared an interest in gardening.

"That was where it all started, in the garden," said Michael. "It was last summer, when I was out trimming the rose bushes in the front yard. Molly said she caught me looking at the house across the street. The widow woman who lives there is younger than we are, maybe 50. We nod and say 'Hi,' but in ten years, I've never even been inside her front door. But Molly said I was taking too long on those rose bushes, that I was waiting for our neighbor—her name is Mrs. Jessup—to come out of the house. Of course, I denied it, but she insisted. Kept talking about it for days."

In the following months, Molly pursued the idea of Michael's supposed extramarital relationship. At first she only suggested that he had been trying to lure Mrs. Jessup out for a meeting. Within a few weeks, she "knew" that they had been together. Still later, this had turned into a sex orgy.

Molly had talked of little else and had begun to incorporate many commonplace observations into her suspicions. A button undone on Michael's shirt meant that he had just returned from a visit with "the woman." The adjustment of the living room venetian blinds tipped her off that he had been trying to semaphore messages the night before. A private detective Molly hired for surveillance only stopped by to chat with Michael, submitted a bill for $50, and resigned.

Molly continued to do the cooking and washing for herself, but Michael now had to take care of his own meals and laundry. She slept normally, ate well, and, when she wasn't with him, seemed to be in good spirits. Michael, on the other hand, was becoming a nervous wreck. She listened in on his telephone calls and steamed open his mail. Once she told him that she would file for divorce, but she "didn't want the children to find out." Twice he had awakened at night to find her wrapped tightly in her bathrobe and standing beside his bed, glowering down at him and waiting for him to make his move. Last week she had strewn the hallway outside his room with thumbtacks, so that he would cry out and awaken her when he sneaked away for one of his late-night sexual rendezvous.

Michael smiled and said sadly, "You know, I haven't had sex with anybody for nearly 15 years. Since I had my prostate operation, I just haven't had the ability."

Evaluation of Molly McConegal

If you compare the criteria for this diagnosis to the basic criteria for Schizophrenia (or any of the other foregoing diagnoses), you will note many differences.

First, consider symptoms. Delusions are the only psychotic symptom allowed to any important degree in Delusional Disorder. The delusion can be any of the six types listed in the Coding Notes. In Molly's case, they were of the Jealous Type, but the Persecutory and Grandiose Types are also common. Note that with the exception of olfactory or tactile hallucinations that reinforce the content of certain delusions, Delusional Disorder patients will never fulfill the "A" criteria for Schizophrenia.

The duration of the delusions need be only one month; however, most patients, like Molly, have been ill much longer by the time they come to professional attention. The consequences are mild for Delusional Disorder. Indeed, outside of the direct effects of the delusion (in Molly's case, her marital harmony), work and social life may not be affected much at all.

However, the exclusions are pretty much the same as for Schizophrenia. Always rule out a **general medical condition** or **cognitive disorder**, especially a **dementia with delusions**, when evaluating delusional patients. This is especially important in older patients, who can be quite crafty at disguising the fact that they are cognitively impaired. **Substance-Induced Psychotic Disorders** can closely mimic Delusional Disorder. This is especially true for **Amphetamine-Induced Psychotic Disorder With Onset During Withdrawal**, in which fully oriented patients may describe how they are being attacked by gangs of pursuers.

Molly McConegal had neither history nor symptoms to support any of the foregoing disorders; however, laboratory and toxicology studies may be needed for many patients. Other than irritability when she was with her husband, she had no symptoms of a **mood disorder**. Even then, her affect was quite appropriate to the content of her thought. However, many of these patients can develop mood syndromes secondary to the delusions. Then the diagnosis depends on the chronology and severity of mood symptoms. Information from relatives or other third parties is often required to determine which came first. Also, the mood symptoms must be relatively mild and brief to sustain a diagnosis of Delusional Disorder.

Although these patients may have associated conditions, including **Body Dysmorphic Disorder**, **Obsessive–Compulsive Disorder**, or **Avoidant, Paranoid**, or **Schizoid Personality Disorder**, there was no evidence for any of these in Molly McConegal. Her diagnosis would be as follows:

Axis I	297.1	Delusional Disorder, Jealous Type
Axis II	V71.09	No diagnosis
Axis III		None
Axis IV		None
Axis V	GAF = 55	(highest level past year)

298.8 Brief Psychotic Disorder

Patients with brief Psychotic Disorder are psychotic for at least one day and return to normal within a month. (As with Schizophreniform Disorder, any patients who remain symptomatic after that period of time have to be given a different diagnosis.) It doesn't matter how many symptoms they have had or whether they have had trouble functioning socially or at work.

Some patients who experience a postpartum psychosis may be given this diagnosis. Even then, it is a rare condition: The incidence of postpartum psychosis is only about 1 or 2 per 1,000 women who give birth. European clinicians are more likely to diagnose this sort of condition. (This doesn't necessarily mean that the condition occurs more frequently in Europe, just that European clinicians may either be more alert to it—or, perhaps, overdiagnose it.) Brief Psychotic Disorder may be more common among young patients (teenagers and young adults) and among patients who are from lower socioeconomic strata or who have pre-existing personality disorders.

In DSM-III-R, this category was called Brief Reactive Psychosis. The name and criteria reflected the notion that it may occur in response to some overwhelmingly stressful event, such as death of a relative. In the DSM-IV criteria, this concept is retained only as a modifier. To decide whether a stressor has caused a psychosis may require interviewing a spouse, relative, or friend to learn about the patient's premorbid adjustment, past history of similar reactions to stress, and the chronological relationship between stressor and the onset of symptoms.

Criteria for Brief Psychotic Disorder

- The patient has at least one of the following that is *not* a culturally sanctioned response:
  ✓ Delusions
  ✓ Hallucinations
  ✓ Speech that is markedly disorganized
  ✓ Behavior that is markedly disorganized or catatonic
- The patient has symptoms from 1 to 30 days and eventually recovers completely.
- The symptoms are not due to a mood disorder, Schizophrenia, or Schizoaffective Disorder.
- This disorder is not directly caused by a general medical condition or the use of substances, including prescription medications.

Coding Notes

Specify whether:

With Postpartum Onset. In a woman, the disorder begins within four weeks of having a baby.

With Marked Stressor(s). The stressors must appear to cause the symptoms, must occur shortly before their onset, and must be severe enough that nearly anyone of that culture would feel markedly stressed.

Without Marked Stressor(s).

If the diagnosis is made without waiting for recovery, the term (Provisional) should be appended.

Do not include any symptom that is a culturally sanctioned response.

Melanie Grayson

This was Melanie Grayson's first pregnancy, and she had been quite apprehensive about it. She had gained thirty pounds and her blood pressure had been slightly too high. But she had needed only a spinal block for anesthesia, and her husband was in the room with her when she delivered a healthy baby girl.

That night she slept fitfully; she was irritable the next day. But she breast-fed her baby and seemed to listen attentively when the nurse practitioner came to instruct her on bathing and other postpartum care.

The next morning, while Melanie was having breakfast, her husband came to take her and the baby home. When she ordered him to turn off the radio, he looked around the room and said he didn't hear one. "You know very well what radio," she yelled, and threw a tea bag at him.

The mental health consultant noted that Melanie was alert, fully oriented, and cognitively intact. She was irritable but not depressed. She kept insisting that she heard a radio playing: "I think it's hidden in my pillow." She unzipped the pillowcase and felt around inside. "It's some sort of a news report. They're talking about what's happening in the hospital. I think I just heard my name mentioned."

Melanie's flow of speech was coherent and relevant. Apart from throwing the tea bag and looking for the radio, her behavior was unremarkable. She denied hallucinations involving any of the other senses. She insisted that the voices she heard could not be imaginary, and she didn't think someone was trying to play a trick on her. She had never used drugs or alcohol, and her obstetrician vouched for her excellent general health. After much discussion, she agreed to remain in the hospital a day or two longer to try to get to the bottom of the mystery.

Evaluation of Melanie Grayson

Despite her obvious psychosis (hallucinations and delusions), the brevity of her symptoms kept Melanie from meeting the "A" criteria for **Schizophrenia**, **Schizophreniform Disorder**, or **Schizoaffective Disorder**. What's left?

Although Melanie remained alert and cognitively intact, any patient with abrupt onset of psychotic symptoms should be carefully evaluated for a possible **delirium**. Many **general medical conditions** can also produce psychotic symptoms. Anyone who becomes psychotic soon after entering the hospital should be evaluated for a **Substance-Induced Psychotic Disorder With Onset During Withdrawal**. Melanie had no prominent mood symptoms; if she had, a diagnosis of a **mood disorder with psychotic features** might have been entertained. Patients with certain **personality disorders** (e.g., **Borderline**) who have very brief psychotic symptoms precipitated by stress do not require a separate diagnosis of Brief Psychotic Disorder.

It is worth noting that many patients who develop psychosis after delivery may have mixtures of symptoms that include euphoria, psychosis, and cognitive changes. Many of these patients have some form of mood disorder (often **Bipolar I Disorder**). Diagnosis should be made with extreme care in all cases of postpartum psychosis; the diagnosis of Schizophrenia should never be made, except in the most obvious and certain of circumstances.

With a very brief duration of psychosis and none of the exclusions, Melanie would fulfill the somewhat undemanding criteria for Brief Psychotic Disorder. Until she recovered, the diagnosis would have to be made provisionally. Her five-axis diagnosis at this time would be as follows:

Axis I	298.8	Brief Psychotic Disorder, With Postpartum Onset (Provisional)
Axis II	V71.09	No diagnosis
Axis III	650	Normal delivery
Axis IV		Childbirth
Axis V	GAF = 40	(current)

297.3 Shared Psychotic Disorder

Extremely rare, Shared Psychotic Disorder is dramatic and is inherently interesting. Previously called Induced Psychotic Disorder, it was known as long ago as 150 years as folie à deux, which means "double insanity." Usually two people are involved, but three, four, or more can be involved. It affects women more often than men, and it usually occurs within families. Isolation may play a role in the development of this strange condition.

One of the persons affected is independently psychotic; through a close (and often dependent) association, the other has come to believe in the delusions and other experiences of the first. The content of the delusion is usually believable; occasionally, the content may be bizarre. Isolating the independently psychotic patient may cure the other(s), but this is by no means an invariable remedy. For one thing, the parties involved are often closely related and reinforce each other for their psychopathology.

Criteria for Shared Psychotic Disorder

• Someone who is closely associated with a delusional person also develops a delusion.

- The content of this new delusion is similar to that of the first person's delusion.
- The disorder is not explained better by another psychotic disorder, such as Schizophrenia or a mood disorder with psychotic features.
- This disorder is not directly caused by a general medical condition or the use of substances, including prescription medications.

Miriam Phillips

Miriam Phillips was 23 when she was hospitalized. She had spent nearly all her life in the Ozarks, where she sometimes attended class in a three-room school. Although she was bright enough, she had little interest in her studies and often volunteered to stay home to care for her mother, who was unwell. When she was in the 12th grade, she dropped out of high school to stay home full-time.

It was lonely living in the hills. Miriam's father, a long-distance trucker, was away most of the time. She had never learned to drive, and there were no close neighbors. Their television set received mostly snow; there was little in the way of mail; and there were no visitors at all. So she was surprised late on a Monday afternoon when two men paid a call.

After identifying themselves as FBI agents, they asked if she was the Miriam Phillips who three weeks earlier had written a letter to the president. When she asked how they had known, they showed her a faxed copy of her own letter:

Dear Mr. President, what do you plan to do about the Cubans? They have been working on mother. Their up to no good. Ive seen the police, but they say Cubans are your job, and I guess their right. You have to do your job or Ill have a dirty job to do. Miriam Phillips.

When Miriam finally figured out that the FBI agents thought she had threatened the president, she relaxed. She hadn't meant that at all. She had meant that if no one else took action, she'd have to crawl under the house to get the gravity machines.

"Gravity machines?" The two agents looked at each other.

She explained. They had been installed under the house by Cuban agents of Fidel Castro after the Bay of Pigs invasion in the 1960s. The machines pulled your body fluids down toward your feet. They hadn't affected her yet, but they had bothered her mother for years. Miriam had seen the hideous swelling in her mother's ankles. Some days it extended almost to her knees.

The two agents listened to her politely, then left. As they passed through town on their way to the airport, they called at the local community mental health clinic. Within a few days, a mental health worker came to interview Miriam, who agreed to enter the hospital voluntarily for a "checkup."

On admission, Miriam appeared remarkably intact. She had a full range of appropriate affect and normal cognitive abilities and orientation. Her reasoning ability seemed good, aside from the story about the gravity machines. As far back as her teens, her mother had told her how the machines came to be installed in the crawlspace under their house. The mother had been a nurse, and Miriam had always accepted her word in medical matters. By some unspoken agreement, the two had never discussed the matter with Miriam's father.

After Miriam had been on the ward for three days, her therapist asked whether she thought any other explanation for her mother's edema was possible. Miriam considered. She had never felt the gravity effects herself. She had believed that her mother told her the truth, but she now supposed that even Mother could have been mistaken.

Though Miriam was given no medication, after a week she stopped talking about gravity machines and asked to be discharged. At the end of their shift that afternoon, two young attendants gave her a lift home. As they walked her to the front door, it was opened by a short woman, quite stout, with salt-and-pepper hair. Her lower legs were neatly wrapped in elastic bandages. Through the partly opened door she darted a glance at the two men.

"Hmmm!" she said. "You look like Cubans."

Evaluation of Miriam Phillips

Miriam had no hallucinations, negative symptoms, or disordered behavior or affect, but the symptom experienced by her and her mother was pretty bizarre. Therefore, **Schizophrenia** could not be ruled out just on the basis of symptoms. However, there was no evidence that her delusions caused any occupational or social dysfunction; her own isolation appeared to have begun at least five years earlier, before the onset of her shared delusion. There was no history or other evidence to support **Substance-Induced Psychotic Disorder** or **Psychotic Disorder Due to a General Medical Condition**. The additional fact that her delusion mirrored her mother's confirmed the diagnosis of Shared Psychotic Disorder.

Miriam's delusions became less prominent after only a few days away from her mother. (If they had persisted for a long time, the diagnosis of another, independent psychosis would have been considered.) In working further with her, a therapist would also want to consider the possibility of a personality disorder, such as **Dependent Personality Disorder**.

Axis I	297.3	Shared Psychotic Disorder
Axis II	799.9	Diagnosis Deferred
Axis III		None
Axis IV		None
Axis V	GAF = 40	(current)

293.8x Psychotic Disorder Due to a General Medical Condition

A psychosis arising in a patient who has a general medical condition shouldn't be especially rare. Many diseases can produce psychosis, and a number of them are relatively common. But few, if any, studies bear on questions of epidemiology. When such patients do appear, they are too often misdiagnosed as having Schizophrenia or some other psychosis. This can lead to real tragedy: A patient who is not appropriately treated early enough may go on to experience (or cause) serious harm.

Criteria for Psychotic Disorder Due to a General Medical Condition

- The patient has prominent delusions or hallucinations.
- History, physical exam, or laboratory findings suggest that a general medical condition has directly caused these symptoms.
- The symptoms don't occur solely during a delirium.
- No other mental disorder better accounts for these symptoms.

Coding Notes

Code, based on the predominant symptoms:

293.81   With Delusions
293.82   With Hallucinations

Use the name of the medical disorder in the Axis I code, not General Medical Condition. On Axis III, also code the specific general medical condition that has caused the psychosis.

If the patient has a preexisting dementia (Alzheimer's or Vascular) and *then* becomes psychotic, do not use code 293.8x. Instead, the cognitive disorder takes precedence, and you would code, for example, 290.42 (Vascular Dementia, With Delusions).

Rodrigo Chavez

After he retired from teaching at age 65, Rodrigo Chavez spent most of his time sitting alone in his room. Sometimes he played the acoustic guitar; once or twice he shot targets at the rifle range. True to his lifelong habit, he never drank. Other than his immediate family, he had few social contacts. "My cigarettes are my best friends," he put it during the forensic examination.

When Rodrigo was nearly 70, an inoperable carcinoma of the lung was diagnosed. After a course of palliative radiotherapy, he declined further treatment and settled down in his apartment to die. Four months later, he first noticed right-sided headaches that would sometimes awaken him in the middle of the night. The doctors had told him he was terminally ill, so he didn't seek medical attention. Then he began to associate the headaches with natural gas, which he smelled coming out of the ventilator duct in his bathroom. When he called to report the problem to his landlady, Mrs. Riordan, she sent around the building's handyman, who could find nothing wrong.

When his headaches and the odors increased, Rodrigo recalled that, weeks before, she had gone out several times to watch while repairmen from the power company dug up the street outside the apartment building. The logical conclusion fairly burst upon him: His landlady was trying to poison him.

As the odor worsened, his anger mounted. It had begun to affect his voice, which had become raspy and high-pitched. He had several shouted arguments with Mrs. Riordan. One of these they carried on through her apartment door at 2 A.M., several weeks after he first noticed the gas. He threatened to report her to the housing authority; she called him "a crazy old coot." After he threatened her ("If I'm not safe, your life isn't worth 15 cents!"), they both made telephone calls to the police, who could find nothing to charge anyone with.

The night he was arrested, Rodrigo sat just inside his open doorway, yelling insults at Mrs. Riordan. When she lumbered to the top of the stairs to investigate, he shot her once, just behind her left ear. The arresting officers noted that he seemed "strangely detached" from the murder of his landlady. One of them wrote down this statement: "It wouldn't matter, just for me. But I couldn't stand her gassing all those other people in the house."

The forensic examiner noted that Rodrigo Chavez was an elderly, slightly built man who was clean-shaven and neatly groomed. He was gaunt, looking as if he has lost considerable weight. His speech was clear, coherent, relevant, and spontaneous, but his voice was high-pitched and gravelly. He appeared calm, and he described his mood as "medium," but he became angry when describing his landlady's attempts to poison him. He was fully oriented to person, place, and time, and he earned a perfect score on the Mini-Mental State Exam. He was fully aware that he had lung cancer. Insight for the fact of his psychosis was nil, and his judgment by recent history had been extremely poor.

X-ray of his chest showed a right lung that was full of tumor; compared with a previous series, skull films suggested a metastatic lesion located in the right frontal lobe.

Evaluation of Rodrigo Chavez

Rodrigo was clearly psychotic: He had prominent olfactory hallucinations and an elaborate delusion about being poisoned. These had been present for several months. (If insight is retained that the hallucinations are a product of the patient's own mind, one would generally not diagnose a psychotic disorder.) Aside from his psychosis, his thinking was clear. He was oriented and he scored well on the Mini-Mental State Exam, so he had no evidence of a **delirium** or a **dementia**. He had had no history of drinking or taking drugs; this would seem to rule out a **Substance-Induced Psychotic Disorder**. His mood had been at times angry, but appropriately so, given the content of his delusion and hallucination, so a **mood disorder with psychotic features** would also seem unlikely. There was no previous history of behavior or personality change that would qualify him for a diagnosis of **Schizophrenia**. Other features atypical for Schizophrenia included the late age of onset and relatively brief duration.

Rodrigo had a history of a cancer that is known to metastasize to the brain; his headaches suggested that it had already done so. His gravelly, high-pitched voice could be due to extension of the growth or to another metastasis within his chest or neck. The findings on chest X-ray and MRI confirmed the diagnosis. Other general medical conditions that can cause psychosis include temporal lobe epilepsy, primary brain tumors (not metastases), endocrine disorder such as thyroid and adrenal disease, vitamin deficiency states, central nervous system syphilis, multiple sclerosis, systemic lupus erythematosus, Wilson's disease, and head trauma.

Although Rodrigo had *both* hallucinations and delusions, the olfactory hallucinations appeared first and seemed to predominate, resulting in the fifth-digit code.

Axis I	293.82	Psychotic Disorder Due to a Metastatic Carcinoma, With Hallucinations
Axis II	V71.09	No diagnosis
Axis III	198.3	Cancer of the lung, metastatic to the brain
Axis IV		Arrested for murder
Axis V	GAF = 15	(current)

Substance-Induced Psychotic Disorder

The category of Substance-Induced Psychotic Disorder includes all psychoses caused by mind-altering substances. The predominant symptoms are usually hallucinations or delusions; depending on the substance, they can occur during withdrawal or acute intoxication. Usually, the course is brief; again, treatment depends on the drug responsible. Although most of these psychoses are self-limiting, early recognition is crucial. Patients have died during Substance-Induced Psychotic Disorders. Several of these disorders can closely mimic endogenous mental diseases such as Schizophrenia. Many diagnoses are possible, if we include all the possible combinations of different substances with the type and duration of psychosis and its relation to intoxication or withdrawal.

Criteria for Substance-Induced Psychotic Disorder

- The patient has prominent hallucinations or delusions. Don't include hallucinations that the patient realizes are caused by substance use.
- History, physical exam, or laboratory data substantiate that *either*:
    - ✓ These symptoms have developed within a month of Substance Intoxication or Withdrawal, *or*
    - ✓ Medication use has caused the symptoms.
- Another, non-substance-induced psychotic disorder does not better account for the symptoms. (See Coding Notes.)
- The symptoms don't occur only in the context of a delirium.

Coding Notes

The codes used for Substance-Induced Psychotic Disorder are somewhat arcane. Different numbers are used to describe a psychosis with delusions and with hallucinations, and the coding for alcohol is different from that for all other substances. If delusions and hallucinations are both present, code the one that dominates the clinical picture. The numbers to use are as follows:

With Delusions:

291.5	Alcohol
292.11	Amphetamine [or Amphetamine-Like Substance]; Cannabis; Cocaine; Hallucinogen; Inhalant; Opioid; Phencyclidine [or Phencyclidine-Like Substance]; Sedative, Hypnotic, or Anxiolytic; Other [or Unknown] Substance

With Hallucinations:

291.3	Alcohol
292.12	Amphetamine [or Amphetamine-Like Substance]; Cannabis; Cocaine; Hallucinogen; Inhalant; Opioid; Phencyclidine [or Phencyclidine-Like Substance]; Sedative, Hypnotic, or Anxiolytic; Other [or Unknown] Substance

When criteria are met for Substance Intoxication or Withdrawal (see p. 81, 72), specify whether:

With Onset During Intoxication

With Onset During Withdrawal

DSM-IV suggests several instances in which a non-substance-related disorder may better explain the symptoms of psychosis:

- Psychotic symptoms begin before the onset of the substance use.
- Psychotic symptoms persist long after (a month or more) the substance use stops.
- Psychotic symptoms are more severe than you would expect from the amount and extent of substance use.
- The patient has had previous psychotic episodes independent of substance use.

Use this diagnosis instead of Substance Intoxication or Withdrawal only (1) when the symptoms exceed those you would expect from a syndrome of intoxication or withdrawal, *and* (2) when they are serious enough by themselves to require clinical care.

Psychoses caused by most medications taken in therapeutic doses are coded as follows, for example:

Axis I   292.12   Estrogen-Induced Psychotic Disorder, With Hallucinations, With Onset During Intoxication

Axis III E932.2   Ovarian hormones

In such a case, the symptoms must not instead be caused by a Psychotic Disorder Due to a General Medical Condition. If you cannot be sure, you can temporarily resort to Psychotic Disorder Not Otherwise Specified until the medication is changed or more information is gathered.

Danny Finch

Danny Finch put up with the ear problem for three days before he finally called for an appointment. The doctor poked at this and that, and worried a little over his tremor.

"You don't drink, do you?"

"A little. But what about my ear?"

"It's perfectly normal."

"But I hear something. It's like someone chanting. I can almost make out what they're saying. You're sure no one's put something in there, a hearing aid?" He dug at the ear with his little finger.

"Nope, clean as a whistle. Here, don't do that!" The doctor scribbled a referral to the mental health clinic down the hall. That was late on a Friday afternoon, and the clinic was closed by then.

On Monday afternoon, when he finally got to his appointment, Danny could once again write his name legibly. He was also eating solid food again, and the voices were in full throat. As he talked with the interviewer, he could hardly concentrate because they were screaming at him, "Don't tell about the drinking!" and "Why don't you just kill yourself?" He was so terrified that he accepted with relief a voluntary commitment to the mental health ward, where his admitting diagnosis was Schizophrenia. Twice a day he was given a potent neuroleptic medication, which he tucked under his tongue and discarded in a tissue when he pretended to blow his nose.

Danny slept soundly at night and cleaned his plate at every meal while the voices screamed on. At the end of the week, he was visited by a consultant who learned that the voices came from about two feet behind him and talked in sentences. Reluctantly, he admitted that they told him not to talk about his drinking.

A rapid review of Danny's chart revealed no mention of drinking problems, but a little coaxing soon pried loose the whole story. Since his early 20s, there had been heavy drinking, loss of two jobs (he had a shaky hold on his present one), and a divorce, all related to his fondness for bourbon. Most recently he had been drinking more than a pint each evening, often a fifth on the weekends. Usually he managed to taper off; this time, he had quit suddenly after a bout of what he called "the stomach flu."

Evaluation of Danny Finch

Danny's auditory hallucinations had been present far too briefly for **Schizophrenia**, though he described them in terms closely resembling it. A **Brief Psychotic Disorder** might be possible, except that a **Substance-Induced Psychotic Disorder** must not better explain the symptoms. He had just been seen by a physician, who pronounced him fit; there was no evidence of any other **general medical condition**. The fact that he was fully oriented and maintained his attention would rule out **delirium** and other **cognitive disorders**. He seemed appropriately frightened by his experiences, but he presented no evidence of **mood disorder**.

Danny's psychosis, formerly called *alcoholic auditory hallucinosis*, is a disorder of withdrawal that usually occurs only after weeks or months of heavy drinking. By about a four-to-one ratio, it is much more common in men than women; this approximates the ratio of male to female alcoholics. Auditory hallucinosis is sometimes misidentified as **Alcohol Withdrawal Delirium**, though the criteria for the latter make the differences clear (see p. 21).

Withdrawal from other drugs can also produce psychosis. **Barbiturates**, which have many of the same effects as alcohol, are the most notorious of these. Some patients experience prolonged psychoses after the use of **hallucinogens** such as LSD. The risk may be greater in those with pre-existing personality disorders.

Danny's symptoms were clearly more serious than would be expected in **Alcohol Withdrawal With Perceptual Disturbances** (which would be diagnosed if he had retained insight). Hence his diagnosis would be as follows:

Axis I	291.3	Alcohol-Induced Psychotic Disorder, With Hallucinations, With Onset During Withdrawal
Axis II	V71.09	No diagnosis
Axis III		None
Axis IV		None
Axis V	GAF = 35	(on admission
	GAF = 70	(at discharge)

298.9 Psychotic Disorder Not Otherwise Specified

The category of Psychotic Disorder Not Otherwise Specified should be used for symptoms or syndromes that do not meet the criteria for any of the disorders described above. Some of these are as follows:

Charles Bonnet syndrome. In this disorder (first described in 1790!), elderly people report complex visual hallucinations (scenes, people) but no other hallucinations or delusions. They also have insight that what they "see" is unreal.

Postpartum psychosis. This includes conditions that *don't* meet criteria for Brief Psychotic Disorder or other more specific disorders.

Auditory hallucinations. This pertains only to hallucinations that persist without the presence of other symptoms.

Other. Psychotic Disorder Not Otherwise Specified is the category to use when your patient is psychotic, but the information is conflicting or too inadequate to permit a definitive diagnosis.

CHAPTER 5

Mood Disorders

Quick Guide to the Mood Disorders

DSM-IV uses three groups of criteria sets to diagnose mental problems related to mood: (1) mood episodes, (2) mood disorders, and (3) specifiers describing most recent episode and recurrent course . I'll cover each of them in this Quick Guide. As usual, the page number following each item below refers to the point where a more detailed discussion begins.

Mood Episodes

Simply expressed, *a mood episode* refers to any period of time when a patient feels abnormally happy or sad. Mood episodes are the "building blocks" from which many of the codable mood disorders are constructed. Most mood disorder patients will have one or more of these four types of episode: Major Depressive, Manic, Mixed, and Hypomanic. Without additional information, none of these types of mood episode is a codable diagnosis.

Major Depressive Episode. For at least two weeks, the patient feels depressed (or cannot enjoy life) and has problems with eating and sleeping, guilt feelings, loss of energy, trouble concentrating, and thoughts about death (p. 191).

Manic Episode. For at least one week, the patient feels elated (or sometimes only irritable) and may be grandiose, talkative, hyperactive, and distractible. Bad judgment leads to marked social or work impairment; often patients must be hospitalized (p. 195).

Mixed Episode. In this case, the patient has fulfilled the symptomatic criteria for both a Manic *and* a Major Depressive Episode, but it has lasted as briefly as a week (p. 199).

Hypomanic Episode. This is much like a Manic Episode, but it is briefer and less severe. Hospitalization is not required (p. 200).

Mood Disorders

A *mood disorder* is a pattern of illness due to an abnormal mood. Nearly every patient who has a mood disorder experiences depression at some time, but some also have highs of mood. Many, but not all, mood disorders are diagnosed on the basis of a mood episode. Most patients with mood disorders will fit into one of the codable categories listed below.

Depressive Disorders

Major Depressive Disorder. These patients have had no Manic or Hypomanic Episodes, but have had one or more Major Depressive Episodes. Major Depressive Disorder will be either Recurrent or Single Episode (p. 203).

Dysthymic Disorder. This type of depression is not severe enough to be called a Major Depressive Episode. Dysthymic Disorder lasts much longer than Major Depressive Disorder, and there are no high phases (p. 223).

Depressive Disorder Not Otherwise Specified. Use this category when a patient has depressive symptoms that do not meet the criteria for the depressive diagnoses above or for any other diagnosis in which depression is a feature (p. 236).

Bipolar Disorders

Approximately 25% of mood disorder patients experience Manic or Hypomanic Episodes. Nearly all of these patients will also have episodes of depression. The severity and duration of the highs and lows determine the specific bipolar disorder.

Bipolar I Disorder. There must be at least one Manic Episode; most Bipolar I patients have also had a Major Depressive Episode (p. 210).

Bipolar II Disorder. This diagnosis requires at least one Hypomanic Episode plus at least one Major Depressive Episode (p. 219).

Cyclothymic Disorder. Cyclothymic patients have had repeated mood swings, but none that are severe enough to be called Major Depressive Episodes or Manic Episodes (p. 226).

Bipolar Disorder Not Otherwise Specified. Use this category when a patient has bipolar symptoms that do not meet the criteria for the bipolar diagnoses above (p. 238).

Other Mood Disorders

Mood Disorder Due to a General Medical Condition. Either highs or lows of mood can be caused by various types of physical illness (p. 229).

Substance-Induced Mood Disorder. Alcohol or other substances can cause high or low moods that may not meet criteria for any of the above-mentioned episodes or disorders (p. 233).

Mood Disorder Not Otherwise Specified. Use this category for patients who do not fit neatly into *any* of the mood disorder categories mentioned above (p. 238).

Other Causes of Depressive and Manic Symptoms

Schizoaffective Disorder. In these patients, symptoms suggestive of Schizophrenia coexist with a Major Depressive or a Manic Episode (p. 164).

Cognitive disorders with depressed mood. The qualifier With Depressed Mood can be coded into the diagnosis of Dementia of the Alzheimer's Type (p. 30) or Vascular Dementia (p. 35). A delirium can also often begin with depression, anxiety, or other expressions of dysphoria. In evaluating patients with altered mood, especially in a hospital setting, be sure to consider the cognitive disorders.

Adjustment Disorder With Depressed Mood. This term codes one way of adapting to a life stress (p. 454).

Personality disorders. Dysphoric mood is specifically mentioned in the criteria for Borderline Personality Disorder (p. 478), but depressed mood can accompany Avoidant, Dependent, and Histrionic Personality Disorders.

Bereavement. Sadness at the death of a relative or friend is a common experience. When symptoms last longer than two months, the patient may have a mood disorder (p. 540).

Other disorders. Depression can accompany many other mental disorders, including Schizophrenia, the eating disorders, Somatization Disorder, and the sexual and gender identity disorders. Mood symptoms are likely in patients with an anxiety disorder (especially Panic Disorder, Obsessive–Compulsive Disorder, Phobic Disorder, and Posttraumatic Stress Disorder).

Specifiers

Two special sets of descriptions can be applied to a number of the mood episodes and mood disorders.

Specifiers Describing Most Recent Episode

These descriptors help characterize the most recent Major Depressive Episode; the second two can also apply to a Manic Episode. (Note that the DSM-IV specifiers for severity and chronicity are described following the criteria for the mood episodes to which they apply; these others are described separately.)

With Atypical Features. These patients eat a lot and gain weight, sleep excessively, and have a feeling of leaden paralysis. They are often excessively sensitive to rejection (p. 239).

With Melancholic Features. This term applies to Major Depressive episodes characterized by some of the "classical" symptoms of severe depression. These patients awaken early, feeling worse than they do later in the day. They lose appetite and weight, feel guilty, are either slowed down or agitated, and do not feel better when something happens that they would normally like (p. 240).

With Catatonic Features. There are features of either motor hyperactivity or inactivity. Catatonic features can apply to Major Depressive Episodes and to Manic Episodes (p. 240).

With Postpartum Onset. A Manic or Major Depressive Episode (or a Brief Psychotic Episode) can occur in a woman within a month of having a baby (p. 241).

Describing Course of Recurrent Episodes

These describe the overall *course* of a mood disorder, not just the form of an individual episode.

With or Without Full Interepisode Recovery. These designations describe the presence (or absence) of symptoms between Manic, Hypomanic, Mixed, or Major Depressive Episodes (p. 242).

With Rapid Cycling. Within one year, the patient has had at least four episodes (in any combination) meeting criteria for Major Depressive, Manic, Mixed and/or Hypomanic Episodes (p. 243).

With Seasonal Pattern. These patients regularly become ill at a certain time of the year, such as fall or winter (p. 244).

Introduction

Mood refers to a sustained emotion that colors the way we view life. Recognizing mood disorders is extremely important, because as many as 20% of adult women and 10% of adult men may have one. Their prevalence seems to be increasing in both sexes, and they account for as much as 50% of a typical mental health practice. Mood disorders can occur in people from any race or social class, but they are more common among those who are single and who have no "significant other." A mood disorder is also more likely in someone who has relatives with similar problems.

The mood disorders have many diagnoses, qualifiers, and levels of severity. Although they may seem complicated, they can be reduced to a few main principles.

TIPS A few years ago, the mood disorders were referred to as *affective disorders*; many clinicians still use the older term. Note by the way, that the term *affect* covers more that just a patient's statement of emotion. It also takes in how the patient *appears* to be feeling, as shown by facial expression, posture, eye contact, tearfulness, and other physical clues.

Unfortunately, clinicians (including some mental health specialists) commonly make two sorts of mistakes when evaluating patients with depression:

First, clinicians may focus on a patient's anxiety, alcoholism, or psychotic symptoms and ignore underlying symptoms of depression or dysthymia. An important rule to remember is this: *Always* look for a mood disorder in any new patient, even if the chief complaint is something else.

Second, clinicians may diagnose depression and fail to notice the presence of alcoholism or another disorder (e.g., Somatization Disorder). This suggests another, equally important rule: *Never* assume that a mood disorder is your patient's only Axis I or Axis II problem.

Using DSM-IV Codes for Mood Disorders

The following numbered steps suggest an organized approach to the recognition and diagnosis of the elements described in the Quick Guide.

1. Identify the current and past mood episodes: Major Depressive, Manic, Mixed, or Hypomanic. Again, these are not coded themselves, but serve as the "building blocks" for the actual diagnosis. If your patient's symptoms do not conform to those for one of these basic mood episodes, skip to step 8.

2. Using the building blocks, choose the appropriate type of mood disorder: Bipolar or Major Depressive Disorder. If the diagnosis is Bipolar II, the fourth and fifth digits are already assigned; skip to step 5. If the diagnosis is Cyclothymic Disorder, the five-digit code is already assigned and you are finished.

3. If in step 2 you diagnosed a Bipolar I or Major Depressive Disorder, examine the course of your patient's history to select the appropriate fourth-digit designation. For Major Depressive Disorder, this will be either Single Episode or Recurrent. For Bipolar I Disorder, it will be one of the following bipolar subtypes: Single Manic Episode or Most Recent Episode Manic, Hypomanic, Depressed, Mixed, or Unspecified. (For criteria for the various subtypes, see the discussions of these diagnoses.)

4. Assign the fifth-digit severity code, using the criteria supplied for Manic, Major Depressive, or Mixed Episodes that are appended to the episode criteria. (Note that Bipolar I Disorder, Most Recent Episode Hypomanic, does not have any severity criteria; the full code number is automatically 296.40.)

5. Consult Table 5.1 (p. 244). If the most recent episode is Major Depressive, use the specifier Chronic if it is appropriate.

6. As appropriate, add other episode specifiers from Table 5.1 that describe your patient's current episode. These modifiers are With Atypical Features, With Catatonic Features, With Melancholic Features, and With Postpartum Onset.

7. From the table, add any course specifiers relevant to your patient's disorder. These include With or Without Interepisode Recovery, With Rapid Cycling, and With Seasonal Pattern.

8. If your patient's symptoms do not qualify as a mood episode, consider these mood disorders: Dysthymic Disorder, Mood Disorder Due to a General Medical Condition, and Substance-Induced Mood Disorder. Each of them has its own set of criteria independent of any mood episode. If you diagnose one of these disorders, the coding stops here.

9. If your patient does not fit into any of the categories mentioned above, turn to Depressive Disorder Not Otherwise Specified, Bipolar Disorder Not Otherwise Specified, or Mood Disorder Not Otherwise Specified. There you will find discussions of some mood disorders that are not spelled out fully in the DSM-IV criteria, but that may describe your patient.

MOOD EPISODES

I describe the various mood episodes in this section. You will find case vignettes illustrating each one in the mood disorders sections, which follow.

Major Depressive Episode

Major Depressive Episode is not a codable diagnosis; it is one of the "building blocks" of the mood disorders. You will use it often—it is one of the most common problems for which patients seek help. Apply it carefully after considering a patient's full history and mental status exam. Of course, clinicians should be careful using every label and every diagnosis. I mention this caution here because some clinicians tend to use the Major Depressive Episode label without carefully considering the criteria.

A Major Depressive Episode must meet five criteria. There must be (1) a quality of depressed mood (or loss of interest or pleasure) that (2) has existed for a minimum period of time, (3) is accompanied by a required number of symptoms, (4) has resulted in disability, and (5) does not violate any of the listed exclusions.

Quality of mood

Depression is usually experienced as a lowering of mood from normal (patients may describe it as feeling "unhappy," "down in the dumps," or many other terms expressing sadness). Several problems can interfere with the recognition of depression:

Not all patients can recognize or accurately describe how they feel.

Clinicians and patients who come from different cultural backgrounds may have difficulty agreeing that the problem is depression.

The presenting symptoms of depression may vary greatly. One patient may be slowed down and crying; another will smile and deny that anything is wrong. Some sleep and eat too much; others complain of insomnia and anorexia.

Some patients don't really feel depressed; they experience depression only as a loss of pleasure or reduced interest in their usual activities (including sex).

It is crucial to diagnosis that the episode must represent a noticeable change from the patient's usual level of functioning. If the patient does not notice it (some are too ill to pay attention or too apathetic to care), family or friends may report that there has been a change.

Duration

The patient must have felt bad most of the day, nearly every day, for at least two weeks. This requirement is meant to ensure that Major Depressive Episodes are differentiated from the transient "down" spells that most of us sometimes feel.

Symptoms

The patient must have at least five of the symptoms listed in the criteria below. One of those five must be either depressed mood or loss of pleasure. (*Depressed mood* is self-explanatory; *loss of pleasure* is nearly universal among depressed patients). Many patients will have lost *appetite and weight*. More than three-fourths report trouble with *sleep*. Typically, they awaken early in the morning, long before it is time to arise. However, some patients eat and sleep more than usual; these patients would qualify for the With Atypical Features specifier (p. 239).

Depressed patients will usually complain of *fatigue*, which they may express as tiredness or loss of energy. Their speech or movements may be *slowed down*; sometimes there is a marked pause before answering a question or initiating an action that has been requested. This is called psychomotor retardation. Speech may be very quiet, sometimes inaudible. Some patients simply stop talking completely, except in response to a direct question. At the extreme, complete muteness may ensue.

At the other extreme, some depressed patient feel so anxious that they become *agitated*. Agitation may be expressed as hand wringing, pacing, or an inability to sit still. The ability of depressed patients to evaluate themselves objectively plummets, and this shows up as low self-esteem or guilt. They may develop *trouble with concentration* (real or perceived) so severe that sometimes a misdiagnosis of dementia may be made. Thoughts of death, *death wishes*, and *suicidal ideas* are the most serious depressive symptoms of all, because there is a significant risk that they will be successfully acted upon.

In general, the more symptoms a patient has from this list, the more reliable will be the diagnosis of Major Depressive Episode. It should be noted, however, that depressed patients can have many symptoms besides those listed in the DSM-IV criteria. These may include crying spells, phobias, obsessions, and compulsions. Patients may admit to feeling hopeless, helpless, or worthless. Anxiety symptoms, especially Panic Attacks (see p. 251) can be so prominent that they blind clinicians to the underlying depression. Many patients drink more (occasionally, less) alcohol when they become depressed; this can lead to difficulty in sorting out the differential diagnosis (which should be treated first, the depression or the drinking?). Some patients lose contact with reality and develop delusions or hallucinations. These psychotic features can be either *mood-congruent* (e.g., a depressed man feels so guilty that he imagines he has committed some awful sin) or *mood-incongruent* (e.g., a depressed woman believes she is being persecuted by the FBI; this is not a typical theme of depression).

There are two situations in which you should *not* count a symptom toward a diagnosis of Major Depressive Episode. The first case is when a symptom is fully explained by a general medical condition. For example, you would not count fatigue as a symptom in a patient who is recovering from major surgery—in that situation, you expect fatigue. The second case is when a symptom results from mood-incongruent delusions or hallucinations. For example, don't count insomnia that is a response to hallucinated voices that scream political slogans throughout the night.

Impairment

The episode must have been severe enough to cause material distress or impairment in the patient's work (or school) performance, social life (withdrawal or discord), or some other area of functioning (such as sex). Of the various consequences of mental illness, the effect on work may the hardest to detect. Perhaps this is because earning a livelihood is so important that most people will go to great lengths to hide symptoms that could threaten their employment.

Exclusions

Regardless of the severity or duration of symptoms, Major Depressive Episode should not be diagnosed in the face of clinically important substance use or a general medical disorder, or if the patient has been bereaved within the last two months. (There is even an exclusion for the bereavement exclusion: If the symptoms are unusually severe, a Major Depressive Episode may be diagnosed regardless of the time elapsed since the death of a friend or relative.)

Criteria for Major Depressive Episode

- In the same two weeks, the patient has had five or more of the following symptoms, which are a definite change from usual functioning. Either depressed mood or decreased interest or pleasure must be one of the five.
  - ✓ Mood. For most of nearly every day, the patient reports depressed mood or appears depressed to others.
  - ✓ Interests. For most of nearly every day, interest or pleasure is markedly decreased in nearly all activities (as noted by the patient or by others).
  - ✓ Eating and weight. Although the patient is not dieting, there is a marked loss or gain of weight (such as 5% in one month) or appetite is markedly decreased or increased nearly every day.
  - ✓ Sleep. Nearly every day the patient sleeps excessively or not enough.
  - ✓ Observable Psychomotor activity. Nearly every day others can see that the patient's activity is speeded up or slowed down.
  - ✓ Fatigue. Nearly every day there is tiredness or loss of energy.

    ✓ Self-worth. Nearly every day the patient feels worthless or inappropriately guilty. These feelings are not just about being sick; they may be delusional.

    ✓ Concentration. As noted by the patient or by others, nearly every day the patient is indecisive or has trouble thinking or concentrating.

    ✓ Death. The patient has had repeated thoughts about death (other than the fear of dying), or about suicide (with or without a plan), or has made a suicide attempt.

- These symptoms cause clinically important distress or impair work, social, or personal functioning.
- They don't fulfill criteria for Mixed Episode.
- This disorder is not directly caused by a general medical condition or the use of substances, including prescription medications.
- Unless the symptoms are severe (defined as severely impaired functioning, severe preoccupation with worthlessness, ideas of suicide, delusions or hallucinations, or slowed psychomotor activity), the episode has not begun within two months of the loss of a loved one (Bereavement).

Coding Notes

Use the following codes (including Chronic) for the current or most recent Major Depressive Episode in Major Depressive, Bipolar I, or Bipolar II Disorders.

    Fifth-digit severity codes for Major Depressive Episode:

    .x1 Mild. Symptoms barely meet the criteria and result in little distress or interference with the patient's ability to work, study, or socialize.

    .x2 Moderate. Intermediate between Mild and Severe.

    .x3 Severe Without Psychotic Features. The number of symptoms well exceeds the minimum for diagnosis, *and* they markedly interfere with patient's work, social, or personal functioning.

    .x4 Severe With Psychotic Features. The patient has delusions or hallucinations, which may be mood-congruent or mood-incongruent. Specify, if possible:

        Severe With Mood-Congruent Psychotic Features. The content of the patient's delusions or hallucinations is completely consistent with the typical themes of depression: death, disease, guilt, nihilism (nothingness), low self-worth, or punishment that is deserved.

        Severe With Mood-Incongruent Psychotic Features. The content of the patient's delusions or hallucinations is not consistent with the typical themes of depression. Mood-incongruent themes include delusions of control, persecution, thought broadcasting, and thought insertion.

.x5 In Partial Remission. Use this code for patients who formerly met full criteria for Major Depressive Episode and now either (1) have fewer than five symptoms *or* (2) have had no symptoms for less than two months.

.x6 In Full Remission. The patient has had no material evidence of Major Depressive Episode during the past two months.

.x0 Unspecified.

Chronicity specifier: Chronic. Full criteria for a Major Depressive Episode have been met without interruption for the previous two years or longer. (The Chronicity specifier can be used with any of the severity specifiers above except In Partial Remission or In Full Remission. It carries no code number.)

When the criteria are applied to children or adolescents, the abnormal mood can be irritable instead of depressed, and there can be failure to gain weight rather than actual weight loss.

Don't count a symptom that is obviously explained by a general medical condition or by a mood-incongruent delusion or hallucination.

No diagnosis of Major Depressive Episode can be given if it was superimposed onto a Dysthymic Disorder and the full criteria are no longer present. Then only diagnose Dysthymic Disorder. See also page 224.

Examples of Major Depressive Episode are included in the following diagnoses: Major Depressive Disorder, Single Episode (p. 203); Major Depressive Disorder, Recurrent (p. 207); Bipolar I Disorder, Most Recent Episode Manic (p. 212); Hypersomnia Related to an Axis I Disorder (p. 428); Insomnia Related to an Axis I Disorder (p. 425); Amnestic Disorder Due to a General Medical Condition (p. 46).

Manic Episode

The second "building block" of the mood disorders, Manic Episode has been recognized for at least 150 years. The classic triad of manic symptoms consists of heightened self-esteem, increased motor activity, and pressured speech. These symptoms are obvious and often outrageous, so Manic Episode is not often overdiagnosed; however, when psychotic symptoms are florid, Manic Episode has sometimes been misdiagnosed as Schizophrenia. This tendency to misdiagnosis may have decreased since 1980, when the DSM-III criteria increased clinicians' awareness.

Manic Episode is much less common than Major Depressive Episode, perhaps affecting 1% of all adults. Men and women are about equally likely to have mania.

The list of features that must be present in order to make a diagnosis of Manic Episode is identical to that for depressive episode: There must be (1) a mood quality that (2) has existed for a required period of time, (3) is attended by a required number of symptoms, (4) has resulted in a considerable degree of disability, and (5) does not violate any of the listed exclusions.

Quality of Mood

The quality of mood in a Manic Episode is most often euphoric and expansive, though a few patients will be only irritable. Sometimes euphoria and irritability are present together.

Duration

The patient must have had symptoms for a minimum of one week. This time requirement helps to differentiate Manic Episode from Hypomanic Episode.

Symptoms

At least three of the symptoms listed in the criteria below must be present to an important degree during this one-week period. (Note that if the patient's *abnormal mood* is only irritable, without any euphoric component, four symptoms are required.) Some patients seem to feel quite jolly; this bumptious good humor can be quite infectious and may make others feel like laughing with them. But as the mania worsens, this humor becomes less cheerful. It takes on a "driven," unfunny quality that is uncomfortable for both patient and listener.

Heightened *self-esteem* can become grandiose to the point that it is delusional. Then patients believe that they can advise presidents and solve the problem of world hunger, in addition to more mundane tasks such as doing psychotherapy and running the very medical facilities where they are currently patients. Because such delusions are in keeping with the euphoric mood, they are called *mood-congruent*.

Manic patients typically report feeling rested on *little sleep*. Sleep time seems wasted; they prefer to pursue their many projects. In its early stages, this heightened activity may be goal-directed and useful; manic patients who are only moderately ill can accomplish quite a lot in a 20-hour day. But as they become more and *more active*, agitation ensues, and they may begin many projects they never complete. At this point they have lost *judgment* for what is reasonable and attainable. They may become involved in risky business ventures, indiscreet sexual liaisons, and questionable religious or political activities.

These patients are eager to tell anyone who will listen about their ideas, plans, and work, and they do so in speech that is loud and difficult to interrupt. Manic *speech* is often rapid and pressured, as if there were too many dammed-up words trying to get out through too small a valve. The resulting speech may exhibit *flight of ideas*, in which one thought triggers another to which it bears only a marginally logical association. As a result, a patient may wander far afield from where the conversation (or monologue) started. Manic patients may also be *easily distracted* by sounds or movements that other people would ignore.

Some manic patients retain insight and seek treatment, but many will deny that anything is wrong. They often rationalize that no one who feels so well or productive could possibly be ill. Manic behavior therefore continues until it ends spontaneously or the patient is hospitalized or jailed.

Some symptom presentations not specifically mentioned in the DSM-IV criteria are worth noting here as well. First, even during an acute Manic Episode, many patients have brief periods of depression. These "microdepressions" are relatively common; depending on the symptoms associated with them, they may indicate a Bipolar I Disorder, Most Recent Episode Mixed (see p. 215). Second, patients may use substances (especially alcohol) in an attempt to relieve the uncomfortable, driven feeling that accompanies a severe Manic Episode. When clinicians become confused about which came first, the substance use or the mania, the question can usually be sorted out with the help of informants. Less often, the substance use temporarily obscures the symptoms of the mood episode. Finally, catatonic symptoms occasionally occur in a Manic Episode, sometimes causing the episode to seem like Schizophrenia. But a history (obtained from informants) of acute onset and previous episodes with complete recovery can help clarify the diagnosis.

Impairment

Manic Episodes typically wreak havoc on the lives of patients and all those who associate with them. Although productivity at work (or school) may initially improve, as mania worsens a patient becomes less and less able to complete projects. Friendships are strained by arguments. Sexual entanglements can result in disease and unwanted pregnancy. Even when the episode has resolved, guilt and recriminations remain behind.

Exclusions

The exclusions for Manic Episode are the same as for Major Depressive Episode. General medical conditions such as hyperthyroidism can produce hyperactive behavior; patients who misuse certain psychoactive substances (especially amphetamines) will appear speeded up and may also report feeling strong, powerful, and euphoric.

Criteria for Manic Episode

- For at least one week (or less, if the patient has to be hospitalized), the patient's mood is abnormally and persistently high, irritable, or expansive.
- To a material degree during this time, the patient has persistently had three or more of these symptoms (four if the only abnormality of mood is irritability):
  ✓ Grandiosity or exaggerated self-esteem
  ✓ Reduced need for sleep
  ✓ Increased talkativeness
  ✓ Flight of ideas or racing thoughts
  ✓ Easy distractibility
  ✓ Speeded-up psychomotor activity or increased goal-directed activity (social, sexual, work, or school)
  ✓ Poor judgment (as shown by spending sprees, sexual adventures, foolish investments)
- Symptom severity results in at least one of these:
  ✓ Causes psychotic features
  ✓ Requires hospitalization to protect the patient or others
  ✓ Impairs work, social, or personal functioning.
- The symptoms don't fulfill criteria for Mixed Episode.
- They are not directly caused by a general medical condition or the use of substances, including prescription medications.

Coding Notes

Fifth-digit severity codes for Manic Episode (use these codes for the current or most recent episode of a Bipolar I Disorder):

   .x1 Mild. Symptoms barely meet the criteria.

   .x2 Moderate. There is an extreme increase in either activity level or impaired judgment.

   .x3 Severe Without Psychotic Features. The patient requires nearly constant supervision to avert physical harm to self or to others.

   .x4 Severe With Psychotic Features. The patient has delusions or hallucinations, which may be mood-congruent or mood-incongruent (specify, if possible):

      Severe With Mood-Congruent Psychotic Features. The content of the patient's delusions or hallucinations is completely consistent with typical themes of mania: exaggerated ideas of identity, knowledge, power, self-worth, or relationship to God or someone famous.

Severe With Mood-Incongruent Psychotic Features. The content of the patient's delusions or hallucinations is not consistent with typical themes of mania. Mood-incongruent delusions include control, persecution, thought broadcasting, and thought insertion.

.x5 In Partial Remission. Use this code for patients who formerly met criteria for Manic Episode and now either (1) have fewer than the required number of symptoms *or* (2) have had no symptoms for less than two months.

.x6 In Full Remission. These patients formerly met criteria for Manic Episode but have had no material evidence of mania for at least two months.

.x0 Unspecified.

If a patient's Manic Episode has been precipitated by somatic therapy (such as ECT, antidepressants, or bright light), it cannot be used as evidence of Bipolar I Disorder.

Elisabeth Jacks had a Manic Episode; her history is given in the section on Bipolar I Disorder, Most Recent Episode Manic (p. 212).

Mixed Episode

Clinicians as far back as Kraepelin recognized that mixed forms of mania and depression could exist. What no one has done yet is agree on the definition that should be employed. Mixed Episodes are especially common in younger people and in those over 60. Males may outnumber females.

I won't try to list again the five qualities that typify Mixed Episodes—it would be a rehash of the qualities typical of Manic, Depressive, and Hypomanic Episodes.

Criteria for Mixed Episode

- The patient has fulfilled symptom criteria for both a Major Depressive Episode and a Manic Episode nearly every day for a week or more.
- Symptom severity results in one or more of these:
  ✓ Causes psychotic features
  ✓ Requires hospitalization to protect the patient or others
  ✓ Impairs work, social, or personal functioning
- The symptoms are not directly caused by a general medical condition or the use of substances, including prescription medications.

Coding Notes

Fifth-digit severity codes for Mixed Episode (use these codes for the current or most recent episode of a Bipolar I Disorder):

.x1 Mild. Symptoms barely meet criteria for both Manic and Major Depressive Episodes.

.x2 Moderate. Intermediate between Mild and Severe.

.x3 Severe Without Psychotic Features. The patient requires nearly constant supervision to avert physical harm to self or to others.

.x4 Severe With Psychotic Features. The patient has delusions or hallucinations, which may be mood-congruent or mood-incongruent. Specify, if possible:

> Severe With Mood-Congruent Psychotic Features. The content of the patient's delusions or hallucinations is completely consistent with the typical themes of depression or mania.

> Severe With Mood-Incongruent Psychotic Features. The content of the patient's delusions or hallucinations is not consistent with the typical themes of depression or mania.

.x5 In Partial Remission. Use this code for patients who formerly met full criteria for Mixed Episode and now either (1) have too few symptoms to fulfill the criteria or (2) have had no symptoms for less than two months.

.x6 In Full Remission. The patient has had no material evidence of Mixed Episode for at least two months.

.x0 Unspecified.

If a patient's Mixed Episode has been precipitated by somatic therapy (such as ECT, antidepressants, or bright light), it cannot be used as evidence of Bipolar I Disorder.

Winona Fisk had a Mixed Episode. Her story is given in the section on Bipolar I Disorder, Most Recent Episode Mixed (p. 215).

Hypomanic Episode

Hypomanic Episode is the last of the four mood disorder "building blocks." Comprising the same symptoms as Manic Episode, it is Manic Episode writ small. Left without treatment, some patients with Hypomanic Episode may become manic later on. But many, especially those who have Bipolar II Disorder, have repeated Hypomanic Episodes. Hypomanic Episode isn't codable as a diagnosis; it forms the basis for Bipolar II Disorder and (debatably) for Cyclothymic Disorder. (Regarding Cyclothymic Disorder, see the Tip, p. 228)

Hypomanic Episode requires (1) a mood quality that (2) has existed for a required period of time, (3) is attended by a required number of symptoms, (4) has resulted in some degree of disability, and (5) does not violate any of the listed exclusions.

Quality of Mood

The quality of mood in Hypomanic Episode is usually euphoric, usually without the driven quality present in Manic Episode. However, irritability can also be a feature. Whatever the mood description, it is clearly different from the patient's usual nondepressed mood.

Duration

The patient must have had symptoms for a minimum of four days—a marginally shorter time requirement than that for Manic Episode.

Symptoms

The same number of symptoms from the same list are required as for Manic Episode: at least three of the symptoms must be present to an important degree during this four days. If the patient's *abnormal mood* is only irritable, four symptoms are required. Heightened *self-esteem* is never so grandiose that it becomes delusional. By definition, hypomanic patients are never psychotic.

The *sleep* of hypomanic patients may be brief, and *activity level* increases, sometimes to the point of agitation. Although the degree of agitation is less than in a Manic Episode, hypomanic patients can also feel driven and uncomfortable. *Judgment* deteriorates, and may lead to untoward consequences for finances or for work or social life. *Speech* may become rapid and pressured; *racing thoughts* or *flight of ideas* may be noticeable. *Easy distractibility* can be a feature of Hypomanic Episode. (In addition to the DSM-IV criteria, note that in Hypomanic Episode, as in Manic Episode, substance use is common.)

Impairment

How severe can the impairment be without qualifying as a Manic Episode? This is to some extent left to the judgment of the practitioner. Lapses of judgment, such as spending sprees and sexual indiscretions, can occur in either Manic or Hypomanic Episodes, but by definition, only the patient who is truly manic will be seriously impaired. If behavior becomes so extreme that hospitalization is needed, the label must be changed.

Exclusions

The exclusions are the same as those for Manic Episode. General medical conditions such as hyperthyroidism can produce hyperactive behavior; patients who misuse certain substances (especially amphetamines) will appear speeded up and may also report feeling strong, powerful, and euphoric.

Criteria for Hypomanic Episode

- For at least four days the patient has a distinct, sustained mood that is elevated, expansive, or irritable. This is different from the patient's usual nondepressed mood.
- During this time, the patient has persistently had three or more of the following symptoms (four if the only abnormality of mood is irritability); they have been present to an important degree:
  ✓ Grandiosity or exaggerated self-esteem
  ✓ Reduced need for sleep
  ✓ Increased talkativeness
  ✓ Flight of ideas or racing thoughts
  ✓ Easy distractibility
  ✓ Speeded-up psychomotor activity or increased goal-directed activity (social, sexual, work, or school)
  ✓ Poor judgment (as shown by spending sprees, sexual adventures, foolish investments)
- The patient has no features of psychosis (delusions, hallucinations, bizarre behavior or speech).
- These symptoms represent a distinct change from the patient's usual functioning.
- Other people can notice the change in mood and functioning.
- The episode does not require hospitalization or markedly impair work, social, or personal functioning.
- The symptoms are not directly caused by a general medical condition or the use of substances, including prescription medications.

Coding Notes

If a patient's Hypomanic Episode has been precipitated by somatic therapy (such as ECT, antidepressants, or bright light), it cannot be used as evidence of Bipolar II Disorder.

There are no severity codes for Hypomanic Episode.

MOOD DISORDERS BASED ON THE MOOD EPISODES

From this point, the format of my presentation differs somewhat from that of the DSM-IV and of the Quick Guide at the beginning of the chapter. Instead of discussing first the depressive and then the bipolar disorders, I discuss the mood disorders according to the degree to which their diagnosis involves one or more of the mood episode "building blocks" (Major Depressive, Manic, Mixed, and/or Hypomanic Episodes). In this section of the chapter, I discuss the disorders whose diagnosis depends on the involvement of mood episodes: Major Depressive Disorder, Single Episode and Recurrent; the various Bipolar I Disorders; and Bipolar II Disorder. The section following this covers the disorders that do *not* crucially involve these episodes.

296.2x Major Depressive Disorder, Single Episode

When a patient has had only one Major Depressive Episode and has never had a Manic or Hypomanic Episode, the diagnosis is Major Depressive Disorder. Of course, a patient who has a single episode today may have another episode months or years from now. Then the diagnosis would have to be changed to Major Depressive Disorder, Recurrent—or to Bipolar I Disorder, Most Recent Episode Depressed, or Bipolar II Disorder, if there has been a Manic or Mixed (Bipolar I) or Hypomanic (Bipolar II) Episode between the two Major Depressive Episodes.

Major Depressive Disorder usually begins in the middle to late 20s, but it can occur at any time of life, from childhood to old age. The onset may be sudden or gradual. Although episodes last on average from six to nine months, they range from a few weeks to many years. The cases of Adelaide Turner (p. 429) and Gerald Pratt (p. 47) also present patients who had a single episode of Major Depressive Disorder.

Criteria for Major Depressive Disorder, Single Episode

- The patient has one Major Depressive Episode.
- Schizoaffective Disorder doesn't explain the episode better, and it isn't superimposed on Schizophrenia, Schizophreniform Disorder, Delusional Disorder, or Psychotic Disorder Not Otherwise Specified.
- If the patient has ever had Manic, Mixed, or Hypomanic Episodes, *all* were directly precipitated by substance use or by antidepressant therapy (e.g., with ECT, medication, or bright light).

Coding Note

From Table 5.1, include any specifiers that apply to this Major Depressive Episode.

Brian Murphy

Brian Murphy had inherited a small business from his father and built it into a large one. When he sold out a few years later, he invested most of his money; with the rest, he bought a small almond farm in northern California. With his tractor, he handled most of the farm chores himself. Most years the farm earned a few hundred dollars, but as Brian was fond of pointing out, it really didn't make much difference. If he never made a dime, he felt he got "full value from keeping busy and fit."

When Brian was 55, his mood, which had always been normal, slid into depression. Farm chores seemed increasingly to be a burden; his tractor sat undriven in its shed.

As his mood blackened, Brian's body functioning seemed to deteriorate. Although he was constantly fatigued, often falling into bed by 9 P.M., he would invariably awaken at 2 or 3 A.M. Then obsessive worrying kept him awake until sunrise. Mornings were worst for him. The prospect of "another damn day to get through" seemed overwhelming. In the evenings he usually felt somewhat better, though he'd sit around working out sums on a magazine cover to see how much money they'd have if he "couldn't work the farm" and they had to live on their savings. His appetite deserted him. Although he never weighed himself, he had to buckle his belt two notches smaller than he had several months before.

"Brian just seemed to lose interest," his wife reported the day he was admitted to the hospital. "He doesn't enjoy anything any more. He spends all his time sitting around and worrying about being in debt. We owe a few hundred dollars on our credit card, but we pay it off every month!"

During the previous week or two, Brian had begun to ruminate about his health. "At first it was his blood pressure," his wife said. "He'd ask me to take it several times a day. I still work part-time as a nurse. Several times he thought he was having a stroke. Then yesterday he became convinced that his heart was going to stop. He'd get up, feel his pulse, pace around the room, lie down, put his feet above his head, do everything he could to 'keep it going.' That's when I decided to bring him here."

"We'll have to sell the farm." That was the first thing Brian said to the mental health clinician when they met. Brian was casually dressed and rather rumpled. He had prominent worry lines on his forehead, and he kept feeling for his pulse. Several times during the interview, he seemed unable to sit still; he would get up from the bed where he was sitting and pace over to the window.

His speech was slow but coherent. He talked mostly about his feelings of being poverty-stricken and his fears that the farm would have to go on the block. He denied having hallucinations, but admitted to feeling tired and "all washed up— not good for anything any more." He was fully oriented, had a full fund of information, and scored a perfect 30 on the Mini-Mental State Exam. He admitted that he was depressed, but he denied having thoughts about death. Somewhat reluctantly, he agreed that he needed treatment.

Evaluation of Brian Murphy

In the following (somewhat lengthy) discussion, the paragraph numbers refer to the steps in diagnosis of a mood disorder that I have listed beginning on p. 189.

1. The first step is to try to identify the current (and any previous) mood episodes. Brian Murphy had been ill much longer than two weeks. He had at least six of the symptoms (five necessary) for a Major Depressive Episode: low mood, loss of interest, fatigue, sleeplessness, low self-esteem, loss of appetite, and agitation. He was so seriously stressed that he required hospitalization. Although we do not have the results of his physical exam and laboratory testing, the vignette provides no history that would suggest a **general medical condition** (e.g., pancreatic carcinoma) or **substance use**. (His clinician should definitely ask about this—many people drink more when they are depressed.) He had not been recently **bereaved**. He was clearly severely depressed and different from his usual self. He would thus easily fulfill the criteria for **Major Depressive Episode**.

2. Next, what type of mood disorder did Brian have? There had been no Manic or Hypomanic Episodes, ruling out any form of **Bipolar I or II Disorder**. His delusions of poverty would suggest a psychotic disorder (such as **Schizoaffective Disorder**), but he had too few psychotic symptoms. He was deluded but had no other of the "A" criteria for Schizophrenia (see p. 144). His mood symptoms would rule out **Brief Psychotic Disorder** and **Delusional Disorder**. He would thus fulfill the criteria for Major Depressive Disorder.

3. There are just two subtypes of Major Depressive Disorder: **Single Episode** and **Recurrent**. Although Brian Murphy might subsequently have other episodes of depression, this was the only one so far. Therefore, the first part of his Axis I diagnosis would be: 296.2x (Major Depressive Disorder, Single Episode). Patients who have had only depressive episodes, but more than one, should be evaluated for Major Depressive Disorder, Recurrent (see the next diagnosis). If a patient who has been diagnosed as having Major Depressive Disorder, Single Episode, later

has a Manic, Hypomanic or Mixed Episode, the diagnosis will have to be changed to some form of Bipolar I or II Disorder. These are discussed later.

4. Now, consider the severity of Brian Murphy's depression (see the Coding Notes for Major Depressive Episode). Although he had most of the required symptoms, he was not suicidal (he feared death, but didn't want it). His delusion that he was poor and would have to sell the farm was mood-congruent—that is, in keeping with the usual cognitive themes of depression. (However, the thought that his heart would stop and the pulse checking were probably not delusional. They signified the overwhelming anxiety he felt about the state of his health.) The delusion would establish his depression as Severe With Psychotic Features. His Axis I coding would now be 296.24 (Major Depressive Disorder, Single Episode, Severe With Mood-Congruent Psychotic Features).

5. The Major Depressive Episode had been present for less than two years, so it would not be specified as Chronic.

6. Now consider the specifiers for the most recent episode, which are discussed at the end of this chapter. Brian had had no abnormalities of movement that would qualify him for With Catatonic Features; nor did his depression have Atypical Features (e.g., he didn't have increased appetite or sleep too much). Of course, he would not qualify for With Postpartum Onset. But his wife complained that he didn't "enjoy anything any more," suggesting that he might qualify for With Melancholic Features. He was agitated when interviewed (marked psychomotor slowing would have also qualified for this criterion), and he had lost considerable weight. He reported awakening early on many mornings (terminal insomnia). The interviewer did not ask him whether this episode of depression differed qualitatively from how he felt when his parents died, but it's a good bet that he would have agreed that it did. The Axis I diagnosis would now be 296.24 (Major Depressive Disorder, Single Episode, Severe With Mood-Congruent Psychotic Features, With Melancholic Features).

7. Because Brian had had only one episode, he could not qualify for any of the course specifiers—With or Without Full Interepisode Recovery, With Rapid Cycling, or With Seasonal Pattern. These criteria are also discussed at the end of the chapter. So the coding for Axis I would be complete as given above.

Although the prospect of using four different sets of criteria to code one patient may seem daunting, taking it one step at a time simplifies matters. The process is really quite logical and, once you get the hang of it, quick. The same basic methods should be applied to all examples of depression.

Some patients with severe depression also report many of the symptoms typical of **Panic Disorder, Generalized Anxiety Disorder**, or some other **anxiety disorder**. In such a case, two diagnoses may be made. Usually the mood disorder is listed first; it is often considered the primary diagnosis, with anxiety symptoms occurring as a part of the overall picture of Major Depressive Disorder.

The complete diagnosis for Brian Murphy would be as follows:

Axis I	296.24	Major Depressive Disorder, Single Episode, Severe With Mood-Congruent Psychotic Features, With Melancholic Features
Axis II	V71.09	No diagnosis
Axis III		None
Axis IV		None
Axis V	GAF = 51	(on admission)

296.3x Major Depressive Disorder, Recurrent

Roughly half the patients who have one Major Depressive Episode will have another. At the point of their developing a second episode, they are rediagnosed as having Major Depressive Disorder, Recurrent (at one time this was called *recurrent unipolar depression*). Perhaps 25% of these patients will eventually develop a Manic Episode, thereby requiring another rediagnosis: Bipolar Disorder. But most will have only depressions.

In a given patient, symptoms of depression remain pretty much the same from one episode to the next. These patients will have an episode about every four years; there is some evidence that the frequency of episodes increases with age. Multiple episodes of depression greatly increase the likelihood of suicide attempts and completed suicide. Patients with recurrent episodes are also much more likely than those with a single episode to be impaired by their disease.

Criteria for Major Depressive Disorder, Recurrent

- The patient has had at least two Major Depressive Episodes.
- Schizoaffective Disorder doesn't explain these episodes better, and they aren't superimposed on Schizophrenia, Schizophreniform Disorder, Delusional Disorder, or Psychotic Disorder Not Otherwise Specified.
- If the patient has ever had Manic, Mixed, or Hypomanic Episodes, *all* were precipitated by substance use or by antidepressant therapy (e.g., ECT, medication, or bright light).

Coding Notes

From Table 5.1, include any specifiers that apply to these Major Depressive Episodes.

To count as more than one, episodes must be separated by at least a two-month period during which the criteria for Major Depressive Episode are not fulfilled.

Aileen Parmeter

"I just know it was a terrible mistake to come here." For the third time, Aileen Parmeter got out of her chair and walked to her window. A wiry five feet two inches, this former Marine master sergeant (she had supervised a steno pool) weighed a scant 100 pounds. Through the slats of the venetian blinds she peered longingly at the freedom of the parking lot below. "I just don't know whatever made me come."

"You came because I asked you to," her therapist explained. "Your nephew called and said you were getting depressed again. It's just like last time."

"No, I don't think so. I was just upset," she explained patiently. "I had a little cold for a few days and couldn't play my tennis. I'll be fine if I just get back to my little apartment."

"Have you been hearing voices or seeing things this time?"

"Well, of course not." She seemed rather offended. "You might as well ask if I've been drinking."

After her last hospitalization, Aileen had been well for about 10 months. Although she had taken her medicine for only a few weeks, she had remained active until three weeks ago. Then she stopped seeing her friends and wouldn't play tennis because she "just didn't enjoy it." She worried constantly about her health and had been unable to sleep. Although she didn't complain of decreased appetite, she had lost about 10 pounds.

"Well, who wouldn't have trouble? I've just been too tired to get my regular exercise." She tried to smile, but it came off crooked and forced.

"Miss Parmeter, what about the suicidal thoughts?"

"I don't know what you mean."

"I mean, each time you've been here—last year, and two years before that—you were admitted because you tried to kill yourself."

"I'm going to be fine now. Just let me go home."

But her therapist, whose memory was long, had Aileen committed for observation and ordered a private room so she could be observed one-on-one.

At 3 A.M. Aileen got up, smiled wanly at the attendant, and went in to use the bathroom. Looping a strip she had torn from her sweatsuit over the top of the door, she tried to hang herself. As the silence lengthened, the attendant called out softly, then tapped on the door, then opened it and sounded the alarm.

The code team responded with no time to spare.

The following morning the therapist was back at her bedside. "Why did you try to do that, Miss Parmeter?"

"I didn't try to do anything. I must have been confused." She gingerly touched the purple bruises that ringed her neck. "This sure hurts. I know I'd feel better if you'd just let me go home."

Aileen remained hospitalized for 10 days. Once her sore neck would allow, she began to take her antidepressant medication again. Soon she was sleeping and eating normally, and she made a perfect score on the Mini-Mental State Exam. She was released to go home to her apartment and tennis, still uncertain why everyone had made such a fuss about her.

Evaluation of Aileen Parmeter

Aileen never acknowledged feeling depressed, but she had lost interest in her usual activities. This change had lasted longer than two weeks. As in previous episodes, her other symptoms included fatigue, insomnia, loss of weight, and suicidal behavior. (Although she reproached herself for entering the hospital, these feelings referred exclusively to her being ill and would not be scored as guilt.) She was sick enough to require hospitalization, fulfilling the criterion of impairment.

Aileen could have a **Mood Disorder Due to a General Medical Condition**, and this would have to be pursued by her therapist, but the history of recurrence would make this seem unlikely. Symptoms of apathy and memory can sometimes raise the question of dementia, but Aileen's Mini-Mental State Exam showed no evidence of memory impairment. She denied alcohol consumption, so **Substance-Induced Mood Disorder** would also appear unlikely (although this too would need to be pursued). She clearly met the criteria for **Major Depressive Episode**.

There was no evidence that Aileen had ever had a mania, hypomania, or psychosis; this would rule out **Bipolar I or II Disorder**. She would thus fulfill the criteria for some form of Major Depressive Disorder. She had had more than one episode separated by substantially more than two months, which would satisfy the requirement for the term Recurrent. Her preliminary Axis I diagnosis would thus be 296.3x (Major Depressive Disorder, Recurrent).

Next, consider the severity of her depression. It is always a problem how best to score someone with so little insight. Even with the suicide attempt, Aileen *appeared* barely to meet the five symptoms needed for Major Depressive Episode. According to the rules, she would receive a severity coding of no greater than Moderate. However, this would be inaccurate and possibly dangerous, for a patient this ill; one of her symptoms, suicidal behavior, was very severe indeed. The coding instructions are meant to be guides, not shackles. Aileen's depression should be coded as Severe.

Even though Aileen required hospitalization and made a serious suicide attempt, she emphatically denied delusions and hallucinations, so she would not qualify for Severe With Psychotic Features. Her Axis I diagnosis would now be 296.33 (Major Depressive Disorder, Recurrent, Severe Without Psychotic Features).

Aileen would not qualify for any of the specifiers for the most recent episode—perhaps because her lack of insight prevented her from providing full information. (With longer observation, she might qualify for With Melancholic Features, however.) The course specifier With Full Interepisode Recovery (p. 242) would also apply.

Other diagnoses are sometimes found in patients with Major Depressive Disorder, whether Single Episode or Recurrent. These include several of the anxiety disorders (especially **Obsessive–Compulsive Disorder**) and the **substance-related disorders** (especially **Alcohol Dependence** or **Abuse**). There is no evidence for any of these here, and Aileen's complete diagnosis would be as follows:

Axis I	296.33	Major Depressive Disorder, Recurrent, Severe Without Psychotic Features, With Full Interepisode Recovery
Axis II	V71.09	No diagnosis
Axis III		None
Axis IV		None
Axis V	GAF = 15	(on admission)
	GAF = 60	(at discharge)

Bipolar I Disorders

Bipolar I Disorder is shorthand for any cyclic mood disorder that includes at least one Manic Episode. Although this nomenclature has only been adopted within the past 20 years or so, the Bipolar I Disorders have been recognized for over a century. Formerly, they were collectively called manic–depressive illness; older clinicians may still refer to them this way. Men and women are about equally affected, for a total of approximately 1% of the general adult population. Bipolar Disorder is strongly hereditary.

DSM-IV mentions two technical points in evaluating episodes of Bipolar I (and II) Disorders. First, for an episode to count as a new episode, it must either represent a change of polarity (e.g., from Major Depressive Episode to Manic or Mixed Episode) or be separated from the previous one by a normal mood that lasts at least two months. Secondly, a Manic, Mixed, or Hypomanic Episode will occasionally seem to be precipitated by the treatment of a depression. Antidepressant drugs, ECT, or bright light (used to treat seasonal depression) may cause a patient to move rapidly from depression into a full-blown

Manic Episode. The bipolar disorders are defined by the occurrence of *spontaneous* depressions, manias, and hypomanias; therefore, any treatment-induced mood episode cannot be used to help make the diagnosis of a Bipolar I (or Bipolar II) condition.

Each of the six following brief sets of criteria includes the warning that the mood episodes must not be superimposed on a psychotic disorder—specifically Schizophrenia, Schizophreniform Disorder, Delusional Disorder, or Psychotic Disorder Not Otherwise Specified. Because the longitudinal course of a Bipolar I Disorder differs strikingly from those of the psychotic disorders, this should only rarely cause diagnostic problems.

> **TIP** Carefully inquire about symptoms of Alcohol Dependence in Bipolar I patients; alcoholism is diagnosed in as many as 30%. Often, the alcohol-related symptoms are the ones that are first apparent.

296.0x Bipolar I Disorder, Single Manic Episode

Having a single Manic Episode is not unusual, especially early in the course of Bipolar I Disorder. Of course, the vast majority of such patients will later have subsequent Major Depressive Episodes, as well as additional Manic Episodes. Bipolar males are more likely than females to have a Manic Episode as the first one. No patient vignette will be given here; the symptoms should be very similar to those of any other Manic Episode.

Criteria for Bipolar I Disorder, Single Manic Episode

- The patient has had just one Manic Episode and no Major Depressive Episodes.
- Schizoaffective Disorder doesn't explain the Manic Episode better, and it isn't superimposed on Schizophrenia, Schizophreniform Disorder, Delusional Disorder, or Psychotic Disorder Not Otherwise Specified.

Coding Notes

Specify Mixed: If a single episode meets the criteria for Mixed Episode (see p. 199), it would be recorded, for example, as 296.02 (Bipolar I Disorder, Single Manic Episode, Mixed, Moderate).

From Table 5.1, include any specifiers that apply to this Manic Episode.

> **TIP** Older patients who develop a mania for the first time may have a comorbid neurological disorder. They may also have a higher mortality. First-episode mania in the elderly may be quite a different illness from recurrent mania in the elderly, and should probably be given a different diagnosis, such as 296.80 (Bipolar Disorder Not Otherwise Specified).

296.4x Bipolar I Disorder, Most Recent Episode Manic

The Most Recent Episode category is for patients who are currently manic and have had at least one previous Manic, Major Depressive, or Mixed Episode. Usually this episode will be current, and the patient will have been admitted to a hospital. Occasionally, you might use this category for a new patient who is on lithium.

Criteria for Bipolar I Disorder, Most Recent Episode Manic

- The patient's most recent episode is a Manic Episode.
- The patient has had at least one previous Major Depressive, Manic, or Mixed Episode.
- Schizoaffective Disorder doesn't explain these episodes better, and they aren't superimposed on Schizophrenia, Schizophreniform Disorder, Delusional Disorder, or Psychotic Disorder Not Otherwise Specified.

Coding Notes

From Table 5.1, include any specifiers that apply to this Manic Episode or to the overall course of the disorder.

Elisabeth Jacks

Elisabeth Jacks was 38 years old and ran a catering service with her second husband, Donald, who was the main informant.

Elisabeth already had two grown children, so Donald could understand why this pregnancy might have upset her. But she had seemed unnaturally sad. From about her fourth month of pregnancy, she spent much of each day in bed. She didn't arise until afternoon, when she began to feel a little less tired. Her appetite, voracious during her first trimester, fell off, so that by the time of delivery she was several pounds lighter than usual for a full-term pregnancy. She had to give up keeping the household and business accounts, because she couldn't focus her attention long enough to add a column of figures. Still, the only time Donald became really alarmed was one evening at the beginning of Elisabeth's ninth month, when she told him that she had been thinking for days that she wouldn't survive childbirth and he would have to rear the baby without her. "You'll both be better off without me, anyway," she had said.

After their son was born, Elisabeth's mood brightened almost at once. The crying spells and the hours of rumination disappeared; briefly, she seemed almost her normal self. Late one Friday night, however, when the baby was three weeks old, Donald returned from catering a banquet to find Elisabeth dressed in nothing but bra and panties, icing a cake. Two other just-iced cakes were lined up on the counter, and the kitchen was littered with dirty pots and pans.

"She said she'd made one for each of us, and she wanted to party," Donald told the clinician. "I started to change the baby—he was howling in his basket—but she wanted to drag me off to the bedroom. She said 'Please, sweetie, it's been a long time.' I mean, even if I hadn't been dead tired, who could concentrate with the baby crying like that?"

On Saturday, Elisabeth was out all day with girlfriends, leaving Donald home with the baby. On Sunday she spent nearly $300 "for Christmas presents" at an April garage sale. She seemed to have boundless energy, sleeping only two or three hours a night before arising, rested and ready to go. On Monday she decided to open a bakery; by telephone, she tried to charge over $1,600 worth of kitchen supplies to their VISA card. She'd have done the same the next day, but she talked so fast that the person she called couldn't understand her. She hung up in frustration.

Elisabeth's behavior became so erratic that for the next two evenings Donald stayed off work to care for the baby, but his presence only seemed to provoke her sexual demands. Then there was the marijuana. Before Elisabeth became pregnant, she would have an occasional toke (she called it her "herbs"). During the past week, not all the smells in the house had been fresh-baked cake, so Donald thought she might be at it again.

Yesterday Elisabeth had shaken him awake at 5 A.M. and announced, "I am becoming God." That was when he had made the appointment to bring her for an evaluation.

Elisabeth herself could hardly sit still when she talked to the interviewer. In a burst of speech, she described her renewed energy and plans for the bakery. She volunteered that she had never felt better in her life. In rapid succession she then described how she was feeling (ecstatic), how it made her feel when she put on her best silk dress (sexy), where she had purchased the dress, how old she had been when she bought it, and to whom she was married at the time.

Evaluation of Elisabeth Jacks:

Elisabeth's case vignette provides a fairly typical picture of manic excitement. Her mood was definitely elevated. Aside from the issue of marijuana smoking (which appeared to be a symptom, not a cause), her relatively late age of onset was the only other symptom that was at all atypical.

For at least a week Elisabeth had had this high mood, accompanied by most of the other typical symptoms: reduced need for sleep, talkativeness, flight of ideas (a sample run is given in the vignette), and poor judgment (buying Christmas gifts at the April garage sale). Her disorder caused considerable distress, for her family if not for her; this is usual for patients with Manic Episode. The severity of the symptoms (not their number or type) and the degree of impairment were what would differentiate her full-blown **Manic Episode** from a **Hypomanic Episode**.

The issue of a **general medical condition** is not addressed in the vignette. Medical problems such as hyperthyroidism, multiple sclerosis, and brain tumors would have to be ruled out by the admitting clinician before a definitive diagnosis could be made. Although Elisabeth may have been smoking **marijuana**, misuse of this substance would never be confused with mania. Although the depression that occurred early in her pregnancy would have met the criteria for **Major Depressive Episode**, her current Manic Episode would obviate a **Major Depressive Disorder**. Because the current episode was too severe for hypomanic symptoms, she could not have **Cyclothymic Disorder**. Therefore, the diagnosis would have to be a **Bipolar I Disorder** (it could not be **Bipolar II**, because she was hospitalized).

The Bipolar I subtypes, as described earlier, are based upon the nature of the most recent episode. Elisabeth would meet the criteria for 296.4x (Bipolar I Disorder, Most Recent Episode Manic).

Next, score the severity of Elisabeth's mania (see the Coding Notes for Manic Episode). With slight changes, these severity codes are almost identical to those describing Major Depressive Episode. They are satisfactorily self-explanatory, though the clinician must differentiate among Mild, Moderate, and Severe With and Without Psychotic Features. Whether Elisabeth was actually psychotic is not made clear in the vignette. If it is taken literally, she thought she was becoming God, in which case she would qualify for Severe With Psychotic Features. These would be judged Mood-Congruent because grandiosity was quite in keeping with her exalted mood.

The only episode specifier that Elisabeth would qualify for would be With Postpartum Onset. She developed her Manic Episode within a few days of delivery. **Delirium** must be ruled out for any postpartum patient, but she was able to focus her attention well. Thus, the complete diagnosis would be as follows:

Axis I	296.44	Bipolar I Disorder, Most Recent Episode Manic, Severe With Mood-Congruent Psychotic Features, With Postpartum Onset
Axis II	V71.09	No diagnosis

Axis III	None
Axis IV	Childbirth
Axis V GAF = 25	(current)

296.40 Bipolar I Disorder, Most Recent Episode Hypomanic

In any given patient, symptoms of mood disorder tend to remain the same from one episode to the next. However, it is possible that after an initial Manic Episode, a subsequent mood upswing may be less severe, and therefore only Hypomanic. (By definition, the first episode of a Bipolar I Disorder cannot be Hypomanic.) I have provided no vignette for this disorder. However, I have described a Hypomanic Episode in the case of Iris McMaster, a patient with Bipolar II Disorder (see p. 219).

Criteria for Bipolar I Disorder, Most Recent Episode Hypomanic

- The patient's most recent episode is a Hypomanic Episode.
- The patient has previously had one or more Manic or Mixed Episodes.
- The symptoms cause clinically important distress or impair work, social, or personal functioning.
- Schizoaffective disorder doesn't explain the above episodes better, and they aren't superimposed on Schizophrenia, Schizophreniform Disorder, Delusional Disorder, or Psychotic Disorder Not Otherwise Specified.

Coding Note

From Table 5.1, include any specifiers that apply to the overall course of the disorder.

296.6x Bipolar I Disorder, Most Recent Episode Mixed

Mixed forms of mania and depression were described as far back as 1921 by Emil Kraepelin. The Mixed Episode designation may be used less often than it should be. Studies have shown that many manic patients have depressive features, but experts still argue about whether this really makes these patients different.

Criteria for Bipolar I Disorder, Most Recent Episode Mixed

- The patient's most recent episode is a Mixed Episode.
- The patient has had at least one Major Depressive, Manic, or Mixed Episode.
- Schizoaffective Disorder doesn't explain these episodes better, and they aren't superimposed on Schizophrenia, Schizophreniform Disorder, Delusional Disorder, or Psychotic Disorder Not Otherwise Specified.

Coding Note

From Table 5.1, include any specifiers that apply to this Mixed Episode or to the overall course of the disorder.

Winona Fisk

By the time she was 21, Winona Fisk had already had two lengthy mental health hospitalizations, one each for mania and depression. Then she was well for a year on maintenance lithium, which she discontinued abruptly in the spring of her junior year in college. She said she did it because she "felt so well." When two brothers brought her to the hospital 10 days later, she had been suspended for repeatedly disrupting classes with her boisterous behavior.

On the ward, Winona's behavior was mostly a picture of manic excitement. She spoke nonstop and was constantly on the move, often rummaging through other patients' purses and lockers. But many of the thoughts flooding her mind were so sad that for 8 or 10 days she often spontaneously wept for several minutes at a time. She said she felt depressed and guilty, not for her behavior in class, but for being such a burden to her family. During these brief episodes, she claimed to hear the heart of her father beating from his grave. She often expressed the wish to join him in death. She ate little and lost 15 pounds; she often awakened weeping at night and was unable to get back to sleep.

Nearly a month's treatment with lithium, carbamazepine, and neuroleptics was largely futile. Her mood disorder eventually yielded to six bilateral ECT sessions.

Evaluation of Winona Fisk:

Winona's two previous episodes of Bipolar I Disorder would make that diagnosis crystal clear. The only remaining tasks would be to decide about the most recent episode and code its severity.

Typically enough, Winona's episode began with feeling "too good" to be ill; that got her into trouble with her lithium. Once she was hospitalized, her symptoms fulfilled criteria for Manic Episode. But at times throughout the day, she did have "microdepressions" during which she experienced several depressive symptoms. If the time requirement could be ignored, these would be enough to qualify for a diagnosis of Major Depressive Episode. This would fulfill the criteria for a Mixed Episode.

The severity of Winona's episode could be judged on the basis of either the dominant symptoms or the worst symptoms, depending on which set conveyed more information. For most of the day Winona was manic, but during her depressive episodes she had mood-congruent psychotic symptoms (hearing the heartbeat of her dead father). Her clinician felt that coding the psychotic symptoms would give more information about severity.

What about the episode and course specifiers? With Melancholic Features might apply to Winona (she awakened early, felt guilty, and lost weight). However, this qualifier is supposed to describe only a Major Depressive Episode, and we have already established that most of the time the symptoms of her current episode were manic. As for the course specifiers, the vignette notes that she was well for a year between her second and her current hospitalizations, so With Full Interepisode Recovery would apply.

Winona's five-axis diagnosis would be as follows:

Axis I	296.64	Bipolar I Disorder, Most Recent Episode Mixed, Severe With Mood-Congruent Psychotic Features, With Full Interepisode Recovery
Axis II	V71.09	No diagnosis
Axis III		None
Axis IV		Suspended from school
Axis V	GAF = 25	(on admission)

296.5x Bipolar I Disorder, Most Recent Episode Depressed

Most Recent Episode Depressed will be one of the most frequently used of the Bipolar I subtypes; nearly all Bipolar I patients will receive this diagnosis at some point during their lifetimes. The depressive symptoms will be very much like those of Brian Murphy (p. 204) and Aileen Parmeter (p. 208), each of whom had Major Depressive Disorder. Elisabeth Jacks (p. 212), whose current episode was manic, was depressed just before she became manic.

TIP Investigators who have followed bipolar patients for many years report that some have only manias. The concept of "unipolar mania" has been debated off and on for a long time. There may be some such patients who will never have a depression, but most will, if followed long enough. I have known of patients who had seven episodes of mania over a 20-year period before finally having a first attack of depression. The importance here is that all Bipolar I (and II) patients should be warned to watch out for depressive symptoms, which can be deadly!

Criteria for Bipolar I Disorder, Most Recent Episode Depressed

- The patient's most recent episode is a Major Depressive Episode.
- The patient has had at least one previous Manic or Mixed Episode.
- Schizoaffective Disorder doesn't explain these episodes better, and they aren't superimposed on Schizophrenia, Schizophreniform Disorder, Delusional Disorder, or Psychotic Disorder Not Otherwise Specified.

Coding Note

From Table 5.1, include any specifiers that apply to this Major Depressive Episode or to the overall course of the disorder.

296.7 Bipolar I Disorder, Most Recent Episode Unspecified

A patient's Bipolar I Disorder might be coded Most Recent Episode Unspecified if the coder (e.g., a medical records clerk) had insufficient information to specify a more precise subtype. Mental health professionals should themselves have little occasion to use this code. Note that it has only four digits. Because the episode type is unknown, no episode specifiers can apply.

Criteria for Bipolar I Disorder, Most Recent Episode Unspecified

- Other than duration, the patient currently or recently meets criteria for a Major Depressive, Manic, Mixed, or Hypomanic Episode.
- The patient has had at least one previous Manic or Mixed Episode.
- These symptoms cause clinically important distress or impair work, social, or personal functioning.
- Schizoaffective Disorder doesn't explain these episodes better, and they aren't superimposed on Schizophrenia, Schizophreniform Disorder, Delusional Disorder, or Psychotic Disorder Not Otherwise Specified.
- The symptoms are not directly caused by a general medical condition or the use of substances, including prescription medications.

Coding Note

From Table 5.1, include any specifiers that apply to the overall course of the disorder.

296.89 Bipolar II Disorder

Bipolar II Disorder is not only a recent term; the *concept* itself was little known until the past two decades. Bipolar I and Bipolar II patients have very similar symptoms. The important distinction is the degree of disability and discomfort imposed by the high phase, which, by definition, never leads to psychosis and never requires hospitalization in Bipolar II. Bipolar II patients have recurrent Major Depressive Episodes interspersed with Hypomanic Episodes.

Like Bipolar I, Bipolar II must be diagnosed on the basis of mood episodes that arise spontaneously. Don't count Hypomanic Episodes precipitated by antidepressants, ECT, or bright light therapy. (In such a case, ask the patient and informants whether there has been another Hypomanic Episode that wasn't precipitated by treatment—many patients will have had one.)

Women may be more prone than men to develop Bipolar II Disorder (the sexes are about equally represented in Bipolar I Disorder); fewer than 1% of the general adult population are affected. Sal Camozzi was another patient with Bipolar II Disorder; his history is given in the section on Insomnia Related to an Axis I Disorder (p. 426).

Criteria for Bipolar II Disorder

- The patient has had at least one Major Depressive Episode.
- The patient has had at least one Hypomanic Episode.
- There have been no Manic or Mixed Episodes.
- Schizoaffective Disorder doesn't explain these episodes better, and they aren't superimposed on Schizophrenia, Schizophreniform Disorder, Delusional Disorder, or Psychotic Disorder Not Otherwise Specified.
- These symptoms cause clinically important distress or impair work, social, or personal functioning.

Coding Notes

Specify current or most recent episode:

Hypomanic

Depressed

From Table 5.1, include any specifiers that apply to the most recent episode if it is Major Depressive, or to the overall course of the disorder.

Iris McMaster

"I'm a writer," said Iris McMaster. It was her first visit to the interviewer's office, and she wanted to smoke. She fiddled with a cigarette and didn't seem to know what to do with it. "It's what I do for a living. I should be home doing it now—it's my life. Maybe I'm the finest creative writer since Dostoevsky. But my friend Charlene said I should come in, so I've taken time away from working on my play and my comic novel, and here I am." She finally put the cigarette back into the pack.

"Why did Charlene think you should come?"

"She thinks I'm high. Of course I'm high. I'm always high when I'm in my creative phase. Only she thinks I'm too nervous." Iris was slender and of average height; she wore a bright pink spring outfit. She looked longingly at her pack of cigarettes. "God, I need one of those."

Her speech could always be interrupted, but it was salted with bon mots, neat turns of phrase, and original similes. But Iris was also able to give a coherent history. She was 45, was married to an engineer, and had a daughter who was nearly 18. And she really was a writer who had sold articles about a wide variety of subjects to women's magazines over the last several years.

For three or four months Iris had been in one of her high phases, cranking out an enormous volume of essays on wide-ranging topics. Her "wired" feeling was uncomfortable in a way, but it hadn't troubled her because she felt so productive. Whenever she was creating, she didn't need much sleep. A two-hour nap would leave her rested and ready for another 10 hours at the word processor. At those times, her husband would fix his own meals and kid her about having "a one-track mind."

Iris never ate much during her high phases, and she lost weight. But she didn't get herself into trouble: no sexual indiscretions, no excessive spending ("I'm always too busy to shop"). And she volunteered that she had never "seen visions, heard voices or had funny ideas about people following me around." She had never spent time "in the funny farm."

As Iris paused to gather her thoughts, her fingers clutched the cigarette package. She shook her head almost imperceptibly. Without uttering another word, she grabbed her purse, arose from her chair, and swooped out the door. It was the last the interviewer saw of her for a year and a half.

In November of the following year, a person who seemed like an impostor announced herself as Iris McMaster and dropped into the office chair. She had gained 30 or 40 pounds, which she had stuffed into ill-fitting, tacky slacks and a bulky knit sweater.

"As I was saying," were the first words she uttered. Just for a second, the corners of her mouth twitched up. But for the rest of the hour she soberly talked about her latest problem: writer's block. About a year ago, she had finished her play and was well into her comic novel when the muse deserted her. For months now, she had been arising around lunchtime and spending long afternoons staring at her word processor. "Sometimes I don't even turn it on!" she said. She couldn't focus her thinking sharply enough to create anything that seemed worth saving. Most nights she tumbled into bed at 9. She felt tired and heavy, as if her legs were made of bricks.

"It's cheesecake, actually," was the way Iris explained her weight gain. "I have it delivered. For months I haven't been interested enough to cook for myself." She hadn't been suicidal, but the only time she felt much better was when Charlene took her out to lunch. Then she ate and made conversation pretty much as she used to. "I've done that quite a lot recently, as anyone can see." Once she returned home, the depression quickly returned.

Finally, Iris apologized for walking out a year and a half ago. "I didn't think I was the least bit sick," she said, "and all I really wanted to do was get back to my computer and get your character on paper!"

Evaluation of Iris McMaster

This discussion will focus on the episode of elevated mood Iris had during her first visit. There are two possibilities for such an episode: Manic and Hypomanic Episodes. As far as the time requirement was concerned, Iris could have had either type of episode—Hypomanic requires four days, Manic one week. She admitted that she felt "wired," and this feeling had apparently been sustained for several months. It was also abnormal for her. During her high phase, she had at least four symptoms (three required): high self-esteem, decreased need for sleep, talkativeness, and increased goal-directed activity (writing).

The elevated mood of a Manic Episode is described as "abnormally and persistently" elevated, whereas that of a Hypomanic Episode need be only "sustained" and "different from the usual nondepressed mood" (see the criteria sets). This distinction has perhaps too little difference, and requires some judgment on the part of the clinician. The real distinction between hypomania and mania consists in the effects of the mood disturbance upon patient and surroundings. Manic Episodes cause marked impairment of functioning, whereas Hypomanic Episodes do not. During her high spells, Iris's writing productivity actually increased, and her social relationships (those with her husband and friends) did not appear to suffer.

Assuming that Iris had no **general medical condition** or **Substance-Induced Mood Disorder**, she could have one of three mood disorders: Bipolar I, Bipolar II, or Cyclothymic Disorder. Judged from lack of hospitalizations and of psychosis, Iris had never had a true mania; this would rule out **Bipolar I Disorder**. Also, her mood swings were relatively few, not numerous, as would be required for a diagnosis of **Cyclothymic Disorder**.

The only remaining category, then, would be **Bipolar II Disorder**. But to qualify for that diagnosis, there must be at least one Major Depressive Episode. On Iris's second visit to the clinician, her depressive symptoms included feeling depressed most of the time, weight gain, hypersomnia, fatigue, and poor concentration (her "writer's block"), which would fulfill criteria for Major Depressive Episode. If her depression had not met the criteria for Major Depressive Episode, her diagnosis would have been **Mood Disorder Not Otherwise Specified**. This diagnosis would also be appropriate for a patient who had never had a depression but had been interviewed after only one Hypomanic Episode.

In coding Bipolar II Disorder, clinicians are asked to specify the most recent episode. Iris's was a depression. Although Bipolar II Disorder allows no room for a fifth-digit severity code, her clinician wanted to describe the severity of her depressive episode. This would provide a baseline from which to judge later improvement. She had only the minimum number of symptoms needed for Major Depressive Episode, but her work had been seriously impaired. A severity of Moderate seemed appropriate (this is mirrored in her GAF score). If further interview revealed additional (or more serious) symptoms, Severe Without Psychotic Features should be considered. These specifiers leave leeway for the clinician's judgment.

None of the course specifiers applied, but Iris had a number of symptoms of the episode specifier With Atypical Features. Her mood seemed to brighten when she was having lunch with her friend; she also gained weight, slept excessively, and had a sensation of heaviness in her limbs. With a total of four of these symptoms (only three are required), at the time of the second interview her full diagnosis would read:

Axis I	296.89	Bipolar II Disorder, Depressed, Moderate, With Atypical Features
Axis II	V71.09	No diagnosis
Axis III		None
Axis IV		None
Axis V	GAF = 60	(current)

ADDITIONAL MOOD DISORDERS

As I have shown up to this point, many of the mood disorder patients seen in a mental health practice can be diagnosed by referring to Manic, Hypomanic, Mixed, and Major Depressive Episodes. These four types of mood episodes must be ruled out for any patient with mood symptoms. Several other conditions that do not involve these episodes will be considered next.

300.4 Dysthymic Disorder

Dysthymic patients are chronically depressed. They have many of the same symptoms that are found in Major Depressive Episodes, including low mood, fatigue, hopelessness, trouble concentrating, and problems with appetite and sleep. Absent from the criteria are thoughts of death or suicidal ideas. We aren't allowed to diagnose Dysthymia if the patient has ever had a Manic or Hypomanic Episode. These patients typically regard their chronic low mood as normal, and their disorder sometimes used to be called *depressive personality disorder* or *depressive neurosis*.

In the course of their lifetimes, perhaps 6% of adults have Dysthymic Disorder. Because they suffer quietly and are not severely disabled, such individuals often don't come to light until a Major Depressive Episode supervenes. This is the fate of many dysthymic patients, who often seem to have a personality change after beginning treatment. In 1993 this phenomenon was recounted in a book that made the *New York Times* best-seller list: *Listening to Prozac*. However, the astonishing response to medication this book reported is by no means limited to one drug.

TIP A patient who has Dysthymic Disorder for two years, then develops Major Depressive Episode, can be given both diagnoses. (A patient can also have had a *previous* Major Depressive Episode, provided that there was a full recovery—no important symptoms—for at least two months before the Dysthymic Disorder began.) These situations are sometimes called *double depression*.

Criteria for Dysthymic Disorder

- On the majority of days for two years or more, the patient reports depressed mood or appears depressed to others for most of the day.
- When depressed, the patient has two or more of these:
  - ✓ Appetite decreased or increased
  - ✓ Sleep decreased or increased
  - ✓ Fatigue or low energy
  - ✓ Poor self-image
  - ✓ Reduced concentration or indecisiveness
  - ✓ Hopeless feelings
- During this two-year period, the above symptoms are never absent longer than two consecutive months.
- During the first two years of this syndrome, the patient has not had a Major Depressive Episode.

- The patient has had no Manic, Hypomanic, or Mixed Episodes.
- The patient has never fulfilled criteria for Cyclothymic Disorder.
- The disorder does not exist *solely* in the context of a chronic psychosis (such as Schizophrenia or Delusional Disorder).
- The symptoms are not directly caused by a general medical condition or the use of substances, including prescription medications.
- The symptoms cause clinically important distress or impair work, social, or personal functioning.

Coding Notes

Specify whether:

Early Onset, if it begins by age 20.

Late Onset, if it begins at age 21 or later.

From Table 5.1, the only specifier that can apply is With Atypical Features.

In children, the abnormal mood may be one of irritability, and the time required is only one year.

A Major Depressive Episode may precede Dysthymic Disorder if it has remitted for a full two months before Dysthymic Disorder begins. Also, Dysthymic Disorder may begin first, if it lasts at least two years before a Major Depressive Disorder begins. In this case, the two diagnoses may be made together.

Noah Sanders

For Noah Sanders, life had never seemed much fun. He was 18 when he first noticed that most of the time he "just felt down." Although he was bright and studied hard, throughout college he was often distracted by thoughts that he didn't measure up to his classmates. He landed a job with a leading electronics firm, but turned down several promotions because he felt that he could not cope with added responsibility. It took dogged determination and long hours of work to compensate for this "inherent second-rateness." The effort left him chronically tired. Even his marriage and the birth of his two daughters only relieved his gloom for a few weeks at a time, at best. His self-confidence was so low that, by common consent, his wife always made most of their family's decisions.

"It's the way I've always been. I am a professional pessimist," Noah told his family doctor one day when he was in his early 30s. The doctor replied that he had a depressive personality.

For many years that description seemed to fit. Then, when Noah was in his early 40s, his younger daughter left home for college; after this, he began to feel increasingly that life had passed him by. Over a period of several months, his depression deepened. He had worsened to the point that he now felt he had never really been depressed before. Even visits from his daughters, which had always cheered him up, failed to improve his outlook.

Usually a sound sleeper, Noah began awakening at about 4 A.M. and ruminating over his mistakes. His appetite fell off and he lost weight. When for the third time in a week his wife found him weeping in their bedroom, he confessed that he had felt so guilty about his failures that he thought they'd all be better off without him. She decided that he needed treatment.

Noah was started on an antidepressant medication. Within two weeks, his mood had brightened and he was sleeping soundly; at one month, he had "never felt better" in his life. Whereas he had once avoided oral presentations at work, he began to look forward to them as "a chance to show what I could do." His chronic fatigue faded, and he began jogging to use up some of his excess energy. In his spare time, he started his own small business to develop and promote some of his engineering innovations.

Noah remained on his medication. On the two or three occasions when he and his therapist tried to reduce it, he found himself relapsing into his old, depressive frame of mind. He continues to operate his small business as a sideline.

Evaluation of Noah Sanders:

For most of his adult life, Noah's mood symptoms were chronic, rather than acute or recurring. He was never without these symptoms for longer than a few weeks at a time, and they were present most days. They included general pessimism, low self-esteem, and chronic tiredness. His indecisiveness encouraged his wife to assume the role of family decision maker. The way he felt was not different from his usual self; in fact, he said it was the way he had always been. That and the duration are the main features that differentiate Dysthymic Disorder from a **Major Depressive Episode**.

The differential diagnosis of Dysthymic Disorder is essentially the same as for Major Depressive Disorder. **Mood Disorder Due to a General Medical Condition** and **Substance-Induced Mood Disorder** must be ruled out. The remarkable chronicity and poor self-image invite speculation that Noah's difficulties might be explained by a personality disorder, such as **Avoidant** or **Dependent Personality Disorder**. The vignette does not address all the criteria that would be necessary to make those diagnoses. However, an important diagnostic principle holds that the more treatable conditions should be diagnosed (and treated) *first*. If, despite relief of the mood disorder, Noah continued to be shy and awkward and to have a negative self-image, an Axis II diagnosis would be considered.

Noah would also qualify for a diagnosis of **Major Depressive Disorder,**

Single Episode. According to the Coding Notes, both diagnoses could be made because Dysthymic Disorder had been present well over two years before the Major Depression began. Without psychotic features, he had quite a number of depressive symptoms (including thoughts about death) which would suggest that he was severely ill. None of the course specifiers would apply to Noah's Major Depressive Disorder, but the following symptoms would meet the criteria for the episode specifier With Melancholic Features: He no longer reacted positively to pleasurable stimuli (being with his daughters); he described his mood as a definite change from normal; and he reported guilt feelings, early morning awakening, and loss of appetite.

Once treated, Noah seemed to undergo a personality change. His mood lightened and his behavior changed to the point that, by contrast, he seemed almost hypomanic. However, these symptoms were not "unequivocal" for a Hypomanic Episode, so a diagnosis of Dysthymic Disorder would not be excluded. (Also, remember that a Hypomanic Episode precipitated by treatment does not count *toward* a diagnosis of Bipolar II Disorder. It should not count *against* the diagnosis of Dysthymic Disorder, either.)

Noah's Dysthymic Disorder had been present since late adolescence, so it should be coded as Early Onset. The only other possible qualifier would be With Atypical Features, which he did not have.

The full diagnosis of Noah Sanders would be as follows:

Axis I	296.23	Major Depressive Disorder, Single Episode, Severe Without Psychotic Features, With Melancholic Features
	300.4	Dysthymic Disorder, Early Onset
Axis II	799.9	Diagnosis deferred
Axis III		None
Axis IV		None
Axis V	GAF = 50	(on admission)
	GAF = 90	(at discharge)

301.13 Cyclothymic Disorder

Cyclothymic patients are chronically either elated or depressed, but they never fulfill criteria for a Manic, Mixed, or Major Depressive Episode. Cyclothymic Disorder was at one time regarded as a personality disorder. This may have been partly due to the fact that it begins so gradually and lasts such a long time. Studies of genetics and treatment response suggest that, like Dysthymic Disorder, it is more accurately (and safely, because it can often be treated easily with medication) classified with the bipolar mood disorders.

Criteria for Cyclothymic Disorder

- For at least two years, the patient has had many periods of hypomanic symptoms (see p. 200) and many periods of low mood that don't fulfill criteria for a Major Depressive Episode.
- The longest the patient has been free of mood swings during this period is two months.
- During the first two years of this disorder, the patient has not fulfilled criteria for a Manic, Mixed, or Major Depressive Episode.
- Schizoaffective Disorder doesn't explain the disorder better, and it isn't superimposed on Schizophrenia, Schizophreniform Disorder, Delusional Disorder, or Psychotic Disorder Not Otherwise Specified.
- The symptoms are not directly caused by a general medical condition or the use of substances, including prescription medications.
- These symptoms cause clinically important distress or impair work, social, or personal functioning.

Coding Notes

In children and adolescents, the time required is only one year.

After the required two years (one for children), a Manic, Mixed, or Major Depressive Episode may be superimposed on the Cyclothymic Disorder. Then a Bipolar I or II diagnosis may be made concomitantly with the Cyclothymic Disorder diagnosis.

Honey Bare

"I'm a yo-yo!"

Without her feathers and sequins, Honey Bare looked anything but provocative. She had begun life as Melissa Schwartz, but she loved using her stage name. The stage in question was Hoofer's, one of the bump-and-grind joints that thrived near the waterfront. The billboard proclaimed that it was "Only a Heartthrob Away" from the Navy recruiting station. Ever since she'd dropped out of college four years before, Honey had been a front-liner in the four-girl show at Hoofer's. Every afternoon on her way to work she passed right by the mental health clinic, but this was her first visit inside.

"In our current gig, I play the Statue of Liberty. I receive the tired, the poor, and the huddled masses. Then I take off my robes."

"Is that a problem?" the interviewer wanted to know.

Most of the time, it wasn't. Honey liked her little corner of show biz. When the fleet was in, she played to thunderous applause. "In fact, I enjoy just about everything I do. I don't drink much, and I never do drugs, but I go to parties. I sing in our church choir, go to movies—I enjoy art films quite a bit." When she felt well, she slept little, talked a lot, started a hundred projects, and even finished some of them. "I'm really a happy person—when I'm feeling up."

But every couple of months there'd be a week or two when Honey didn't enjoy much of anything. She'd go to work and paste a smile on her face, but when the curtain rang down, the smile came off with her makeup. She was never suicidal, and her sleep and appetite didn't suffer; her energy and concentration were normal. But it was as if all the fizz had gone out of her ginger ale. She could see no obvious cause for her mood swings, which had been going on for years. She could count on the fingers of her hands the number of weeks she had been "just normal."

Lately Honey had acquired a boyfriend, a chief petty officer who wanted to marry her. He said he loved her because she was so vivacious and enthusiastic, but he had only seen her when she was bubbly. Always before, when she was depressed, he had been out to sea. Now he had written that he was being transferred to shore duty, and she feared it would be the end of their relationship. At the thought, two large tears trickled down her cheeks through the mascara.

Four months and several visits later, Honey was back, wearing a smile. The lithium carbonate, she reported, seemed to be working well. The peaks and valleys of her moods had smoothed out to rolling hills. She was still playing the Statue of Liberty down at Hoofer's.

"My sailor's been back for nearly three months," she said with a smile, "and he's still carrying the torch for me."

> **TIP** DSM-IV is uncharacteristically coy as to whether the hypomanic periods in Cyclothymic Disorder must meet the *criteria* for Hypomanic Episode, as opposed to only having some of the *symptoms*. It is implied by the note (p. 365 of DSM-IV) explaining that after two years Bipolar II Disorder may also be diagnosed if a Major Depressive Episode develops. Of course, if the patient did not meet criteria for a Hypomanic Episode, this would not be possible.

Evaluation of Honey Bare

The first and most obvious question is this: Had Honey ever met the criteria for either a Manic or a Major Depressive Episode? From the vignette, the answer would appear to be "No." When feeling down, she had no vegetative symptoms (problems with sleep or appetite) of **Major Depressive Episode**. She had normal concentration, had never been suicidal, and did not complain of feeling worthless. When she was "up," she had hypomanic symptoms (talkative, more active than at other times), and would meet the criteria for Hypomanic Episode.

Honey would fulfill criteria for **Cyclothymic Disorder**. She has had many mood swings; only infrequently was her mood neither high nor low. Because she was never psychotic, she could not qualify for a diagnosis such as **Schizoaffective Disorder**. She didn't use drugs or alcohol, ruling out a **Substance-Induced Mood Disorder**. **Bipolar I, Bipolar II**, and **Major Depressive Disorders** are ruled out due to the lack of Manic and Major Depressive Episodes. However, because they too involve so many swings of mood, either **Bipolar I** or **II With Rapid Cycling** can sometimes be confused with Cyclothymic Disorder.

By definition, Cyclothymic Disorder is relatively mild. Because its phases shift so rapidly, no attempt is made to characterize its most recent episode as hypomanic or depressed. Therefore, additional fourth- and fifth-digit coding is unnecessary. Episode and course specifiers are not relevant to this diagnosis. Honey's complete diagnosis would be as follows:

Axis I	301.13	Cyclothymic Disorder
Axis II	V71.09	No diagnosis
Axis III		None
Axis IV		None
Axis V	GAF = 70	(on admission)
	GAF = 90	(current)

293.83 Mood Disorder Due to a General Medical Condition

Many medical conditions can cause depression; some can cause manic symptoms as well. It is vital always to consider general medical conditions when evaluating a mood disorder. This is not only because they are treatable—with today's therapeutic options, most mood disorders are highly treatable. It is because some of the general medical conditions themselves, if left inadequately treated too long, have serious consequences (including death). The following vignette illustrates the importance of keeping in mind medical conditions as possible causes of a mood disorder.

Criteria for Mood Disorder Due to a General Medical Condition

- The patient's clinical presentation is dominated by a mood disorder that persists and is characterized by *either or both* of these:
  ✓ Depressed mood *or* markedly decreased interest or pleasure in nearly all activities, *or*

✓ Mood that is elevated, expansive, or irritable.
- History, physical exam, or laboratory findings suggest a general medical condition that seems likely to have directly caused these symptoms.
- No other mental disorder (such as Adjustment Disorder With Depressed Mood secondary to having a medical disorder) better accounts for these symptoms.
- The symptoms don't occur solely during a delirium.
- These symptoms cause clinically important distress or impair work, social, or personal functioning.

Coding Notes

Specify whether:

With Manic Features. Mood is mainly elevated or irritable.

With Depressive Features. Mood is mainly depressed, but criteria for a Major Depressive Episode are not fulfilled.

With Major Depressive-Like Episode. All criteria for a Major Depressive Episode (other than the general medical condition exclusion) are fulfilled.

With Mixed Features. Manic and depressive symptoms are present in about equal proportions.

Depression associated with the general medical condition of Alzheimer's or Vascular Dementia is designated as part of the Axis I code for that dementia (see pp. 30 and 35). Depression that occurs with other dementias must be coded separately on Axis I.

On Axis III, code the specific general medical condition that has caused the mood disorder. The name of the specific general medical condition also goes into the Axis I diagnosis.

Lisa Voorhees

By the time she arrived at the mental health clinic, Lisa Voorhees had already seen three doctors. All of them thought that her problems were entirely mental. Although she had "been 39 for several years," she was slender and smart, and she knew that she was attractive to men.

She intended to stay that way. Her job as personal secretary to the chairman of the Department of English and Literature at a large Midwestern university introduced her to a lot of eligible males. And that was where Lisa first noticed the problem that made her think she was losing her mind.

"It was this gorgeous assistant professor of Romance languages," she told the interviewer. "He was always in and out of the office, and I'd done everything short of sexual harassment to get him to notice me. Then one day last spring, he asked me out to dinner and a show. And I turned him down! I just wasn't interested. It was as if my sex drive had gone on strike!"

For several weeks she continued to feel uninterested in men, and then one morning she "woke up next to some odious creep from the provost's office" she'd been avoiding for months. She felt disgusted with herself, but they made love again, anyway, before she kicked him out.

For the next several months, Lisa's sexual appetite would suddenly change every two or three weeks. Privately, she had begun to call it "The Turn of the Screw" and wondered if she was going mad. During her active phase, she felt airy and light, and could pound away at her word processor 12 hours a day. But the rest of the time, nothing pleased her. She was a grouch at the office, slept badly (and alone), and joked that her keyboard was conspiring to make her feel clumsy.

Even Lisa's wrists felt weak. She had bought a wrist rest to use when she was typing, and that helped for a while. But she could find neither splint nor tonic for the fluctuations of her sex drive. One doctor told her it was "the change" and prescribed estrogen; another diagnosed "manic–depression" and offered lithium. A third suggested pastoral counseling, but instead she had come to the clinic.

In frustration, Lisa arose from her chair and paced to the window and back.

"Wait a minute—do that again," the interviewer ordered.

"Do what? All I did was walk across the room."

"I know. How long have you had that limp?"

"I don't know. Not long, I guess. What with the other problems, I hardly noticed. Does it matter?"

It proved to be the key. Three visits to a neurologist, some X-rays, and an MRI later, Lisa's diagnosis was multiple sclerosis. The neurologist explained that multiple sclerosis sometimes caused mood swings, and referred her back to the mental health clinic for therapy.

Evaluation of Lisa Voorhees

On paper, the various criteria sets make reasonably clear-cut the differences between mood disorders with "emotional" causes and those caused by general medical conditions or substance use. In practice, it is not always obvious.

Lisa's mood symptoms alternated between periods of highs and lows. Although they lasted two weeks or longer, none of these extremes was severe enough to qualify as a **Manic**, **Hypomanic**, or **Major Depressive Episode**. The depressed period was too brief for **Dysthymic Disorder**; the whole episode had not lasted long enough for **Cyclothymic Disorder**; and there was no evidence of a **Substance-Induced Mood Disorder**.

Mood Disorder Due to a General Medical Condition must fulfill two important criteria. The first criterion is that symptoms must be directly produced by physiological mechanisms of the illness itself, not simply by an emotional reaction to having the illness. For example, patients with illnesses such as multiple sclerosis and cancer of the head of the pancreas are known to have a special risk of depression, and not just as a reaction to the news or continuing stress of having a serious medical problem.

Several lines of evidence could bear on a causal relationship between a medical condition and mood symptoms. A connection may exist if the mood disorder is more severe than the general medical symptoms seem to warrant or than the psychological impact would be on most people. However, such a connection would *not* be presumed if the mood symptoms begin before the patient learns of the general medical condition. Similar mood symptoms developing upon the disclosure of a *different* medical problem would argue against a diagnosis of Mood Disorder Due to a General Medical Condition. By contrast, arguing for a connection would be clinical features different from those usual for a primary mood disorder (such as atypical age of onset). None of these conditions obtained in the case of Lisa Voorhees.

A known pathological mechanism that can explain the development of the mood symptoms in physiological terms obviously argues strongly in favor of a causal relationship. Multiple sclerosis, affecting many areas of the brain, would appear to satisfy this criterion. A high percentage of patients with multiple sclerosis have reported mood swings. Periods of euphoria have also been reported in these patients; anxiety may be more common still.

Many other medical conditions can cause depression. Examples include **medications**, such as reserpine and methyldopa, and other **toxins**. **Endocrine disorders** are also important causes: Hypothyroidism and hypoadrenocorticalism are associated with depressive symptoms, whereas hyperthyroidism and hyperadrenocorticalism are linked with manic or hypomanic symptoms. **Infectious diseases** can cause depressive symptoms (many otherwise normal people have noted lassitude and low mood when suffering from a bout of the flu). **Space-occupying lesions of the brain** (tumors and abscesses) have also been associated with depressive symptoms, as have **vitamin deficiencies**. Finally, about one-third of patients with Alzheimer's disease, Huntington's disease, and stroke may develop serious depressive symptoms.

The second major criterion for Mood Disorder Due to a General Medical Condition is that the mood symptoms must not occur only during the course of a **delirium**. Delirious patients can have difficulties with memory, concentration, lack of interest, episodes of tearfulness, and frank depression that closely resemble Major Depressive Disorder. Lisa presented no evidence that suggested delirium.

Further coding would be needed to specify whether Lisa's mood disorder occurred With Manic, Depressive, or Mixed Features. At different times, Lisa had both extremes of mood; neither predominated. The code and name of the general medical condition would be included on Axis III, as follows:

Axis I	293.83	Mood Disorder Due to Multiple Sclerosis, With Mixed Features
Axis II	V71.09	No diagnosis

Axis III   340   Multiple sclerosis
Axis IV   None
Axis V   GAF = 70   (current)

Substance-Induced Mood Disorder

Substance use is an especially common cause of mood disorder. Intoxication with cocaine or amphetamines can precipitate manic symptoms, and depression is particularly likely to be caused by withdrawal from cocaine, amphetamines, alcohol, or barbiturates. The presence of mood symptoms is enough to make the diagnosis; they need not fulfill criteria for Major Depressive, Manic or, Hypomanic Episodes.

Health care professionals often fail to recognize Substance-Induced Mood Disorder. This is a cautionary tale, one that is probably replayed hundreds of times every working day in therapists' offices around the world.

Criteria for Substance-Induced Mood Disorder

- The patient's clinical presentation is dominated by a mood disorder that persists and is characterized by *either or both* of these:
  ✓ Depressed mood *or* markedly decreased interest or pleasure in nearly all activities, *or*
  ✓ Mood that is elevated, expansive, or irritable.
- History, physical exam, or laboratory data substantiate that *either*
  ✓ These symptoms have developed within a month of Substance Intoxication or Withdrawal, *or*
  ✓ Medication use has caused the symptoms.
- The symptoms cause clinically important distress or impair work, social, or personal functioning.
- This disorder does not occur *solely* during a delirium.
- A non-substance-induced mood disorder does not better explain the symptoms.

Coding Notes

Code according to the specific substance involved:

291.8   Alcohol
292.84   Amphetamine [or Amphetamine-Like Substance]; Cocaine; Hallucinogen; Inhalant; Opioid; Phencyclidine [or Phencyclidine-Like Substance]; Sedative, Hypnotic, or Anxiolytic; Other [or Unknown] Substance

Specify the type:

With Depressive Features. Mood is mainly depressed.

With Manic Features. Mood is mainly elevated or irritable.

With Mixed Features. Manic and depressive symptoms are present in about equal proportions

When criteria are met for Substance Intoxication or Withdrawal, specify whether:

With Onset During Intoxication

With Onset During Withdrawal

Use this diagnosis instead of Substance Intoxication or Substance Withdrawal only (1) when the symptoms exceed those you would expect from a syndrome of intoxication or withdrawal *and* (2) when they are serious enough by themselves to require clinical care.

Although the diagnosis of Substance-Induced Mood Disorder has no time or symptom requirements, there must be no non-substance-induced mood disorder that better explains the symptoms. Look for these indications of a non-substance-induced mood disorder:

Previous episodes of Bipolar I or II Disorder or Major Depressive Disorder, Recurrent

Symptoms that are much worse than would be expected for the amount and duration of the substance use

Mood disorder symptoms that precede onset of substance use

Mood disorder symptoms that continue long (at least a month) after intoxication or withdrawal stops

Strong family history of mood disorder

Mood disorders caused by most medications taken in therapeutic doses would be coded as follows, for example:

Axis I	292.84	Reserpine-Induced Mood Disorder, With Depressive Features
Axis III	E942.6	Reserpine

Rachel Inouye

"It doesn't seem fair—first the accident and now this." Rachel Inouye's mother seemed near tears as she talked with the interviewer. Rachel herself sat quietly in her wheelchair. "I guess any normal 16-year-old is likely to feel depressed with a fractured pelvis, but our surgeon said this might be manic–depression."

Until five months ago, Rachel had seemed pretty much like any other adolescent girl—moody at times, but generally outgoing and friendly. A bad fall during gymnastics class had left her with a fractured pelvis and bladder problems. Although her doctors had assured the family that she would eventually recover, a body cast had kept her at home for five months. To keep up with her schoolwork, she relied on a home tutor to help her with the assignments her friends brought.

For the first several weeks, Rachel's grades actually improved slightly. But then her moodiness had worsened dramatically. For a day or two she would be high-spirited, giggling and talking rapidly; during these times, she slept little and was full of plans about what she would do when she finally escaped her wheelchair. These phases would alternate with times when she was irritable, tearful, and uncommunicative. Although she could not be accurately weighed, she had probably lost about 10 pounds; to her mother, she looked thin and gaunt. Regardless of whether her mood was up or down, she complained of difficulty sleeping. A week ago she had frightened her mother by saying that she "might as well be dead." That precipitated the call to their surgeon and the mental health referral.

Throughout her mother's recitation, Rachel had remained completely silent. Now, with her mother out of the room, she proved surprisingly communicative. Although she admitted making the remark about being better off dead, she denied that she ever felt suicidal. She was "pretty damned sick" of living in a wheelchair, and her interests and energy were often low. Questions about her social life and relationship with her parents produced little useful information. Finally, the subject of drug use was brought up.

"Why is that important?" asked Rachel.

"Drugs can sometimes cause mood swings like you've been having."

After a long pause, Rachel began to relate the story of her boyfriend, who once or twice a week brought her a supply of cocaine. Snorting it several times a day, she felt euphoric and energetic; once it ran out, she became depressed.

The interviewer remarked that it sounded like an expensive gift.

"Oh, he can afford it. He deals it. He sells to half the kids in the school. You're not going to tell my mom, are you?"

Evaluation of Rachel Inouye

It is all too easy to identify mood symptoms and make a double leap—first to a diagnosis of Major Depressive Episode, then to Bipolar I or II Disorder. This tendency could have been strengthened by Rachel's physical disability; it is hard to visualize substance use in someone who is confined to a wheelchair.

Even so, Rachel had not had symptoms that were severe enough to qualify for a diagnosis of either **Major Depressive Episode** or **Manic Episode**; therefore, no diagnosis of **Major Depressive Disorder** or **Bipolar I or II Disorder** could be made. The mood swings she reported had not lasted long enough (two years required) for **Cyclothymic Disorder** or **Dysthymic Disorder**. Her physical injuries were not the sort that would cause a **Mood Disorder Due to a General Medical Condition**. **Mood Disorder Not Otherwise Specified** should only be diagnosed as a last resort. All patients who withdraw from cocaine have depressive symptoms; Rachel's were more severe than usual, warranting a diagnosis of cocaine mood disorder instead of Cocaine Intoxication or Withdrawal.

None of the conditions that would suggest a non-substance-induced mood disorder (see Coding Notes) applied to Rachel.

In addition to her mood disorder, Rachel's cocaine use must also be scored on Axis I. She did not fulfill criteria for Cocaine Dependence (she only had withdrawal symptoms), so Cocaine Abuse was diagnosed. It would be listed first, because it was the underlying reason she needed mental health care. No episode or course specifiers apply to Substance-Induced Mood Disorder. Neither Cocaine Intoxication nor Withdrawal would be specified in the Axis I code, because both phases were implicated in her symptoms. Some indication of severity may be given on Axis V, the GAF Scale; it can also be designated as an Axis I qualifier.

Any patient who misuses substances should also be evaluated for a personality disorder; no such evidence is presented in this vignette.

Rachel's full diagnosis would be as follows:

Axis I	305.60	Cocaine Abuse
	292.84	Cocaine-Induced Mood Disorder, With Mixed Features, Mild
Axis II	V71.09	No diagnosis
Axis III	808.8	Fracture of pelvis
Axis IV	None	
Axis V	GAF = 61	(current)

311 Depressive Disorder Not Otherwise Specified

The Depressive Disorder Not Otherwise Specified category includes depressive disorders that are not (yet?) well enough recognized to be given code numbers of their own. They must also not fulfill criteria for an Adjustment Disorder With Depressed Mood or With Mixed Anxiety and Depressed Mood (see p. 454). Here are a few examples:

Minor depressive disorder. This is a term for use with patients who have had two or more weeks of depression, but fewer than the five symptoms required for a Major Depressive Episode by DSM-IV. Suggested criteria for this proposed disorder are presented beginning on page 719 of DSM-IV.

Postpsychotic depressive disorder of Schizophrenia. Once the acute psychosis has subsided, many patients who have been diagnosed as having schizophrenia develop depression. It can be coded here. A more detailed list of suggested criteria is presented beginning on page 711 of DSM-IV.

Major Depressive Episode superimposed on a psychosis. The psychosis could be Delusional Disorder, Psychotic Disorder Not Otherwise Specified, or even an acute episode of Schizophrenia. The difference between this and the preceding diagnosis is timing: In this case, the depression occurs *with* the psychosis.

> **TIP** Clinicians who encounter patients with postpsychotic depressive disorder of Schizophrenia or with a Major Depressive Episode superimposed on a psychosis should think carefully about the diagnosis. Likewise, the occurrence of a Manic Episode in a patient who was formerly diagnosed as psychotic (see below) should cause one to wonder whether the original diagnosis was correct. In both cases, some of these patients may actually have a Bipolar I Disorder, and not Schizophrenia or another psychotic disorder at all.

Premenstrual Dysphoric Disorder. This condition occurs exclusively in women. The symptoms begin not long after ovulation and include depressed or anxious mood, pronounced lability of mood (sudden tearfulness, anger, sadness), and loss of interest in usual activities. It materially interferes with social or occupational activities and affects the patient during most of her menstrual cycles. Suggested criteria for this proposed disorder are given beginning on page 715 of DSM-IV.

Recurrent Brief Depressive Disorder. At least once a month for the past year, the patient has had an episode of depression that lasts anywhere from 2 to 14 days and is *not* associated with the menstrual cycle. Suggested criteria for this proposed disorder are presented beginning on page 721 of DSM-IV.

Undiagnosed Depression. This term could apply to any patient who appears to have a depressive disorder for which the clinician can't determine the cause. Of course, this term should only be used as an interim diagnosis; it should be changed as soon as additional information clarifies the nature of the cause. Such a depression might eventually be rediagnosed as Mood Disorder Due to a General Medical Condition, Substance-Induced Mood Disorder, or Major Depressive Disorder.

296.80 Bipolar Disorder Not Otherwise Specified

Patients with bipolar symptoms that do not meet criteria for any better-defined bipolar disorder can be coded as having Bipolar Disorder Not Otherwise Specified.

Recurrent Hypomanic Episodes. These episodes occur without intervening Major Depressive Episodes.

Manic Episode superimposed on a psychosis. These psychoses could include Delusional Disorder, Psychotic Disorder Not Otherwise Specified, or Schizophrenia, Residual Type.

Undiagnosed mania. This category could be used for any patient who appears to have a mania for which the clinician can't determine the cause. This mania could eventually be rediagnosed as Mood Disorder Due to a General Medical Condition, Substance-Induced Mood Disorder, or a bipolar disorder. Of course, this term should also only be used as an interim diagnosis.

296.90 Mood Disorder Not Otherwise Specified

The Mood Disorder Not Otherwise Specified category is provided for any patient whose symptoms do not clearly belong either to Depressive Disorder Not Otherwise Specified or Bipolar Disorder Not Otherwise Specified. Any patient coded here will have been seen briefly or evaluated incompletely—in other words, there is too little information to know whether there have ever been manic symptoms. For example, a patient who is currently depressed and too ill to give a complete history might not be able to state whether there has been an earlier hospitalization for mania. This code will be used infrequently; like most Not Otherwise Specified categories, it should be changed to a more specific one as soon as you can obtain the additional relevant information.

SPECIFIERS THAT DESCRIBE THE MOST RECENT EPISODE

The episode specifiers describe features of the patient's *current* or *most recent* episode of illness. No additional code number is assigned for these features. (DSM-IV also places the severity specifiers here. However, because they are specific to their respective episodes of illness—Major Depressive, Manic, Mixed, and Hypomanic—I have placed them with those criteria, earlier in this chapter.) Each of the following special qualifiers can apply to a Major Depressive Episode in Major Depressive, Bipolar I, and Bipolar II Disorders. With Catatonic Features can also apply to a Manic Episode.

With Atypical Features

Not all seriously depressed patients have the classical vegetative symptoms typical of melancholia (see below). Atypical patients have the reverse: Instead of sleeping and eating too little, they sleep and eat too much. This pattern is especially common among younger patients (teenagers and college-age patients).

Two reasons make it important to specify With Atypical Features: (1) Because such patients' symptoms often include anxiety and sensitivity to rejection, they risk being mislabeled as having an anxiety disorder or a personality disorder. (2) They may respond differently to treatment than do patients With Melancholic Features. Atypical patients may respond to specific antidepressants (monoamine oxidase inhibitors), and may also show a favorable response to bright light therapy for seasonal (winter) depression.

Iris McMaster was a patient whose Bipolar II Disorder was diagnosed as With Atypical Features p. 220).

Criteria for With Atypical Features

For the most recent two weeks or more of a Major Depressive Episode, *or* predominating during the most recent two years of Dysthymic Disorder:

- The patient experiences mood reactivity, with improved mood when something good happens or seems about to happen (e.g., presence of friends).
- At least two of the following occur:
  - ✓ There is a material increase in appetite or weight.
  - ✓ There is excessive sleeping.
  - ✓ Arms or legs feel heavy, leaden.
  - ✓ Work or interpersonal relations are impaired by sensitivity to rejection that is long-standing and not limited to periods of depression.
- During the same episode, the patient does *not* qualify for With Melancholic Features or With Catatonic Features.

With Catatonic Features

With Catatonic Features can be added to the diagnosis of patients with Major Depressive, Manic, or Mixed Episodes. However, these episode features are seldom encountered. A clinician who works with very sick inpatients may encounter only a small handful of these patients in a lifetime. The catatonic features usually associated with mania include hyperactivity, impulsivity, *and* combativeness. These patients may also refuse to keep their clothes on.

The catatonic features associated with depression include markedly reduced mobility (even to the point of stupor), mutism, negativism, mannerisms, and stereotypies. *Negativism* is diagnosed when the patient offers resistance to passive movement or repeatedly turns away from the examiner. *Mannerisms* are repeated movements that appear to have no purpose; *stereotypies* are repeated movements that are a nonessential part of goal-directed behavior.

Catatonic symptoms are essentially the same, whether they occur in patients with mood disorders or with Schizophrenia. Some of them are described further in the case of Edward Clapham, a patient with Schizophrenia, Catatonic Type (p. 152).With Catatonic Features cannot be applied to Hypomanic Episode.

Criteria for With Catatonic Features

- Two or more of the following dominate the clinical picture:
  ✓ Immobility (catalepsy or waxy flexibility) or stupor
  ✓ Apparently purposeless hyperactivity not influenced by external stimuli
  ✓ Mutism or extreme negativism
  ✓ Prominent posturing, stereotypies, mannerisms, or grimacing
  ✓ Echolalia (repeating words or phrases someone else has just said) or echopraxia (mimicking another's gestures)

With Melancholic Features

The With Melancholic Features specifier refers to the classical "vegetative" symptoms of severe depression and a negative view of the world. Melancholic patients awaken too early in the morning, feeling worse than they do later in the day. They also have reduced appetite and lose weight. They take little pleasure in their usual activities (including sex) and are not cheered by the presence of people whose company they normally enjoy. DSM-IV notes that this loss of pleasure is not merely relative, but total or nearly so. Brian Murphy (see p. 204) was one such patient.

Melancholic features are especially common among patients who first develop severe depression in midlife. This condition used to be called *involutional melancholia*, from the observation that it seemed to occur in patients who were in middle to old age (the so-called *involutional period*). However, it is now recognized that melancholic features can affect patients of any age; they are particularly likely to occur in psychotic depressions. Depression with melancholia is especially responsive to somatic treatments such as antidepressant medication and ECT. Contrast this picture with that given for With Atypical Features (see above).

With Melancholic features can be applied to any Major Depressive Episode that is the patient's most recent mood episode in Major Depressive Disorder or Bipolar I or II Disorder.

Criteria for With Melancholic Features

- When symptoms of a Major Depressive Episode are most severe, the patient has *either or both* of these:
  ✓ Loses pleasure in nearly all activities
  ✓ Feels no better when something good happens (e.g., when in the company of friends, when given a raise)
- The patient has three or more of the following:
  ✓ Different quality of depressed mood from what would be experienced at the death of a relative
  ✓ Diurnal variation of mood, in which the depression is consistently worse in the mornings
  ✓ Terminal insomnia, awakening at least two hours early
  ✓ Markedly speeded-up or slowed psychomotor activity
  ✓ Marked loss of appetite or weight
  ✓ Guilt feelings that have been inappropriate or excessive

With Postpartum Onset

Over half of all women have "baby blues" after giving birth. They feel sad and anxious, cry, complain of poor attention, and have trouble sleeping. This lasts a week or two and is usually of little consequence. But only about 10% of these women have enough symptoms to be diagnosed as having a depressive disorder; they often have a personal history of mental disorder. Only about 2 out of 1,000 new mothers actually become psychotic.

The With Postpartum Onset specifier has the briefest "set" of criteria in DSM-IV. After she gave birth, Elisabeth Jacks had a Manic Episode (see p. 212), but Major Depressive Episodes are much more common postpartum events. With Postpartum Onset can apply to Bipolar I and Bipolar II Disorders, to either type of Major Depressive Disorder, or to Brief Psychotic Disorder.

Criterion for With Postpartum Onset

- An episode of the disorder begins within four weeks after childbirth.

SPECIFIERS FOR COURSE OF RECURRENT EPISODES

The course specifiers for mood disorders are yet another way for clinicians to code variations on the themes of mania and depression. These specifiers require the clinician to step back from the patient's current symptoms and examine the full history—for several years back, in the cases of With Rapid Cycling and With Seasonal Pattern. As with the other episode specifiers, no additional code number goes with the course specifiers, only more words.

With and Without Full Interepisode Recovery

With and Without Full Interepisode Recovery apply to the intervals between two mood episodes of any type. Note that the interepisode period must be at least two months for the second episode to qualify as a separate episode. These specifiers can be used with Major Depressive Disorder, Recurrent, and with Bipolar I or Bipolar II Disorders. (Although most bipolar patients recover completely between episodes, about one-quarter continue to have some problems with work or social life during interepisode periods.) In patients who have Dysthymic Disorder, they can be used if the criteria for Major Depressive Disorder are otherwise alternately fulfilled and resolved.

Criteria for With and Without Full Interepisode Recovery

Specify if:

With Full Interepisode Recovery. There is a full remission between the two most recent episodes.

Without Full Interepisode Recovery. There isn't.

With Rapid Cycling

Typically, the bipolar disorders follow a more or less indolent course: a number of months (perhaps three to nine) of depression, followed by somewhat fewer months of mania or hypomania. Other than their number, the individual episodes meet full criteria for Major Depressive, Manic, Mixed, or Hypomanic Episodes. Although as patients age the entire cycle tends to speed up, most patients have no more than one cycle per year, even after five or more complete cycles. But some patients, especially women, cycle much more rapidly than this: They may go from mania to depression to mania again within a few weeks. Recent research suggests that patients who cycle rapidly are more likely to originate from higher socioeconomic classes; in addition, a past history of rapid cycling predicts that this pattern will continue in the future. Patients who cycle rapidly may be more difficult than other patients to manage with standard maintenance regimens. With Rapid Cycling can apply to Bipolar I and Bipolar II Disorders.

Criterion for With Rapid Cycling

• In the past year, there have been four or more episodes that meet criteria for Major Depressive Episode, Manic Episode, Mixed Episode, or Hypomanic Episode. The boundaries of these episodes are indicated by a switch between high and low or by a period of remission.

Coding Note

For an episode to count as a separate episode, it must be marked by a partial or full remission for at least two months or by a change in polarity (such as from Manic to Major Depressive).

With Seasonal Pattern

With Seasonal Pattern is yet another specifier of mood disorders that has only been recognized in the last 20 years or so. In the usual pattern, depressive symptoms (often these are also Atypical) appear during fall or winter months and remit in the spring and summer. Winter depression patients may report other difficulties, such as Pain Disorder symptoms or a craving for carbohydrates, during their depressed phase. Winter depressions occur more commonly in polar climates, especially in the far North. With Seasonal Pattern can apply to Bipolar I and Bipolar II Disorders and to Major Depressive Disorder, Recurrent Type.

Sal Camozzi was a patient whose Bipolar II Disorder was described as With Seasonal Pattern. His history is presented in the chapter on sleep disorders (p. 426).

Table 5.1 Specifiers That Apply to the Mood Disorders

Disorder	Severity Specifiers	Chronicity	With Atypical Features	With Catatonic Features	With Melancholic Features	With Postpartum Onset	With/Without Full Interepisode Recovery	With Rapid Cycling	With Seasonal Pattern
Major Depressive, Single Episode	p. 194	p. 195	p. 239	p. 240	p. 240	p. 241			
Major Depressive, Recurrent	p. 194	p. 195	p. 239	p. 240	p. 240	p. 241	P. 242		p. 244
Dysthymic			p. 239						
Bipolar I, Single Manic Episode	p. 198			p. 240		p. 241			
Bipolar I, Most Recent Episode Depressed	p. 194	p. 195	p. 239	p. 240	p. 240	p. 241	p. 242	p. 243	p. 244
Bipolar I, Most Recent Episode Manic	p. 198			p. 240		p. 241	p. 242	p. 243	p. 244
Bipolar I, Most Recent Episode Mixed	p. 200			p. 240		p. 241	p. 242	p. 243	p. 244
Bipolar I, Most Recent Episode Hypomanic							p. 242	p. 243	p. 244
Bipolar I, Most Recent Episode Unspecified							p. 242	p. 243	p. 244
Bipolar II, Hypomanic							p. 242	p. 243	p. 244
Bipolar II, Depressed	p. 194	p. 195	p. 239	p. 240	p. 240	p. 241	p. 242	p. 243	p. 244
Cyclothymic									

Note. This table can help you to arrange the sometimes lengthy string of names, codes, and modifiers for the mood disorders. Just start reading from left to right in the table, putting in any modifiers that apply in the order you come to them. Not all diagnoses can utilize all the possible descriptors listed here; those that do apply are indicated by the page number where they can be found. Criteria for severity and chronicity specifiers are provided with the criteria for the various types of episodes, early in this chapter. Criteria for the remaining specifiers are provided at the end of the chapter. You will notice that none of these qualifiers applies to Cyclothymic Disorder. Bear in mind also that Substance-Induced Mood Disorder and Mood Disorder Due to a General Medical Condition have their own lists of specifiers.

Note. Adapted by permission from the *Diagnostic and Statistical Manual of Mental Disorders*, 4th ed. (pp. 376, 388), by the American Psychiatric Association, 1994, Washington, DC: Author. Copyright 1994 by the American Psychiatric Association.

Criteria for With Seasonal Pattern

- Major Depressive Episodes regularly begin at a particular season of the year.
- Complete recovery or change of polarity also occurs regularly during a particular season.
- These seasonal changes have occurred in each of the previous two years, during which no other nonseasonal Major Depressive Episodes have occurred.
- Over the patient's lifetime, seasonal Major Depressive Episodes materially outnumber nonseasonal episodes.

Coding Note

Disregard examples where there is a clear seasonal cause, such as being unemployed every summer.

Anxiety Disorders

Quick Guide to the Anxiety Disorders

One or more of the following conditions may be diagnosed in patients who present with prominent anxiety symptoms; a single patient may have more than one anxiety disorder. Most anxiety disorders begin when the patient is relatively young. As in earlier chapters, the page number following each item indicates where a more detailed discussion begins.

Anxiety "Building Blocks"

Agoraphobia and Panic Attacks are not codable disorders in and of themselves. They are the "building blocks" from which several of the codable anxiety disorders are constructed.

Agoraphobia. Patients with this condition fear situations or places such as entering a store, where they might have trouble obtaining help if they become anxious (p. 247).

Panic Attack. This is a brief episode in which a patient feels intense dread accompanied by a variety of physical and other symptoms; it begins suddenly and peaks rapidly (p. 251).

Anxiety Disorders

The codable anxiety disorders include the following:

Panic Disorder. These patients experience repeated Panic Attacks, together with worry about having additional attacks and other mental and behavioral changes related to them. Panic disorder usually occurs with Agoraphobia (p. 255), but it is sometimes diagnosed Without Agoraphobia (p. 258).

Agoraphgobia Without History of Panic Disorder. This is a codable form of Agoraphobia related to fear of developing panic-like symptoms, in which the full criteria for Panic Disorder are not met (p. 250).

Specific Phobia. In this condition, patients fear specific objects or situations, such as animals, storms, heights, blood, airplanes, being closed in, or any situation that may lead to vomiting, choking, or developing an illness (p. 259).

Social Phobia. These patients imagine themselves embarrassed when they speak, write, or eat in public, use a public urinal, or the like (p. 262).

Obsessive-Compulsive Disorder. These patients are bothered by repeated thoughts or behaviors that appear senseless, even to them (p. 265).

Posttraumatic Stress Disorder. These patients repeatedly relive a severely traumatic event, such as combat or a natural disaster (p. 269).

Acute Stress Disorder. This condition is much like Posttraumatic Stress Disorder, except that it begins during or immediately after the stressful event and lasts a month or less (p. 273).

Generalized Anxiety Disorder. Although they experience no episodes of acute panic, these patients feel tense or anxious much of the time (p. 276).

Anxiety Disorders Due to a General Medical Condition. Panic Attacks or generalized anxiety symptoms can be caused by numerous medical conditions (p. 280).

Substance-Induced Anxiety Disorder. Various substances can lead to anxiety symptoms that don't necessarily fulfill criteria for any of the above-mentioned disorders (p. 282).

Anxiety Disorder Not Otherwise Specified. Use this category to code disorders with prominent anxiety symptoms that do not fit neatly into any of the groups above (p. 285).

Other Causes of Anxiety Symptoms

Avoidance behavior that is associated with sexual aversion is classified with the sexual dysfunctions (p. 338).

Anxiety symptoms can be found in patients with almost any Axis I disorder. They are especially prevalent in patients with Major Depressive Episode (p. 191) and Somatization Disorder (p. 294).

Introduction

The conditions discussed in this chapter are characterized by anxiety and by behavior calculated to ward it off. A certain level of anxiety is not only normal; it is even adaptive. For example, a person about to take an examination or speak in public is spurred on to prepare adequately by the fear of failure.

Anxiety is also a symptom found in nearly all mental disorders. But when it is the main symptom or experience that requires the help of a mental health clinician, DSM-IV places it in a class by itself. Collectively, anxiety disorders are the most common of all the mental disorders.

Notice the careful choice of wording above: ". . . that requires the help of a mental health clinician . . . " This is meant to emphasize the fact that patients often complain of anxiety, when the root of the difficulty is a general medical condition or a different Axis I problem (such as a mood, somatoform, cognitive, or substance-related disorder). These conditions should be considered for *any* patient who presents with anxiety or avoidance behavior.

Agoraphobia

In Greek, *agoraphobia* literally means "fear of the marketplace." But in contemporary usage it refers to the fear some people have of any situation or place where escape seems difficult (or embarrassing) or help unavailable if they should have anxiety symptoms. Open or public places such as theaters and crowded supermarkets qualify; so does travel. The patients either avoid the feared place or situation, or, if they must confront it, suffer intense anxiety or require the presence of a companion. Most Agoraphobia involves such situations as being away from home, standing in a crowd, staying home alone, being on a bridge, or traveling by bus, car, or train.

Agoraphobia can develop in the wake of a series of Panic Attacks (see p. 251), when fear of recurrent attacks causes the patient to avoid leaving home or participating in other activities. In other patients, Agoraphobia develops without any preceding Panic Attacks. As noted earlier, Agoraphobia is not coded by itself. It is a "building block" used to help define (either by its inclusion or exclusion) several DSM-IV diagnoses.

Note that in this part of the chapter, the order of presentation differs somewhat both from that in the DSM and that in the Quick Guide, above. First, I discuss the noncodable Agoraphobia and the codable Agoraphobia Without History of Panic Disorder in connection with the same patient. I then discuss the noncodable Panic Attack and the codable Panic Disorder in connection with the second patient.

Criteria for Agoraphobia

- The patient has anxiety about being in a place or situation from which *either* or *both*
  - ✓ Escape could be difficult or embarrassing, *or*
  - ✓ If a panic attack occurred, help might not be available.
- The patient:
  - ✓ Avoids these situations or places (restricting travel), *or*
  - ✓ Endures them, but with material distress (a panic attack might occur), *or*
  - ✓ Requires a companion when in the situation.
- Other mental disorders don't explain the symptoms better.

Coding Notes

By itself, Agoraphobia is not a codable DSM-IV diagnosis. Code the particular disorder of which the Agoraphobia is a part.

The other disorders referred to above (see third bullet) include Social Phobia (e.g., the patient avoids public eating for fear of embarrassment), Specific Phobia (the patient avoids certain limited situations, such as telephone booths), Obsessive–Compulsive Disorder (e.g., the patient avoids dirt for fear of contamination), and Posttraumatic Stress Disorder (e.g., the patient avoids movies about Vietnam). Children who avoid leaving home should be evaluated for Separation Anxiety Disorder.

Lucy Gould

"I'd rather have her with me, if that's all right." Lucy Gould was responding to the clinician's suggestion that her mother wait outside the office. "By now, I don't have any secrets from her."

Since age 18, Lucy hadn't been anywhere without her mother. In fact, in those six years she'd hardly been anywhere at all. "There's no way I could go out by myself—it's like entering a war zone. If someone's not with me, I can barely stand to go to doctor appointments and stuff like that. But I still feel awfully nervous."

The nervousness Lucy complained of had never included actual panic attacks; she never felt she couldn't breathe or was about to die. This was an intense motor agitation that had caused her to flee from shopping malls, supermarkets, and movie theaters. Neither could she ride on public transportation—buses and trains both terrified her. She had the feeling, vague but always present, that something awful would happen there. Perhaps she would become so anxious that she would pass out or wet herself, and no one would be able to help her. She hadn't been alone in public since the week before her high school commencement. She had only been able to go up onto the platform to receive her diploma because she was with her best friend, who would know what to do if she needed help.

Lucy had always been a timid, rather sensitive girl. For the first week of kindergarten, she cried each time her mother left her by herself at school. But her father had insisted that she "toughen up," and within a few weeks she had nearly forgotten her terror. She subsequently maintained a nearly perfect attendance record at school until her father died of leukemia, shortly after her 17th birthday. Her terror of being away from home had begun within a few weeks of his funeral.

To make ends meet, her mother had sold their house and they had moved into a condominium across the street from the high school. "It's the only way I got through my last year," Lucy explained.

For several years, Lucy had kept house while her mother assembled circuit boards at an electronics firm outside of town. Lucy was perfectly comfortable in that role, even though her mother was away for hours at a time. Her physical health had been good; she had never used drugs or alcohol; and she had never had depression, suicidal ideas, delusions, or hallucinations. But a year ago Lucy had developed insulin-dependent diabetes, which required frequent trips to the doctor. She had tried to take the bus by herself, but after several failures (once, in the middle of traffic, she had forced the rear door open and sprinted for home), she had given up. Now her mother was applying for disability assistance so that she could remain at home to provide the aid and attendance Lucy required.

Evaluation of Lucy Gould

Because of her fears, Lucy avoided a variety of situations and places (supermarkets, malls, buses, and trains), or else she required a companion. She couldn't state exactly what might happen—only that it would be awful and embarrassing, and that help might not be available. It was not unusual that her symptoms only came to light when another problem prevented her from staying at home.

Lucy's symptoms were too varied for **Specific** or **Social Phobia**. (Note also that in Agoraphobia, the perceived danger emanates from the environment; in Social Phobia, it comes from the relationship with other people.) Her problem was not that she feared being left alone, as would be the case with **Separation Anxiety Disorder** (although she clearly had had elements of that diagnosis when she was five). She had not had a major trauma, as would be the case in **Posttraumatic Stress Disorder** (the death of her father was traumatic, but her own symptoms did not focus on reliving this experience). There is no indication that she had **Obsessive–Compulsive Disorder**.

These symptoms fulfill the criteria for Agoraphobia. Coding is discussed below.

300.22 Agoraphobia
Without History of Panic Disorder

Agoraphobia Without History of Panic Disorder has been considered relatively uncommon. Some clinical investigators have recently reported it to be common; other have found that many cases were actually misdiagnosed Specific Phobias. It is clear that the diagnosis occurs, but how often? More research will have to be done before we can answer this question.

Criteria for Agoraphobia
Without History of Panic Disorder

- The patient has Agoraphobia (see above) related to the fear of experiencing panic-like symptoms.
- The patient has never fulfilled the criteria for Panic Disorder (see lists, pp. 255, 258).
- The symptoms are not directly caused by a general medical condition or by the use of substances, including medications.
- If the patient does have a general medical condition, the fears clearly exceed those that usually accompany it.

Coding Note

The "panic-like symptoms" mentioned above (see first bullet) can include any of the Panic Attack symptoms (see criteria, p. 252), plus any other symptoms that could embarrass or incapacitate the patient. For example, the patient may refuse to leave home for fear of losing bladder control.

Further evaluation of Lucy Gould

Agoraphobia can accompany a variety of diagnoses, most important of which are the mood disorders (those including **Major Depressive Episodes**). However, Lucy denied having symptoms of depression (as well as **psychosis** and **substance use**). Although she had diabetes, it developed many years after her Agoraphobia symptoms became apparent; besides, there is no physiological connection between Agoraphobia and diabetes. Her anxiety symptoms were far more extensive than the **realistic concerns** you would expect from the average person with diabetes.

Because Lucy had never experienced an abrupt panic attack, she would not meet the criteria for **Panic Disorder with Agoraphobia**. But her anxiety symptoms included restlessness and the fear of urinary incontinence; she would therefore fulfill criteria for Agoraphobia Without History of Panic Disorder. Her complete diagnosis would be as follows:

Axis I	300.22	Agoraphobia Without History of Panic Disorder
Axis II	V71.09	No diagnosis
Axis III	250.01	Insulin-dependent Diabetes Mellitus
Axis IV		None
Axis V	GAF = 31	(current)

Panic Attack

A person experiencing a panic attack feels foreboding—a sense of disaster that is usually accompanied by cardiac symptoms (such as palpitations, rapid heartbeat) and trouble breathing (shortness of breath, chest pain). The attack usually begins abruptly (within 10 minutes or so) and rapidly builds to a peak. The entire episode usually lasts less than half an hour. Panic Attacks may occur only a few times in the life of the patient or many times per week. Over half of these people awaken at night with Panic Attacks. Many patients change their behavior in reaction to the fear that the attacks mean they are psychotic or physically ill.

Panic Attacks may occur by themselves (when they may qualify for a diagnosis of Panic Disorder) or in connection with a variety of other anxiety conditions or disorders, which may include Agoraphobia, Social and Specific Phobias, or Posttraumatic Stress Disorder. They can be a feature of Anxiety Disorder Due to A General Medical Condition and of Substance-Induced Anxiety Disorder. They can also occur as isolated experiences in normal young adults; pathological panic attacks usually begin in the person's 20s. The lifetime prevalence of Panic Attacks is about 10%.

Panic Attacks are important for several reasons:

They are common (perhaps 30% of all adults have experienced at least one).

They are often easily treated, perhaps only by obtaining a little reassurance or by breathing into a paper bag).

Untreated, they can be severely debilitating.

Sometimes they mask other illnesses that range from severe mood disorders to heart attacks.

Some Panic Attacks are triggered by specific situations, such as passing over a bridge or roaming through a crowded supermarket. Such attacks are said to be *cued* or *situationally bound*. Others have no relationship to a specific stimulus but arise spontaneously, as in Panic Disorder. These are termed *unexpected* or *uncued*. A third type, *situationally predisposed* attacks, are those in which the patient often, but not invariably, becomes panic-stricken when confronted by the stimulus.

Criteria for Panic Attack

- The patient suddenly develops a severe fear or discomfort that peaks within 10 minutes.
- During this discrete episode, four or more of the following symptoms occur:
  ✓ Chest pain or other chest discomfort
  ✓ Chills or hot flashes
  ✓ Choking sensation
  ✓ Derealization (feeling unreal) or depersonalization (feeling detached from self)
  ✓ Dizzy, lightheaded, faint, or unsteady feelings
  ✓ Fear of dying
  ✓ Fears of loss of control or becoming insane
  ✓ Heart pounding, racing, or skipping beats
  ✓ Nausea or other abdominal discomfort
  ✓ Numbness or tingling
  ✓ Sweating
  ✓ Shortness of breath or smothering sensation
  ✓ Trembling

Coding Note

By itself, Panic Attack is not a codable DSM-IV diagnosis. Code the particular disorder of which the Panic Attack is a part.

Shorty Rheinbold

Seated in the clinician's waiting room, Shorty Rheinbold should have been relaxed. The lighting was soft and restful; the sofa on which he was sitting was comfortably upholstered. Angel fish swam lazily in their clean glass tank. But Shorty felt anything but calm. Perhaps it was the receptionist—he wondered whether she was competent to handle an emergency with his sort of problem. She looked something like a badger, holed up behind her word processor. For several minutes he had been feeling worse with every heartbeat.

His heart was the key. When Shorty first sat down, he hadn't even noticed it. It was quietly doing its job inside his chest. But then, without any warning, it had begun to demand his attention. At first it had only skipped a beat or two, but after a minute there had begun a ferocious assault on the inside of his chest wall. Every beat had become a painful, bruising thump that made him clutch at his chest. He tried to do it under his jacket so as not to attract too much attention.

The pounding heart and chest pain could mean only one thing: After two months of attacks every few days, Shorty was beginning to get the message. Then, right on schedule, the shortness of breath began. It seemed to arise from his left chest area, where the heart was doing all its damage. It clawed its way up through his lungs and into his throat, gripping him around the neck so that he could get his breath only in the briefest of gulps.

He was dying! Of course, the cardiologist Shorty had consulted the week before had assured him that his heart was as sound as a brass bell, but this time he was sure it was about to fail. He didn't know why he hadn't died before—he had feared it with almost every attack. Now it seemed impossible that he would survive this attack. He wondered if he even wanted to. That thought made him suddenly feel the need to retch.

Shorty leaned forward so he could grip both his chest and his abdomen as unobtrusively as possible. He could hardly hold anything at all—the familiar tingling and numbness had started up in his fingers, and he could feel his hands shaking as they tried to contain the various miseries that had taken over his body.

He glanced across the room to see whether "Miss Badger" had noticed, but she was still pounding away at her keyboard. No help from that quarter; she hadn't seen a thing. Perhaps all the patients behaved this way. Perhaps—

Suddenly, there *was* an observer. Shorty was watching *himself*. Some part of him had floated free and seemed to hang suspended, halfway up the wall. From this vantage point, he could look down and view with pity and scorn the quivering flesh that was, or had been, Shorty Rheinbold.

Now the Spirit Shorty saw that Shorty's face had become hot and fiery red. Hot air had filled his head, which seemed to expand with every gasp. He floated farther up the wall and the ceiling melted away; he soared out into the brilliant sunshine. He squeezed his eyes shut but could not keep out the blinding light.

Evaluation of Shorty Rheinbold

Shorty's Panic Attack was quite typical: it began suddenly, developed rapidly, and included more than the four required symptoms. His shortness of breath and heart palpitations are classical Panic Attack symptoms; he also had chest pain, lightheadedness, and numbness in his fingers. Shorty's fear that he would die is typical of the fears that patients have during an attack. The sensation of watching himself (*depersonalization*) is a less common panic symptom.

Shorty's Panic Attack was *uncued*, which means that it seemed to happen spontaneously. He was unaware of any event, object, or thought that triggered it. Uncued attacks are typical of **Panic Disorder**, but *cued* (also called *situationally bound*) attacks can occur as well. The Panic Attacks that develop in **Social Phobia** or **Specific Phobia** are cued to the stimuli that repeatedly and predictably provide the trigger.

Panic Attacks can be found in several **general medical conditions**. One of these is acute myocardial infarction (MI), the very condition many panic patients fear the most. Of course, patients with symptoms like Shorty's should be evaluated for MI and other medical disorders, when indicated. These include low blood sugar, irregular heartbeat, mitral valve prolapse, temporal lobe epilepsy, and a tumor called pheochromocytoma. Intoxication with several **psychoactive substances** often produce panic attacks: these include **amphetamine**, **marijuana**, and **caffeine**. Some patients misuse alcohol or sedative drugs in an effort to reduce the severity of their panic attacks.

There is no code number associated with Panic Attack. As Major Depressive Episode is to the mood disorders, it is a "building block" that is associated with several of the anxiety disorders. Shorty's complete diagnosis is given later.

Panic Disorder

Panic Disorder is a common anxiety disorder in which the patient experiences Panic Attacks (usually many, but always more than one) and worries about having another. These Panic Attacks are usually *uncued*, though *situationally predisposed* attacks and *cued/situationally bound* attacks can also occur (see definitions, just above). Perhaps half of Panic Disorder patients also have symptoms of Agoraphobia, though many do not. From this distinction have come the two types of diagnosable Panic Disorder—With and Without Agoraphobia. The relationship is usually as follows.

Panic Attacks are such excruciating experiences that patients will do nearly anything to avoid them. Many patients develop such fear of having another that they avoid situations or circumstances that they associate with Panic Attacks. The Agoraphobia usually develops within just a few weeks. Often patients find that staying home helps prevent further Panic Attacks. But other Panic Disorder patients don't have Agoraphobia.

Panic Disorder typically begins during when the patient is young. It is one of the most common anxiety disorders, found in as many as 3% of the general adult population (as opposed to the 10% figure for Panic Attacks in general). It is especially common among women.

TIP Depressions are so often found in patients who complain of recurrent Panic Attacks that the association cannot be overemphasized. Some studies suggest that over half of Panic Disorder patients can also be diagnosed as having Major Depressive Disorder. Clearly, every patient who presents with panic symptoms must be carefully evaluated for symptoms of a mood disorder.

300.21 Panic Disorder with Agoraphobia

When Agoraphobia occurs in patients who have Panic Attacks, it usually develops within the first year. Thereafter, the two conditions may wax and wane together, or the Agoraphobia may continue even though the Panic Attacks are reduced. Whenever a patient complains about symptoms of either Agoraphobia or a Panic Attack, be sure to inquire carefully for symptoms of the other condition; they often occur together.

Criteria for Panic Disorder With Agoraphobia

- The patient has recurrent Panic Attacks that are not expected.
- For a month or more after at least one of these attacks, the patient has had one or more of these:
  ✓ Ongoing concern that there will be more attacks
  ✓ Worry as to the significance of the attack or its consequences (for health, control, sanity)
  ✓ Material change in behavior, such as doing something to avoid or combat the attacks
- The patient also has Agoraphobia.
- The Panic Attacks are not directly caused by a general medical condition or by the use of substances, including medications.
- The Panic Attacks are not better explained by another anxiety or mental disorder.

Coding Note

DSM-IV specifically notes that Panic Attacks can occur in the following anxiety disorders, which should be ruled out before diagnosing Panic Disorder With Agoraphobia: Social Phobias, Specific Phobias, Obsessive–Compulsive Disorder, and Posttraumatic Stress Disorder. Children who have Panic Attacks on leaving home should be evaluated for Separation Anxiety Disorder.

Shorty Rheinbold Again

Shorty opened his eyes to discover that he was lying on his back on the waiting room floor. Two people were bending over him. One was the receptionist. He didn't recognize the other, but he guessed it must be the mental health clinician who was supposed to interview him.

"I feel like you saved my life," he said.

"Not really," the clinician replied. "You're just fine. Does this happen often?"

"Every two or three days now." Shorty cautiously sat up. After a moment or two, he allowed them to help him to his feet and into the inner office.

Just where his problem began wasn't quite clear at first. Shorty was 24 and had spent four years in the Coast Guard. Since his discharge, he'd knocked around a bit, and then moved in with his folks while he worked in construction. Six months ago, he'd gotten a job as cashier in a filling station.

That was just fine, sitting in a glassed-in booth all day making change, running credit cards through the electronic scanner, and selling chewing gum. The wages weren't exciting, but he didn't have to pay rent. Even with eating out almost every evening, Shorty still had enough at the end of the week to take his girl out on Saturday nights. Neither one of them drank or used drugs, so even that didn't set him too far back.

The problem began one day after Shorty had been working for a couple of months, when the boss told him to go out on the wrecker with Bruce, one of the mechanics. They had stopped along the eastbound Interstate to pick up a Buick Skylark with a blown head gasket. For some reason they had trouble getting it into the sling. Shorty was on the traffic side of the truck, trying to manipulate the hoist in response to Bruce's shouted directions. Suddenly, a caravan of tractor-trailer trucks roared past. The noise and the blast of wind caught Shorty off guard. He spun around into the side of the wrecker, fell, and rolled to a stop, inches from huge tires rolling by . . .

Shorty's color and heart rate had returned to normal. The remainder of his story was easy enough to tell. He continued to go out on the truck, even though he felt scared, nearly panicking every time he did so. He'd only go when Bruce was along, and he carefully avoided the traffic side of the vehicles.

But that wasn't the worst of the problem—he could always quit and get another job. Lately, Shorty had been having these attacks at other times, when he was least expecting them. When he was shopping last week, he had had to abandon the cart full of groceries he was buying for his mother. Nothing seemed to trigger the attacks; they just happened, though not when he was at home or in his glass cage at work. Now he didn't even want to go to the movies with his girl. For the last few weeks he had suggested that they spend Saturday night at her place watching TV instead. She hadn't complained yet, but he felt that it was only a matter of time.

"I have just about enough strength to tough it out through the work day," Shorty said. "But I've got to get a handle on this thing. I'm too young to spend the rest of my life like a hermit in a cave."

Further evaluation of Shorty Rheinbold

The fact of Shorty's Panic Attacks has already been established. They were originally associated with the specific situation of working around the wrecker. More recently, he feared all sorts of other situations that involved being away from home: driving, shopping, even going to the movies. As a result, he either avoided them or had to be accompanied by Bruce or his girlfriend. Shorty's life space had already begun to contract as a result of his fears; without treatment, it would seem to be only a matter of time before he would have to quit his job. These symptoms are typical (and fulfill criteria for Agoraphobia). The combination of Panic Attacks with Agoraphobia would qualify Shorty for the codable diagnosis Panic Disorder with Agoraphobia, provided that other causes of his symptoms could be ruled out.

A number of **general medical conditions** can cause Panic Attacks, and might thereby conceivably be related to Agoraphobia; however, a cardiologist had recently pronounced Shorty to be medically fit. **Substance-Induced Anxiety Disorder** is also eliminated by the history: Shorty didn't use drugs or alcohol. (However, watch out for Panic Disorder patients who "medicate" themselves with drugs or alcohol.) The diagnosis of a **Specific Phobia** or **Social Phobia** would seem unlikely, because the focus of Shorty's anxiety was not a single situation (such as enclosed places) or a social situation. **Somatization Disorder** patients may also complain of anxiety symptoms, but this is an unlikely diagnosis for a generally healthy man.

Although the vignette does not address this possibility, **Major Depressive Disorder** can accompany Panic Disorder in over half of the cases, as noted earlier. The danger lies in the often dramatic anxiety symptoms overshadowing subtle depressive symptoms, so that the clinician overlooks them completely. When the criteria for both an anxiety and a mood disorder are met, they should both be listed on Axis I. Other anxiety disorders can also be found in Panic Disorder patients; these include **Generalized Anxiety Disorder** and **Specific Phobia**.

Shorty's mood was anxious, not depressed or irritable. Therefore, his diagnosis would be as follows:

Axis I	300.21	Panic Disorder With Agoraphobia
Axis II	V71.09	No diagnosis
Axis III		None
Axis IV		None
Axis V	GAF = 61	(current)

TIP Differentiating Panic Disorder With Agoraphobia from other anxiety disorders that involve avoidance (especially Specific and Social Phobias) can be difficult. The final decision often comes down to clinical judgment, though the following sorts of information can be helpful:

1. How many Panic Attacks does the patient have, and what type are they (cued, uncued, situationally predisposed)? Uncued attacks suggest

Panic Disorder; cued attacks suggest Specific or Social Phobia.

2. In how many situations do they occur? Limited situations suggest a Specific or Social Phobia; attacks that occur in a variety of situations suggest Panic Disorder with Agoraphobia.

3. Does the patient awaken at night with Panic Attacks? This is typical of Panic Disorder.

4. What is the focus of the fear? If it is having a subsequent Panic Attack, Panic Disorder may be the correct diagnosis—unless the Panic Attacks occur only when the patient is, say, riding in an airplane, in which case you might correctly diagnose Specific Phobia, Situational Type.

5. Does the patient constantly worry about having Panic Attacks, even when in no danger of facing a feared situation (such as taking an elevator)? This would suggest Panic Disorder with Agoraphobia.

Good luck.

300.01 Panic Disorder Without Agoraphobia

When Panic Disorder occurs alone, the symptoms are very similar to those already described in the case of Shorty Rheinbold. Clinicians who have worked extensively with anxiety disorder patients report that relatively few have Panic Disorder Without Agoraphobia. However, it may be more common than we realize—these patients are not as as disabled as those with Agoraphobia (they don't become housebound), and are therefore less likely to come to the attention of health care professionals. In this group, women outnumber men two to one.

Criteria for Panic Disorder Without Agoraphobia

- The patient has recurrent Panic Attacks that are not expected.
- For a month or more after at least one of these attacks, the patient has had one or more of these:
  ✓ Ongoing concern that there will be more attacks
  ✓ Worry as to the significance of the attack or its consequences (for health, control, sanity)
  ✓ Material change in behavior, such as doing something to avoid or combat the attacks
- The patient does not have Agoraphobia.
- The Panic Attacks are not directly caused by a general medical condition or by the use of substances, including medications.
- The Panic Attacks are not better explained by another anxiety or mental disorder.

Coding Note

DSM-IV specifically notes that Panic Attacks can occur in the following anxiety disorders, which should be ruled out before diagnosing Panic Disorder Without Agoraphobia: Social Phobias, Specific Phobias, Obsessive–Compulsive Disorder, and Posttraumatic Stress Disorder. Children who have Panic Attacks on leaving home should be evaluated for Separation Anxiety Disorder.

TIP You can make more than one Axis I diagnosis. Suppose that your patient has a Major Depressive Disorder and symptoms of Panic Disorder. Record both diagnoses, if both sets of criteria are fulfilled. But don't diagnose Panic Disorder unless for at least a month the patient has been concerned about having further attacks.

300.29 Specific Phobia

Patients with Specific Phobias have unwarranted fears of specific objects or situations. The best recognized are phobias of animals, blood, heights, travel by airplane, being closed in, and thunderstorms. The anxiety produced by exposure to one of these stimuli may be a Panic Attack or more generalized anxiety, but it is always directed at something specific. (However, these patients can also worry about what they might do—faint, panic, or lose control—if they have to confront whatever it is they are afraid of.) Usually, the closer they are to the feared stimulus (and the more difficult it would be to escape), the worse they feel. Patients with Specific Phobias involving blood, injury, or injection often experience what is called a *vasovagal response*; this means that reduced heart rate and blood pressure actually do cause the patients to faint.

A person who must face one of these feared activities or objects will immediately begin to feel nervous or panicky, a condition known as *anticipatory anxiety*. The degree of discomfort is often mild, however, so most people do not seek professional help. When it causes a patient to avoid feared situations, anticipatory anxiety can be a major inconvenience; it can even interfere with working.

Among the general population, Specific Phobia is one of the most frequently reported of the anxiety disorders. Perhaps 10% of U.S. adults have suffered to some degree from one of these Specific Phobias (formerly called Simple Phobias), though by no means would all of these people qualify for a DSM-IV diagnosis. Onset is usually in the late teens or early 20s; women far outnumber men.

Criteria for Specific Phobia

- The patient experiences a strong, persistent fear that is excessive or unreasonable. It is set off (cued) by a specific object or situation that is either present or anticipated.
- The phobic stimulus almost always immediately provokes an anxiety response, which may be either a Panic Attack or symptoms of anxiety that do not meet criteria for a Panic Attack.
- The fear is unreasonable or out of proportion, and the patient realizes this.
- The patient either avoids the phobic stimulus or endures it with severe anxiety or distress.
- Patients under the age of 18 must have the symptoms for six months or longer.
- Either there is marked distress about this fear, or it markedly interferes with the patient's usual routines or social, job, or personal functioning.
- The symptoms are not better explained by another anxiety or mental disorder.

Coding Notes

Specify type:

    Situational Type (airplane travel, being closed in)

    Natural Environment Type (thunderstorms, heights, for example)

    Blood–Injection–Injury Type

    Animal Type (spiders, snakes)

    Other Type (situations that might lead to illness, choking, vomiting)

The types of Specific Phobia are arranged in descending order of frequency (as found in adults). If more than one type is present, code them all.

Children with Specific Phobia may express the anxiety response by clinging, crying, freezing, or having tantrums. They may not have insight that their fear is unreasonable or out of proportion. Other Type in children can include avoiding loud noises or people in costumes.

DSM-IV specifically notes some of the other anxiety disorders that should be ruled out before diagnosing Specific Phobia: Social Phobia (the patient avoids public eating or other activities for fear of embarrassment); Obsessive–Compulsive Disorder (the patient fears dirt or contamination); Posttraumatic Stress Disorder (e.g., the patient avoids movies about Vietnam); and Agoraphobia (With or Without Panic Disorder). Children who avoid leaving home should be evaluated for Separation Anxiety Disorder.

Esther Dugoni

A slightly built woman of nearly 70, Esther Dugoni was healthy and fit, though in the last year or two she had developed a tremor characteristic of early

Parkinson's disease. For the several years since she had retired from her job teaching horticulture in junior college, she had concentrated on her own garden. At the flower show the year before, her rhododendrons had won first prize.

But 10 days earlier, her mother had died in Detroit, over halfway across the country. She and her sister had been appointed coexecutors. The estate was large, and she would have to make a number of trips to probate the will and dispose of the house. That meant flying, and this was why she had sought help from the mental health clinic.

"I can't fly!" she had told the clinician. "I haven't flown anywhere for 20 years."

Esther had been reared during the Depression; as a child, she had never had the opportunity to fly. With five children of her own to care for on her husband's schoolteacher pay, she hadn't traveled much as an adult. She had made a few short hops years ago when two of her children were getting married in different cities. On one of those trips, her plane had circled the field for nearly an hour, trying to land in Omaha between thunderstorms. The ride was wretchedly bumpy; the plane was full; and many of the passengers were airsick, including the two men on either side of her. There was no one to help—the cabin attendants had to remain strapped in their seats. She had kept her eyes closed and breathed through her handkerchief to try to filter out the odors that filled the cabin.

They finally landed safely, but it was the last time Esther had ever been up in an airplane. "I don't even like to go to the airport to meet someone," she reported. "Even that makes me feel short of breath and kind of sick to my stomach. Then I get sort of a dull pain in my chest and I start to shake—I feel that I'm about to die, or something else awful will happen. It all seems so silly."

Esther really had no alternatives to flying. She couldn't stay in Detroit until all of the business had been taken care of; it would take months. The train didn't connect, and the bus was impossible.

TIP   Fears involving animals of one sort or another are remarkably common. Children are especially susceptible to animal phobias, and many adults don't much care for spiders, snakes, and cockroaches. But a diagnosis of Specific Phobia, Animal Type, should not be made unless the patient is truly impaired by the symptoms. For example, prisoners serving a life sentence would not be diagnosed as having a phobia of snakes, because they would never have to confront snakes and could not restrict their activities because of the fear of encountering snakes.

Evaluation of Esther Dugoni

Esther's anxiety symptoms were cued by the prospect of airplane travel; even going to the airport always produced anxiety, and she had avoided plane travel for years. She recognized that this fear was unreasonable ("silly"), and it embarrassed her; it was about to interfere with how she conducted her business.

Specific Phobias are not usually associated with any **general medical condition** or **substance-related disorder**. In response to delusions, patients with **Schizophrenia** will sometimes avoid objects or situations (a telephone that is "bugged," food that is "poisoned"), but such patients do not have the required insight that their fears are unfounded. Of course, the fears any patient experiences must be differentiated from the fears associated with other anxiety disorders (see the Coding Notes, above, for the list of disorders to be ruled out). Esther's complete history was enough to enable her clinician to rule out these other diagnoses. Her five-axis diagnosis would thus be as follows:

Axis I	300.29	Specific Phobia, Situational Type
Axis II	V71.09	No diagnosis
Axis III	332.0	Parkinson's disease, primary
Axis IV		Death of a family member
Axis V	GAF = 75	(current)

300.23 Social Phobia

With onset typically in the middle teens, Social Phobia is a fear of appearing clumsy, silly, or shameful, and of having this behavior observed by others. Patients fear such social gaffes as choking when eating in public, trembling when writing, or being unable to perform when speaking or playing a musical instrument. The sexes are about equally represented, but it is men who sometimes fear using a public urinal. Fear of blushing especially affects females, who often cannot say what is so terrible about turning red. Fear of choking is often acquired after an episode of choking on food; this can occur at any time from childhood to old age.

Many men and women with Social Phobias actually do have noticeable physical symptoms: blushing, hoarseness, tremor, and perspiration. Such patients may have actual Panic Attacks. Some patients fear (and avoid) many such public situations.

Recent studies of general populations report a lifetime occurrence of Social Phobias ranging from 4% to as high as 13%. However, when only those patients who are truly inconvenienced by their symptoms are considered, the numbers are probably lower than these. Whatever the actual figure, these findings contradict previous impressions that Social Phobias are rarely encountered. Perhaps interviewers have too often been insensitive to a common, but silently endured, condition.

Criteria for Social Phobia

- The patient strongly, repeatedly fears at least one social or performance situation that involves facing strangers or being watched by others. The patient

specifically fears showing anxiety symptoms or behaving in some other way that will be embarrassing or humiliating.
- The phobic stimulus almost always causes anxiety, which may be a cued or situationally predisposed Panic Attack.
- The patient realizes that this fear is unreasonable or out of proportion.
- The patient either avoids the situation or endures it with severe distress or anxiety.
- Either there is marked distress about having the phobia, or it markedly interferes with the patient's usual routines or social, job, or personal functioning.
- Patients under the age of 18 must have the symptoms for six months or longer.
- The symptoms are not better explained by a different mental disorder, including anxiety disorders, Body Dysmorphic Disorder, a pervasive developmental disorder, or Schizoid Personality Disorder.
- The symptoms are not directly caused by a general medical condition or by the use of substances, including medications.
- If the patient has another mental disorder or a general medical condition, the phobia is not related to it.

Coding Notes

Specify whether: Generalized. The patient fears most social situations. (If the Social Phobia is Generalized, evaluate the patient for an Axis II diagnosis of Avoidant Personality Disorder.)

Children cannot receive this diagnosis unless they have demonstrated the capacity for social relationships. The anxiety must occur not just with adults, but with peers. They may express the anxiety response by clinging, crying, freezing, or withdrawing. They may not recognize that the fear is unreasonable or out of proportion.

Valerie Tubbs

"It starts right here, and then it spreads like wildfire. I mean, like *real* fire." Valerie Tubbs pointed to the right side of her neck, which was carefully concealed in a blue silk scarf. It had been happening for almost 10 years, any time she was with people; it was worse if she was with a lot of people. Then she felt that everybody noticed.

Although she had never tried, Valerie didn't think that her reaction was something she could control. She just blushed whenever she thought people were watching her. It had started during a high school speech class, when she had to give a talk. She had become confused about the difference between a polyp and a medusa, and one of the boys had commented on the red spot that had appeared on her neck. She had quickly flushed all over and had to sit down, to the general amusement of the class.

"He said it looked like a bull's-eye," she said. Since then, Valerie had tried to avoid saying *anything* to more than a handful of people. She had given up her dream of becoming a fashion buyer for a department store because she couldn't tolerate the scrutiny that the job would entail. Instead, for the last five years she had worked dressing mannequins for the same store.

Valerie said that it seemed "stupid" to be so afraid. It wasn't just that she turned red; she turned *beet*-red. "I can feel prickly little fingers of heat crawling out across my neck and up my cheek. My face feels like it's on fire, and my skin is being scraped with a rusty razor." Whenever she blushed, she didn't feel exactly panicky. It was a sense of anxiety and restlessness that made her wish her body belonged to someone else. Even the thought of meeting new people caused her to feel irritable and keyed up.

Evaluation of Valerie Tubbs

Valerie had insight that her fear of blushing was excessive, but with her scarf she avoided exposure to scrutiny. Her phobia also prevented her from working at the job she would have preferred. With no actual Panic Attacks, and in the absence of **Anxiety Due to a General Medical Condition** and **Substance-Induced Anxiety Disorder**, determining her disorder would come down to the differential diagnosis of phobias. In the absence of a typical history, the **Specific Phobias** would be quickly dismissed.

Patients who have **Panic Disorder With Agoraphobia** may avoid dining out because they fear the embarrassment of having a Panic Attack in a public restaurant. Then you would only diagnose a Social Phobia if it had been present prior to the onset of the Agoraphobia and was unrelated to it. (Sometimes even clinicians who specialize in diagnosing and treating the anxiety disorders can have trouble deciding between these two diagnoses.) **Anorexia Nervosa** patients avoid eating, but the focus is on their weight, not on the embarrassment that might result from gagging or leaving food on the lips.

It is important to differentiate Social Phobia from the nonspecific social anxiety that is so common among teenagers and other young people; this explains the criterion that patients under the age of 18 must have had symptoms for at least half a year. Also keep in mind that many people worry about or feel uncomfortable with social activities such as speaking in public (**stage fright** or **microphone fright**). They should not receive this diagnosis unless it materially affects their working or social lives in some way.

Social Phobias are often associated with suicide attempts and **mood disorders**. Anyone with a Social Phobia may be at risk for self-treatment with **drugs** or **alcohol**; Valerie's clinician should ask carefully about these conditions. Social Phobia has elements in common with **Avoidant Personality Disorder**, which is often diagnosed in patients with Social Phobia. This diagnosis might be warranted if Valerie were *generally* inhibited socially, were overly sensitive to criticism, and felt inadequate. There is no indication that her fears involved social situations other than blushing, so the qualifier Generalized would not be used. Her full diagnosis would be as follows:

Axis I	300.23	Social Phobia
Axis II	V71.09	No diagnosis
Axis III		None
Axis IV		None
Axis V	GAF = 61	(current)

300.3 Obsessive-Compulsive Disorder

Obsessions are recurrent thoughts, beliefs, or ideas that dominate a person's thought content. They persist, despite the fact that the person believes they are unrealistic and may try to resist them. *Compulsions* are acts (either physical or mental) performed repeatedly in a way that the person realizes is neither appropriate nor useful. Compulsions may be comparatively simple, such as uttering or thinking a word or phrase of protection against an obsessive thought. But some are almost unbelievably complex—as in the elaborate dressing, washing, or bedtime rituals that can take up hours every day. Most patients have both obsessions and compulsions, which usually result in anxiety and dread. Patients usually recognize them as being irrational and want to resist them.

Obsessive–Compulsive Disorder (OCD) typically begins in adolescent or early adult life; the symptoms may wax and wane. Although it is uncommon as anxiety disorders go, it is clinically important because it is usually chronic and often debilitating. It puts patients at risk for celibacy or marital discord, and interferes with performance at school and work.

There are four major symptom patterns in OCD; their features can sometimes overlap.

- The most common is a fear of contamination that leads to excessive handwashing.
- Doubts ("Did I turn off the cooktop?") lead to excessive checking—the patient returns repeatedly to be sure that the cooktop is really off.
- Obsessions without compulsions constitute a less common pattern.
- Obsessions and compulsions slow some patients down to the point that it can take them hours, for example, just to eat breakfast.

Men and women are equally likely to develop OCD. Its prevalence, which may be as high as 2% in the general population, is reported to be greater among the upper classes and in those of high intelligence. OCD is probably at least in part inherited.

Criteria for Obsessive–Compulsive Disorder

- The patient has obsessions or compulsions, or both.
  - ✓ Obsessions. The patient must have *all* of these:
    - Recurring, persisting thoughts, impulses, or images inappropriately intrude into awareness and cause marked distress or anxiety.
    - These ideas are not just extreme worries about ordinary problems.
    - The patient tries to disregard or suppress these ideas, or to neutralize them by thoughts or behavior.
    - The patient is aware that these ideas are a product of the patient's own mind.
  - ✓ Compulsions. The patient must have *all* of these:
    - The patient feels the need to repeat physical behaviors (checking the stove to be sure it is off, handwashing) or mental behaviors (counting things, silently repeating words).
    - These behaviors occur as a response to an obsession or in accordance with strictly applied rules.
    - The aim of these behaviors is to reduce or eliminate distress or to prevent something that is dreaded.
    - These behaviors are either not realistically related to the events they are supposed to counteract, or they are clearly excessive for that purpose.
- During some part of the illness, the patient recognizes that the obsessions or compulsions are unreasonable or excessive.
- The obsessions and/or compulsions are associated with at least one of these:
  - ✓ They cause severe distress.
  - ✓ They take up time (more than an hour per day).
  - ✓ They interfere with the patient's usual routine or social, work, or personal functioning.
- If the patient has another Axis I disorder, the content of obsessions or compulsions is not restricted to it.
- The symptoms are not directly caused by a general medical condition or by the use of substances, including medications.

Coding Notes

Specify if: With Poor Insight. During most of this episode the patient does not realize that these thoughts and behaviors are unreasonable or excessive. (Neither this specifier nor the insight requirement above applies to children.)

DSM-IV specifies preoccupations typical of other Axis I disorders that must be ruled out: appearance (Body Dysmorphic Disorder); food (eating disorders); being seriously ill (Hypochondriasis); guilt (mood disorders); sexual fantasies or urges (paraphilias); substance use (substance use disorders); and hair pulling (Trichotillomania).

Leighton Prescott

Pausing for a moment, Leighton Prescott leaned forward to straighten the stack of journals on the interviewer's desk. When he leaned back and resumed talking, he folded his hands. The skin was chapped and the color of dusty bricks.

"So I would get this feeling that there could be semen on my hands and that it might be transferred to a woman and get her pregnant, even if I only shook hands with her. I started washing extra carefully each time I masturbated."

Leighton Prescott was a 23-year-old graduate student in plant physiology. He was enormously bright and dedicated to science, but his grades had slipped badly over the past few months. He attributed this to the handwashing rituals. Whenever he had the thought that he might have contaminated his hands with semen, he felt compelled to scrub them thoroughly.

A year earlier, this had only meant three or four minutes with a bar of soap and water as hot as he could stand it. Soon he required a nail brush; still later he was brushing his hands and wrists as well. By now this had evolved into an elaborate ritual. First he scraped under his nails with a blade; then he used the brush on them. He then lathered surgical soap to his elbows and scrubbed with a different brush for 15 minutes per arm. Then he would have to start over with his nails, because semen scrubbed off his arms might have lodged under them. If he had the thought that he had not performed one of the steps exactly right, he would have to start all over again. In recent weeks this had become the norm.

"I know it seems crazy," he said with a glance at his hands. "I'm a biologist. That part of me knows that spermatozoa can't live longer than a few minutes on the skin. But if I don't wash, the pressure just builds up and up, until I *have* to wash—washing is the only thing that relieves the anxiety."

Leighton didn't think he was depressed, though he was appropriately concerned about his symptoms. His sleep and appetite had been normal; he had never felt guilty or suicidal.

"Just stupid, especially when my girl stopped seeing me. I used the bathroom in a restaurant where I took her to eat. After 45 minutes, she had to send the manager in for me." He laughed ruefully. "She said she might see me again, if I'd clean up my act."

Evaluation of Leighton Prescott

Leighton's obsessions and compulsions both easily fulfilled the requirements for OCD. He tried to suppress the recurrent thoughts (about semen), which he recognized were the unreasonable products of his own mind. He felt compelled to ward off these ideas about contamination by repetitive handwashing, which he acknowledged was grossly excessive. By the time he came for help, his symptoms occupied several hours each day, interfered with his schooling and social life, and caused him severe distress. He had no other identifiable Axis I disorder that might account for his symptoms.

An important step in evaluating anyone for OCD is to determine whether the patient's focus of concern is pathological. For example, someone who lives in a ghetto or a war zone might be prudent to triple-lock the doors and check security frequently. Had Leighton been excessively concerned about real-life problems (such as passing his exams or succeeding with his girlfriend), he might instead warrant a diagnosis of **Generalized Anxiety Disorder**.

Although by definition OCD patients recognize their obsessions and compulsions as unreasonable or excessive, some lose insight during much of their illness. Leighton recognized that he was being unreasonable, and his OCD therefore would not be coded as With Poor Insight. When insight is lost to the degree that the obsession becomes delusional, consider a diagnosis of **Delusional Disorder**.

Patients with **general medical conditions** and **substance-related disorders** rarely present with obsessions or compulsions, though repetitive behavior is characteristic of **Tourette's Disorder** and **temporal lobe epilepsy**. Inquire carefully about past or present tics, reported in about one-quarter of all OCD patients; there is also a relationship between OCD and Tourette's Disorder. Obsessional thinking or compulsive behavior can be found in a variety of other mental disorders. People may obsessively pursue any number of activities, such as **gambling**, **drinking**, and **sex**. The differential diagnosis also includes **Body Dysmorphic Disorder** (the patient obsesses about body shape), **Hypochondriasis** (the patient obsesses about health), and other Axis I disorders mentioned above in the Coding Notes.

Perhaps 20% of OCD patients have premorbid obsessional traits. Because of its name, **Obsessive–Compulsive Personality Disorder** (see p. 493) can be confused with OCD. Although the personality disorder often coexists with OCD, they are far from the same. Patients with only the personality disorder do not have obsessions or compulsions at all. They are perfectionistic and become preoccupied with rules, lists, and details. They may accomplish tasks slowly because they keep checking to be sure it is being done exactly right, but they do not have the desire to resist these behaviors. Clinicians who treat many anxiety disorder patients claim that the border zone between OCD and **Schizotypal Personality Disorder** is a common problem in differential diagnosis.

Leighton's full diagnosis would be as follows:

Axis I	300.3	Obsessive–Compulsive Disorder
Axis II	V71.09	No diagnosis
Axis III		None
Axis IV		None
Axis V	GAF = 60	(current)

> TIP As many as half of OCD patients have an accompanying mood disorder. Some only show their obsessional symptoms when they are in the midst of a severe depression. OCD patients are also highly likely to have another anxiety disorder.

309.81 Posttraumatic Stress Disorder

People who survive severely traumatic events often have Posttraumatic Stress Disorder (PTSD). Survivors of combat are the most frequent victims, but it is also encountered in people who have survived other disasters, both natural and man-made. These include rape, floods, abductions, and airplane crashes, as well as the threats that may be posed by a kidnapping or hostage situation. Children can have PTSD as a result of inappropriate sexual experience, whether or not there is actual injury. PTSD can be diagnosed even in those who have learned about severe trauma (or its threat) suffered by someone to whom they are close—children, spouses, other close relatives. Implicitly excluded from the definition are ordinary life experiences such as bereavement, divorce, and serious illness; however, a spouse's sudden, unexpected death or a child's life-threatening illness could qualify as a traumatic event.

After some delay (symptoms do not usually develop immediately after the trauma), the person in some way relives the traumatic event and tries to avoid thinking about it. There are also symptoms of physiological hyperarousal, such as an exaggerated startle response. PTSD patients often feel guilt or personal responsibility ("I should have prevented it").

In general, the worse or more enduring the trauma, the greater the likelihood of developing PTSD. The risk runs to one-quarter of the survivors of heavy combat and two-thirds of former prisoners of war. Those who have experienced natural disasters such as fires or floods are generally less likely to develop symptoms. Older adults are less likely to develop symptoms than are younger ones. About half the patients recover within a few months; others can experience years of incapacity.

Criteria for Posttraumatic Stress Disorder

- The patient has experienced or witnessed or was confronted with an unusually traumatic event that has *both* of these elements:
  - The event involved actual or threatened death or serious physical injury to the patient or to others, *and*
  - The patient felt intense fear, horror, or helplessness.
- The patient repeatedly relives the event in at least one of these ways:
  - ✓ Intrusive, distressing recollections (thoughts, images)
  - ✓ Repeated, distressing dreams

- ✓ Through flashbacks, hallucinations, or illusions, feeling or acting as if the event were recurring (includes experiences that occur when intoxicated or awakening)
- ✓ Marked mental distress in reaction to internal or external cues that symbolize or resemble some part of the event
- ✓ Physiological reactions (such as rapid heart beat, elevated blood pressure) in response to these cues
- The patient repeatedly avoids the trauma-related stimuli and has numbing of general responsiveness (absent before the traumatic event), as shown by three or more of the these:
  - ✓ Tries to avoid feelings, thoughts, or conversations concerned with the event
  - ✓ Tries to avoid activities, people or places that recall the event
  - ✓ Cannot recall an important feature of the event
  - ✓ Experiences marked loss of interest or participation in activities important to the patient
  - ✓ Feels detached or isolated from other people
  - ✓ Experiences restriction in ability to love or feel other strong emotions
  - ✓ Feels life will be brief or unfulfilled (lack of marriage, job, children)
- The patient has at least two of the following symptoms of hyperarousal that were not present before the traumatic event:
  - ✓ Insomnia (initial or interval)
  - ✓ Angry outbursts or irritability
  - ✓ Poor concentration
  - ✓ Excessive vigilance
  - ✓ Increased startle response
- The symptoms above have lasted longer than one month.
- These symptoms cause clinically important distress or impair work, social, or personal functioning.

Coding Notes

Specify whether:

Acute. Symptoms have lasted less than three months.

Chronic. Symptoms have lasted three months or longer.

Specify if: With Delayed Onset. The symptoms did not appear until at least six months after the event.

In children, response to the traumatic event may be agitation or disorganized behavior. Young children may relive the event through repetitive play, trauma-specific re-enactment, or nightmares without recognizable content.

Barney Gorse

"They're gooks! The place is staffed with gooks!"

Someone sitting behind Barney Gorse had dropped a book onto the tile floor, and that had set him off. Now he had backed into a corner in the waiting room of the mental health clinic. His pupils were widely dilated, and perspiration stood out on his forehead. He was panting heavily. He pointed a shaky finger at the Oriental student who stood petrified on the other side of the room. "Get this goddamn gook out of here!" He made a fist and started to lumber in the direction of the student.

"Hang on, Barney. It's okay." Barney's therapist took him firmly by the elbow and led him to a private office. They sat there in silence for a few minutes, while Barney's breathing gradually returned to normal and the therapist reviewed his chart.

Barney Gorse was 39 now, but he had been barely 20 when his draft number came up and he joined the Ninth Infantry Division in Vietnam. At that time President Nixon was "winding down the war," which made it seem all the more painful when Barney's squad was hit by mortar fire from North Vietnamese regulars.

He had never talked about it, even during "anger displacement" group therapy with other veterans. Whenever he was asked to tell his story, he would fly into a rage. But something truly devastating must have happened to Barney that day. The reports mentioned a wound in the upper thigh; he had been the only member of his squad to survive the attack. He had been awarded a Purple Heart and a full pension.

Barney hadn't been able to remember several hours of the attack at all. And he had always been careful to avoid films and television programs about war. He said he'd had enough of it to last everybody's lifetime; in fact, he had gone to some lengths to avoid thinking about it. He celebrated his discharge from the Army by getting drunk, which was how he stayed for six years. When he finally sobered up, he turned to drugs. Even that hadn't been enough to obliterate the nightmares that still haunted him; he awakened screaming several times a week. Sudden noises would startle him into a panic attack.

Now, thanks to disulfiram and a chaplain in the county jail where he had been held as a persistent public nuisance, Barney had been clean and sober for six months. On the condition that he would seek treatment for his drug use, he had been released. The specialists in substance misuse had quickly recognized that he had other problems, and that had led him here.

Last week when they met, Barney's therapist had reminded him again that he needed to dig into his feelings about the past. He had responded that he didn't have any feelings; they'd dried up on him. For that matter, the future didn't look so good, either: "Got no job, no wife, no kids. I just wasn't meant to have a life." He got up and put his hand on the doorknob to leave. "It's no use. I just can't talk about it."

Evaluation of Barney Gorse

Let us summarize the criteria that must be fulfilled before the diagnosis of PTSD can be made.

1. There must be severe trauma. Barney's was the stress of combat, but a variety of civilian stressors are also possible candidates. The important feature is that the stressor must be unusually traumatic. Divorce or death of a spouse, for example, though undeniably stressful, are commonplace and do not qualify for PTSD.

2. The stress must be relived in some way. Barney had flashbacks, during which it seemed to him that he was actually back in Vietnam. Less dramatic forms of recollection include recurrent memories, dreams, and any other reminder of the event that results in distress or physiological symptoms.

3. The patient must attempt (wittingly or unwittingly) to achieve emotional distance from the stressful event. Barney's efforts were quite evident (amnesia, refusing to see movies and TV programs, refusing to talk about Vietnam). Distancing can also be accomplished by a general numbing of emotional responsiveness (isolation from others, inability to love).

4. PTSD patients must have symptoms of increased arousal. Barney suffered from insomnia and a severe startle response; others may have general irritability, poor concentration, or excessive vigilance. As with all symptoms, the clinician would have to determine that these symptoms of arousal had not been apparent before Barney's Vietnam trauma.

The history of severe trauma in combat and the typical symptoms would render any other explanation for Barney's symptoms unlikely. A patient with **Intermittent Explosive Disorder** might become aggressive and lose control, but would not have the history of severe trauma. But clinicians must *always* be alert to the possibility of **Anxiety Disorder Due to a General Medical Condition**, which could be diagnosed instead of or in addition to PTSD. For example, head injuries would be relatively common among veterans of combat or other violent trauma. Brain damage resulting from head injury would be coded on Axis III. **Situational Adjustment Disorder** shouldn't be confused with PTSD: The severity of the trauma would be far less, and the effects would be more transient and less dramatic.

In PTSD, comorbidity is the rule rather than the exception. Barney had used drugs and alcohol; any substance-related disorder would also be coded on Axis I. (Barney's clinician would have gathered additional information about use of other substances.) Of combat veterans who have PTSD, half or more also have a problem with **Substance Dependence** or **Abuse**; **Polysubstance Dependence** is common. Other anxiety disorders (**Phobic Disorder, Generalized Anxiety Disorder**) and mood disorders (**Major Depressive Disorder, Dysthymic Disorder**) are likewise common in this population. Dissociative disorders (**Dissociative Amnesia, Dissociative Fugue**) may also occur. Any coexisting personality disorder would be coded on Axis II. **Malingering** is also a diagnosis that should be investigated whenever there appears to be a possibility of material gain (insurance, disability, legal problems).

Three time qualifiers are possible with PTSD. Although the vignette is not precise on this point, Barney's symptoms probably began by the time he was discharged from the military, so he would not qualify for With Delayed Onset. He had certainly been ill for longer than three months (hence Chronic).

> **TIP** There is still considerable controversy over the qualifier of With Delayed Onset. Many experts deny that symptoms of PTSD can begin many months or years after the trauma. Nonetheless, the qualifier is there to use when it seems appropriate.

Barney's complete diagnosis would read as follows:

Axis I	309.81	Posttraumatic Stress Disorder, Chronic
	303.90	Alcohol Dependence, Early Full Remission
Axis II	V71.09	No diagnosis
Axis III		None
Axis IV		Lives alone
		Unemployed
Axis V	GAF = 35	(current)

308.3 Acute Stress Disorder

A new diagnosis in DSM-IV, Acute Stress Disorder was spawned by the observation that some people briefly develop symptoms immediately after traumatic stress. This is not exactly new information; it was recognized as far back as 1865, after the U.S. Civil War. For many years it was called "shell shock." Like PTSD, Acute Stress Disorder can also be encountered in civilians.

The criteria for Acute Stress Disorder embody all the elements required for PTSD:

- A severe stress that provokes fear, horror, or helplessness
- Re-experiencing of the event in some way
- Numbing of responsiveness
- Hyperarousal (or symptoms of severe anxiety)

If the symptoms last longer than a month, it is no longer an Acute Stress Disorder. At that point, a diagnosis of PTSD might be indicated.

Criteria for Acute Stress Disorder

- The patient has experienced or witnessed or was confronted with an unusually traumatic event that has *both* of these elements:
  - The event involved actual or threatened death or serious physical injury to the patient or to others, *and*
  - The patient felt intense fear, horror, or helplessness.
- Either during the event or just afterward, the patient experiences three or more of these symptoms of dissociation:
  - ✓ Feelings of detachment or numbness, or emotional unresponsiveness
  - ✓ Diminished awareness of surroundings, as in a daze
  - ✓ Derealization
  - ✓ Depersonalization
  - ✓ Amnesia for important aspects of the event
- The patient repeatedly re-experiences the event in one or more of these ways:
  - ✓ Recollections (dreams, flashbacks, illusions, images, thoughts)
  - ✓ The sense of reliving the event
  - ✓ Mental distress as a reaction to reminders of the event
- The patient strongly avoids activities, conversations, feelings, people, places, or thoughts reminiscent of the trauma.
- There are marked symptoms of anxiety or hyperarousal, such as excessive vigilance, insomnia, irritability, poor concentration, restlessness, or increased startle response.
- At least one of the following applies:
  - ✓ The patient feels marked distress as a result of the symptoms.
  - ✓ They interfere with usual social, job, or personal functioning.
  - ✓ They block the patient from doing something important, such as getting legal or medical help or telling family or other supporters about the experience.
- The symptoms begin within four weeks of the trauma and last from two days to four weeks.
- The symptoms are not directly caused by a general medical condition or by the use of substances, including medications.
- They are not merely a worsening of another Axis I or Axis II disorder.
- Brief Psychotic Disorder is ruled out.

Marie Trudeau

Marie Trudeau and her husband, André, sat in the intake interviewer's office. Marie was the patient, but she spent most of the time rubbing the knuckles of one hand and gazing vacantly about the room. André did most of the talking.

"I just can't believe the change in her," he said. "A week ago, she was completely normal. Never had anything like this in her life. Heck, she's never had *anything* wrong with her. Then, all of a sudden, boom! She's a mess."

At André's exclamation, Marie jerked around to face him and rose half out of her chair. For a few seconds she stood there, frozen except for her gaze, which darted from one side of the room to the other.

"Aw, geez, I'm sorry, honey. I forgot." He put his arm around her. Grasping her shoulders firmly but gently, he eased her back into the chair. He held her there until she began to relax her grip on his arm.

A week earlier, Marie had just finished her gardening and was sitting in the back yard with a lemonade, reading a book. When she heard airplane engines, she looked up and saw two small planes flying high overhead, directly above her. "My God," she thought, "they're going to collide!" As she watched in horror, they did collide.

She could see perfectly. The sun was low, highlighting the two planes brilliantly against the deep blue of the late afternoon sky. Something seemed to have been torn off one of the planes—the news media later reported that the right wing of one plane had ripped right through the cockpit of the other. Thinking to call 911, Marie picked up her portable phone, but she didn't dial. She could only watch as two tiny objects suddenly appeared beside the stricken airplanes and tumbled in a leisurely arc toward her.

"They weren't objects, they were people." It was the first time she had spoken during the interview. Marie's chin trembled and a lock of hair fell across her eye. She didn't try to brush it back.

As she continued to watch, one of the bodies hurtled into her yard 15 feet from where she was sitting. It buried itself six inches deep in the soft earth behind her rose bushes.

What happened next, Marie seemed to have blanked out completely. The other body landed in the street a block away. Half an hour later, when the police knocked on her door, they found her in the kitchen peeling carrots for supper and crying into the sink. When André arrived home an hour after that, she seemed dazed. All she would say was "I'm not here."

In the six days since, Marie hadn't improved much. Although she might start a conversation, she would usually trail off in midsentence. She couldn't focus much better on her work at home. Amy, their nine-year-old daughter, seemed to be taking care of *her*. Three nights running Marie had awakened from a dream, trying to cry out but managing only a terrified squeak. She kept the blinds in the kitchen closed, so she wouldn't even have to look into the back yard.

"It's like someone I saw in a World War II movie," André concluded. "You'd think she'd been shell-shocked."

Evaluation of Marie Trudeau

Anxiety and depressive symptoms are nearly universal following a severe stress. Usually these are relatively short-lived, however, and do not include the full spectrum of symptoms required for Acute Stress Disorder. This diagnosis should only be considered when major symptoms last longer than two days after a rare event that would severely traumatize nearly anyone. Such an event was the plane crash Marie witnessed. She was dazed and emotionally unresponsive, and could not recall what had happened during part of the accident. She had nightmares, avoided looking into the back yard, and startled easily. Since the incident, she had been unable to carry on with her work at home.

Would any other diagnosis be possible? According to André, Marie's previous health had been good, reducing the chances that she instead had a **general medical condition**. We aren't told whether she used alcohol or drugs; perhaps the fact that she was drinking only a lemonade at the time of the crash would suggest that she did not. The clinician would have to ask specifically, anyway, to rule out a **substance-related disorder**. Acute Stress Disorder patients can have severe depressive symptoms ("survivor's guilt"), to the point that a concomitant diagnosis of **Major Depressive Disorder** may be justified in some cases.

Marie's five-axis diagnosis would be as follows:

Axis I	308.3	Acute Stress Disorder
Axis II	V71.09	No diagnosis
Axis III		None
Axis IV		None
Axis V	GAF = 61	(current)

300.02 Generalized Anxiety Disorder

Generalized Anxiety Disorder (GAD) can be difficult to diagnose. The symptoms are relatively unfocused; the nervousness is low-key and chronic; and there are no Panic Attacks. Although some patients may be able to state what it is that makes them nervous, others cannot.

The symptoms are also common. Nearly everybody worries, and most people find that worry can sometimes be hard to control. GAD patients typically worry far more about many things ("everything") than objective facts can justify. Many patients have been this way for years, without coming to the attention of a clinician. Perhaps this is because the degree of impairment in GAD is usually not severe.

GAD is found in 3–5% of the general adult population.

Criteria for Generalized Anxiety Disorder

- For more than half the days in at least six months, the patient experiences excessive anxiety and worry about several events or activities.
- The patient has trouble controlling these feelings.
- Associated with this anxiety and worry, the patient has three or more of the following symptoms, some of which are present for over half the days in the past six months:
  ✓ Feelings of being restless, edgy, keyed up
  ✓ Tiring easily
  ✓ Trouble concentrating
  ✓ Irritability
  ✓ Increased muscle tension
  ✓ Trouble sleeping (initial insomnia or restless, unrefreshing sleep)
- Aspects of another Axis I disorder do not provide the focus of the anxiety and worry.
- The symptoms cause clinically important distress or impair work, social, or personal functioning.
- The disorder is not directly caused by a general medical condition or by the use of substances, including medications.
- It does not occur only during a mood disorder, psychotic disorder, Posttraumatic Stress Disorder, or a pervasive developmental disorder.

Coding Notes

Children need fulfill only one of the six checkmarked symptoms above.

Aspects of another Axis I disorder (see fourth bullet) include worry about the following: weight gain (Anorexia Nervosa); contamination (Obsessive–Compulsive Disorder); having a Panic Attack (Panic Disorder); separation from home or relatives (Separation Anxiety Disorder); public embarrassment (Social Phobia); and having physical symptoms (somatoform disorders).

Bert Parmalee

For most of his adult life, Bert had been "a worry-wart." At age 35, he still had dreams that he was flunking all of his college electrical engineering courses. But recently he had felt that he was walking a tightrope. For the past year he had been the administrative assistant to the chief executive officer of a *Fortune* 500 company, where he had previously worked in product engineering.

"I took the job because it seemed a great way to move up the corporate ladder," he said, "but almost every day I have the feeling my foot's about to slip off the rung."

Each of the company's six ambitious vice-presidents saw Bert as a personal pipeline to the chief. His boss was a hard-driving workaholic who constantly sparked ideas and wanted them implemented yesterday. Several times he had told Bert that he was pleased with his performance. In fact, Bert was doing the best job of any administrative assistant he had ever had, but that didn't seem to reassure Bert.

"I've felt uptight just about every day since I started this job. My chief expects action and results. He has zero patience for thinking about how it should all fit together. Our vice-presidents all want to have their own way. Several of them hint pretty broadly that if I don't help them, they'll put in a bad word with the boss. I'm always looking over my shoulder."

Bert had trouble concentrating at work; at night he was exhausted but had trouble getting to sleep. Once he did, he slept fitfully. He had become chronically irritable at home, yelling at his children for no reason. He had never had a panic attack, and he didn't think he was depressed. In fact, he still took a great deal of pleasure in the two activities he enjoyed most: Sunday afternoon football on TV and Saturday night lovemaking with his wife. But recently his wife had offered to take the kids to her mother's for a few weeks, to relieve some of the pressure. This only resurrected some of his old concerns that he wasn't good enough for her—that she might find someone else and leave him for good.

Bert was slightly overweight and balding, and he looked apprehensive. He was carefully dressed and fidgeted a bit; his speech was clear, coherent, relevant, and spontaneous. He denied having obsessions, compulsions, phobias, delusions, or hallucinations. On the Mini-Mental State Exam, he scored a perfect 30. He said that his main problem—his only problem—was his nagging uneasiness.

Valium made him drowsy. He had tried meditating, but found that it only allowed him to concentrate more effectively on his problems. For a few weeks he had tried having a cocktail before dinner; that had both relaxed him and started him worrying about becoming an alcoholic. Once or twice he even went with his brother-in-law to an Alcoholics Anonymous meeting. "Now I've decided to try dreading one day at a time."

Evaluation of Bert Parmalee

Bert's symptoms would fit the inclusion criteria for GAD:

1. He had multiple worries (his job, being an alcoholic, losing his wife); none of these was adequately supported by fact. The excessiveness of his worries would differentiate them from the usual sort of anxiety that is not pathological.

2. Despite repeated efforts (meditation, reassurance, medication), he had been unable to control these fears.

3. He had at least four physical or mental symptoms (three required): trouble concentrating, fatigue, irritability, and sleep disturbance.

4. He had been having difficulty nearly every day for longer than the required six months.

5. His symptoms caused him considerable distress, perhaps even more than is usual for patients with GAD.

One of the difficulties about diagnosing GAD is that so many other conditions must be excluded. A number of **general medical disorders** can produce anxiety symptoms; a complete workup of Bert's anxiety would have to consider these possibilities. From the information contained in the vignette, a **Substance-Induced Anxiety Disorder** would appear unlikely.

Anxiety symptoms can be found in nearly every category of mental disorder, including **psychotic mood** (depressed or manic), **eating**, **somatoform**, and **cognitive disorders**. From Bert's history, none of these would seem remotely likely. An **Adjustment Disorder with Anxiety** would be eliminated because Bert's symptoms met the criteria for another Axis I disorder.

It is important that the patient's worry and anxiety must not focus solely on features of another Axis I disorder, especially another anxiety disorder; specific examples are mentioned in the Coding Notes. Nevertheless, note that a patient can have GAD in the presence of another Axis I disorder if it is not the *sole* focus of the worry. It is not uncommon, for example, to diagnose a **Major Depressive Disorder** along with GAD, provided that the symptoms of GAD existed prior to the onset of the depression. (Look carefully for symptoms of depression in patients with GAD; even mild depressive illnesses can help predict improvement in GAD symptoms with antidepressant medication.) Other **anxiety disorders** and **substance-related disorders** may also be diagnosed with GAD.

Bert's complete diagnosis would be as follows:

Axis I	300.02	Generalized Anxiety Disorder
Axis II	V71.09	No diagnosis
Axis III		None
Axis IV		Difficult work conditions
Axis V	GAF = 70	(current)

TIP It is reasonable to ask this question: Does diagnosing GAD in a depressed patient help with your evaluation? After all, the anxiety symptoms may disappear once the depression has been sufficiently treated. The value, I suppose, is that flagging the anxiety symptoms gives a more complete picture of the patient's pathology. Also, you may have to treat the anxiety symptoms independently later on.

293.89 Anxiety Disorder
Due to a General Medical Condition

Many medical disorders can produce anxiety symptoms. Usually the symptoms will be similar to those of Panic Disorder or GAD, but occasionally they may take the form of obsessions or compulsions. In general, anxiety symptoms will not be caused by a medical disorder, but it is supremely important to identify those that are. The symptoms of untreated medical disorders can evolve from anxiety to permanent disability (consider the dangers of an untreated brain tumor).

As in the following vignette, the most common general medical causes of anxiety symptoms are probably diabetes, hyperthyroidism, and other endocrine disorders. A more complete listing of possible causes is included in Appendix B.

Criteria for Anxiety Disorder
Due to a General Medical Condition

- The patient has prominent anxiety, compulsions, obsessions, or Panic Attacks.
- History, physical exam, or laboratory findings suggest a general medical condition that seems likely to have directly caused these symptoms.
- No other mental disorder better accounts for these symptoms.
- The symptoms cause important clinical distress or impair work, social, or personal functioning.
- The symptoms don't occur solely during a delirium.

Coding Notes

Depending on the dominant symptomatology, specify whether:

With Generalized Anxiety

With Panic Attacks

With Obsessive–Compulsive Symptoms

DSM-IV specifically mentions that an Adjustment Disorder With Anxiety, precipitated by the stress of a serious medical illness, must be ruled out.

In the Axis I diagnosis, include the name of the actual general medical condition (not the term "general medical condition"). On Axis III, code the specific general medical condition.

Millicent Worthy

"I wonder if we could just leave the door open." Millicent Worthy got up from the chair and opened the examining room door. She had fidgeted throughout the first part of the interview. During the last few minutes, she had hardly seemed to be paying attention at all. "I feel better not being so closed in." Once she finally settled down, she told this story.

Millicent was 24 and divorced. She had never touched drugs or alcohol. Until about four months ago, she'd been well all her life. She had visited a mental health clinic only once before, when she was 12: Her parents were having marital problems, and the entire family had gone for family counseling.

She had first felt nervous while tending the checkout counter at the video rental outlet where she worked. She felt cramped, hemmed in, as if she needed to walk around. One afternoon, when she was the only employee in the store and she had to stay behind the counter, her heart began to pound and she perspired and became short of breath. She thought she was about to die.

Over the next several weeks, Millicent gradually became aware of other symptoms. Her hand had begun to shake; she noticed it one day at the end of her shift when she was adding up the receipts from her cash register. Her appetite was voracious, yet in the past six weeks her weight had dropped nearly 10 pounds. She still loved watching movies on video, but lately she felt so tired at night that she could barely keep awake in front of the TV. Her mood had been somewhat irritable.

"As I thought about it, I realized that all this started about the time my boyfriend and I decided to get married. We've been living together for a year, and I really love him. But I'd been burned before, in my first marriage. I thought that might be what was bothering me, so I gave back his ring and moved out. If anything, I feel worse now than before."

Several times during the interview Millicent shifted restlessly in her chair. Her speech was rapid, though she could be interrupted. Her eyes seemed to protrude slightly, and although she had lost weight, a fullness in her neck suggested a goiter. She admitted that she was having trouble tolerating heat. "There's no air conditioner in our store. Last summer it was no problem—we kept the door open. But now it's terrible! And if I wore less clothing to work, they'd have to give me a desk in the adult video section."

Millicent's thyroid function studies proved to be markedly abnormal. Within two months an endocrinologist had brought her hyperactive thyroid under control, and her anxiety symptoms had disappeared completely. Six months later, she and her fiancé were married.

Evaluation of Millicent Worthy

Millicent had at least one Panic Attack; if she had had them repeatedly and if the symptoms of her goiter had been overlooked, she could have been misdiagnosed as having **Panic Disorder Without Agoraphobia**. Her symptoms (restlessness, fatiguability, irritability) could have been misinterpreted as **Generalized Anxiety Disorder**. Panic Attacks and symptoms of generalized anxiety are the two syndromes that are most commonly associated with general medical disorders. (Even Millicent interpreted her own symptoms as psychological.) Such a scenario reinforces the wisdom of placing general medical conditions at the top of the list of differential diagnoses.

Irritability, restless hyperactivity, and weight loss also suggest a **Manic Episode**, but these are usually accompanied by a subjective feeling of high energy, not fatigue. Millicent's rapid speech could be interrupted; in mania, it often cannot. Her lack of previous depressions or manias would also militate against a mood disorder. Her history would rule out a **Substance-Induced Anxiety Disorder**.

Although Millicent had had at least one Panic Attack, she was mainly affected with generalized anxiety symptoms, hence the specifier for her Axis I diagnosis. The Axis IV diagnosis was made not because it seemed a cause of her anxiety symptoms, but because it was felt that her relationship with her fiancé was a problem that should be addressed as part of the overall treatment plan.

Axis I	293.89	Anxiety Disorder Due to Hyperthyroidism, With Generalized Anxiety
Axis II	V71.09	No diagnosis
Axis III	242.0	Hyperthyroidism with goiter
Axis IV		Estrangement from fiancé
Axis V	GAF = 70	(on admission)
	GAF = 85	(at discharge)

Substance-Induced Anxiety Disorder

Many substances can produce anxiety symptoms. These may occur during acute intoxication (or heavy use, as with caffeine) or during withdrawal (as with alcohol or sedatives). The substances most commonly associated with anxiety symptoms are marijuana, amphetamines, and caffeine. See Appendix B, for a summary of the substances for which intoxication or withdrawal can be expected to create anxiety.

Criteria for Substance-Induced Anxiety Disorder

- The patient has prominent anxiety, compulsions, obsessions, or Panic Attacks.
- History, physical exam or laboratory data, substantiate that *either*
    ✓ These symptoms have developed within a month of Substance Intoxication or Withdrawal, *or*
    ✓ Medication use has caused the symptoms.

- No other anxiety disorder better accounts for these symptoms.
- The symptoms cause clinically important distress or impair work, social, or personal functioning.
- The symptoms don't occur solely during a delirium.

Coding Notes

Codes for Substance-Induced Anxiety Disorders:

291.8	Alcohol
292.89	Amphetamine [or Amphetamine-Like Substance]; Caffeine; Cannabis; Cocaine; Hallucinogen; Inhalant; Phencyclidine [or Phencyclidine-Like Substance]; Sedative, Hypnotic, or Anxiolytic; Other [or Unknown] Substance

Depending on the dominant symptomatology, specify whether:

With Generalized Anxiety

With Obsessive–Compulsive symptoms

With Panic Attacks

With Phobic Symptoms

Depending on time of onset, specify:

With Onset During Intoxication

With Onset During Withdrawal

No other anxiety disorder must account for the symptoms better than does substance use (see third bullet). A variety of historical information could suggest that this is the case:

Anxiety disorder symptoms precede the onset of substance use.

There have been previous episodes of an anxiety disorder.

The symptoms are much worse than you would expect for the amount and duration of the substance use.

Anxiety disorder symptoms continue long (at least a month) after Substance Intoxication or Withdrawal stops.

The diagnosis of a Substance-Induced Anxiety Disorder should be made only when the anxiety symptoms considerably exceed what you would expect from an ordinary case of Substance Intoxication or Withdrawal for the specific substance.

An anxiety disorder caused by most medications taken in therapeutic doses would be coded as, for example:

Axis I   292.89   Thyroxin-Induced Anxiety Disorder, With
                     Generalized Anxiety
Axis III E932.7   Thyroid replacement (Thyroxin)

Bonita Ramirez

Bonita Ramirez, a 19-year-old college freshman, was brought to the emergency room by two friends. She was alert, intelligent, and well informed, and she cooperated fully in providing information about her distress.

Bonita's parents both had graduate degrees and were well established in their professions. They lived in a well-to-do suburb of San Diego. Bonita was their oldest child and only daughter. Strictly reared in the Catholic faith, she hadn't been allowed to date until a year ago. Until sorority rush week, the only alcohol she had tasted had been Communion wine. By her account and that of her companions, she had been happy, healthy, and vivacious when she arrived on campus a fortnight earlier.

Two weeks had made a remarkable difference. Bonita now sat huddled on the examination table, feet drawn up beneath her. Her arms were wrapped around her knees, and they trembled noticeably. Although it was only September, she wore a sweater and complained of feeling cold. An emesis basin sat beside her, in case she needed it again.

Her voice quavered as she said that nothing like this had ever happened to her before. "I had some beer last week. It didn't bother me at all, except I had a headache the next morning."

This evening there had been a "big sister, little sister" party at the sorority Bonita had just pledged. She had drunk some beer, and that had prompted her to take a few hits from the marijuana cigarette they were passing around. The beer must have numbed her throat, because she had been able to draw the smoke deep into her lungs and hold it, the way her friends had showed her.

For about 10 minutes Bonita hadn't noticed anything at all. Then her head began to feel tight, as if her hair were a wig that didn't fit right. Suddenly, when she tried to breathe, her lungs seemed to hurt, and she became instantly aware that she was going to die. She tried to run, but her legs became rubbery and refused to move.

The other girls hadn't had much experience with drug reactions, but they called one of the men from the fraternity house next door, who came over and tried to talk Bonita down. After an hour, she still felt the panicked certainty that she would die or go mad. That was when they decided to bring her to the emergency room.

At length she said, "They said it would relax me and expand my consciousness. I just want to contract it again."

Evaluation of Bonita Ramirez

Bonita's typical history—she was healthy until the ingestion of a substance that is known to produce anxiety symptoms, especially in a naïve user—is a dead giveaway for the diagnosis. Other drugs that commonly produce anxiety symptoms include **amphetamines**, which can also produce Panic Attack Symptoms, and **caffeine** when used heavily. However, because anxiety symptoms can be encountered at some point during the use of most substances, you can code an anxiety disorder secondary to the use of nearly any of them, provided that the anxiety symptoms are worse than you would expect for ordinary **Substance Withdrawal or Intoxication**. Because she required emergency evaluation and treatment, we would judge this to be the case for Bonita.

Despite the proximity of the development of her symptoms to substance use, her clinician would want to be sure that she did not have a **general medical condition** (or **treatment with medication** for a general medical condition) that could also explain her anxiety symptoms.

Although she was severely panicked when she arrived at the emergency room, Bonita's GAF rating was high because her symptoms had caused her no disability and were expected to be transient. Other diagnosticians might rate her differently, however.

Axis I	292.89	Cannabis-Induced Anxiety Disorder, With Panic Attacks, With Onset During Intoxication
Axis II	V71.09	No diagnosis
Axis III		None
Axis IV		None
Axis V	GAF = 80	(current)

300.00 Anxiety Disorder Not Otherwise Specified

Patients who have prominent symptoms of anxiety or phobic avoidance that don't meet criteria for any of the specific anxiety disorders can be coded as having Anxiety Disorder Not Otherwise Specified. (Be sure that you don't include anyone here who meets criteria for an Adjustment Disorder With Anxiety or With Mixed Anxiety and Depressed Mood.) DSM-IV suggests several specific categories:

Fear of offensive body odor. This can cause some people to avoid social contact.

Mixed anxiety–depressive disorder. These patients have symptoms of both, but don't meet the criteria for either a specific anxiety or mood disorder. DSM-IV includes suggested criteria for this proposed diagnosis on page 723.

Phobic symptoms due to another disorder. Such a disorder could be either a general medical condition or a mental disorder. Examples would include AIDS, Parkinson's disease, Trichotillomania, and many others.

Other. Use this category when you know the patient has an anxiety disorder but you can't tell what caused it.

Somatoform Disorders

Quick Guide to the Somatoform Disorders

When somatic symptoms are a prominent reason for evaluation by a clinician, the diagnosis will be one of the disorders (or categories) listed below. As usual, the page number following each item indicates where a more detailed discussion begins.

Somatoform Disorders

Somatization Disorder. Multiple, unexplained symptoms (including pain and mood symptoms) characterize this chronic disorder, found almost exclusively in women (p. 294).

Undifferentiated Somatoform Disorder. This is a residual category for patients who don't meet criteria for any other somatoform disorder. It is most often useful for patients who nearly, but not quite, meet criteria for Somatization Disorder (p. 298).

Conversion Disorder. These patients complain of isolated symptoms that seem to have no physical cause (p. 290).

Pain Disorder. The pain in question has no apparent physical or physiological basis, or it far exceeds the usual expectations, given the patient's actual physical condition (p. 299).

Hypochondriasis. An otherwise healthy patient who has the unfounded fear of a serious, often life-threatening illness such as cancer or heart disease may warrant this diagnosis (p. 303).

Body Dysmorphic Disorder. In this rare disorder, physically normal patients believe that parts of their bodies are misshapen or ugly (p. 307).

Somatoform Disorder Not Otherwise Specified. This is a catchall category for patients whose somatoform symptoms fail to meet criteria for *any* of the other disorders, including Undifferentiated (p. 309).

Other Causes of Somatic Complaints

General Medical Condition. As an example, a patient who complains of abdominal pain may be evaluated for appendicitis, gastric ulcer, or gallstones, depending on the exact nature of the pain. If no physical cause for the pain is found, Somatization Disorder or Pain Disorder may be diagnosed.

Mood Disorder. Pain with no apparent physical cause is characteristic of some patients with Major Depressive Disorder (p. 203) or Bipolar I Disorder, Most Recent Episode Depressed (p. 217). Because they are treatable and potentially life-threatening, these possibilities must be investigated early.

Substance Use. Patients who use substances may complain of pain or other physical symptoms. These may result from the effects of Substance Intoxication or Withdrawal, or they may represent an effort to obtain the substance of choice.

Factitious Disorder. Patients who want to occupy the sick role (perhaps they enjoy the attention of being in a hospital) consciously fabricate symptoms to attract attention from health care professionals (p. 312).

Malingering. These patients also fabricate somatic or psychological symptoms, but the motive is some form of material gain: avoiding punishment or work, or obtaining money or drugs (p. 539).

Introduction

For centuries, clinicians have recognized that physical symptoms and concerns about health can have emotional origins. DSM-III and its successors have gathered several alternatives to organic diagnoses under one umbrella. Collectively these are called the *somatoform disorders*, because their symptoms are typical of somatic (bodily) disease. Unlike most of the other groups of disorders discussed in this book, the somatoform disorders are not bound together by common etiologies, family histories, or other factors. This chapter is simply a convenient way of collecting a number of conditions that are concerned primarily with physical symptoms.

Several sorts of problems can suggest a somatoform disorder. These include the following:

- Pain that is excessive or chronic
- Conversion symptoms (see Tip below)
- Chronic, multiple symptoms that do not seem to have an adequate explanation
- Complaints that do not improve, despite the use of treatment that helps most patients
- Excessive concern with health or body appearance

> **TIP** *Conversion symptoms* suggest the presence of a neurological deficit when there is evidence that one does not exist. An example would be a patient who complains of blindness but whose pupils constrict when light shines on them, or who blinks at a rapid motion made toward the eyes. The term *conversion* refers to the supposed transformation of anxiety into a physical symptom. These symptoms are sometimes called *pseudoneurological*; they are discussed in greater detail later.

Patients with somatoform disorders have usually been evaluated (perhaps many times) for somatic disease. These evaluations often lead to testing and treatments that are expensive, time-consuming, ineffective, and sometimes dangerous. Such treatment only reinforces the patients' fearful belief in some nonexistent general medical condition. On the other hand, many (perhaps most) of these patients are referred to mental health clinicians by other health care personnel who recognize that, whatever is wrong with the patients, it has strong emotional underpinnings.

It is important to acknowledge that these patients are *not* faking their symptoms, as in Factitious Disorder, or consciously pretending to be ill, as in Malingering. Somatoform patients often believe that they have something seriously wrong; this belief can cause them enormous anxiety and impairment. Without meaning to, they inflict great suffering on themselves and on those around them.

It is also important to remember that just because a patient has a somatoform disorder, this does not ensure against the subsequent development of a general medical condition. These patients can also develop other forms of mental illness.

300.11 Conversion Disorder

Although both DSM-IV and the Quick Guide above present two other somatoform disorders before Conversion Disorder, I discuss Conversion Disorder first here in order to describe the basis for this disorder—the conversion symptom—in detail. Such a symptom is defined as (1) a change in how the body functions when (2) no causative physical or physiological malfunctioning can be found and (3) an emotional conflict seems to play some role in the development of the symptom. As noted earlier, these symptoms are often called *pseudoneurological*, and they occur in both Somatization Disorder and Conversion Disorder. They are somewhat more likely to be found in patients who are medically unsophisticated and in countries where medical practice and diagnosis are still emerging.

Conversion Disorder requires the clinician to judge that a specific psychological stress has caused the conversion symptom. (Example: A man develops blindness after finding his wife in bed with a neighbor.) Difficulties can arise in getting two clinicians to agree about causation; one may see a "causal link" between nearly any two events, whereas another may strenuously argue that no such link exists.

Although it is rarely diagnosed in mental health patients—perhaps in only 1 of 10,000—Conversion Disorder undoubtedly exists. It is usually a disorder of young people and is probably far more common among women than men. Especially susceptible are relatively uneducated people from low socioeconomic groups. It may be diagnosed more often among patients seen in consultation in a general hospital.

TIP Conversion symptoms are so common that they may not provide a good marker for identifying disease. In lifetime population surveys, up to one-third of adults have had at least one such symptom. Some writers argue that anything this common cannot discriminate between a disease state and health.

Furthermore, having a conversion symptom may not allow meaningful predictions about a patient's future course. Follow-up studies find that many people who have had a conversion symptom do not have mental disorder. Years later, many are well, with no physical or mental disorders. Some have Somatization Disorder or another Axis I mental disorder. (Note: When you encounter a conversion symptom, look carefully for Somatization Disorder, which is far more common than Conversion Disorder). A few turn out to have an actual physical (sometimes neurological) illness, including brain or spinal cord tumors, multiple sclerosis, or a variety of other medical and neurological disorders. Although clinicians have undoubtedly improved in their ability to discriminate conversion symptoms from "real disease," it is still distressingly easy to make mistakes.

Although conversion symptoms are called *pseudoneurological* because they resemble genuine sensory or motor symptoms, they usually do not conform to the anatomical pattern that would be expected for a condition with a well-defined physical cause. An example is *stocking anesthesia*, in which the patient complains of numbness of the foot that ends abruptly in a sharp line (like an anklet) encircling the lower leg. The actual pattern of nerve supply to the foot is quite different; it would not result in numbness that ends in such a neat line. Other examples of sensory conversion symptoms include blindness, deafness, double vision, and hallucinations. Examples of motor deficits that are conversion symptoms include impaired balance or coordination (at one time called *astasia-abasia*), weak or paralyzed muscles, lump in throat or trouble swallowing, loss of voice, and retention of urine. Still other symptoms include seizures that are not due to epilepsy or other physiological factors (fever, toxicity), amnesia or other dissociative symptoms, and loss of consciousness (other than with fainting). A symptom that is limited to pain does not qualify as a conversion symptom in DSM-IV.

Criteria for Conversion Disorder

- At least one symptom or deficit of sensory or voluntary motor function suggests a neurological or general medical condition.
- The deficit or symptom is not limited to pain or sexual dysfunction.
- Appropriate investigation does not identify a neurological or general medical condition or the direct effects of substance use that can fully explain it.
- Conflicts or other stressors that precede the onset or worsening of this symptom suggest that psychological factors are related to it.
- The patient doesn't consciously feign the symptoms for material gain (as in Malingering) or in order to occupy the sick role (as in Factitious Disorder).
- It is not a culturally sanctioned behavior or experience.
- It is serious enough to produce at least one of these:
  - ✓ It warrants medical evaluation, *or*
  - ✓ It causes distress that is clinically important, *or*
  - ✓ It impairs social, work, or personal functioning.
- It does not occur solely during Somatization Disorder, and no other mental disorder better explains it.

Coding Note

Specify type of symptom or deficit:

With Motor Symptom or Deficit

With Seizures or Convulsions

With Sensory Symptom or Deficit

With Mixed Presentation

Rosalind Noonan

Rosalind Noonan came to her university's student health service because of a stutter. This was remarkable because she was 18 and she had only been stuttering for two days.

It had begun on Tuesday afternoon during her women's issues seminar. The class had been discussing sexual harassment, which gradually led to a consideration of sexual molestation. To foster discussion, the graduate student leading the seminar asked each participant to comment. When Rosalind's turn came, she stuttered so badly that she gave up trying to talk at all.

"I still ca-ca-ca-can't understand it," she told the interviewer. "It's the first time I've ever had this pr-pr-pro-pro—difficulty."

Rosalind was a first-year student who had decided to major in psychology, she said, "to help me learn more about myself." What she already knew included the following.

Rosalind had no information about her biological parents. She had been adopted when she was only a week old by a high school physics teacher and his wife, who had no other children. Her father was a rigid and perfectionistic man who dominated both Rosalind and her mother.

As a young child, Rosalind was overly active; during her early school years she had difficulty focusing her attention. She would probably have qualified for a diagnosis of Attention-Deficit/Hyperactivity Disorder, but the only evaluation she had ever had was from their family physician, who thought it was "just a phase" that she would soon outgrow. Despite that lack of diagnostic rigor, when she was 12 she did begin to grow out of it. By the time she entered high school, she was doing nearly straight-A work.

Although she had had many friends in high school and had dated extensively, she had never had a serious boyfriend. Her physical health had been excellent, and her only visits to doctors had been for immunizations. Her mood was almost always bright and cheerful; she had no history of delusions or hallucinations, and she had never used drugs or alcohol. "I g-g-grew up healthy and happy," she protested. "That's why I d-d-d-don't understand this!"

"Hardly anyone reaches adulthood without having some problems." The interviewer paused for a response, but received none, and so continued: "For example, when you were a child, did anyone ever approach you for sex?"

Rosalind's gaze seemed to lose focus as tears trickled from her eyes. Haltingly at first, then in a rush, the following story emerged. When she was 9 or 10, her parents had become friendly with a married couple, both English teachers at her father's school. When she was 14, the woman had suddenly died; subsequently, the man was invited for dinner on a number of occasions. One evening he consumed too much wine and was put to bed on their living room sofa. Rosalind awakened to find him lying on top of her in her bed, his hand covering her mouth. She was never certain whether he actually entered her, but her struggles apparently caused him to ejaculate prematurely. After that, he left her room. He never again returned.

The following day she confided her story to her mother, who at first assured Rosalind that she must have been dreaming. When confronted with the evidence of the stained sheets, her mother urged her to say nothing about the matter to her father. It was the last time the subject had ever been discussed in their house.

"I'm not sure what we thought Daddy would do if he found out," said Rosalind, "but we were both afraid of him. I felt I'd done something to be punished for, and I suppose Mom must have worried he'd attack the other teacher."

Evaluation of Rosalind Noonan

Rosalind's stuttering is a classical conversion symptom: It suggests or mimics a neurological condition. It was not related to pain or sexual dysfunction, and it was not a culturally sanctioned symptom. Many clinicians would agree that it was precipitated by the stress of discussing long-buried sexual abuse. It is this aspect of the disorder—the putative psychological factors related to the symptoms—that differentiates Conversion Disorder from Undifferentiated Somatoform Disorder.

The most serious mistake a clinician can make in this context is to diagnose a Conversion Disorder when the symptom is caused by a **general medical condition**. Some very peculiar symptoms eventually turn out to have a medical basis. However, in an adult the abrupt onset of stuttering is almost certain to have no identifiable organic cause. The fact that Rosalind's difficulty disappeared with discussion would be additional evidence that this was a conversion symptom.

Rosalind stated that her health had always been good, but her clinician would nonetheless be well-advised to ask about all the symptoms of **Somatization Disorder**, in which conversion symptoms are so commonly encountered. The fact that she focused on the symptom, rather than on the fear of having some serious disease, would eliminate **Hypochondriasis** from consideration. By definition, conversion symptoms do not include pain; when pain occurs as a symptom that is caused or increased by psychological factors, the diagnosis is likely to be **Pain Disorder**. The other Axis I condition in which conversion symptoms are sometimes encountered is **Schizophrenia,** but there was no evidence that Rosalind had ever been psychotic. She did not consciously feign her symptom, which would rule out **Factitious Disorder** and **Malingering**.

Rosalind was quite concerned about her stuttering, which is different from the affect of unconcerned indifference (usually called *la belle indifference*) often associated with conversion symptoms, either in Conversion Disorder or in

Somatization Disorder. Although many of these patients will also have an Axis II diagnosis of **Histrionic, Dependent, Borderline,** or **Antisocial Personality Disorder**, there was no evidence for any of these in Rosalind's case. As in Somatization Disorder, **mood, anxiety,** and **dissociative disorders** are often associated with Conversion Disorder.

Four types of Conversion Disorder can be specified (see the Coding Note). Rosalind's stuttering was, of course, a symptom of motor dysfunction. Although she was terribly stressed by the sexual molestation, Axis IV is generally used only to describe *current* stressors. Her overall diagnosis would therefore be as follows:

Axis I	300.11	Conversion Disorder, With Motor Symptom or Deficit
Axis II	V71.09	No diagnosis
Axis III		None
Axis IV		None
Axis V	GAF = 75	(current)

300.81 Somatization Disorder

Patients with Somatization Disorder have a pattern of multiple physical and emotional symptoms that lasts for many years. The symptoms affect various areas of the body and must include, at a minimum, symptoms from these groups: pain, gastrointestinal, sexual, and pseudoneurological.

Somatization Disorder is the great-grandchild of what may be the oldest mental health diagnosis: hysteria. The term *hysteria* was coined over 2,000 years ago by the Greeks, who believed that its symptoms arose from a uterus that wandered throughout the body. In more recent times it has been called *Briquet's syndrome*, named for the French physician who described the disorder's typical polysymptomatic presentation. Somatization Disorder is the best studied of the somatoform disorders.

This disorder begins early in life, usually in the teens or early 20s, and can last for many years—perhaps the patient's entire lifetime. Often overlooked by health care professionals, this condition probably affects about 1% of all women; it only rarely occurs in men. It may account for 7–8% of all women visiting a mental health clinic, and perhaps nearly that percentage of hospitalized female mental health patients. There is a strong tendency for this disorder to run in families. Transmission is probably both genetic and environmental.

Criteria for Somatization Disorder

• Starting before age 30, the patient has had many physical complaints occurring over several years.

- The patient has sought treatment for these symptoms, or they have materially impaired social, work, or personal functioning.
- The patient has at some time experienced a total of at least eight symptoms from the following list, distributed as noted. These symptoms need not be concurrent.
  - Pain symptoms (four or more) related to different sites, such as head, abdomen, back, joints, extremities, chest, or rectum, or related to body functions, such as menstruation, sexual intercourse, or urination.
  - Gastrointestinal symptoms (two or more, excluding pain), such as nausea, bloating, vomiting (not during pregnancy), diarrhea, or intolerance of several foods.
  - Sexual symptoms (at least one, excluding pain), including indifference to sex, difficulties with erection or ejaculation, irregular menses, excessive menstrual bleeding, or vomiting throughout all nine months of pregnancy.
  - Pseudoneurological symptoms (at least one), including poor balance or coordination, weak or paralyzed muscles, lump in throat or trouble swallowing, loss of voice, retention of urine, hallucinations, numbness (to touch or pain), double vision, blindness, deafness, seizures, amnesia or other dissociative symptoms, or loss of consciousness (other than with fainting). None of these is limited to pain.
- For each of the symptoms above, one of these conditions must be met:
  - ✓ Physical or laboratory investigation determines that the symptom cannot be fully explained by a general medical condition or by the use of substances (including medications), *or*
  - ✓ If the patient does have a general medical condition, the impairment or complaints exceed what would generally be expected, based on history, laboratory findings, or physical examination.
- The patient doesn't consciously feign the symptoms for material gain (as in Malingering) or in order to occupy the sick role (as in Factitious Disorder).

Coding Note

Note that in each of the four symptom categories above, the specific symptoms are listed in approximate descending order of frequency.

Cynthia Fowler

When Cynthia Fowler told her story, she cried. At age 35, she was talking with the most recent in her series of health care professionals. Her history was a complicated one; it began in her midteens with arthritis that seemed to move from one joint to another. She had been told that these were "growing pains," but the symptoms had continued to come and go over the intervening 20 years. Although she was subsequently diagnosed as having various types of arthritis, laboratory tests never substantiated any of them. A long succession of treatments had proven fruitless.

In her mid-20s, Cynthia was evaluated for left flank pain, but again nothing was found. Later, abdominal pain and vomiting spells were worked up with gastroscopy and barium X-rays. All these studies were normal. A histamine antagonist was added to her growing list of medications, which by now included various anti-inflammatory agents, as well as prescription and over-the-counter analgesics.

Cynthia had thought at one time that many of her symptoms were aggravated by her premenstrual syndrome, which she had diagnosed in herself after reading about it in a women's magazine. She had invariably been irritable with cramps before her period, which used to be so heavy that she would sometimes stay in bed for several days. When she was 26, therefore, she had had a total hysterectomy. Six months later, persistent vomiting led to endoscopy; other than adhesions, no abnormalities were found. Alternating diarrhea and constipation then caused her to experiment with a series of preparations to regulate her bowel movements.

When she was questioned about sex, Cynthia shifted uncomfortably in her chair. She didn't care much for it and had never experienced a climax. Her lack of interest was no problem to her, but each of her three husbands had complained a lot. When she was a young teenager, something sexual might have happened to her, she finally admitted, but that was a part of her life she really couldn't recall. "It's as if someone cut a whole year out of my diary," she explained.

When she was two and her brother was six months old, Cynthia's father had deserted the family. Her mother subsequently worked as a waitress and lived with a succession of men, some of whom she married. When Cynthia was 12, her mother escaped from one of Cynthia's stepfathers; she then placed the two children in foster care.

One way or another, each of Cynthia's former clinicians had disappointed her. "None of the others knew how to help me. But I just know you'll find out what's wrong. Everyone says you're the best in town." Through her tears, she managed a confident smile.

Evaluation of Cynthia Fowler

As its name suggests, Somatization Disorder mimics actual somatic disease. As for most DSM-IV disorders, a **general medical condition** is the first possibility that must be ruled out. Cynthia had already been worked up for a variety of medical conditions and had been prescribed multiple medications, which had done her little good. Judging by the last paragraph of the vignette, her previous clinicians may have been at a loss to diagnose or treat her effectively.

Cynthia's list of symptoms is typical for Somatization Disorder. Among the medical and neurological disorders to consider are multiple sclerosis, spinal cord tumors, and diseases of the heart and lungs. Her symptoms fulfilled criteria for all four categories required by the DSM-IV criteria: pain (abdomen, flank, joints, menstrual); gastrointestinal (diarrhea, vomiting); sexual (excessive bleeding, sexual indifference); and pseudoneurologic (amnesia).

Of course, many people have had symptoms that appear on the DSM-IV's criteria list. What sets apart patients with Somatization Disorder is (1) the number and variety of their symptoms, and (2) the fact that each symptom has no adequate explanation or exceeds expectations considering the history, lab findings, or physical examination. In addition, none of the treatments that Cynthia received ever seemed to be helpful.

Certain other somatoform disorders can be confused with Somatization Disorder. In **Pain Disorder** the patient focuses on severe, often incapacitating somatic pain. Although Cynthia complained of pain in a variety of locations, these were only a part of a picture of somatic illness that was much broader in scope. **Hypochondriasis** patients can have multiple physical symptoms, but they focus their concern on the fear of having a specific organic disease. Cynthia's amnesia is an example of dissociation; it might qualify for the diagnosis of **Dissociative Amnesia** if it were the predominant problem. Cynthia did not have any classical conversion symptoms (e.g., stocking or glove anesthesia, hemiparalysis), but many Somatization Disorder patients do. This brings **Conversion Disorder** into the differential diagnosis. However, as with Pain Disorder, Conversion Disorder would not be diagnosed in any patient who meets the diagnostic criteria for the more encompassing, better-studied Somatization Disorder.

The clinician should inquire carefully about **substance-related disorders**, which are found in one-quarter or more of Somatization Disorder patients. When patients come to the attention of mental health providers, it is often because of a comcomitant **mood disorder** or **anxiety disorder**.

Many Somatization Disorder patients also have one or more **personality disorders**. Especially prevalent is **Histrionic Personality Disorder**, though others (especially **Borderline** and **Antisocial**) may also be diagnosed. Cynthia's words to the clinician in the last paragraph suggest a personality disorder, but not enough information is available.

Cynthia's full diagnosis would read as follows:

Axis I	300.81	Somatization Disorder
Axis II	799.9	Diagnosis Deferred
Axis III		None
Axis IV		None
Axis V	GAF = 61	(current)

TIP The DSM-IV criteria specify that any symptom scored as positive must be unexplained by known mechanisms (anatomical, biochemical, physiological) or must be excessive for the supposed cause. In the race to collect the required number of symptoms, it is easy to overlook this requirement.

Also, DSM-IV lists the symptoms in the four categories of the criteria, but includes "e.g." or "such as" in the description. Other sorts of pain, gastrointestinal, sexual, and conversion symptoms can presumably be counted in diagnosing Somatization Disorder, provided that the other criteria are met.

Finally, half or more of Somatization Disorder patients have symptoms of anxiety disorders (e.g., Panic Disorder) and mood disorders. There is an ever-present danger that clinicians will make an incomplete diagnosis of one of these and ignore the underlying Somatization Disorder.

300.81 Undifferentiated Somatoform Disorder

The category of Undifferentiated Somatoform Disorder was created to include patients whose clinical picture suggests Somatization Disorder (or another somatoform disorder), but who simply lack sufficient symptoms to justify one of these diagnoses. Most often, it will be used for people who don't quite meet criteria for Somatization Disorder. With time, many of them will develop more symptoms; they can then be reclassified on Axis I as having Somatization Disorder.

Of course, fewer symptoms have less predictive power. At follow-up, some of these patients will be well, and some will have general medical conditions and other mental disorders that explain their symptoms. The only noteworthy difference between this category and Conversion Disorder is that patients with the latter must have some psychological factor (a conflict or some other stressful event) that is judged to be related.

Because of the similarity of symptoms and course to those of Somatization Disorder, I give no case vignette for Undifferentiated Somatoform Disorder here.

Criteria for Undifferentiated Somatoform Disorder

- The patient has at least one physical complaint, such as trouble breathing, chest pain, painful urination, fatigue, or the like.
- For any such symptom to be counted, one of these conditions must be met:
  ✓ Physical or laboratory investigation determines that the symptom can-

not be fully explained by a general medical condition or by the use of substances, (including medications), or

✓ If the patient does have a general medical condition, the impairment or complaints exceed what would generally be expected, based on history, laboratory findings, or physical examination.

- The symptoms cause clinically important distress or impair work, social, or personal functioning.
- This condition has lasted six months or longer.
- It isn't better explained by another mental disorder, such as a psychotic, mood, anxiety, somatoform, or sleep disorder or a sexual dysfunction.
- The patient doesn't consciously feign the symptoms for material gain (as in Malingering) or in order to occupy the sick role (as in Factitious Disorder).

TIP A lot of research has shown that isolated physical symptoms don't predict much of anything. Rather than risk making a diagnosis that sounds final (you could be lulled into believing that your diagnostic work is done), it might be better to use the code 300.9, for Unspecified Mental Disorder (nonpsychotic).

307.8x Pain Disorder

Pain Disorder shares a notable feature with Conversion Disorder: These are the only two conditions in DSM-IV whose criteria require a clinician's judgment that psychological factors play an important role in the development or maintenance of symptoms. The problem is that what seems a psychologically important factor to one clinician may seem irrelevant to another, and objectivity may fall victim to theory. However, Pain Disorder is common and disabling enough to be more important clinically than is Conversion Disorder.

A second problem with this diagnosis stems from the fact that pain is subjective and hard to measure with validity. People experience it differently; by definition, there is no gross anatomical pathology. It is therefore hard to be sure that a patient who complains of chronic or excruciating pain, and does not have adequate objective pathology, is mentally ill at all.

The pain these patients experience is usually severe and often chronic. (In the past it has been called *chronic pain syndrome.*) It can take many forms, but especially frequent are pain in the lower back, head, pelvis, and temporomandibular joint. Psychological factors that may cause or worsen the pain include stress resulting from relationships, work, and finances. Typically, Pain Disorder does not wax and wane with time and does not diminish with distraction; it may respond only poorly to analgesics, if at all.

Pain Disorder is more often diagnosed in women than in men. Usually it begins in the 30s or 40s, often following an accident or some other general medical condition. As its duration grinds on, it often leads to increasing incapacity for work and social life, and sometimes to complete invalidism. Although some form of pain incapacitates many adults in the general population, no one knows just how prevalent Pain Disorder itself is.

Criteria for Pain Disorder

- The patient's presenting problem is clinically important pain in one or more body areas.
- The pain causes distress that is clinically important or impairs work, social, or personal functioning.
- Psychological factors seem important in the onset, maintenance, severity, or worsening of the pain.
- Other disorders (mood, anxiety, psychotic) do not explain the symptoms better, and the patient does not meet criteria for Dyspareunia.
- The patient doesn't consciously feign the symptoms for material gain (as in Malingering) or in order to occupy the sick role (as in Factitious Disorder).

Coding Notes

Code according to the predominant cause of pain:

307.80 Pain Disorder Associated with Psychological Factors. If a general medical condition is present, it does not play the major role in the cause, maintenance, severity, or worsening of the pain. Do not use this code if the patient also meets criteria for Somatization Disorder.

307.89 Pain Disorder Associated with Both Psychological Factors and a General Medical Condition. Both of these types of factors seem important in the onset, maintenance, severity, or worsening of the pain.

For either of these, specify whether:

Acute. Has lasted less than six months.

Chronic. Has lasted six months or longer.

Also code the general medical condition *or* site of the pain on Axis III, if the diagnosis is Pain Disorder Associated with Both Psychological Factors and a General Medical Condition. *The site is coded only if the exact general medical condition is not yet known.* The following Axis III code numbers for site of pain are included for your convenience:

Site	Code	Site	Code
Abdominal	789.0	Joint	719.4
Back	724.5	Limb	729.5
Back, low	724.2	Pelvic	625.9
Bone	733.90	Renal	788.0
Breast	611.71	Sciatic	724.3
Chest	786.50	Shoulder	719.41
Ear	388.70	Throat	784.1
Eye	379.91	Tongue	529.6
Facial	784.0	Tooth	525.9
Headache	784.0	Urinary	788.0

Pain Disorder Associated with a General Medical Condition is the term used for any patient who has pain that is mainly caused, worsened, or maintained by a general medical condition, so long as any psychological factors play at most a minor role. This is not considered to be a mental disorder and is coded only on Axis III. The Axis III code numbers for sites are as given above.

Ruby Bissell

Ruby Bissell placed a hand on each chair arm and shifted uncomfortably. She had been talking for nearly half an hour, and the dull, constant ache had worsened. Pushing up with both hands, she hoisted herself to her feet. She winced as she pressed a fist into the small of her back; the furrows on her face caused her to look 10 years older than her 45 years.

Although Ruby had had this problem for nearly six years, she wasn't sure exactly when it began. It could have started when she helped to move a patient from the operating table to a gurney. But the first orthopedist she ever consulted explained that her pulled ligament was mild, so she continued to work as an operating room nurse for nearly a year. Her back hurt whether she was sitting or standing, so she'd had to resign from her job—she couldn't maintain any position longer than a few minutes at a time.

"They let me do supervisory work for a while," she said, "but I had to quit that, too. My only choices were sitting or standing, and I have to spend part of each hour flat on my back."

From her solidly blue-collar parents, Ruby had inherited a work ethic. She'd supported herself from the age of 17, so her forced retirement had been a blow. But she couldn't say she felt depressed about it. In fact, she had never been very introspective about her feelings and couldn't really explain how she felt about many things. She did deny ever having hallucinations or delusions; aside from her back pain, her physical health had been good. Although she occasionally awakened at night with back pain, she had no real insomnia; appetite and weight had been normal. When the interviewer asked whether she had ever had death wishes or suicidal ideas, she was a little offended and strongly denied them.

A variety of treatments had made little difference in Ruby's condition. Pain medication provided almost no relief at all, and she had quit them all before she could get hooked. Physical therapy made her hurt all the more, and an electrical stimulation unit seemed to burn her skin.

A neurosurgeon had found no anatomical pathology and explained to Ruby that a laminectomy and spinal fusion were unlikely to improve matters. Her own husband's experience had caused her to distrust any surgical intervention. He had been injured in a trucking accident a year before her own difficulty began; his subsequent laminectomy had left him not only disabled for work, but impotent. With no children to support, the two lived in reasonable comfort on their combined disability incomes.

"Mostly we just stay at home," Ruby remarked. "We care a lot for each other. Our relationship is the one part of my life that's really good."

The interviewer asked whether they were still able to have any sort of a sex life. Ruby admitted that they did not. "We used to be very active, and I enjoyed it a lot. After his accident, and he couldn't perform, Gregory felt terribly guilty that he couldn't satisfy me. Now my back pain would keep me from having sex, regardless. It's almost a relief that he doesn't have to bear all the responsibility."

Evaluation of Ruby Bissell

For several years Ruby had complained of severe pain that had markedly affected her life. Several psychological factors might have been important in causing, worsening, or maintaining her pain. These included her perception of her husband's feeling about his impotence, her anxiety at being left as the sole breadwinner, and possibly her own resentment at having worked since she was a teenager. (Many patients' disorders have multiple psychological determinants.)

Could her pain have been caused by a **general medical condition**? From the vignette, it would appear not: She had been thoroughly evaluated by her orthopedist, who determined that she did not have pathology adequate to account for the severity of her symptoms. Even if she did have some defined pathology, a somatoform disorder might also be suspected if the distribution, timing or description of the pain was atypical of a general medical condition. Could Ruby have been **Malingering**? This question is especially relevant to anyone who receives compensation for a work-related injury. However, Ruby's suffering seemed genuine, and the vignette gives no indication that she was physically more able at leisure that at work. Her referral had not been made within a legal context, and she cooperated fully with the examination. Furthermore, Malingering would not seem consistent with her long-held work ethic.

Pain is often a symptom of depression; indeed, many practitioners will automatically recommend a course of antidepressant medication for nearly anyone who complains of severe or chronic pain. Although Ruby denied feeling especially depressed, her pain symptoms could still be a stand-in for a **mood disorder**. But she had no suicidal ideas or disturbance of sleep or appetite to support such a diagnosis. Although patients with **substance-related disorders** will sometimes fabricate (or imagine) pain in order to obtain medications, she had been careful to avoid becoming dependent on analgesics.

Several other somatoform disorders should be briefly considered. Ruby could not have had **Somatization Disorder**, because she was too old (39) when the pain began and her physical health was otherwise good. People with **Hypochondriasis** tend to have symptoms other than pain, and they fluctuate with time. According to the DSM-IV definition, pain cannot be a criterion for **Conversion Disorder**.

Because Ruby's pain had been present far longer than six months, it would be subtyped as Chronic. In assigning the exact code, you must judge whether a patient has, in addition to psychological factors, a physiological or anatomical basis for the pain. If Ruby had had some X-ray and laboratory changes consistent with arthritis, even if these were insufficient to explain the severity of her disability, her Axis I disorder might have been diagnosed as 307.89 (Pain Disorder Associated with Both Psychological Factors and a General Medical Condition). In that case, an Axis III diagnosis for cause or site of pain would have been in order. This was not the case, so her final diagnosis would be as follows:

Axis I	307.80	Pain Disorder Associated with Psychological Factors, Chronic
Axis II	V71.09	No diagnosis
Axis III		None
Axis IV		Health problems in husband
Axis V	GAF = 61	(current)

TIP Occasional patients will be completely unable to describe the emotional component of their pain. This inability has been termed **alexithymia** (Greek: "without expression of mood").

300.7 Hypochondriasis

From time to time most adults notice physical sensations (e.g., a cough, skipped heartbeats, or minor pain), physical abnormalities (e.g., a sore or a mole), and other, often vague symptoms suggesting that not all is well with their bodies. If these symptoms occur occasionally and do not worsen with time, most of us ignore them; we generally accept the word of a physician that they are not serious.

People with Hypochondriasis experience this sort of symptom as evidence of some serious illness. This fearful belief persists despite medical evidence and reassurance. Common examples include fear of heart disease (resulting from occasional chest pain or heart palpitations) and fear of cancer (resulting from benign skin moles). These patients are not psychotic: They may agree temporarily that their symptoms could be emotional in origin, though they quickly revert to their obsessional fears. However, at any suggestion that they do not have physical disease, they may become outraged and reject the idea of a mental health consultation.

Although the diagnosis of Hypochondriasis has been around for centuries, it has never yet been well studied; for example, it is not known whether it runs in families. By all accounts, however, it is fairly common, especially in the offices of non-mental health practitioners. It is about as frequent in males as in females. It tends to begin in the 20s or 30s; the prevalence peaks at about 30 or 40. Occasionally, patients will have demonstrable organic disease, but their hypochondriacal symptoms are out of proportion to the seriousness of the actual general medical condition. Although they do not have high rates of current medical illnesses, hypochondriacal patients report a high prevalence of childhood illness.

Historically, Hypochondriasis has been a source of fun for cartoonists and playwrights (read Moliere's *The Imaginary Invalid*), but the disorder causes genuine misery. Although it can resolve completely, it more often runs a chronic course, interfering with work and social life. Many patients go from doctor to doctor in the effort to find someone who will relieve them of the serious disorders they feel sure they have; for a few, it can lead to complete invalidism.

Criteria for Hypochondriasis

- Because of misinterpreting bodily symptoms, the patient becomes preoccupied with ideas or fears of having a serious illness.
- Appropriate medical investigation and reassurance do not relieve these ideas.
- These ideas are not delusional (as in Delusional Disorder) and are not restricted to concern about appearance (as in Body Dysmorphic Disorder).
- They cause distress that is clinically important or impair work, social, or personal functioning.
- They have lasted six months or longer.
- These ideas are not better explained by Generalized Anxiety Disorder, Major Depressive Episode, Obsessive–Compulsive Disorder, Panic Disorder, Separation Anxiety Disorder, or a different somatoform disorder.

Coding Note

Specify when: With Poor Insight. During most of this episode, the patient does not realize that the preoccupation is excessive or unreasonable.

Wally Graham

"The news is good," announced Wally Graham's clinician. "Your X-rays and the other tests show nothing wrong—no cancer, no ulcer, not even gastritis."

Wally Graham did not look pleased. "I don't understand it."

"It means you're okay. There's nothing wrong."

"I mean I don't understand why I'm still having the pain and why I'm throwing up nearly every morning." He slowly began to put on his shirt.

The clinician leafed through his chart. "I checked with your previous HMO. They said you'd had the same set of tests done there six months ago. And the year before that."

"Yes, I told you all about that, last time I was here. I haven't held anything back." Wally had begun to sound angry. "This has been going on for four or five years now. I don't like being this way, you know."

"No, of course not," said the clinician. "I didn't mean that. I meant that for years you've had stomach pains, nausea, vomiting, and diarrhea, and for years you've been afraid you have cancer. You've had at least four workups by excellent clinicians; they've all reassured you that there's nothing wrong. Only you don't feel reassured. Last week you were even gastroscoped by our gastroenterologist. That's the most definitive test you can get. There weren't even enough findings to diagnose an upset stomach! I'm not saying that you don't have pain, but I think your problem is somewhere besides your stomach. I'd like to check out some other possibilities, to see if we can get to the bottom of this."

"I hope so." Wally Graham was less angry, but he still sounded unconvinced. Fully dressed now in his tie and sports jacket, he looked somehow smaller than he had before. He was a 42-year-old, unmarried accountant who worked for a branch of one of the large national firms that advertised on TV. He liked his job (except during tax season, which nobody liked), but several days a month he had to stay in bed with abdominal pains. His supervisor was becoming restive.

Of course, Wally had been worried, maybe even a little depressed. He had felt that way occasionally throughout his ordeal of the past several years. But his concentration had been good, and his interest in work and leisure activities had been high. Any problems with sleep or appetite had been due to the abdominal distress, which only lasted for a few days each time. He had never had suicidal ideas.

Wally had never tried street drugs; for years he had avoided alcohol in any form. Except for his abdominal distress, his health was good. He denied everything on an impressively long list of symptoms that included headache, dizziness, chest pain, painful urination, and musculoskeletal and neurological complaints. Over the years he had had quite a lot of anxiety about having cancer, but he had never experienced a full-blown Panic Attack. He had never heard voices or seen visions, nor did he believe that people were plotting or talking about him behind his back.

The first few times a clinician told Wally he didn't have cancer, he felt relieved. But after a few days the symptoms would start again and he would worry. What if the lab had switched somebody else's test with his? Suppose the radiologist misread the film? "Or perhaps I didn't have cancer then, but I've developed it since the tests were made. How's anyone going to reassure me about that?"

Evaluation of Wally Graham

As for any other somatoform disorder, the first items on the list of things to rule out are **general medical conditions**. They can be easy to miss, especially if the patient has had a long history of complaints that seem to have no physical basis. However, Wally's symptoms had been evaluated for years, to the point that there was little danger anything had been missed. But, despite reassurance, he continued to fear that he had cancer. His distress often caused him to miss work, and he had been ill far longer than the six-month minimum required for this diagnosis.

Hypochondriacal concerns can occur in other Axis I disorders, but some differences can help you discriminate. Hypochondriasis cannot be diagnosed if the symptoms occur *only* in the course of another somatoform disorder (e.g., **Body Dysmorphic Disorder**, **Somatization Disorder**, or **Pain Disorder**) or an anxiety disorder (e.g., **Generalized Anxiety Disorder**, **Panic Disorder**, or **Obsessive–Compulsive Disorder**). Wally had no symptoms suggesting any of these. When somatic delusions occur in **Schizophrenia**, they tend to be bizarre ("I have a computer chip in my nose"). In **Major Depressive Disorder, Severe with Psychotic Features**, they are ego-syntonic but may be influenced by melancholia ("My bowels have turned to cement").

The requirement that hypochondriacal preoccupations not be of delusional intensity can cause difficulty. This is because the dividing line between a delusion and an overvalued idea (such as having cancer) can be extremely fine. Although many of these patients will agree that their symptoms could have an emotional basis, some do not recognize how ill-founded their concerns are. Wally indicated to his clinician that reassurance helped for a time (though his doubts always returned), but some patients never develop even this much insight. They would be coded with the additional specification of **With Poor Insight**. In extreme cases, the diagnosis of **Delusional Disorder** should be considered. This does not appear to apply to Wally, whose overall diagnosis would be as follows:

Axis I	300.7	Hypochondriasis
Axis II	V71.09	No diagnosis
Axis III		None
Axis IV		None
Axis V	GAF = 65	(current)

300.7 Body Dysmorphic Disorder

Patients with Body Dysmorphic Disorder are concerned that there is something wrong with the shape or appearance of a body part. Most often this involves breasts, genitalia, hair, or the nose or some other portion of the face. The ideas these patients have about their bodies are not delusional; as in Hypochondriasis, they are overvalued ideas. At one time the disorder was called dysmorphophobia. Some clinicians still call it that, though it is not a phobia at all (the patient doesn't have a persistent, irrational fear of anything).

This disorder can be devastating. Although they often request medical procedures (e.g., dermabrasion) or plastic surgery to correct their imagined defects, patients are often dissatisfied with the results; such procedures are usually contraindicated in these patients, as in those with other somatoform disorders. Patients may also seek reassurance (which helps only briefly), try to hide their perceived deformities with clothing or body hair, avoid social situations, and even become housebound. Suicide attempts and completions are not unknown.

Little is known about Body Dysmorphic Disorder. Distinctly uncommon, it is rarely encountered in a mental health population, though it may account for as many as 2% of patients who consult a dermatologist. These patients are relatively young; both men and women can be afflicted. (What happens to them as they age?) In addition to the concern about physical appearance, they may also be depressed or anxious.

Criteria for Body Dysmorphic Disorder

- The patient is preoccupied with an imaginary defect of appearance, or is excessively concerned about a slight physical anomaly.
- This preoccupation causes clinically important distress or impairs work, social, or personal functioning.
- Another mental disorder (such as Anorexia Nervosa) does not better explain the preoccupation.

Cecil Crane

Cecil Crane was only 24 when he was referred by a plastic surgeon. "He came in here last week asking for a rhinoplasty," said the referring surgeon on the telephone, "but his nose looks perfect to me. I told him that, but he insisted there was something wrong with it. I've seen this kind of patient before—if I operate, they're never satisfied. It's a lawsuit waiting to happen."

When Cecil appeared a few days later, he had, apart from one or two Greek statues, the most beautiful nose the clinician had ever seen. "What seems to be wrong with it?"

"I was afraid you'd ask that," said Cecil. "Everybody *says* that."

"But you don't believe it?"

"Well, they look at me funny. Even at work—I sell suits at Macy's—I sometimes feel that the customers notice. I think it's this bump here."

Viewed from a certain angle, the spot Cecil pointed out bore the barest suggestion of a convexity. He complained that it had cost him his girlfriend, who always said it looked fine to her. But she was tired of Cecil's going on about plastic surgery all the time, and had finally sought greener pastures.

Cecil felt unhappy, but not depressed. He admitted that he was making a mess of his life, but he had nevertheless maintained his interests in reading and going to the movies. He thought his sex interest was good, though he'd had no chance to test it since the departure of his girlfriend. His appetite was good and his weight was about average for his height. His flow of thought was unremarkable; its content, outside of his concern for his nose, seemed quite ordinary. He even admitted that it was possible that his nose was less ugly than he feared, though he thought it unlikely.

Cecil couldn't say exactly when his worry about his nose began. It may have been about the time he started shaving. He recalled frequently gazing at a silhouette of his profile that had been cut from black paper during a seashore vacation with his family. Although numerous relatives and friends had remarked that it was a good likeness, something about the nose had bothered him. One day he had taken it down from the wall and with a pair of scissors had attempted to put it to rights. Within five minutes the nose lay in snippets on the kitchen table, and Cecil was grounded for a month.

"I sure hope the plastic surgeon is a better artist than I am," he commented.

Evaluation of Cecil Crane

The criteria for Body Dysmorphic Disorder are straightforward. Cecil was preoccupied with his nose, which caused him enough distress to seek surgery. More than one person tried to assure him that his nose was rather ordinary, so his distress evidently exceeded **normal concerns regarding appearance**. There are several disorders in the differential diagnosis to consider, however.

In **Hypochondriasis**, it is not appearance that preoccupies the patient; rather, it is fear of having a disease. In **Anorexia Nervosa**, the patient also has a distorted self-image, but it is only in the context of concern about overweight. In **Delusional Disorder, Somatic Type**, patients lack insight that their complaints might be unreasonable, whereas Cecil was willing to entertain the notion that others might see his nose differently. Complaints from patients with **Schizophrenia** about appearance are often bizarre (one woman reported that when she looked into the mirror, she noticed that her head had been replaced by a mushroom). In **Transsexualism**, patients' complaints are limited to the conviction that they should have been born as persons of the opposite sex.

None of these was the focus of Cecil's concern. However, his clinician would do well to look carefully for **Social Phobia, Obsessive–Compulsive Disorder**, and **Major Depressive Disorder**, all of which may be comorbid with Body Dysmorphic Disorder. Pending investigation for these disorders, Cecil's five-axis diagnosis would be as follows:

Axis I	300.7	Body Dysmorphic Disorder
Axis II	V71.09	No diagnosis
Axis III		None
Axis IV		None
Axis V	GAF = 70	(current)

TIP Patients who have ideas of *delusional* intensity about their bodies should receive a diagnosis of Delusional Disorder (see p. 169) as well as the somatoform diagnosis. Such patients may believe that they have offensive body odor or that they are infested by parasites. Recent work suggests that delusional ideas of this sort and nondelusional Body Dysmorphic Disorder are forms of the same illness. (DSM-V committee, take note.) These delusional ideas and Body Dysmorphic Disorder were all at one time called forms of *monosymptomatic hypochondriasis*—a term that is too broad to have much meaning.

300.81 Somatoform Disorder Not Otherwise Specified

The Somatoform Disorder Not Otherwise Specified category is for patients whose somatic symptoms do not meet criteria for any of the somatoform disorders discussed above. The diagnoses suggested here have not as yet been studied very well and are not formally included in DSM-IV. Any patient who receives a diagnosis in this category should be thought of as provisionally diagnosed. You should keep in mind that with more information, such a patient may qualify for another diagnosis.

Pseudocyesis. The word *pseudocyesis* means "false pregnancy," and it refers to patients who incorrectly believe that they are pregnant. They develop signs of pregnancy such as protruding abdomen, nausea, amenorrhea, breast engorgement, and even labor pains.

Transient hypochondriacal states. These would include conditions that meet criteria for Hypochondriasis, except that they have not lasted for the required six months.

Total environmental allergy syndrome. These patients claim to be allergic to most or all foods, gases, apparel, and other materials with which they come into contact. In the past few years this condition has achieved some notoriety; newspapers have reported interviews with people who have resorted to living in the wilderness, far from civilization.

Chronic fatigue syndrome. People with this disorder, also called *fibromyalgia*, report long-standing fatigue states for which there are few laboratory findings and fewer effective treatments.

Other. Unexplained physical symptoms lasting less than six months may be categorized here.

Factitious Disorder

Quick Guide to Factitious Symptoms

You would think that this would be a *very* quick guide, inasmuch as Factitious Disorder totals only one entry (unless you count the ubiquitous Not Otherwise Specified). But other conditions present with symptoms that are either made up or look as though they were. Once again, the page number following each item indicates where a more detailed discussion begins.

Manufactured Symptoms

Factitious Disorder. These patients make up symptoms for the purpose, in DSM-IV language, of assuming the sick role. They do *not* appear to have material gain in mind (p. 312).

Malingering. These people devise symptoms for material gain: obtaining money or drugs, avoiding work or punishment (p. 539).

Symptoms That May Look Manufactured

Conversion Disorder. These patients complain of isolated symptoms that seem to have no physical cause (p. 290).

Somatization Disorder. Multiple, unexplained symptoms (including pain and mood symptoms) characterize this chronic disorder, found almost exclusively in women (p. 294).

Introduction

Factitious means that something does not occur naturally. In the context of mental health patients, it means that a disorder looks like real disease, but isn't. Patients accomplish this by simulating *symptoms* (e.g., making complaints of pain) or physical *signs* (e.g., warming a thermometer in coffee or submitting a urine specimen that has sand in it). Sometimes they will complain of psychological symptoms, including depression, hallucinations, delusions, anxiety, suicidal ideas, and disorganized behavior. Manufactured symptoms can be very hard to detect because they are subjective.

According to DSM-IV, patients do not behave this way for material gain (such as insurance payments); they do so because of a wish to occupy the sick role. Thus, Factitious Disorder differs profoundly from Malingering. Malingerers may also silt a urine specimen or embellish the subjective reports of their suffering, but they do these things to qualify for financial compensation, to obtain drugs, or to avoid work, punishment, or prosecution for crimes. The motivation in Factitious Disorder is more complex: These patients need the feeling of being cared for or of duping medical personnel. For whatever reason, they manufacture physical or psychological symptoms in a way that they often claim they cannot control.

Patients' symptoms can be quite dramatic, with outright lying about the severity of the distress. The overall pattern of signs and symptoms is generally not typical for the alleged illness, and some patients change their stories upon retelling. Others, however, know a lot about medical terminology; this makes their behavior harder to detect. The individuals may willingly undergo many procedures, some of them painful or dangerous, to continue in the patient role. With therapy that is ordinarily adequate, their symptoms either do not remit or evolve into new complications.

Once hospitalized, the patients complain bitterly and often, and argue frequently with staff members. They characteristically are hospitalized a few days, have few if any visitors, and leave against medical advice once their tests prove negative. Many travel from city to city in the quest for medical care. The most persistent travelers and confabulators among these are sometimes said to have *Münchausen syndrome*, named for the fabled Baron von Münchausen, who told outrageous lies about his adventures.

The diagnosis of Factitious Disorder is made by excluding physical disease and other Axis I disorders. (Although it is possible that a patient could manufacture a personality disorder, I know of no such cases.) However, many patients with Factitious Disorder also have genuine personality disorders.

This disorder begins early in life. No one knows how rare it is, though it is probably more common in males than in females. Often it starts with a hospitalization for genuine physical problems. It results in severe impairment: These patients are often unemployed and do not maintain close ties with family or friends. The lives of these patients are complicated (and sometimes put at risk) by tests, medications, and unnecessary surgical procedures.

TIP Factitious Disorder patients tend to take on symptoms of new (and often poorly investigated) illnesses—the "disorder *du jour*" syndrome. The criteria for the diagnoses are not very specific, and the patients are difficult to manage and often disagreeable. It is far too easy to dismiss them with a diagnosis of Factitious Disorder; it is vital to rule out every other possible physical and Axis I disorder before making this diagnosis.

Criteria for Factitious Disorder

• The patient intentionally feigns physical or mental signs or symptoms.
• The patient's apparent motive for this behavior is to occupy the sick role.
• There are no other motives, such as those found in Malingering (financial gain, revenge, or avoiding legal responsibility).

Coding Note

Code based on predominant symptom:

300.16	With Predominantly Psychological Signs and Symptoms
300.19	With Predominantly Physical Signs and Symptoms
300.19	With Combined Psychological and Physical Signs and Symptoms. Neither predominates

Jason Bird

Jason Bird was a 47-year-old man who was admitted to a cardiac intensive care unit despite having no health care card—he claimed he had lost his billfold to a mugger a few hours earlier. He came to the emergency room of a Midwestern hospital late one Saturday night, complaining of crushing substernal chest pain. Although his electrocardiogram (EKG) was markedly abnormal, it did not show the changes typical of an acute myocardial infarction (MI). The cardiologist on call, noting his ashen pallor and obvious distress, ordered him admitted and then waited for the cardiac enzyme results.

The following day, Jason's EKG was unchanged and the serum enzymes showed no evidence of heart muscle damage. His chest pain continued. He complained loudly that he was being ignored. The cardiologist urgently requested a mental health consultation.

Jason was a slightly built man with a bright, shifting gaze and a four-day growth of beard. He spoke with a nasal Boston accent. His right shoulder bore the tattoo of a boot and the legend "Born To Kick Ass." Throughout the interview he frequently complained of chest pain, but he had no difficulty breathing or talking, and he showed no signs of anxiety about his medical condition.

He said he had grown up in Quincy, Massachusetts, the son of a physician. After high school he had attended college for several years, but found he was "too creative" for a profession or a conventional job. Instead, he had turned to inventing medical devices, and numbered among his successes a positive-pressure respirator that bore his name. Although he had made several fortunes, he had lost nearly everything to his penchant for playing the stock market. He had been visiting in the area, relaxing, when the chest pain struck.

"And you've never had it before?" asked the interviewer, looking through the chart.

Jason denied that he'd had any previous heart trouble. "Not even a twinge. I've always been blessed with good health."

"Ever been hospitalized?"

"Nope. Well, not since a tonsillectomy when I was a kid."

Further questioning was similarly unproductive. As the interviewer left, Jason was demanding extra meal service.

Playing a hunch, the interviewer began telephoning emergency room physicians in the Boston area to ask about a patient with Jason's name or peculiar tattoo. The third try struck pay dirt.

"Jason Bird? I wondered when we'd hear from him again. He's been in and out of half the facilities in the state. His funny-looking EKG—probably an old MI—looks pretty bad, so he always gets admitted, but there's never any evidence that anything acute is going on. I don't think he's addicted. A couple of years ago he was admitted for a genuine pneumonia and got through a week without pain medication and with no withdrawal symptoms. He'll stay in the ICU a couple of days and rag on the staff. Then he'll split. He seems to enjoy needling medical people."

"He told me that he was the son of a physician and that he was a wealthy inventor."

The physician on the other end of the line chuckled. "The old respirator story. I checked into that one when he was admitted here for the third time. That was a different Bird altogether. I don't know that Jason's ever invented anything in his life. As for his father, I think he was a chiropractor."

Returning to the ward to add a note to the chart, the interviewer discovered that Jason had discharged himself against medical advice and departed, leaving behind a complaining letter to the hospital administrator.

Evaluation of Jason Bird

Jason illustrates the principal difficulty of diagnosing Factitious Disorder: The criteria depend heavily on the clinician's ability to infer motive and intent. Jason's EKG did not change and his cardiac enzymes were not elevated, so his interviewer presumed that Jason was feigning or markedly exaggerating his chest pain. There was no evidence that he was seeking some kind of material gain, so the interviewer concluded that he must want to occupy the role of a sick person. Both of these assertions may have been correct, but they were supported not by proof, only by reports from the emergency room.

The list of differential diagnoses is predictable. Most important, of course, Factitious Disorder must be differentiated from **general medical conditions**. This had already been accomplished in Jason's case. In patients presenting with psychological signs and symptoms, **other Axis I disorders** must be ruled out. Patients with somatoform disorders, especially **Somatization Disorder**, may also complain of symptoms that have no apparent organic basis. Those with **Antisocial Personality Disorder** may lie about symptoms, but they usually have some material gain in mind (to avoid punishment, to obtain money). **Schizophrenia** patients may have a bizarre lifestyle that could be confused with the wanderings of the classical Münchausen patient. Patients who feign psychological symptoms may look as though they have **dementia** or **Brief Psychotic Disorder**. None of these disorders could be supported by Jason's history or cross-sectional presentation.

Several other disorders may accompany Factitious Disorder. These include **substance-related disorders** (sedatives and analgesics) and **Dependent, Histrionic**, and **Borderline Personality Disorders**. Patients with the psychological form of Factitious Disorder usually have a serious personality disorder.

Ganser's syndrome, in which the patient gives answers that appear deliberately false (Q: "How many legs does a cow have?" A: "Five!") was once considered a type of Factitious Disorder. Now it is classified as a Dissociative Disorder Not Otherwise Specified (see p. 330).

Jason's symptoms were of a physical disorder, so he would be coded with that specifier:

Axis I	300.19	Factitious Disorder, With Predominantly Physical Signs and Symptoms
Axis II	799.9	Diagnosis Deferred
Axis III		None
Axis IV		None
Axis V	GAF = 41	(current)

300.19 Factitious Disorder Not Otherwise Specified

The Factitious Disorder Not Otherwise Specified category is for patients who have symptoms that are not classifiable under the criteria above.

Factitious disorder by proxy. In this unusual disorder, one person will seek access to medical care by intentionally producing signs or symptoms of illness in someone else. When this second person is a child, the disorder is presumptive evidence of child abuse. Suggested criteria for this proposed diagnosis are given on page 725 of DSM-IV.

Dissociative Disorders

Quick Guide to Dissociation

Dissociative symptoms are principally covered in this chapter, but there are some conditions (especially involving loss or lapse of memory) that are classified elsewhere. As always, the page number following each item indicates where a more detailed discussion begins.

Dissociative Disorders

Dissociative Amnesia. The patient cannot remember important information that is usually of a personal nature. This is usually stress-related (p. 319).

Dissociative Fugue. The patient suddenly travels away from home and cannot remember important details about the past (p. 322).

Dissociative Identity Disorder. One or more additional identities intermittently seize control of the patient's behavior (p. 325).

Depersonalization Disorder. There are episodes of detachment, as if the patient is observing the patient's own behavior from outside. In this condition, the patient does not actually have memory loss (p. 328).

Dissociative Disorder not Otherwise Specified. Patients who have symptoms suggestive of any of the disorders above, but who do not meet criteria for any one of them, may be categorized here (p. 330).

Other Causes of Severe Memory Loss

When dissociative symptoms are encountered in the course of other mental diagnoses, a separate diagnosis of a dissociative disorder is not ordinarily given.

Posttraumatic Stress Disorder. A month or more following a severe trauma, the patient may not remember important aspects of personal history (p. 269).

Acute Stress Disorder. Immediately following a severe trauma, patients may not remember important aspects of personal history (p. 273).

Substance-Induced Disorders. Use of alcohol or other substances may produce blackouts, in which the patient does not recall what happened while intoxicated. Alternatively, there may be state-dependent learning: Important information learned while intoxicated is only recalled the next time the patient is intoxicated (p. 62).

Somatization Disorder. Patients who have a long history of many somatic symptoms that cannot be explained on the basis of known disease mechanisms can also forget important aspects of personal history (p. 294).

Sleepwalking Disorder. Sleepwalking resembles the dissociative disorders, in that there is amnesia for purposeful behavior. But it is classified elsewhere in order to keep all the sleep disorders together (p. 421).

Malingering. Some patients consciously feign symptoms of memory loss. Their object is material gain, such as avoiding punishment or obtaining money or drugs (p. 539).

Introduction

Dissociation occurs when one group of normal mental processes becomes separated from the rest. According to DSM-IV, it is a "disruption in the usually integrated functions of consciousness, memory, identity, or perception of the environment" (p. 477). Basically, some of the patient's thoughts, feelings, or behaviors are removed from conscious awareness and control; for example, an otherwise healthy college student cannot recall any of the events of the previous two weeks. There is a close connection between the phenomena of dissociation and hypnosis.

The dissociative disorders have several features in common:

- They usually begin and end suddenly.
- Although clinicians do not generally agree as to their etiology, episodes are often precipitated by psychological conflicts.

- Although they are generally regarded as rare, their numbers may be increasing.
- In most (except Depersonalization Disorder), there is a profound disturbance of memory.
- Impaired functioning or a subjective feeling of distress is required only for Dissociative Amnesia, Dissociative Fugue, and Depersonalization Disorder.

> **TIP** Conversion symptoms (typical of the somatoform disorders) and dissociation tend to involve the same psychic mechanisms. Whenever you encounter a patient who dissociates, consider whether a diagnosis such as Somatization Disorder is also warranted.

300.12 Dissociative Amnesia

Formerly called Psychogenic Amnesia, Dissociative Amnesia has two main requirements: (1) The patient has forgotten something important, and (2) other Axis I disorders have been ruled out. Of course, the central feature is the inability to remember significant events. Clinicians as far back as Pierre Janet, 100 years ago, recognized several patterns in which this forgetting can occur:

Localized (or Circumscribed). The patient has recall for none of the events during a particular time, often a calamity such as wartime or a natural disaster.

Selective. Certain portions of a time period have been forgotten, such as the birth of a child. This type is less common.

The last three types are much less common, and may eventually lead to a diagnosis of Dissociative Identity Disorder:

Generalized. All of the experiences during the patient's entire lifetime have been forgotten.

Continuous. The patient forgets all events from a given time forward to the present. This is extremely rare now.

Systematized. The patient has forgotten certain classes of information, such as that relating to family or to work.

Dissociative Amnesia begins suddenly, usually following severe stress such as physical injury, guilt about an extramarital affair, abandonment by a spouse, or internal conflict over sexual issues. Sometimes the patient wanders aimlessly near home. After a variable time, the amnesia suddenly ends with complete recovery of memory. Reportedly, it is rare for Dissociative Amnesia to occur again in the same individual. Because other disorders have been ruled out, the clinician may presume that the cause is some overwhelming psychological stress; however, the DSM-IV criteria stop short of saying so.

Dissociative Amnesia has been little studied, so not much is known about demographic patterns, family occurrence, and the like. It is most commonly reported in young women.

Criteria for Dissociative Amnesia

- The patient's main problem is at least one episode of inability to recall important personal information. This information usually concerns trauma or stress, and it is more extensive than could be explained by common forgetfulness.
- These symptoms cause clinically important distress or impair work, social, or personal functioning.
- It does not occur solely during Dissociative Identity Disorder, Dissociative Fugue, Posttraumatic Stress Disorder, Acute Stress Disorder, or Somatization Disorder.
- The symptoms are not directly caused by a general medical condition or by the use of substances, including medications.

Holly Kahn

A mental health clinician presented the following dilemma to a medical center ethicist.

A single, 38-year-old woman had been seen several times in the outpatient clinic. She had complained of depression and anxiety, both of which were relatively mild. These symptoms seemed focused on the fact that she was 38 and unmarried, and "her biological clock was ticking." She had had no problems with sleep, appetite, or weight gain or loss, and had not thought about suicide.

For many months Holly had greatly desired a child, to the point that she intentionally became pregnant by her boyfriend. When he discovered what she had done, he broke off contact with her. The following week she miscarried. Stuck in what she perceived as a boring, unrewarding job as a salesclerk in a store that specialized in teachers' supplies, she had come to the clinic for help in "finding meaning for her life"

The oldest girl in a Midwestern family, Holly had spent much of her adolescence caring for younger siblings. Although she had attended college for two years during her mid-20s, she had come away without a degree, career, or husband to show for it. In the last decade she had lived with three different men; her latest relationship had lasted the longest and had seemed the most stable. She had no history of drug abuse or alcoholism and was in good physical health.

The clinician's verbal description was of a plain, no longer young (and never youthful), heavy-set woman with a square jaw and stringy hair. "In fact, she looks quite a lot like this." The clinician produced a drawing of a woman's head and shoulders. It was somewhat indistinct and smudged, but the features did fit the verbal description. The ethicist recognized it as a flyer that had recently been widely distributed. The copy below the picture read: "Wanted by FBI on suspicion of kidnapping—$5,000 reward for information leading to arrest and successful prosecution."

A day-old infant had been abducted from a local hospital's maternity ward. The first-time mother, barely out of her teens, had handed the baby girl to a woman wearing an operating room smock. The woman had introduced herself as a nursing supervisor and said she needed to take the baby for a final weighing and examination before the mother could take her home. That was the last time anyone could remember seeing either the woman or the baby. The picture had been drawn by a police artist from a description given by the distraught mother. The reward had been offered by the baby's grandparents.

"The next-to-last time I saw my patient, we were trying to work on ways she could take control over her own life. She seemed quite a bit more confident, less depressed. The following week she came in late, looking dazed. She claimed to have no memory of anything she had done for the past several days. I asked her whether she'd been ill, hit on the head, that sort of thing. She denied all of it. I started probing backward to see if I could jog her memory, but she became more and more agitated and finally rushed out. She said she'd return the next week, but I haven't seen her since. It wasn't until yesterday that I noticed her resemblance to the woman in this picture."

The therapist sat gazing at the flyer for a few seconds, then said: "Here's my dilemma. I think I know who committed this really awful crime, but I have a privileged relationship with the person I suspect. Just what is my ethical duty?"

Evaluation of Holly Kahn

Whether Holly took the baby is not the diagnostic issue here. At issue is the cause of her amnesia, which was her most pressing recent problem. She had been under stress because of her desire to have a baby, and this could have provided the stimulus for Dissociative Amnesia.

There is no information provided in the vignette that might support other (mostly biological) causes of amnesia. Specifically, there was no **head trauma** that might have induced an **Amnestic Disorder Due to Concussion. Substance-Induced Persisting Amnestic Disorder** would be ruled out by Holly's history of no substance use. Her general health had been good and there was no history of abnormal physical movements, reducing the likelihood of **epilepsy**. Although she had had a miscarriage, too much time had passed for a **postabortion psychosis** to be a possibility. Some patients with amnesia are also mute; they may be misdiagnosed as having **Catatonic Disorder Due to a General Medical Condition** or **Schizophrenia, Catatonic Type**.

There was no history of a recent, massive trauma that might indicate an **Acute Stress Disorder**. Holly had no confusion about her personal identity and did not travel from home, so she would not qualify for **Dissociative Fugue** (although the two conditions do share the same sort of amnesia). If she was **Malingering**, she did it without an obvious motive (had she been trying to avoid punishment for a crime, simply staying away from the medical center would have served her better). Her five-axis diagnosis would thus be as follows:

Axis I	300.12	Dissociative Amnesia
Axis II	V71.09	No diagnosis
Axis III		None
Axis IV		None
Axis V	GAF = 31	(current)

300.13 Dissociative Fugue

In Dissociative Fugue (formerly called Psychogenic Fugue), the patient suddenly leaves home (or previous activity) and goes on a journey. This often follows a severe stress, such as marital strife or disasters. The travel is purposeful; it is not the aimless wandering that can be encountered in Dissociative Amnesia. There may be disorientation and a sense of confusion. Some patients will assume a new identity and name; they may even take up a new occupation at which they work for months. However, in most instances the episode is brief, lasting a few hours or a few days, and limited to travel. Occasionally, there may be outbursts of violence. Recovery is usually sudden; afterwards, there is amnesia for the episode.

Dissociative Fugue is another of those extraordinarily interesting, rare disorders—the stuff of novels and motion pictures—about which there has been little in the way of recent research. For example, essentially nothing is known about sex ratio or family history.

Criteria for Dissociative Fugue

• The main problem is that the patient suddenly and unexpectedly travels from home or usual workplace and cannot recall personal history.

- The patient may be confused about identity or assume a new identity; these experiences can be partial or complete.
- These symptoms do not occur solely as a part of Dissociative Identity Disorder.
- They are not directly caused by a general medical condition or by the use of substances, including medications.
- They cause clinically important distress or impair work, social, or personal functioning.

John Doe

When the man first walked into the homeless shelter, he hadn't a thing to his name, including a name. He'd been referred from a local hospital's emergency room, but he told the clinician on duty that he'd only gone there for a place to stay. As far as he was aware, his physical health was good. His problem was that he didn't remember a thing about his life prior to waking up on a park bench at dawn that morning. Later, when filling out the paperwork, the clinician had penciled in "John Doe" as the patient's name.

Aside from the fact that he could give a history spanning only about eight hours, John Doe's mental status exam was remarkably normal. He appeared to be in his early 40s. He was dressed casually in slacks, a pink dress shirt, and a nicely fitting corduroy sports jacket with leather patches on the elbows. His speech was clear and coherent; his affect was generally pleasant, though he was obviously troubled at his loss of memory. He denied having hallucinations or delusions ("as far as I know"), though he pointed out logically enough that he "couldn't vouch for what kind of crazy ideas I might have had yesterday."

John Doe appeared intelligent, and his fund of information was good. He could name five recent presidents in order, and he could discuss recent national and international events. He could repeat eight digits forward and six backwards. He scored 29 out of 30 on the Mini-Mental State Exam, failing only to identify the county in which the shelter was located. Although he surmised (he wore a wedding ring) that he must be married, after half an hour's conversation he could remember nothing pertaining to his family, occupation, place of residence, or personal identity.

"Let me look inside your sports jacket," the clinician said.

John Doe looked perplexed, but unbuttoned his jacket and held it open. The label gave the name of a men's clothing store in Cincinnati, some 500 miles away.

"Let's try there," suggested the clinician. Several telephone calls later, the Cincinnati Police Department identified John Doe as an attorney whose wife had reported him missing two days earlier.

The following morning John Doe was on a bus for home, but it was several days before the clinician heard the rest of the story. A 43-year-old specialist in wills and probate, John Doe had been accused of co-mingling the accounts of clients with his own. He had protested his innocence and hired his own attorney, but the Ohio State Bar Association stood ready to proceed against him. The pressure to straighten out his books, maintain his law practice, and defend himself in court and against his own state bar had been enormous. Two days before he disappeared, he had told his wife, "I don't know if I can take much more of this without losing my mind."

Evaluation of John Doe

Although John Doe's case is not quite a classical example of Dissociative Fugue (he did not assume a new identity and adopt a new life), his confusion about his identity is more typical of this diagnosis. He did travel far from home and purposefully set about trying to seek shelter.

Neither at the time of evaluation nor at follow-up was there evidence of alternative Axis I disorders. John had not switched repeatedly between identities, which would rule out **Dissociative Identity Disorder** (the two disorders cannot be diagnosed together). Other than the obvious amnesia, there was no evidence of a cognitive disorder such as **dementia**. At age 43, a new case of **temporal lobe epilepsy** would be unlikely, but a complete evaluation should include a neurological workup. Any mobility in **Dissociative Amnesia** takes the form of aimless wandering, not purposeful travel, as was the case for John. Of course, any patient who has episodes of amnesia must be evaluated for **substance-related disorders** (especially **alcohol-related disorders**).

Conscious imitation of amnesia in **Malingering** can be very difficult to discern from the amnesia involved in Dissociative Fugue. However, although John Doe did have legal difficulties, these would not have been relieved by his feigning amnesia. (When Malingering appears to be a possibility, collateral history from relatives or friends of previous such behavior or of **Antisocial Personality Disorder** can help.) A history of lifelong multiple medical symptoms might suggest **Somatization Disorder**. John had no cross-sectional features that would suggest either **Manic Episode** or **Schizophrenia**, in each of which wandering and other bizarre behaviors can be encountered.

TIP Epilepsy is always mentioned in the differential diagnosis of the dissociative disorders. However, epilepsy and dissociation should not be hard to tell apart in practice, even without the benefit of an EEG. Epileptic episodes usually last no longer than a few minutes and involve speech and motor behavior that are repetitive and apparently purposeless. Dissociative behavior, on the other hand, may last for days or longer and involves complex speech and motor behavior that appear purposeful.

The full diagnosis in this case would be as follows:

Axis I	300.13	Dissociative Fugue
Axis II	V71.09	No diagnosis
Axis III		None
Axis IV		Investigation by State Bar Association
Axis V	GAF = 55	(current)

300.14 Dissociative Identity Disorder

In Dissociative Identity Disorder (DID), which has previously achieved fame as Multiple Personality Disorder, the person possesses at least two distinct personalities or personality states. The number of these can range as high as 200. DSM-IV (p. 770) defines *personality* as "enduring patterns of perceiving, relating to, and thinking about the environment and oneself."

These personalities may have their own names, which may not even be of the patient's own gender. Some may be symbolic, such as "The Worker." They can vary widely in age and style: If the patient is normally shy and quiet, one personality may be outgoing and even boisterous. The personalities may be aware of one another to some degree, though only one interacts with the environment at a time. The transition from one personality to another is usually sudden, often precipitated by stress. Most of the personalities are aware of the loss of time that occurs when another personality is in control.

DID is diagnosed much more commonly by clinicians in North America than in Europe. For some years there has been a hotly running dispute about this. European clinicians (naturally) claim that the disorder is rare, and that by paying so much attention to patients who dissociate, North American clinicians actually encourage the development of cases. The dispute remains unresolved at this writing.

The onset of this fascinating disorder is usually in childhood, though it is not commonly recognized then. Most of the patients are female, and many may have been sexually abused. DID runs a chronic course. It may run in families, but the question of genetic transmission is also unresolved.

Criteria for Dissociative Identity Disorder

- The patient has at least two distinct identities or personality states. Each of these has its own, relatively lasting pattern of sensing, thinking about, and relating to self and environment.
- At least two of these personalities repeatedly assume control of the patient's behavior.

- Common forgetfulness cannot explain the patient's extensive inability to remember important personal information.
- This behavior is not directly caused by substance use (as in alcoholic blackouts) or by a general medical condition.

Coding Note

In children, the symptoms cannot be attributed to fantasy play, including imaginary playmates.

Effie Jens

On her first visit to the mental health clinic, Effie cried and talked about her failing memory. She pointed out that at 26 she was too young for senility, but that on some days she actually felt senile. For several months she had noticed "holes in her memory"—sometimes these lasted for two or three days. Her recall wasn't just spotty; for all she knew about her activities on those days, she might as well have been under anesthesia. However, from telltale signs such as food that had disappeared from her refrigerator and recently arrived letters that had been opened, she knew she must have been awake and functioning during these times.

Effie lived alone in a small apartment on the proceeds of the property settlement from her recent divorce; her family lived in a distant state. She enjoyed quiet things—reading and watching television. She was shy and had trouble meeting people; there was no one she saw often enough to help her account for the missing time.

For that matter, Effie wasn't all that clear about the details of her earlier life. She was the second of three daughters of an itinerant preacher. Her early childhood memories were a jumble of labor camps, cheap hotel rooms, and Bible-thumping sermons. By the time she reached age 13, she had attended 15 different schools.

Late in the interview, she revealed that she had virtually no memory of the entire year she was 13. Her father's preaching had been moderately successful, and they had settled for a while in a small town in southern Oregon. She believed this was the only time she had ever started and finished a year in the same school. But what had happened to her during the intervening months? Of that time she recalled nothing whatsoever.

The following week Effie came back, but she was different. "Call me Liz," she said as she dropped her shoulder bag onto the floor and leaned back in her chair. Without further prompting, she launched into a long, detailed, and dramatic recounting of her activities of the last three days. She had gone out for dinner and dancing with a man she had met in the grocery store, and afterwards they had hit a couple of bars together.

"But I only had ginger ale," she said, smiling and crossing her legs. "I never drink. It's terrible for the figure."

"Are there any parts of last week you can't remember?"

"Oh, no. She's the one who has amnesia."

She was Effie Jens, whom Liz clearly regarded as a person quite different from her own self. Liz was gay, carefree, and sociable; Effie was introspective and preferred solitude. "I'm not saying that she isn't a decent human being," Liz conceded, "but you've met her—don't you think she's just a tad mousy?"

Although for many years she had "shared living space" with Effie, it wasn't until after the divorce that Liz had begun to "come out," as she put it. At first this had happened for only an hour or two, especially when Effie was tired or depressed and "needed a break." Recently Liz had taken control for longer and longer periods of time; once she had done so for three days.

"I've tried to be careful, it frightens her so much," Liz said with a worried frown. "I've begun to think seriously about taking control for all time. I think I can do a better job. I certainly have a better social life."

Besides being able to recount her activities during the blank times that had driven Effie to seek care, Liz could give an eyewitness account of all of Effie's conscious activities as well. She even knew what had gone on during Effie's "lost" year, when she was 13.

"It was Daddy," she said with a curl of her lip. "He said it was part of his religious mission to 'practice for a re-enactment of the Annunciation.' But it was really just another randy male groping his own daughter, and worse. Effie told Mom. At first, she wouldn't believe her. And when she finally did, she made Effie promise never to tell. She said it would break up the family. All these years, I'm the only other one who's known about it. No wonder she's losing her grip—it even makes me sick."

Evaluation of Effie Jens

Effie's two personalities are fairly typical of DID: One was quiet and unassuming, almost mousy, whereas the other was much more assertive. What happened when Liz was in control was unknown to Effie, who experienced these episodes as amnesia. This difficulty with recall was vastly more extensive than would be expected from common forgetfulness. (Effie's history was atypical in that many personalities, not just two, are the rule.)

A number of other causes of amnesia should be considered in the differential diagnosis of this condition. Of course, any possible general medical condition must first be ruled out, but Effie/Liz had no history suggestive of either a **seizure disorder** or **substance use**. Without travel from home, **Dissociative Fugue** cannot be diagnosed; even if Effie (or Liz) had engaged in purposeful travel, DID is a more pervasive disorder and thus would take diagnostic precedence. Obviously, **Dissociative Amnesia** also involves amnesia, but it is not recurrent and does not involve multiple, distinct personalities.

Schizophrenia has often been confused with DID, primarily by lay people who equate "split personality" (which is how many have come to think of Schizophrenia) with Multiple Personality Disorder, the old name for DID. However, although bizarre behavior may be encountered in DID, none of the personalities is typically psychotic. As in other dissociative disorders, the discrimination of **Malingering** can be difficult; information from informants about possible material gain remains the most valuable discriminator. Effie's history was not typical for either of these diagnoses.

Often DID patients will also have **Borderline Personality Disorder**. The danger is that only the personality disorder will be diagnosed by a clinician who mistakes alternating personae for the unstable mood and behavior typical of Borderline Personality Disorder. **Substance-related disorders** sometimes occur with DID.

Axis I	300.14	Dissociative Identity Disorder
Axis II	799.9	Diagnosis Deferred
Axis III		None
Axis IV		Divorce
Axis V	GAF = 55	(current)

300.6 Depersonalization Disorder

Depersonalization can be defined as a sense of being cut off or detached from one's self. This feeling may be experienced as viewing one's own mental processes or behavior; some patients feel as if they are in a dream. When a patient is repeatedly distressed by episodes of depersonalization, and there is no other disorder that better accounts for the symptoms, you can diagnose Depersonalization Disorder. It is important to note that about half the general population has had at least one such episode; no diagnosis should be made unless the symptoms are persistent or recurrent, and unless they cause distress or impair functioning.

People with Depersonalization Disorder also commonly experience derealization, which can be defined as a feeling that the sense that the exterior world is unreal or odd. Patients may notice that the size or shape of objects has changed, or that other people seem robotic or even dead.

Episodes of Depersonalization Disorder are often precipitated by stress; they begin and end suddenly. The disorder begins in the teens or early 20s; usually it is chronic. Because it has been poorly studied, there is no reliable information about demographics, such as sex distribution. We don't even know how common it is.

Criteria for Depersonalization Disorder

- There is a lasting or recurring feeling of being detached from the patient's own body. The patient feels like an outside self-observer, as if in a dream.
- Throughout the experience, the patient knows that this is not really the case (reality testing is intact).
- This phenomenon causes clinically important distress or impairs work, social, or personal functioning.
- This experience doesn't occur solely in the course of another mental disorder, such as Acute Stress Disorder, Panic Disorder, Schizophrenia, or a different dissociative disorder.
- The disorder is not directly caused by a general medical condition or by the use of substances, including medications.

Francine Parfit

"It feels like I'm losing my mind." Francine Parfit was only 20 years old, but she had already worked as a bank teller for nearly two years. Having received several raises during that time, she felt that she was good at her job—conscientious, personable, healthy, and reliable. But she had been increasingly troubled by her "out-of-body experiences," as she called them.

"I'll be standing behind my counter and, all of a sudden, I'm also standing a couple of feet away. I seem to be looking over my own shoulder as I'm talking with my customer. And in my head I'm commenting to myself on my own actions, as if I were a different person I was watching. Stuff like, 'Now she'll have to call the Assistant Manager to get approval for this transfer of funds.' I came to the clinic because I saw something like this on television a few nights ago, and the person got shock treatments. That's when I began to worry something really awful was wrong."

Francine denied that she had ever had blackout spells, convulsions, blows to the head, severe headaches, or dizziness. She had smoked pot a time or two in high school, but otherwise she was drug- and alcohol-free. Her physical health had been excellent; her only visits to physicians had been for immunizations, Pap smears, and a pre-employment physical exam two years ago.

Each episode began suddenly, without warning. First Francine would feel quite anxious; then she'd notice that her head seemed to bob up and down slightly, out of her control. Occasionally she felt a warm sensation on the top of her head, as if someone had cracked a half-cooked egg that was dribbling yolk down through her hairline. The episodes seldom lasted longer than a few minutes, but they were becoming more frequent—several times a week now. If they occurred while she was at work, she could often take a break until they passed. But several times it had happened when she was driving. She worried that she might lose control of the car.

Francine had never heard voices or had hallucinations of other senses; she denied ever feeling talked about or plotted against in any way. She had never had suicidal ideas and didn't really feel depressed.

"Just scared," she concluded. "It's so spooky to feel that you've sort of died."

Evaluation of Francine Parfit

The sensation of being an outside observer of yourself can be quite unsettling; it is one that many people who are not patients have had a time or two. What made Francine's experience stand out was the fact that it recurred often enough and forcibly enough to cause her considerable distress. Notice that she described her experience "as if I were a different person," not "I am a different person." This tells us that she retained contact with reality.

Francine's experiences and feelings were much like those of Shorty Rheinbold, except that his were symptoms of **Panic Disorder** (see p. 254). A variety of conditions include depersonalization as a symptom: **anxiety**, **cognitive**, **mood**, **personality**, and **substance-related disorders**, as well as **Schizophrenia** and **epilepsy**. However, Francine did not complain of Panic Attacks or have symptoms of other disorders that could account for the symptoms.

> **TIP** A collection of symptoms called the phobic anxiety depersonalization syndrome sometimes occurs, especially in young women. In addition to depression, such patients, not surprisingly, have phobias, anxiety, and depersonalization. This condition may be a variant of depressive episode, with atypical features.

Francine's full diagnosis would read as follows:

Axis I	300.6	Depersonalization Disorder
Axis II	V71.09	No diagnosis
Axis III		None
Axis IV		None
Axis V	GAF = 70	(current)

300.15 Dissociative Disorder Not Otherwise Specified

The Dissociative Disorder Not Otherwise Specified category is for patients whose symptoms represent a change in the normally integrative function of identity, memory, or consciousness, but who do not meet criteria for one of the specific dissociative disorders listed above. Here are some examples:

Derealization without depersonalization. Both of these terms are defined on p. 328.

Brainwashing. People who have been indoctrinated may develop dissociative states.

Coma or loss of consciousness. These can be dissociative when they are not due to a general medical condition.

Conditions similar to Dissociative Identity Disorder. Some patients may not fully meet the criteria for DID. For example, they may not have two fully formed personality states, or they do not have amnesia as a part of the syndrome.

Ganser's syndrome. The syndrome of approximate answers, also known by the German word *vorbeireden* (which means "talking past the point"), has been described as a form of dissociation known as Ganser's syndrome. It was at one time classified as a Factitious Disorder. It is described briefly on p. 315.

Dissociative trance disorder. This proposed diagnostic category covers certain dissociative conditions not generally encountered in Western societies. These include amok, koro, latah, pibloktoq, and others. These and other culture-bound syndromes are briefly discussed in DSM-IV, beginning on page 843. It states suggested research criteria for dissociative trance disorder beginning on page 727.

Sexual and Gender Identity Disorders

Quick Guide to the Sexual and Gender Identity Disorders

As in earlier chapters, the page number following each item indicates where a more detailed discussion begins.

Sexual Dysfunctions

With the exception of those that bear gender-specific names, any of the sexual dysfunctions can apply to both males and females.

Low Sexual Desire Disorders

Complaints by the patient (or partner) of inadequate desire for sex may indicate one of these problems:

Hypoactive Sexual Desire Disorder. The patient isn't much interested in sex, though performance may be adequate once sexual activity has been initiated (p. 338).

Sexual Aversion Disorder. The patient finds the idea of genital sexual contact repugnant (p. 338).

Sexual Arousal Disorders

In the arousal disorders, the patient may be interested in sex but doesn't become stimulated enough to complete the sex act.

Female Sexual Arousal Disorder. A woman doesn't lubricate adequately to permit vaginal sex (p. 341).

Male Erectile Disorder. A man's erection isn't sufficient to begin or complete sexual relations (p. 343).

Orgasmic Disorders

In the orgasmic disorders, there is a failure (complete or partial) to achieve climax, even though the patient may be both interested in sex and adequately aroused.

Female Orgasmic Disorder. Despite a normal period of sexual excitement, a woman's climax either is delayed or does not occur at all (p. 346).

Male Orgasmic Disorder. Despite a normal period of sexual excitement, a man's climax is either delayed or does not occur at all (p. 348).

Premature Ejaculation. A man experiences repeated instances of climax before, during, or just after penetration (p. 350).

Sexual Pain Disorders

Dyspareunia. In a woman or man, genital pain occurs at some point during sexual intercourse, often during insertion (p. 352).

Vaginismus. Severe vaginal spasm causes pain for a woman and interferes with penetration (p. 354).

Secondary and Other Sexual Dysfunctions

Sexual Dysfunction Due to a General Medical Condition. Many of the sorts of problems noted above can be caused by anatomical or other physical problems (p. 357).

Substance-Induced Sexual Dysfunction. Many of these sorts of problems can also be caused by intoxication or withdrawal from alcohol or other substances (p. 358).

Sexual Dysfunction Not Otherwise Specified. Use this category when you aren't sure why a patient has a sexual dysfunction (p. 360).

Nonsexual Mental Disorders. Many patients develop sexual dysfunction as a result of other mental disorders. Lack of interest in sex may be encountered especially in Somatization Disorder, Major Depressive Disorder, and Schizophrenia.

Paraphilias

The paraphilias include a variety of sexual behaviors that most people reject as distasteful, unusual, or abnormal. Nearly all of them are practiced largely, perhaps exclusively, by males.

Exhibitionism. The patient has urges to expose the genitals to a stranger who does not expect it (p. 362).

Fetishism. The patient has sexual urges related to the use of inanimate objects (p. 364).

Frotteurism. The patient has urges related to rubbing the genitals against a person who has not consented to this (p. 366).

Pedophilia. The patient has urges involving sexual activities with children (p. 368).

Sexual Masochism. The patient has sexual urges related to being injured, bound, or humiliated (p. 372).

Sexual Sadism. The patient has sexual urges related to inflicting suffering or humiliation on someone else (p. 372).

Transvestic Fetishism. A heterosexual man has sexual urges related to cross-dressing (p. 376).

Voyeurism. The patient has urges related to viewing some unsuspecting person disrobing, naked, or engaging in sexual activity (p. 378).

Paraphilia Not Otherwise Specified. There are quite a few paraphilias that are not widely practiced or that have received too little clinical attention to warrant codes of their own. They include sexual urges involving dead people, animals, feces, urine, enemas, and making obscene phone calls (p. 380).

Gender Identity Disorders

Gender Identity Disorders. Patients strongly identify with the opposite gender and are uncomfortable with their assigned gender roles. Some request sex reassignment surgery to relieve this discomfort (p. 381).

Gender Identity Disorder Not Otherwise Specified. This category is especially for intersex conditions ("hermaphrodites") and people with ambiguous sexual assignment (p. 385).

Other

Sexual Disorder Not Otherwise Specified. This is a catch-all category for sexual problems that do not meet the criteria for any of the foregoing sexual or gender identity disorders (p. 386).

Introduction

Depending on the principal type of pathology, DSM-IV divides the sexual and gender identity disorders into three groups: (1) sexual dysfunctions, (2) paraphilias, and (3) gender identity disorders. As with most other DSM-IV diagnoses, patients can have multiple sexual and gender identity disorders, which can coexist with other Axis I and Axis II diagnoses.

SEXUAL DYSFUNCTIONS

DSM-IV classifies the sexual dysfunctions into four main categories, three of which include a variety of behaviors that represent loss of function from the accepted stages of the normal cycle of sexual response. The activities in these stages vary markedly from one person to the next, and there are many differences between men and women. The stages are as follows:

1. Appetitive. The person desires sexual activity and may have fantasies about it. During this phase occur the sexual desire disorders (beginning on p. 338).

2. Excitement. The individual experiences a feeling of pleasure and physiological change. In the male, the principal such change is penile erection; in the female there is enlargement and lubrication of the vagina, tumescence of the nipples, and swelling of the vulva. Associated with this phase are the sexual arousal disorders (beginning on p. 341).

3. Orgasm. At the peak of sexual excitement, both males and females experience a release of sexual tension with rhythmic contraction of muscles and reproductive organs. The male ejaculates semen. In this phase occur the orgasmic disorders (beginning on p. 345).

4. Resolution. There is general relaxation and a sense of well-being. During a refractory period that can last minutes or longer, the male cannot experience erection or ejaculation. Sexual disorders are only rarely related specifically to the resolution phase.

In addition, there are the sexual pain disorders, which can occur at any stage of the sexual response cycle (they begin on p. 352).

> **TIP** Hypersexuality (excessive interest in sex) is nowhere defined, described, or categorized in DSM-IV; yet it can occur as a symptom in such disorders as Manic Episode, Schizophrenia, cognitive disorders, and personality disorders.

The sexual dysfunctions usually begin in early adulthood, though some may not appear until later in life. Most of them are quite common. Any of them can be caused by psychological or biological factors or by a combination of these.

Also, any of these dysfunctions can be lifelong or acquired. Lifelong (also called primary) means that this dysfunction (e.g., Premature Ejaculation) has been present since the beginning of active sexual functioning. Acquired means that at some time the patient has not had that particular dysfunction. A lifelong dysfunction is vastly more resistant to therapy.

Furthermore, the sexual dysfunctions may be either generalized or situational (i.e., limited to specific situations). For example, a man may experience Premature Ejaculation when with his wife but not with another woman. Some dysfunctions may not even require that the patient have a partner—they can occur during masturbation, for example. (There are a few obvious exceptions: Dyspareunia, Sexual Aversion Disorder, Premature Ejaculation.)

There are no set rules about how much dysfunction must be shown before a diagnosis can be made. Nor do the criteria for sexual dysfunctions specify a minimum time duration. The criteria for all of the sexual dysfunctions specify only that they must cause significant distress or interpersonal difficulties. This leaves you with room for judgment, based on how long the problem has existed and how severely the problem affects patient and partner. This judgment will be influenced by the circumstances surrounding the particular sex activity, the amount of that activity, and with whom it occurs. For example, Female Sexual Arousal Disorder should not be diagnosed if it occurs only with a partner the patient does not like or if intercourse is attempted after little or no foreplay.

You should also not use one of these diagnoses if the behavior occurs only in the course of another Axis I disorder. The criteria likewise explicitly prohibit diagnosis of a sexual dysfunction if it stems entirely from general medical or substance-induced conditions. You can make a diagnosis if its cause appears to be a V-code marital problem or an Axis II personality disorder.

Although they are quite common, the sexual dysfunctions are often ignored by clinicians who do not specialize in their evaluation and treatment; most commonly, clinicians just don't ask. The alert clinician may be able to make a diagnosis of one or more of these conditions in a patient who comes for consultation regarding an unrelated mental health problem.

Type Codes That Apply to Sexual Dysfunctions

In any patient, all of the sexual dysfunctions *can* be coded to reflect three aspects of history: the cause, the duration, and the specificity.

Type Codes for the Sexual Dysfunctions

- Specify one of these:
   Due to Psychological Factors or
   Due to Combined Factors (psychological factors and a general medical condition)
- Specify one of these:
   Lifelong Type (it has occurred throughout the patient's active sexual life) or
   Acquired Type (there has been a time when the patient did not have this sexual dysfunction)
- Specify one of these:
   Generalized Type (the disorder occurs with all partners and in all situations) or
   Situational Type (the disorder occurs only with certain partners or in some situations)

Coding Notes

Although I have picked Female Sexual Arousal Disorder as the example here, the following notes apply to many of the sexual disorders discussed in the following pages.

A patient who has a general medical condition (e.g., diabetes mellitus) that partly, but not completely, accounts for a problem with arousal would be diagnosed as follows:

| Axis I | 302.72 | Female Sexual Arousal Disorder, Due to Combined Factors |
| Axis III | 250.01 | Insulin-dependent diabetes mellitus |

A patient who uses drugs and who has arousal problems due partly, but not solely, to the direct effects of drug use, would be diagnosed as follows (other specifiers would also apply):

| Axis I | 302.72 | Female Sexual Arousal Disorder, Due to Combined Factors |

Patients whose arousal problems are due solely to a combination of substance use (such as heroin intoxication) and a general medical condition (such as diabetes mellitus) should be given two Axis I diagnoses:

| Axis I | 625.8 | Other Female Sexual Dysfunction Due to Diabetes Mellitus |
| | 292.89 | Heroin-Induced Sexual Dysfunction, With Impaired Arousal, With Onset During Intoxication |

Of course, you would have to supply the appropriate Axis I and Axis III codes for each of the examples above.

SEXUAL DESIRE DISORDERS

In the category of sexual desire disorders are two conditions that express abnormality of fantasies about sex and the desire for it.

302.71 Hypoactive Sexual Desire Disorder

and

302.79 Sexual Aversion Disorder

Sexual desire depends upon a number of factors, including the patient's inherent drive and self-esteem, previous sexual satisfaction, an available partner, and a good relationship with the partner in areas other than sex. Sexual desire may be suppressed by long abstinence.

Manifestations of Hypoactive Sexual Desire Disorder can be very variable. It may present as infrequent sexual activity, as a perception that the partner is unattractive, or as actual complaints of low sexual desire. Even though initially uninterested, the person may be able to perform once involved. It is more common among women, but can affect people of both sexes. It affects as much as 20% of the population.

Sexual Aversion Disorder may be experienced as loathing of any genital contact or of certain aspects of genital sexual contact. It can result from painful intercourse, feelings of guilt, or rape or other sexual trauma occurring in childhood or early during the patient's sexual life. The line between this disorder and the preceding one is often blurred; both diagnoses may be appropriate. There is usually low frequency of sexual contact. Sexual Aversion Disorder is probably far less common than Hypoactive Sexual Desire Disorder.

Criteria for Hypoactive Sexual Desire Disorder

- Desire for and fantasy about sexual activity are chronically or recurrently deficient or absent. The clinician judges this on the basis of the patient's age and other life circumstances that may affect sexual functioning.
- This behavior causes marked distress or interpersonal problems.
- Except for another sexual dysfunction, no other Axis I disorder explains the dysfunction better.
- It is not directly and exclusively caused by the use of substances (including medications) or by a general medical condition.

Coding Note

From the section on type codes (p. 337), choose the codes that apply. Also consider the Coding Notes there.

Criteria for Sexual Aversion Disorder

• To an extreme degree, the patient dislikes and avoids all or nearly all genital contact with a sex partner.
• Except for another sexual dysfunction, no other Axis I disorder explains the dysfunction better.
• It causes marked distress or interpersonal problems.

Coding Note

From the section on type codes (p. 337), choose the codes that apply. Also consider the Coding Notes there.

Ernestine Paget

"She hardly ever wants to do it," said James Paget to the marriage therapist.

"That's not quite accurate," Ernestine responded. "The truth is, I never want to do it. It's disgusting."

When they got married three years earlier, Ernestine had been uninterested in sex, though receptive to the idea of it. "It seemed to mean a lot to him, so I put up with it," she explained. "But he was never satisfied. No matter how often we made love, a few days later there he was, wanting more. It got old fast."

"It is the usual expectation," her husband remarked dryly, "and it's not my fault how she was brought up."

In Ernestine's family, like so many others, sex was never discussed and nudity was not allowed. Ernestine could never remember having much curiosity about sex, let alone interest. She had been an only child. "I assume her parents only did it once," offered James.

For the first few months, Ernestine would simply lie still and think about other things, enduring what was a basically boring activity for her because it was important to her new husband. Her gynecologist had assured her that as far as her anatomy and hormones were concerned, she was completely normal. Unless she was figuring out whether it was time to start taking her new prescription of birth control pills, she never thought about sex.

"God knows, I never dream about it," Ernestine said. "Maybe if he'd led up to it more, it would have helped. His idea of foreplay is half an hour of David Letterman and a slap on the butt." She had once tried to explain this to James, but he had only called her "frigid." That was the last word they had exchanged on the subject until now.

Now James pretty much ignored Ernestine. She undressed in the closet; they slept on the two edges of their king-sized bed. She didn't know where he was getting his sex these days, but it wasn't at home and she said she didn't care.

"At least he doesn't have to worry that I'd try to cut it off, like that Bobbitt woman," Ernestine said. "I don't even like to look at it, let alone touch it with a 10-inch knife."

Evaluation of Ernestine Paget

Ernestine's low sex interest was shown not just by absent desire; she denied even fantasizing about it. This is an important point: Some patients may reject the idea of sex with a current (or with any) partner, yet still harbor an abstract interest in sex or in sex with some hypothetical person. When Ernestine began her sexual life with her husband, she was merely uninterested in sex. It was only with experience that she became intolerant of the very idea of sexual contact. The abhorrence of sexual contact could also meet the criteria for **Specific Phobia;** however, no additional diagnosis of Specific Phobia is necessary.

Ernestine's clinician needed to ascertain that she had no other Axis I disorder, such as **Major Depressive Disorder**, **Somatization Disorder**, or **Obsessive–Compulsive Disorder**, that could explain her antipathy to sex. In the presence of any of these, she could only receive the additional diagnosis of a disorder of sexual desire if her sexual symptoms disappeared once the other Axis I pathology had been eliminated. Similar arguments would hold for **substance use** or a **general medical condition**.

Although Ernestine had never had an orgasm, she would not be diagnosed as having **Female Orgasmic Disorder** because she did not experience a normal excitement phase (see the list of the stages of normal sexual response, beginning on p. 335). She could not be diagnosed as having **Female Sexual Arousal Disorder** because she had never experienced sexual excitement.

Both of Ernestine's sexual desire disorders would appear to have lasted throughout her sexual life. Neither was due even in part to a general medical condition. The clinician lacked sufficient information to determine whether these disorders were generalized or confined to specific situations.

The Pagets were also having severe problems with other aspects of their marriage. Had these been the principal focus for treatment, a diagnosis of Partner Relational Problem would have been listed on Axis I. Since this was not the case, it would go on Axis IV as a psychosocial/environmental problem.

Ernestine's complete diagnosis would be as follows:

Axis I	302.71	Hypoactive Sexual Desire Disorder, Lifelong Type, Due to Psychological Factors
	302.79	Sexual Aversion Disorder, Lifelong Type, Due to Psychological Factors
Axis II	V71.09	No diagnosis
Axis III		None
Axis IV		Partner relational problem (withdrawal)
Axis V	GAF = 61	(current)

SEXUAL AROUSAL DISORDERS

Even when they are interested in sex, some men and women may have difficulty becoming sufficiently aroused to complete a sex act. Sexual arousal disorders are often associated with orgasmic disorders, discussed later.

302.72 Female Sexual Arousal Disorder

Female Sexual Arousal Disorder is common; up to one-third of women may be affected. Many of them may also have Dyspareunia and Hypoactive Sexual Desire Disorder. The principal symptom of this disorder is lubrication insufficient to sustain sexual activity through to its conclusion. As with most other sexual disorders, this can be lifelong (always the case) or acquired (developing later in the woman's active sex life).

A number of biological factors that would prevent a diagnosis of Female Sexual Arousal Disorder have been identified. Among the medications that can contribute are antihistamines and anticholinergics. Postmenopausal females may need more foreplay to lubricate to the same degree than they did when they were younger. Female Sexual Arousal Disorder should also not be diagnosed if the problem is present only in the context of another Axis I condition, such as Major Depressive Disorder or Somatization Disorder. However, it can be diagnosed in conjunction with another sexual condition, such as Female Orgasmic Disorder.

Criteria for Female Sexual Arousal Disorder

- Chronically or recurrently, the patient cannot lubricate enough to complete the sexual activity.
- Except for another sexual dysfunction, no other Axis I disorder explains the dysfunction better.
- It is not directly and exclusively caused by the use of substances (including medications) or by a general medical condition.
- It causes marked distress or interpersonal problems.

Coding Note

From the section on type codes (p. 337), choose the codes that apply. Also consider the Coding Notes there.

Julianna Pendergast

"He's the best husband in the world, and he tries so hard. Well, we both do." Julianna Pendergast was 28 and had been married almost five years. Her husband did not accompany her to this interview, though he had agreed to a later interview.

Julianna described their relationship as being close and loving. Although she had never had a climax, she didn't dislike sex. In fact, she looked forward to it and enjoyed the extra sense of closeness that intercourse added. "He always falls asleep on me afterwards," she said. "It's awfully sweet."

When she was 17, Julianna had become sexually active with the captain of the high school football team. It had been interesting and fun "in a wicked sort of way," but she hadn't climaxed, then or ever. "It always hurt a little," she commented. It didn't matter which man she was with (there had been five); she always stayed "kind of dry down there."

With her husband, there had been long sessions of foreplay—three and a half hours one rainy Saturday morning—but even that hadn't helped much. Sex magazines and porn videos only made matters worse. Even before they were married, they had finally come to rely on that old stand-by, petroleum jelly. "Now it doesn't hurt any more," she commented dryly, "but it still all comes to nothing."

Julianna had been thoroughly evaluated by an internist and her gynecologist. Each had given her a clean bill of health. She was taking no medications and had no history of hypertension or diabetes. Her sexual anatomy was normal.

"I'm pretty happy this way, actually," she concluded. "I feel that I get quite a lot out of our sexual relationship. It's my husband who wants to give me more."

Evaluation of Julianna Pendergast

Julianna did not lack interest in sex; in fact, she enjoyed it and looked forward to it for the closeness it brought with her husband. Her principal problem was that she did not become aroused, even when foreplay lasted far longer than normal. She herself noted that she didn't lubricate enough to facilitate intercourse; for years she and her husband had resorted to artificial lubrication.

In part, Juliana's problems with lubrication conditioned her to expect pain, and that led to a second sexual problem: complete anorgasmia. However, DSM-IV criteria quite explicitly reject the diagnosis of **Female Orgasmic Disorder** when there has not been a normal sexual excitement phase. That was certainly the case for Julianna, so only the first diagnosis could be made.

From the testimony of two physicians, no **general medical disorder** or **substance use** contributed to Juliana's difficulty. (Examples of the former would include reduced lubrication due to diabetes mellitus and atrophy of the vaginal mucosa due to menopause.) Her trouble lubricating had been lifelong, and it appeared not to be limited to specific situations (or men). Julianna's diagnosis would therefore be as follows:

Axis I	302.72	Female Sexual Arousal Disorder, Life-long Type, Generalized Type, Due to Psychological Factors
Axis II	V71.09	No diagnosis
Axis III		None
Axis IV		None
Axis V	GAF = 70	(current)

TIP Disorders of female sexual arousal and orgasm are often highly correlated. Among health care clinicians, you may encounter less than slavish adherence to the exact criteria used for these disorders.

302.72 Male Erectile Disorder

Male Erectile Disorder, otherwise known as impotence, can be partial or complete. In either case, the erection is not adequate to complete the sexual activity. Impotence can also be situational, in which case the patient can achieve an erection only under certain circumstances (e.g., with prostitutes). It is probably the most prevalent male sexual disorder, occurring in perhaps 8% of all men. Of all the sexual dysfunctions, this is the one most likely to occur for the first time later in life.

A variety of emotions can play a role in the development or maintenance of this disorder. These include fear, anxiety, anger, guilt, and distrust of the sexual partner. Any of these feelings can so preoccupy a man's attention that he cannot focus adequately on feeling sexual pleasure. Even a single failure may lead to anticipatory anxiety, which then precipitates another round in the circle of failure. Masters and Johnson also talk about an additional factor that they call *spectatoring*, in which the patient evaluates his performance so constantly that he cannot concentrate on the enjoyment of sex. Such a patient may have an erection with foreplay but lose it upon penetration.

Male Erectile Disorder should not be diagnosed if biological factors are the principal cause. This is unlikely if erections occur spontaneously, with masturbation, or with other partners. Some authorities now estimate that half or more of patients who complain of impotence have a biological cause. When biological and psychological factors are both present, as is often the case, the diagnosis can be made with the appropriate additional code (see p. 337).

Like most of the other sexual dysfunctions, Male Erectile Disorder can be either lifelong or acquired; the former is rare and hard to treat.

Criteria for Male Erectile Disorder

- Chronically or repeatedly, the patient cannot get or keep an erection sufficient to complete the sexual activity.
- Except for another sexual dysfunction, no other Axis I disorder explains the dysfunction better.
- It is not directly and exclusively caused by the use of substances (including medications) or by a general medical condition.
- It causes marked distress or interpersonal problems.

Coding Note

From the section on type codes (p. 337), choose the codes that apply. Also consider the Coding Notes there.

Parker Flynn

"I think I must be over the hill."

If you didn't count the three counseling sessions he had had while sifting through the wreckage of his first marriage, this was Parker Flynn's first visit ever to a mental health professional. At age 45 he had been a bridegroom for only two months, and he was afraid he was losing his sexual potency.

Everything had been fine before the wedding, but the first evening of their honeymoon Parker had been unable to get enough of an erection to do either him or his wife much good. He supposed he'd had too much champagne—normally he didn't touch alcohol. His wife had also been married before and knew a thing or two about men. She hadn't criticized; she'd even said it would be all right. But she was attractive and 10 years younger than he, and he was worried.

"It's what happens when you get older," Parker insisted. "And I'm definitely older."

Before he popped the question, he had undergone a complete physical examination. Other than being a few pounds overweight—Parker was devoted to chocolate ice cream—he was given a clean bill of health. Besides the ice cream, he denied any other addictions, including alcohol, drugs, and tobacco.

"I get so nervous when it's time to make love," Parker explained. "I can get a pretty good erection when we're fooling around, but when it's time to get serious, I lose it. Her first husband was something of a stud, and I keep wondering how my performance measures up to his."

Evaluation of Parker Flynn

Parker's interest in sex seemed to be just fine; he gave every indication (normal erections) that there was nothing wrong with the excitatory phase. But because he worried about maintaining his erection, he did have difficulty. His problem was exacerbated by the phenomenon of spectatoring (see above), in which he wondered how he was doing while he was doing it.

Parker's physical condition was good, ruling out **Sexual Dysfunction Due to a General Medical Condition**. Some patients with impotence may suffer from **sleep apnea**; of course, it is vital to explore this possibility, because of the potentially lethal nature of this disorder. No previous mental health problems would preclude the diagnosis. His difficulty may have begun with an alcohol-related incident, but from his history, **substance use** played no role in its maintenance. Also note that, as they age, men may require more stimulation to achieve erection than they did when younger; such a physiological change should not constitute evidence of Male Erectile Disorder. **Sporadic erectile problems** that don't cause important distress also should not be given this diagnosis.

Parker's problem was not lifelong but acquired; the vignette provides no evidence that it applied only in specific situations, so neither Situational nor Generalized Type was specified. His diagnosis would thus read as follows:

Axis I	302.72	Male Erectile Disorder, Acquired Type, Due to Psychological Factors
Axis II	V71.09	No diagnosis
Axis III		None
Axis IV		None
Axis V	GAF = 70	(current)

ORGASMIC DISORDERS

There is a great deal of normal variation in the time it takes individuals to achieve climax. Clinicians must judge when a patient's difficulty is serious enough to warrant a diagnosis. (Note that the experience of climax, like that of arousal, may change with advancing age.) Inhibited orgasm is much more common in women than in men.

302.73 Female Orgasmic Disorder

Achieving a climax is a problem for about 30% of women. A few general medical conditions, including hypothyroidism, diabetes, and vaginal damage, can contribute to this diagnosis (it used to be called Inhibited Female Orgasm). Orgasm can also be inhibited by medications such as antihypertensives, central nervous system stimulants, tricyclic antidepressants, and monoamine oxidase inhibitors. Possible psychological factors include fear of pregnancy, hostility of the patient toward her partner, and guilty feelings about sex. Age, previous sexual experience, and the adequacy of foreplay must also be considered in making this diagnosis.

Once learned, a woman's ability to achieve orgasm persists, often increasing throughout life. It is unusual for this disorder to be acquired in the absence of other sexual dysfunctions.

Criteria for Female Orgasmic Disorder

- After a normal phase of sexual excitement, the woman's orgasm is persistently or repeatedly delayed or absent. The clinician's judgment of this is based on her sexual experience, adequacy of foreplay, and norms for her age.
- Except for another sexual dysfunction, no other Axis I disorder explains the dysfunction better.
- It is not directly and exclusively caused by the use of substances (including medications) or by a general medical condition.
- It causes marked distress or interpersonal problems.

Coding Note

From the section on type codes (p. 337), choose the codes that apply. Also consider the Coding Notes there.

Fiona Freebairn

It was almost a year before Fiona Freebairn stopped mourning her husband. Adam had died in an automobile crash not long after they both graduated from college. They had been extraordinarily close, sharing everything and enjoying an unusually rich and varied sex life. But months of cooking for one and sleeping alone finally persuaded her to rejoin the world of the living. Almost immediately, she met Mark.

"Of course, he isn't Adam. But then Adam wasn't Mark, either," she observed practically. "I'll always love Adam, but Mark's special, too."

The problem was with their sex life—Fiona wondered if they would even prove to be "incompatible." It wasn't that she found Mark unattractive. In fact, she thought about him quite a lot. And when they were making love, she found that she became very interested.

"After 20 or 30 minutes of lovemaking, I feel like I could just explode," she said. "Only I don't."

Mark was a considerate lover who offered Fiona plenty of foreplay and a great deal of cuddling and warmth. But, although she responded eagerly and lubricated thoroughly, she had never had an orgasm with him. The only relief from her frustration had been to masturbate to climax when she was alone again.

"When I'm with Mark, I somehow find myself thinking about Adam. When that happens, I just can't get over the top. After a while, Mark can't hold out any longer, and then he feels bad. And all I get for my efforts is a bucket load of guilt."

> **TIP** Antidepressants and other psychotropic medications sometimes cause Substance-Induced Sexual Dysfunction With Impaired Orgasm. The diagnosis is easily confirmed by discontinuing the medication.

Evaluation of Fiona Freebairn

Fiona clearly became sexually excited; inability to achieve the release of orgasm had only developed after her husband's death. Although women can have considerable variability in the type and intensity of stimulation they need (many have **sporadic orgasmic problems** that do not justify a diagnosis), most clinicians would regard her problem as far outside the boundaries of normal variation.

Aside from **general medical conditions** and **substance use** that can inhibit orgasm (there was no evidence of either in her case), the Axis I diagnosis **Somatization Disorder** must also be considered. But as far as we know, Fiona was in good health and had been sexually active (and orgasmic) with Adam. These facts point to psychological factors as the basis for her difficulty. Her ability to climax with masturbation would justify the modifier Situational Type.

Axis I	302.73	Female Orgasmic Disorder, Acquired Type, Situational Type, Due to Psychological Factors
Axis II	V71.09	No diagnosis
Axis III		None
Axis IV		None
Axis V	GAF = 71	(current)

302.74 Male Orgasmic Disorder

Men with orgasmic disorder achieve erection without difficulty but have problems coming to orgasm. Some only take a long time; others may not be able to ejaculate into a partner at all. Because of the prolonged friction, partners of these patients may complain of soreness. Anxiety about performance may cause secondary impotence in the patient himself. At one time this diagnosis was called Inhibited Male Orgasm.

Even when it has been present on a lifelong basis, the man can usually ejaculate by masturbating (alone or with the help of his sex partner). The personalities of patients with lifelong Male Orgasmic Disorder have been described as rigid and puritanical; some seem to equate sex with sin. The disorder may be acquired from interpersonal difficulties, fear of pregnancy, or lack of sexual attractiveness of the partner. Retarded ejaculation is somewhat more common in patients with Obsessive–Compulsive Disorder. Note that there is a difference between this diagnosis and absence of ejaculation.

Male Orgasmic Disorder is probably uncommon. When men do have problems with retarded (or absent) climax, there is often a medical cause; examples include hyperglycemia, prostatectomy, abdominal aortic surgery, Parkinson's disease, and spinal cord tumors. Some men have a physical abnormality that, upon orgasm, causes semen to be expelled into the urinary bladder (retrograde ejaculation). Drugs like alphamethyldopa (an antihypertensive) and thioridazine (a neuroleptic), as well as alcohol, have also been implicated. As the sole cause, none of these instances would be coded as an Axis I disorder.

Criteria for Male Orgasmic Disorder

- After a normal phase of sexual excitement, the man's orgasm is persistently or repeatedly delayed or absent. The clinician's judgment of this is based on the man's age and the adequacy of duration, focus, and intensity of sexual activity.
- Except for another sexual dysfunction, no other Axis I disorder explains the dysfunction better.
- It is not directly and exclusively caused by the use of substances (including medications) or by a general medical condition.
- It causes marked distress or interpersonal problems.

Coding Note

From the section on type codes (p. 337), choose the codes that apply. Also consider the Coding Notes there.

> **TIP** The drug thioridazine, which can inhibit a man's ability to have orgasm, is sometimes used to treat patients with Premature Ejaculation (see the next diagnosis).

Rodney Stensrud

Rodney Stensrud and his girlfriend, Frannie, had come to the clinic seeking relief for Rodney's "performance problem." They had been together for nearly a year, and they disagreed as to the extent of the problem.

Rodney was frankly worried. It had always taken him a long time to have a climax, and now, after 40 minutes or so of vigorous intercourse, he sometimes found himself wilting under pressure. Frannie was more sanguine. Her previous boyfriend had never been able to last longer than five minutes, and that often left her unsatisfied.

"Now I almost always come more than once," she said with an air of satisfaction. Recently Rodney had been taking even longer, and she admitted that she was getting pretty sore. "Maybe if we could get it back down to about half an hour," she suggested.

Rodney's parents had reared him strictly. Throughout his childhood, he had attended parochial school. In his words, he was "pretty clear on the concept of good versus evil." He admitted that he felt guilty that he and Frannie were living together without benefit of clergy, but she wasn't ready to take that step yet. She used to laugh and tell him that she wanted to "save something for after the baby came."

Before meeting Frannie, Rodney's only experience had been with two prostitutes he had encountered while he was in the Navy. It had taken him hardly any time at all with either of them. In fact, he felt that the one with the mouth had rather shortchanged him. "There sure wasn't any delay involved," he said. Neither had he experienced any particular problem masturbating, either when he was an adolescent or more recently when Frannie was gone on an extended business trip.

Rodney had been referred by a urologist, who had found nothing physically wrong. The couple's only drinking was an occasional glass of white wine. At one time Rodney had occasionally used marijuana at parties, but Frannie was death on drugs so he had given it up a year ago.

Evaluation of Rodney Stensrud

After apparently normal appetitive and excitation phases, Rodney took an inordinately long time to reach climax. From the vignette, this does not appear to have been a lifelong problem. His problem was causing him distress, and he was already headed down the road to secondary impotence.

Rodney's problem was situational; he experienced no ejaculatory delay when with a prostitute or when masturbating. His referring physician had noted no **general medical conditions** that might account for his disorder, and there was no significant **substance use**. His upbringing was somewhat puritanical, reinforcing the impression that the basis of his disorder was psychological, not physical. There was no evidence of any **other Axis I disorder** that might be diagnosed instead.

Frannie's reaction to Rodney's disorder was perhaps somewhat atypical. Female partners sometimes complain of discomfort from prolonged intercourse necessary to achieve climax. Would the fact that Frannie found value in Rodney's disorder present a possible problem for therapy? Although it would not seem readily codable on Axis IV, Rodney's clinician should keep this factor in mind when working with the couple.

Rodney's complete diagnosis would be as follows:

Axis I	302.74	Male Orgasmic Disorder, Acquired Type, Situational Type, Due to Psychological Factors
Axis II	V71.09	No diagnosis
Axis III		None
Axis IV		None
Axis V	GAF = 65	(current)

302.75 Premature Ejaculation

In Premature Ejaculation, as the name implies, the man climaxes too quickly—sometimes just as he and his partner reach the point of insertion. The results are disappointment and a sense of failure for both; secondary impotence sometimes ensues as well. Stress in a relationship can exacerbate the condition, which of course promotes more stress. However, some women may value Premature Ejaculation, because it decreases their exposure to unwanted sexual activity or pregnancy.

Premature Ejaculation is a commonplace disorder; it accounts for nearly half the men treated for sexual disorders. It is especially frequent among men with more education—presumably they are sensitized to the issue of partner satisfaction. Whereas anxiety is often a factor, physical abnormalities rarely cause this problem. DSM-IV does not even include a statement about general medical conditions in the criteria.

Criteria for Premature Ejaculation

• With minimal sexual stimulation, the patient often ejaculates earlier than he wants to (before, during, or just after penetration). The clinician should evalu-

ate age, novelty of partner or situation, frequency of sexual activity, and other factors that can affect duration of the excitement phase.
- It is not directly and exclusively caused by the use of substances.
- It causes marked distress or interpersonal problems.

Coding Note

From the section on type codes (p. 337), choose the codes that apply. Also consider the Coding Notes there.

Claude Campbell

Claude Campbell could remember, in embarrassing detail, the first time it ever happened. He had been a very young Marine second lieutenant stationed in Vietnam in the last year of the war. Suddenly granted leave to go to town, he had had to borrow a pair of trousers from the battalion chaplain.

Claude and two friends were seated at a sidewalk table, drinking a mixture that the military called a "Bombs Away," when a prostitute sat down next to him. When she set to work warming her hand between his thighs, it only took a few moments before he felt himself lose control. A crimson blush spread across his face as a stain darkened the front of the chaplain's khaki trousers.

"That was one of the worst times, but it sure wasn't the last," said Claude. After he left the Marines, he finished college and got a job selling computers. He soon married a girl he had dated during high school. Their wedding night, and most of their other nights, were never quite the disaster of the Vietnam bar, but he could never last longer than a minute or two after insertion.

"Not that it bothered her," commented Claude ruefully. "She never enjoyed sex much, anyway. She was always glad to get it over with in a hurry. I know now why she insisted on 'saving it' for after we were married. She never wanted to spend it in the first place."

Claude always hoped that his problems had been largely due to his first wife's prudery and disapproval, but several months into his new marriage things hadn't improved much. "She's being very patient," he said, "but we're both beginning to get desperate."

Evaluation of Claude Campbell

Claude's difficulty had been with him ever since his sex life began. Although a few such incidents might be dismissed in a youngster or in any man with a new partner, in a mature adult (we don't know exactly how old Claude is) who has been in a lasting relationship with frequent sexual activity, it must be considered pathological. Claude's difficulty was clearly causing him distress, so he would fully meet the criteria. **General medical conditions** do not play a significant role in the development of Premature Ejaculation, as noted earlier. Claude's problem was not situational (it had occurred with both of his wives and with the prostitute).

Axis I	302.75	Premature Ejaculation, Lifelong Type, Generalized Type, Due to Psychological Factors
Axis II	V71.09	No diagnosis
Axis III		None
Axis IV		None
Axis V	GAF = 70	(current)

SEXUAL PAIN DISORDERS

Symptoms of the sexual pain disorders can occur at any time during sexual activity. However, they are usually focused on the time of actual insertion during intercourse. Although a man may complain of pain with sex, this is rare; nearly all of these patients are women.

302.76 Dyspareunia

Dyspareunia (the word is Greek, and it means "painful intercourse") may be experienced as an ache, a twinge, or a sharp pain. Anxiety can produce tension in the vaginal mucosa and thereby produce pain. Soon anxiety comes to replace sexual enjoyment.

Dyspareunia is both a symptom and a diagnosis. As a symptom, it is quite common in women, and it often coincides with Vaginismus (see below). It can have a variety of causes. Nearly a third of women who have had gynecological surgery will experience some degree of dyspareunia. Infections, scars, and pelvic inflammatory disease have also been reported as causes. If the sexual pain is due entirely to failure of lubrication, Dyspareunia would not be diagnosed. When it is a symptom of a general medical condition, dyspareunia is never listed as an Axis I diagnosis.

In men, dyspareunia (the symptom) is rare and almost always associated with some general medical condition, such as Peyronie's disease (a lateral bend in the erect penis), prostatitis, or infections (e.g., gonorrhea and herpes).

Criteria for Dyspareunia

- The patient often experiences genital pain with sexual intercourse.
- It is due neither to Vaginismus nor to inadequate lubrication.
- Except for another sexual dysfunction, no other Axis I disorder explains the dysfunction better.
- It is not directly and exclusively caused by the use of substances (including medications) or by a general medical condition.
- It causes marked distress or interpersonal problems.

Coding Note

From the section on type codes (p. 337), choose the codes that apply. Also consider the Coding Notes there.

Mildred Frank

Mildred Frank and her twin sister, Maxine Whalen (see next diagnosis), had been having problems with pain during intercourse. Their symptoms were different and quite personal, but they had always discussed everything with each other. Now they made the joint decision to seek help. The gynecologist had referred both of them to the mental health clinic.

"It's sort of a burning," was how Mildred described her difficulty. "When it's bad, it feels like your hands do if you're sliding down a rope. It's awful! Even if I use Vaseline, it still bothers me."

The referral letter noted that she'd had surgery for a prolapsed uterus but was otherwise healthy. "I could have told you that," she said. "I've never even been to a doctor, except to have my babies."

On close questioning, Mildred admitted that the pain didn't occur often. But during the past year or two she had always been afraid it would hurt, and that made her tense up when she was having intercourse with her husband. She had had some vaginal infections, but these had been largely under control during the last few months; the gynecologist didn't think that they caused the pain she complained of. The letter also noted that her physical exam had been completed easily, with no evidence of vaginal spasm.

"Maybe I do overreact," she said. "At least that's what my husband tells me. He says I'm too excitable, that I should just relax."

Evaluation of Mildred Frank

Many women have **sporadic pain with intercourse**, in which case diagnosis is usually not warranted. The pain Mildred experienced with intercourse produced enough distress to qualify for a diagnosis of Dyspareunia; the real problem would be ruling out other causes.

First, **Vaginismus** would be ruled out because the gynecologist was able to insert a speculum without causing spasm. Of course, Mildred might have had spasm only when faced with the necessity of intercourse, but she described the pain as burning, not cramping. (Also, she had compared notes with her sister, Maxine, who did have Vaginismus; see below.) Mildred had pain even when she used petroleum jelly, so her problem would not appear to be a matter of **inadequate lubrication**. She described herself as otherwise healthy, and her gynecologist made no mention of a **general medical problem**. Her clinician would have to determine that there was no **substance-induced** condition, though this would seem unlikely.

Although sexual dysfunctions can be expected with a number of Axis I disorders (**anxiety disorders**, **mood disorders**, **psychotic disorders**), there is only one for which the criteria specifically mention painful intercourse; this is **Somatization Disorder**. Mildred claimed that she had been otherwise healthy, which would greatly reduce the likelihood of this diagnosis. However, she should be evaluated carefully for this troubling condition.

Although Mildred's pain with intercourse was acquired fairly recently and only occurred occasionally, it did cause her to seek treatment. She had had no other partners than her husband, though nothing in the vignette suggests that she would have fared better with another partner. Although she had had some vaginal infections, the doctor felt that they couldn't completely account for her pain; this would be the reason for the last specifier listed. Although insufficient symptoms were noted to warrant a personality disorder, her clinician felt that certain of her behaviors justified mention on Axis II.

Axis I	302.76	Dyspareunia, Acquired Type, Due to Combined Factors
Axis II	V71.09	No diagnosis; histrionic personality features
Axis III		None
Axis IV		None
Axis V	GAF = 71	(current)

306.51 Vaginismus

In Vaginismus, the patient experiences a cramping contraction of her vaginal muscles when she attempts to have sexual intercourse. The resulting pain can be severe enough to prevent consummation of a marriage, sometimes for years. Some patients can't even use a tampon; some require anesthesia for a vaginal exam. Although these patients may respond to oral stimulation, many come to avoid all sex. Frustration and loss of self-esteem are the results. The partner may feel rejected; his performance anxiety can result in impotence.

Vaginismus can be associated with other sorts of sexual dysfunction, including absence of interest, arousal, or orgasm. General medical conditions and substance-induced conditions do not play a significant role in Vaginismus. Although it may not be as uncommon as some authorities have assumed, little is known about its occurrence and other demographic features.

Criteria for Vaginismus

- The woman repeatedly has spasms of the vaginal muscles that interfere with sexual intercourse.
- It causes marked distress or interpersonal problems.
- Except for another sexual dysfunction, no other Axis I disorder explains the dysfunction better.
- It is not directly and exclusively caused solely by a general medical condition.

Coding Note

From the section on type codes (p. 337), choose the codes that apply. Also consider the Coding Notes there.

Maxine Whalen

Maxine Whalen and her twin sister, Mildred Frank (see preceding diagnosis), had been having problems with pain during intercourse; as noted above, they made a joint decision to seek help. Finding no anatomical causes for either of them, the gynecologist had referred both to the mental health clinic.

Maxine wasn't married yet, and she didn't think she wanted to be. "It's not that I don't get horny," she explained. "And I love foreplay. I could do it all night. But every time a man has tried to enter me—well, both times, actually—something inside me clamps down like a trap. I couldn't even get a pencil inside, let alone a penis. I can't even use a tampon."

Maxine usually relieved her frustration by masturbating, which reliably produced a climax. Oral sex had also worked. "Not many men are likely to be satisfied with that for long," she remarked. "It makes me feel like a freak."

The spasms that contracted Maxine's vaginal muscles produced severe, cramping pain. They were so extreme that her gynecologist had had to insert the speculum under general anesthesia. The exam revealed no physical abnormalities.

On her second visit, Maxine remembered something that Mildred apparently hadn't known. When the girls were four, they had been molested in some way. Even Maxine wasn't sure exactly what had happened. She only knew that some man—she thought it might be the Uncle Max for whom she had been named—had taken the girls to a tavern, stood them on the bar, and allowed the other patrons to "play" with them.

Evaluation of Maxine Whalen

Maxine's history of severe pain and obstructed penetration suggested the diagnosis of Vaginismus. The fact that the spasm was reproduced by the attempted introduction of the gynecologist's speculum was diagnostic. Unless a patient is both unattached and content to refrain from intercourse, it is axiomatic that Vaginismus will produce distress or interpersonal difficulty.

Maxine's history did not indicate that there had ever been a time since she became sexually active when she was free of vaginal spasm; therefore, it was lifelong. Her gynecologist found no physical cause (no surprise there; none are usually reported). By elimination, it would have to be attributed to psychological factors. It also occurred in a variety of contexts, so it was generalized rather than situational.

Axis I	306.51	Vaginismus, Lifelong Type, Generalized Type, Due to Psychological Factors
Axis II	V71.09	No diagnosis
Axis III		None
Axis IV		None
Axis V	GAF = 65	(current)

TIP Note that Vaginismus and Dyspareunia are not diagnosed in the same patient. Although pain with intercourse is a feature of both, the presence of vaginal spasm marks the difference between the two conditions.

SECONDARY AND OTHER SEXUAL DYSFUNCTIONS

Sexual Dysfunction Due to a General Medical Condition

The criteria for all of the foregoing sexual problems, with the exception of Sexual Aversion Disorder and Premature Ejaculation, contain statements that they cannot be diagnosed if the symptoms can be completely accounted for by a general medical condition. Here is the section wherein such dysfunctions should be coded. Some of these (generally, those you are more likely to encounter) have their own specific codes; others are covered by the catch-all coding, Other [Male or Female] Sexual Dysfunction Due to a General Medical Condition. For example, patients whose ability to have orgasm is inhibited by one of many general medical conditions would have to be placed in this catch-all subcategory.

I have not provided a vignette for these conditions; they are too numerous, and their symptoms will be pretty much like those already described. Do note, however, that these patients will have symptoms not only of the sexual problem but of the specific general medical condition.

Appendix B provides a partial listing of the general medical disorders that have reportedly produced sexual dysfunctions. Some of these disorders affect large number of Americans. Take Male Erectile Disorder as an example. It is estimated that it is caused by diabetes in some 2,000,000 men, by other endocrine disorders in 300,000, by vascular disease in 1,500,000, by multiple sclerosis in 180,000, by trauma (such as spinal cord injuries) in 400,000, and by the effects of radical surgery in 650,000.

Criteria for Sexual Dysfunction Due to a General Medical Condition

- Clinically important sexual dysfunction dominates the clinical picture.
- It causes marked distress or interpersonal problems.
- History, physical exam, or laboratory findings suggest that the direct physiological effects of a general medical condition can fully explain these symptoms.

- Another mental disorder (such as Major Depressive Disorder) cannot better explain the sexual dysfunction.

Coding Notes

Coding of these conditions depends on the predominant type of dysfunction. The specific general medical condition must also be coded on Axis III.

607.84	Male Erectile Disorder Due to [State the general medical condition]
608.89	Male Dyspareunia Due to [State the general medical condition]
608.89	Male Hypoactive Sexual Desire Disorder Due to [State the general medical condition]
608.89	Other Male Sexual Dysfunction Due to [State the general medical condition]
625.0	Female Dyspareunia Due to [State the general medical condition]
625.8	Female Hypoactive Sexual Desire Disorder Due to [State the general medical condition]
625.8	Other Female Sexual Dysfunction Due to [State the general medical condition]

Review the Coding Notes in the section on type codes (p. 337) for further information about combining codes for problems due to general medical conditions and substance use. Note that type codes (p. 337) do *not* apply to Sexual Dysfunction Due to a General Medical Condition.

> **TIP** In a mental health practice, it will be unusual to see a patient whose sexual problems are due exclusively to a general medical condition. Most mental health clinicians will probably find more utility in other, more explicit diagnostic codes that include the specifier Due to Combined Factors.

Substance-Induced Sexual Dysfunction

As general medical conditions, a substantial number of psychoactive substances can affect the sexual abilities of men and women. Information for some of these substance classes is summarized in Chapter 3, Table 3.1. Note that you would substitute this diagnosis for the specific type of Substance Intoxication only when the patient's problems in that area exceed those you would expect in the usual course of Substance Intoxication.

The same reasons that apply to the general medical conditions have prompted me not to include a vignette in this section.

Criteria for Substance-Induced Sexual Dysfunction

- Clinically important sexual dysfunction dominates the clinical picture.
- It causes marked distress or interpersonal problems.
- History, physical exam or laboratory data substantiate that substance use fully explains the symptoms, as shown by either of these:
  ✓ These symptoms have developed within a month of Substance Intoxication, or
  ✓ Medication use has caused the symptoms.
- No other sexual dysfunction better explains these symptoms.

Coding Notes

Assign a code number based on the specific substance:

291.8	Alcohol
292.89	All others, including Amphetamine [or Amphetamine-Like Substance]; Cocaine; Opioid; Sedative, Hypnotic, or Anxiolytic; Other [or Unknown] Substance

Based upon the predominant feature, specify whether:

With Impaired Desire

With Impaired Arousal

With Impaired Orgasm

With Sexual Pain

Also specify if: With Onset During Intoxication.

Substance-Induced Sexual Dysfunction should be diagnosed instead of Substance Intoxication only if the sexual symptoms are serious enough to warrant independent clinical evaluation and exceed those that would be expected for a syndrome of intoxication.

DSM-IV suggests several types of evidence that a non-substance-induced sexual dysfunction better explains the symptoms. These include the following:

The symptoms begin before the onset of the substance use.

The symptoms persist long (a month or more) after the substance use stops.

The symptoms are more severe than would be expected from the amount and extent of substance use.

The patient has had previous episodes of the disorder, independent of substance use.

Although the type codes that apply to other sexual dysfunctions do not apply here, see the Coding Notes in that section (p. 337) for information about combining those that are substance-induced with those caused by a general medical condition. Note that type codes (p. 337) do *not* apply to Substance-Induced Sexual Dysfunctions.

302.70 Sexual Dysfunction Not Otherwise Specified

Use the Sexual Dysfunction Not Otherwise Specified category to code patients whose sexual dysfunctions don't qualify for any of the specific sets of criteria spelled out above. DSM-IV specifically mentions the following two examples:

Absent erotic feelings. A patient has apparently normal arousal and orgasmic phases, but little in the way of erotic feelings.

Undiagnosed. You believe that the patient has a sexual dysfunction, but you don't know the cause.

PARAPHILIAS

Literally, *paraphilia* means "abnormal or unnatural attraction." The sexual relationships of these people differ from normal in regard to their preferred sexual objects or in the ways they relate to those objects. Their sexual activities revolve around the themes of (1) objects or nonhuman animals; (2) humiliation or suffering of the patient or partner; or (3) nonconsenting persons, including children. Mere desires or fantasies about these sexual activities can upset some patients sufficiently to warrant a diagnosis, but far more commonly patients act upon their desires. In descending order, the most common paraphilias are Pedophilia, Exhibitionism, Voyeurism, and Frotteurism. All the rest are encountered much less frequently.

In many patients, the paraphilic behavior may be present much of the time, though other patients may indulge in it only occasionally (e.g., when under stress). Although the criteria specify gender for only one of the paraphilias (Transvestic Fetishism), almost all paraphilia patients are male. Many patients have multiple paraphilias (the average is three or four). Most fantasize sexual contact with their victims.

Several of these behaviors are illegal. Patients who practice Frotteurism, Voyeurism, or Exhibitionism are acutely aware of this and usually take pains to avoid detection or to secure an escape route. Pedophiles often delude themselves that what they are doing is for the children's good, but nonetheless caution their victims not to tell their parents or the authorities. Often patients come to the attention of a mental health professional because they have run afoul of the law.

It should be noted that many people are sexually excited by images or ideas (such as women's panties and bras), but do not act upon their ideas and are not distressed by them. In such cases, a paraphilia should not be diagnosed. On the other hand, some patients are not distressed by their paraphilias, apart from the anxiety they may experience when they come to legal attention. Still others may experience a great deal of guilt and remorse whether or not they are apprehended, despite which they persist in pursuing their activities.

The paraphilias are hardly ever due to a general medical condition. However, unusual sexual behavior may be encountered in several Axis I disorders: Schizophrenia, bipolar mood disorders, Mental Retardation, and Obsessive-Compulsive Disorder. Of course, Axis II pathology is frequently a feature of paraphilia patients.

TIP Although none of these criteria sets specify age limits, most paraphilias begin during adolescence. This is also the time when people begin to discover and explore their sexuality; teenage boys, in particular, typically experiment with a variety of sexual behaviors. However, any teenager so involved with paraphilic behavior as to meet the diagnostic criteria that appear below should also be considered a candidate for diagnosis.

It should also be noted that the boundaries of what is considered normal in human sexual behavior are not sharply drawn. Certainly Pedophilia is universally condemned, even among populations of imprisoned felons. But for most other paraphilias, one can find parallel behaviors in the general population. Revealing oneself, watching, and touching constitute part of everyday sexual experience. Even coercion and pain (in moderation) figure in the sexual activities of many people who would be considered fairly conventional. Cross-dressing has for centuries been an important part of theater. I admit that I have trouble imagining contexts within which Fetishism might be considered normal, however.

302.4 Exhibitionism

Although no one knows just how many exhibitionists there are in the world, Exhibitionism is one of the most commonplace sexual offenses. These patients are almost invariably male, and their victims are nearly always child or adult females. Men who prefer to expose themselves to children have a higher rate of recidivism than do those who choose only adult women as their victims. In most cases unsuspecting strangers are the victims. (DSM-IV states that this is always the case; however, a small percentage of exposures are made to women known to the exhibitionist.)

Exhibitionism begins before the age of 18, but it may persist until the patient is in his 30s or later. These patients don't attempt to have other contact with their victims, and they are hardly ever physically dangerous. Many of them have mates and relatively normal sex lives. Often, the urge to exhibit comes in waves: The patient may yield daily for a week or two, then remain inactive for weeks or months. Exhibitionistic behavior most often occurs when the patient is either under stress or has free time. The use of alcohol is seldom a factor.

An exhibitionist tends to follow the same pattern with each offense. He may fantasize while driving around looking for a victim (often he is careful to leave himself an escape route to use if he is detected by someone other than the victim). One may expose himself with an erection; another may be flaccid. A third may be quite aggressive, savoring the look of shock or terror he produces. The person may masturbate when he shows himself to the woman or when he relives the scene in his imagination later on. Many will fantasize having sex with their victims, but most exhibitionists do not attempt to enact these fantasies. However, some exhibitionists may also engage in rape, Frotteurism, Voyeurism, or Pedophilia.

Criteria for Exhibitionism

- Repeatedly for at least six months, the patient has intense sexual desires, fantasies, or behavior concerning genital self-exposure to an unsuspecting stranger.
- This causes clinically important distress or impairs work, social, or personal functioning.

Ronald Spivey

Ronald Spivey was a 39-year-old attorney who occasionally served as a judge pro tem in the municipal court of his home city. He referred himself because of the anxiety symptoms he developed after a woman threatened to report him for showing her his erect penis at the swimming pool of the apartment complex where they both lived.

"I thought she had been looking at me in an interested way," he said, smoothing back his toupee. "She was wearing a very skimpy bikini, and I thought she was inviting me to reveal myself. So I sat in such a way that she could look up the leg of my swimming trunks."

Ronald had gone to law school on a scholarship. He had grown up in an inner-city neighborhood, not far from Hoofer's, a strip-tease joint not far from the Navy recruiting station. When he was in grade school, his friends and he sometimes sneaked in through a side door to watch part of the show. On a dare when he was 15, he pulled down his pants in front of two strippers who had just left the building. The women laughed and applauded; later, he masturbated as he fantasized that they were fondling him.

From time to time after that, through college and law school, Ronald would occasionally drive around "trolling," as he called it—looking for a girl or young woman walking by herself in a secluded area. As he drove, he would masturbate. When he found the right combination of circumstances (a woman who took his fancy in a secluded location, with no one else around), he would hop out of his car and confront the woman with his erection. Often, the look of surprise on her face would cause him to ejaculate.

With his marriage, which coincided with his graduation from law school, Ronald's exhibitionistic activity subsided for a time. Although sexual intercourse with his wife was fully satisfactory to both of them, he continued to imagine showing himself to a stranger, with whom he would then have intercourse. As a practicing lawyer, he sometimes had afternoons when a continued court case left him at loose ends. Then he might go trolling again, sometimes several times in a month. At other times he might go months without activity.

About the woman at the apartment complex pool, Ronald said, "I really think she did want to." Her bikini had been very revealing, and he'd been thinking for several days about having sex with her. He contrived to sit so that she was virtually sure to glance between his thighs. When she noticed what he had intended her to see, her response was, "That confirms what I've always thought about lawyers!" Since then he had been in near panic at the thought that she would notify the state bar association.

Evaluation of Ronald Spivey

Ronald's history of exhibiting himself dated to his teenage years and had persisted for at least two decades. If he were apprehended, he could lose his livelihood, if not his liberty. The fact that he continued this illegal behavior despite its possible consequences showed the strength of his urge. (Note that, whereas "trolling" is typical behavior for an exhibitionist, exposing himself to a woman whom the exhibitionist might meet again is not.)

Ronald's assumption that the woman wanted him to "reveal" himself is fairly typical of the cognitive distortion to which these patients fall prey. It would take a pretty unusual woman to have any interest at all in a relative stranger who bared himself to her at a public swimming pool.

Although it is possible that an Axis I disorder could present together with Exhibitionism, it is unlikely that either **Schizophrenia** or **Bipolar I Disorder** would have been present for over 20 years without detection. Of course, **Mental Retardation** would have prevented Ronald from entering, much less completing, law school.

The clinician noted "Diagnosis deferred" as a reminder to search for personality disorders at a later interview.

Ronald's complete diagnosis would be as follows:

Axis I	302.4	Exhibitionism
Axis II	799.9	Diagnosis Deferred
Axis III		None
Axis IV		None
Axis V	GAF = 65	(current)

302.81 Fetishism

In its original sense, a fetish was an idol or other object that had magical significance. In the context of sexual activity, it refers to something that excites an individual's sexual fantasies or desires. Such objects include underwear, shoes, stockings, and other inanimate objects. The definition of Fetishism excludes cross-dressing that is not sexually exciting (as in Transvestic Fetishism) and objects designed for use during sex, such as dildoes or vibrators. Bras and panties are probably the most common objects used as fetishes.

Some people collect great numbers of their preferred fetishes; some resort to stealing (from stores or clotheslines) to get them. They may smell, rub, or handle these objects while masturbating, or they may ask sex partners to wear them. Without a fetish, such a person may be unable to get an erection.

The onset of Fetishism is usually in adolescence, although many patients report similar interests even in childhood. Although some women may show a degree of Fetishism, nearly all fetishists are men. The disorder tends to be a chronic condition. With time, a patient may use a fetish to replace more usual (human) love objects.

Criteria for Fetishism

• Repeatedly for at least six months, the patient has intense sexual desires, fantasies, or behavior concerning the use of inanimate objects (such as shoes or underwear).

- This results in clinically important distress or impairs work, social, or personal functioning.
- The objects are not used solely in cross-dressing (as female clothing is used in Transvestic Fetishism) and are not equipment intended to stimulate the genitals (such as a vibrator).

Corky Brauner

When he was 13, Corky Brauner found a pair of his older sister's panties that his mother had absent-mindedly put away with his own underwear. They were embroidered with flowers and the word "Saturday," and he found them peculiarly exciting. He slept with them under his pillow for a couple of nights and masturbated with them twice before sneaking them back into his sister's drawer Friday evening. From time to time throughout the balance of his adolescence, when he was alone in the house, Corky would appropriate various items of his sister's underwear.

He lived alone when he went to college, so he was able to collect and keep a small wardrobe of lingerie without worrying that it would be discovered. Although he had a few bras and slips, he preferred panties. By his senior year he owned several dozen. Some of these he had purchased, but he preferred those he could persuade a woman to leave behind after a date. He had even stolen one or two pairs from backyard clotheslines, but that was dangerous and he didn't do it often.

When Corky wasn't entertaining company, which was often, he would take one or more of the pairs of panties out of the drawer and play with them. He would smell them, rub them on his face, and masturbate with them. During these activities, he would pretend he was making love to the original owner of the panties. If he did not know her, he would imagine what she might have looked like.

Corky was driven into treatment by the laughter of his most recent girlfriend when he found that he had to put her underwear under his pillow in order to get an erection when they were making love. "I've gotten totally fixated on panties," he said during his initial interview. "I seem to prefer them to women."

Evaluation of Corky Brauner

Corky's interest in panties is a typical example of Fetishism. It had persisted for years—more than long enough to meet the criteria. This interest had developed to the point that he had amassed quite a collection, obtained from a variety of sources.

Corky's distress stemmed not from his own perception of his behavior, but from the fact that a girlfriend criticized his behavior. In this way he learned that he preferred panties to people—not an infrequent progression for fetishists.

The differential diagnosis of Fetishism can include **Transvestic Fetishism**, in which men are stimulated by wearing and viewing themselves in women's clothing. Fetishists may put on clothing of the opposite sex, but wearing it is incidental to the sexual gratification they derive from the clothing itself. They do not fantasize about their own attractiveness when so attired. Corky showed no interest in cross-dressing.

Many fetishists have also been involved in **rape, Exhibitionism, Frotteurism, Pedophilia,** or **Voyeurism**, but none of these behaviors are mentioned in Corky's vignette. The clinician working up his case should inquire carefully about these and other paraphilias. Pending the outcome of such an inquiry, Corky's full diagnosis would be as follows:

Axis I	302.81	Fetishism
Axis II	V71.09	No diagnosis
Axis III		None
Axis IV		None
Axis V	GAF = 61	(current)

TIP Some patients are sexually stimulated by portions of the human body, including feet, noses, breasts, and buttocks. Although some clinicians consider such behavior to be a type of Fetishism, DSM-IV calls it partialism, a type of Paraphilia Not Otherwise Specified (see p. 380).

302.89 Frotteurism

Frotteurism (the term is derived from the French word frotter, meaning "to rub") usually takes place on crowded sidewalks or public transportation. (Having a means of escape is a concern to the frotteur.) The victim is attractive to the patient and usually wears tight clothing. The frotteur rubs his genitals against her thighs or buttocks, or he may fondle her breasts or genitalia with his hands. Ejaculation usually occurs within the time it takes to get from one bus or subway stop to the next.

Frotteurs often fantasize about an ongoing intimate relationship with the victim. The victim typically does not make an immediate outcry, because she hopes that she is mistaken about what appears to be happening. Note that it is the act of touching or rubbing, not the coercion involved, that is exciting to the frotteur. However, some also have a history of involvement in rape, Exhibitionism, Pedophilia, Sexual Sadism, or Voyeurism.

This condition usually begins in adolescence; it is sometimes precipitated by observing others engage in frottage. Most acts occur when the frotteur is between the ages of 15 and 25; frequency gradually declines thereafter. No one appears to know how common this condition is, and it may be underreported.

Criteria for Frotteurism

- Repeatedly for at least six months, the patient has intense sexual desires, fantasies, or behaviors that involve touching and rubbing against a person who doesn't consent to this behavior.
- This causes clinically important distress or impairs work, social, or personal functioning.

Henry McWilliams

Henry McWilliams had been born in London. Dressed in his short gray pants, white shirt, and school tie, he rode the London Underground every day to his exclusive school. One day, when he was nine, he saw a man rubbing up against a woman on the Underground.

Henry was small when he was nine, and even in the crowded subway car he had an excellent eye-level view. The woman (she was an adult, though Henry had no idea how old) was a bit overweight and dressed in a tight-fitting miniskirt. She was facing away from the man, who allowed the weight of the crowd surging through the doors to press him up against her. The man tugged at his crotch, and then, as the train began to move, rubbed himself against her.

"I never saw her face, but I could tell she didn't like it," said Henry. "She tried to push him away, she tried to move, but there was no place for either of them to go. Then the train stopped and he ran out the door."

Henry the adult, age 24, had now referred himself for treatment. He had moved with his parents to the United States when he was 15. Since his graduation from high school, he had worked as a messenger for a large legal firm. Many days he spent several hours on the subway in his official capacity. He guessed that he had rubbed against 200 women in five years. He was seeking help at the insistence of one of the partners in his law firm, who the week before had happened to ride the same train and had watched him in action.

When Henry was in need, he would go into the men's room and put on a condom so as not to stain his trousers. Then he would roam up and down the outskirts of a crowd on a subway platform until he found a woman who interested him. This would be someone who was youngish but not young ("They're less likely to scream"), and well-rounded enough to stretch tight the material of her skirt or slacks. He especially liked it if the material was leather. He would board after she did, and if she did not turn around, would rub his erect penis up and down against her buttocks as the train began to roll.

Henry was very sensitive, so it didn't take much pressure. Sometimes the woman didn't even seem to realize what was going on, or maybe she didn't want to admit it, even to herself. He usually climaxed within a minute. Then he would bolt out the door at the next stop. In the event that he was interrupted, he would hang around the platform until he spotted another woman in another crowd.

"It helps if I imagine that we're married or engaged," he explained. "I'll pretend that she's wearing my ring, and I've come home for a quickie."

Evaluation of Henry McWilliams

Henry's method of operation was fairly typical for frotteurs, most of whom tend to follow the same pattern each time they offend. Like most, he had had many episodes of this behavior over the years and fantasized having an intimate relationship with each victim. Henry was not especially upset about his own behavior; he came for treatment because that was what his employers demanded.

Although patients with **Schizophrenia** or **Mental Retardation** will sometimes engage in sexual behavior that is inappropriate to the context, Henry bore no evidence whatsoever of either condition. His five-axis diagnosis would be as follows:

Axis I	302.89	Frotteurism
Axis II	V71.09	No diagnosis
Axis III		None
Axis IV		None
Axis V	GAF = 70	(current)

302.2 Pedophilia

Pedophilia is a term derived from the Greek meaning "love of children"; in the context of a paraphilia, of course, it means sex with children. Pedophilia is far and away the most common of the paraphilias that involve actual contact. Estimates vary, but by the age of 18, up to 20% of American children have been sexually molested in some way. The perpetrator is usually a relative, friend, or neighbor, not a stranger. The vast majority of pedophiles are men, but Pedophilia has been occasionally reported in women; however, adequate studies are lacking.

The types of acts vary. Some pedophiles will only look; others want to touch or undress a child. But most acts involve oral sex or touching of the genitals of the child or perpetrator. In cases other than incest, most pedophiles don't require actual penetration. When they do, however, they may use force to achieve it. Victims are usually age 12 or under.

This behavior usually begins in later teenage years, though some pedophiles do not start until midlife. It may be more common among persons who were themselves abused as children. Once Pedophilia has begun, it tends to run a chronic course. A large minority (up to 50%) of pedophiles use alcohol as a prelude to their contacts with children.

Many pedophiles "specialize" in children (this type of Pedophilia is called *exclusive*); they often confine themselves to children of a particular sex and age range. Others, however, are also attracted to adults (this type of Pedophilia is called nonexclusive). Like other paraphilic individuals, pedophiles may develop a degree of cognitive distortion about their activities: They tell themselves that sexual experience is important for children's development or that children enjoy it. Most pedophiles do not force their attentions on children, but depend on guile, friendship, and persuasion. A number of studies suggest that children who are lonely or otherwise uncared for may be at special risk for accepting the advances of a pedophile.

Overall, perhaps 15–25% of those convicted reoffend within a few years of their release from prison. Alcohol use and trouble forming intimate relationships with adult women increase the chances of recidivism. Men who prefer boys are about twice as likely to reoffend as are those who prefer girls.

Criteria for Pedophilia

- Repeatedly for at least six months, the patient has intense sexual desires, fantasies, or behaviors concerning sexual activity with a sexually immature child (usually age 13 or under).
- This causes clinically important distress or impairs work, social, or personal functioning.
- The patient is 16 or older and at least five years older than the child.

Coding Notes

State whether:

Sexually Attracted to Males

Sexually Attracted to Females

Sexually Attracted to Both

Specify if: Limited to Incest.

State whether:

Exclusive Type (aroused only by children)

Nonexclusive Type

Exclude from this diagnosis a late adolescent who has an ongoing sexual relationship with a child who is 12 or 13 years old.

TIP One aspect of the criteria that can be confusing is the required five-year age difference between perpetrator and victim. As the Coding Notes indicate, a late adolescent having a sexual relationship with someone 12 or 13 years old would not be diagnosed as having Pedophilia. A 20-year-old male having an affair with a 14-year-old consenting girl would, however.

Raymond Boggs

At age 58, Raymond Boggs—his orange prison jumpsuit stretched tightly over his pear-shaped body—seemed an unlikely convict. In contrast to the swagger of the younger inmates, he shuffled, head down, along the corridor to the interview room.

Raymond recalled becoming interested in sex at an early age. One of his earliest memories was of sex play with a teenage girl who was babysitting him and his younger sister. As an adult, the sight of little girls' bodies particularly fascinated him. He remembered as a child of seven or eight watching his sister having her bath. He would hang around until his mother had to shoo him from the bathroom. When they were teenagers, he had watched outside his sister's window at night, trying to get a glimpse of her as she undressed for bed. When she entered puberty, his evening vigils stopped. "It was the body hair. It seemed so coarse and disgusting. That was when I discovered that I only really liked girls who were—um, smooth."

Despite these tastes, in his mid-20s Raymond married the daughter of the foreman in the printing shop where he worked. During the early years of their marriage, the couple maintained an active sex life. Usually he would try to fantasize that he was making love with a young girl. Once he persuaded his wife to shave off all her pubic hair, but as it grew back she complained of itching and refused to do it again. They had three children, all sons. In retrospect, their gender seemed a minor miracle: Little boys didn't tempt him at all.

As the years went by, Raymond acquired a small stack of pornographic magazines featuring children. He kept them hidden under a pile of rags in his tool shed. When his sexual tension became too high, he would masturbate while he imagined himself frolicking with the naked children in these pictures.

By his early 50s, Raymond's life had taken a turn for the worse. His sons had all left home, and a series of pelvic operations caused his wife to reject his sexual advances, sometimes for months at a time. To fill his time, he took up photography. Especially over the long summer months, he found ready subjects in the neighborhood children he befriended. Some of the little girls he could persuade to pose partly or completely disrobed.

He preferred those who were five or six years old, but on occasion he would photograph a girl as old as eight. (The older children were more independent and harder to persuade.) These sessions occurred principally in a secluded spot behind his tool shed. He used candy and quarters as bait, afterwards reminding each child that her parents wouldn't like it if she told.

"I'm not proud of it," he said as he tried to ease the bulging waistband of his jumpsuit. "It was just something I couldn't resist. The feeling I'd get when she'd slip down her panties—it was anxiety and ecstasy and butterflies in my stomach. Sort of the way you'd feel if you won the lottery. But I never touched one; all I did was look. And I never thought it might hurt them any."

Raymond had been looking and taking pictures for the better part of 10 years when he was discovered by a 12-year-old boy who had ventured behind the tool shed to collect specimens of native plants for a science exhibit. The boy told his father, who called the girl's mother, who called the police. The trial—a three-week media feeding frenzy—featured the corroborative testimony of no fewer than seven neighborhood girls, now in varying stages of adolescence, who had at one time or another been victimized by Raymond Boggs.

Sentenced to 5 to 10 years in the penitentiary, Raymond still faced millions of dollars in civil lawsuits. The day after he was arrested, his wife filed for divorce and entered therapy. One of his sons broke off contact with him; another moved out of the state.

TIP DSM-IV does not have a specific category for incest. Some of these may be pedophiles, but many men (most incestuous adults are male) only become interested in daughters or stepdaughters who have reached puberty.

Evaluation of Raymond Boggs

When the facts of the case are clear, there is little to dispute the diagnosis of Pedophilia. Occasionally an alcoholic who is **intoxicated** may perpetrate an isolated incident of fondling a child, but then it is usually evident that this is not a frequent sexual outlet. As an example of their overall defective judgment, patients with **Mental Retardation** or **Schizophrenia** may sometimes fall into this mode of sexual release. Occasionally, a parent (usually a celebrity) is accused of child molestation as a part of a messy divorce; the facts often do not bear out the allegations.

The legal facts were indisputable in the case of Raymond Boggs, and he freely admitted to his long-standing behavior. He also insisted that his behavior was strictly visual, never tactile. This is typical of a large number of such patients.

Exhibitionists may show themselves to children, but they don't approach the victims for further sexual activity. Some pedophiles may also practice **Sexual Sadism**; if so, both diagnoses should be made.

DSM-IV asks the clinician to choose several specifiers to help pinpoint the patient's pathology. Raymond was sexually attracted only to females; although he worried about what might have happened if he had had daughters, none of his offenses were incestuous. He had also been sexually active with his wife for many years, so the specifier Nonexclusive Type would apply.

Axis I	302.2	Pedophilia, Sexually Attracted to Females, Nonexclusive Type
Axis II	V71.09	No diagnosis
Axis III		None
Axis IV		Incarceration
		Alienation from family
Axis V	GAF = 55	(current)

Sexual Masochism and Sexual Sadism

Sexual Masochism and Sexual Sadism have a great deal in common besides the experience of pain during the sex act. Both conditions begin in childhood; both are usually chronic. Their methods include bondage, blindfolding, spanking, cutting, and humiliation (by defecation, urination, or forcing the submissive partner to imitate an animal). Some form of beating is probably the most commonly used. As time goes on, patients in both of these groups often need to increase the severity of the torture to produce the same degree of sexual satisfaction. In this sense, their behavior resembles the addictions.

I discuss these disorders a bit differently from the others in this part of the chapter. First, I present a case vignette describing a pair of individuals who illustrate these two complementary diagnoses. I then describe each diagnosis and its criteria in turn, and present the evaluation of each individual following the criteria.

Martin Allingham and Samuel Brock

"We're perfectly suited," said Samuel Brock. "I like to do it, he likes it done."

He and Martin Allingham had come to medical attention the night Martin almost died. In their bedroom they had devised an elaborate contraption of pulleys, ropes, collars, and shackles that they used to turn Martin upside down and partly strangle him while Sam applied the whip.

"I get the most beautiful orgasm when I'm about to pass out," reported Martin.

Sam and Martin had been in school together. Sam was a jock; Martin was the class wimp. How perfectly this suited them they didn't realize until one Saturday afternoon on the deserted playground when they were 15. The two were fighting, and Sam began sitting on Martin, twisting his fingers into pretzels. Although Martin cried, the growing urgency of his erection was evident as the pain increased. After they parted, Sam had masturbated while recalling the sensation of absolute control.

Without discussing it much, by common consent Sam and Martin met again two weeks later. When they were 19, they got an apartment together; they had been living together ever since. Now they were 28.

Martin didn't have to be hurt to enjoy sex, but it greatly enhanced the pleasure. He had tried spanking and bondage, but asphyxia was the best. When he was younger he had played the field and tried other partners. But most of them had either hurt him too much or not enough; besides, he and Sam were both afraid of AIDS. For the last several years they had worked at the same department store and had been faithful to each other.

The night of the accident, Sam was at work and Martin got himself into the harness. He apparently cinched the noose a shade too tight and lost consciousness, though he didn't remember that. When Sam found Martin, he had no pulse and wasn't breathing. Fortunately, Sam had learned CPR in the Boy Scouts. He called 911, and Martin made a full recovery.

A police report was made, and a pair of officers interviewed Sam. He admitted that their sex life had recently become increasingly violent, even death-defying. But that hadn't been his idea; it was Martin who had needed more to produce the same effects. Sam admitted that he "got off" on pain, but some pain seemed to do about as well as a lot.

"I wouldn't want to really hurt him," he said. "I love him."

302.83 Sexual Masochism

Many people derive sexual pleasure from some degree of pain. This even includes females, a small minority of whom admit that they enjoy being spanked in conjunction with sex. By the best estimates, about 5% of sexual masochists are women. Sexual Masochism is thus the only paraphilia in which any appreciable number of women participate.

By choking, pricking, or shocking, some masochists inflict pain upon themselves. Perhaps 30% of them also participate in sadistic behavior at times. A few pursue an especially dangerous form of masochism, called *hypoxyphilia*. This is a method that masochists sometimes use to produce sexual arousal. It is near-asphyxiation, which they induce by placing a noose around the neck, by putting an airtight bag over the head, or by using amyl nitrite ("poppers"). Some masochists, like Martin Allingham, report that the reduced oxygen level promotes an especially intense sexual high. One or two accidental deaths occur per million people in the general population each year from these practices.

Although masochists derive sexual gratification from feeling pain or degradation, they do not necessarily surrender control. Many sadomasochistic relationships are carefully planned; often the partners agree upon a secret word by which the masochist can indicate that it really is time to stop. It should be noted that some prostitutes will accept pain, within limits, because the pay is better than that for standard sex. Such individuals should not be diagnosed as having Sexual Masochism unless they derive pleasure from the practice.

Criteria for Sexual Masochism

- Repeatedly for at least six months, the patient has intense sexual desires, fantasies, or behaviors concerning real acts of being beaten, bound, humiliated, or otherwise made to suffer.
- This causes clinically important distress or impairs work, social, or personal functioning.

Evaluation of Martin Allingham

Martin's sexual behavior included elements of inflicted pain. Bondage was one of these elements, as was the practice of hypoxyphilia, which Martin used to enhance his own sexual pleasure. Martin had acted on these urges far longer than the six-month minimum required by DSM-IV; he would therefore amply fulfill the criteria for Sexual Masochism.

Masochists will sometimes cross-dress in response to the demands of a sadistic partner. If the act of wearing clothing of the opposite gender also produces sexual excitement (and not just the humiliation of cross-dressing), then **Transvestic Fetishism** should also be diagnosed. Many patients with Sexual Masochism also meet criteria for a personality disorder. The vignette is silent on this issue, but Martin's clinician should thoroughly explore the possibility of Axis II disorders; they could significantly affect therapy. Martin's full diagnosis at this point would be as follows:

Axis I	302.83	Sexual Masochism
Axis II	799.9	Diagnosis Deferred
Axis III		None
Axis IV		None
Axis V	GAF = 25	(current)

302.84 Sexual Sadism

Much of the behavior of sadists is complementary to that of masochists; the difference is that sadists are the perpetrators rather than the recipients. Inflicting pain or humiliation is sexually stimulating to them; the suffering of others arouses them sexually. They experience fantasies of dominance and restraint. They usually limit themselves to only a few partners; most sadists have a willing partner.

Sadists will sometimes use nonconsenting victims, and they may indulge in rape. When they do, it can be brutally different from ordinary rape—sadists will use even more force than is necessary. However, fewer than 10% of rapists are sadists.

Although Sam was homosexual, most sexual sadists are heterosexual.

Criteria for Sexual Sadism

• Repeatedly for at least six months, the patient has intense sexual desires, fantasies, or behaviors concerning real acts of causing physical or psychological torment or otherwise humiliating another person.
• This causes clinically important distress or impairs work, social, or personal functioning.

Evaluation of Samuel Brock

By his own admission, Sam derived sexual pleasure from producing pain. He had acted on his urges, which had been present for over 10 years, and would therefore qualify for a diagnosis of Sexual Sadism. Unlike Martin, however, he was content to continue at the same level of intensity; he didn't need to increase the level of his activity to obtain sexual satisfaction.

Would Sam warrant any other diagnosis? A personality disorder should probably be considered in the differential diagnosis of anyone with Sam's proclivities. **Antisocial Personality Disorder** would be the logical choice, but it is doubtful that Sam would qualify: He had finished high school, had worked at the same job for a number of years, and had been faithful to his partner. His complete diagnosis at this point would thus be the following:

Axis I	302.84	Sexual Sadism
Axis II	V71.09	No diagnosis
Axis III		None
Axis IV		None
Axis V	GAF = 71	(current)

302.3 Transvestic Fetishism

Transvestic fetishists are defined as heterosexual males who cross-dress in order to achieve sexual excitement; they experience frustration when this behavior is interfered with. There is much variability in the amount of cross-dressing. Some will do it occasionally, while alone; others frequently go out in public. Some limit it to underwear; others get togged out completely. They may spend up to several hours a week getting dressed and wearing women's clothing. Many will masturbate or have intercourse when they cross-dress. They may fantasize about themselves as girls and keep a collection of female clothing, often wearing it under their normal male attire.

The onset of Transvestic Fetishism is usually during adolescence, or even in childhood. Most of these individuals were not effeminate boys. Like other types of Fetishism, this behavior often gradually replaces normal sex. Through videos, magazines, or personal interaction, there may be considerable involvement in the transvestite subculture. A small number of these men gradually feel increasingly comfortable dressed as women and become transsexual. Such gender dysphoria may be the stimulus to seek treatment. Some patients have been previously involved in rape, Exhibitionism, or Pedophilia.

Although the vast majority of all paraphilics are men, Transvestic Fetishism is the only paraphilia that DSM-IV expressly limits to males, and heterosexual males at that. As with all other aspects of DSM-IV, this is not done for ideological reasons; it is simply that the condition has been seldom, if ever, encountered in women. However, some authorities report that a very few female transvestites have been found.

Criteria for Transvestic Fetishism

- Repeatedly for at least six months, a heterosexual male has intense sexual desires, fantasies, or behavior concerning cross-dressing.
- This causes clinically important distress or impairs work, social, or personal functioning.

Coding Note

Specify if: With Gender Dysphoria. The patient is persistently uncomfortable with gender identity or role.

Paul Castro

When Paul Castro was seven, his parents began to employ their teenage neighbor to babysit. Julie was precocious and imaginative; she would persuade Paul to play dress-up in her clothing, which she would remove for the occasion. At first Paul only tolerated this, but later he would become excited at the sensation of her silky panties as he drew them up over his skinny thighs.

When Julie acquired a steady boyfriend and lost interest in Paul, he would sometimes borrow a bra and panties from his mother to dress up in. By his late teens he had collected a small wardrobe of women's underwear, which he would put on as often as once or twice a week. Standing in front of a mirror wearing a bra, its cups attractively padded, he might fantasize himself being embraced—sometimes by a man, sometimes a woman. A time or two he tried on lipstick and an old dress his mother hardly ever wore. But those made him look silly and conspicuous, he thought, and he subsequently limited himself to lingerie. However, he never felt any sense of discomfort at being male or any desire to change his gender.

After a year of junior college, Paul got a job as a clerk in a bookstore and moved into his own apartment. Some days he would wear his panties and bra (without the padding) to work under his sport shirt and slacks. Then he might masturbate in the men's room during lunch hour, imagining himself making love to a beautiful woman, both of them dressed in their silk underwear. If he was otherwise occupied during lunch, throughout the afternoon he would enjoy the delicious sensation of silk next to his skin and the anticipation of release while looking at himself in the mirror that evening.

Paul was so attired when he was discovered by paramedics who picked him up after he was clipped by a passing bus on his way to work one morning. He awakened to find his right upper arm in a splint and passers-by agog over his size 40C Maidenform bra. It was his shame over this episode that finally drove him into treatment when he was 24.

Evaluation of Paul Castro

Western society tolerates some cross-dressing and even considers it normal. Female impersonation has had a long and honorable history in the theater (stage and film); Halloween apparel also comes to mind.

In **Sexual Masochism**, patients may be forced to cross-dress to excite a sadistic lover; if they do not also experience sexual excitement, Transvestic Fetishism cannot be diagnosed. And patients with **Gender Identity Disorder** (transsexualism) often dress in clothing appropriate to the opposite sex, but without the slightest degree of stimulation. Homosexual males may wear dresses and makeup; some manage to pass for women. However, this behavior is intended to enhance their appeal to other gay men; it does not provide direct sexual stimulation.

Obviously, Paul's behavior fit none of these alternative explanations. In fact, other than his interest in lingerie, he had fairly conventional heterosexual interests (judged by his fantasies when masturbating). He therefore would not receive the specifier With Gender Dysphoria.

Axis I	302.3	Transvestic Fetishism
Axis II	V71.09	No diagnosis
Axis III	810.00	Fractured clavicle
Axis IV		None
Axis V	GAF = 71	(current)

302.82 Voyeurism

Watching people engaged in private activities is sexually arousing to voyeurs. Of course, this is even true of many people who do not have a paraphilia, such as those who enjoy pornographic films. The difference is that a voyeur's gratification derives from viewing ordinary people who do not realize they are being watched and would probably not permit it if they did.

The victims of these "peeping Toms" are almost always strangers. Most voyeurs will usually masturbate while they are watching. Afterwards, they may fantasize having sex with the target, though activity with the target is rarely sought. Some voyeurs prefer this method of sexual gratification, but most have normal sex lives otherwise. Like exhibitionists, they take precautions to avoid detection.

Nearly all of these patients are men. They usually begin their peeping careers in their teens—almost always by age 15. Once begun, this tends to be a chronic disorder.

Criteria for Voyeurism

- Repeatedly for at least six months, the patient has intense sexual desires, fantasies, or behaviors concerning the act of watching an unsuspecting person who is naked, disrobing, or having sex.
- This causes clinically important distress or impairs work, social, or personal functioning.

Rex Collingwood

This referral came at the request of a judge of the superior court, who had been displeased to find Rex Collingwood brought before the bench for the second time in less than a year. This time, at age 23, Rex had been caught literally with his pants down, masturbating outside the master bedroom window of a house on a quiet suburban street. He had been so fascinated by the aspect of the woman inside removing her underwear that he failed to notice the approach of her husband, who was walking the dog.

When Rex was growing up, his family had lived near the campus of a small Midwestern college. He had made friends with the caretaker at the student union—a gangly philosophy major named Rollo, who, in exchange for minor custodial work, lived rent-free in a room on the second floor. When Rex was 14, Rollo showed him the tiny hole he had discovered in the floorboards immediately above the women's toilet. Intermittently for some weeks, Rex and Rollo had squatted in the dark above the peephole, waiting for women to enter. Because they were looking straight down, they couldn't see much, but the images provided plenty of grist for Rex's fantasy life.

When he graduated from high school, Rex went to work in an auto body shop. The bookkeeper, Darlene, was a year or two older than he, and they soon began living together. Rex and Darlene made love four or five times a week; they each expressed satisfaction with the arrangement. Rex sometimes wondered whether he was "oversexed" because he still occasionally had the urge to "go looking." He had tried X-rated videos, but it wasn't the same—those people knew they were being watched, and they were paid, besides.

So every two or three months Rex would spend a couple of evenings driving on dark, quiet streets, seeking the right venue. Catching a glimpse of naked flesh was titillating, but watching a woman undressing added the delicious suspense of not knowing how much would be revealed. Whatever he saw, Rex would add to the stock of images to conjure up when he made love with Darlene.

Best of all was watching people have sex. He had carefully memorized the locations of several such encounters, and he returned to them again and again when the urge struck. Summertime was best, for then people were less likely to get under the covers. He had once or twice stood in the bushes for as long as two hours, watching while his targets worked up their passion and his. That was what had drawn him back to the house where he was apprehended, although it was less than four blocks from where he had been arrested a year before.

"I suppose I should feel ashamed," Rex told the interviewer, "but I'm not. I think it's normal to be interested. And if they really cared about their privacy, they'd close their curtains, wouldn't they?"

Evaluation of Rex Collingwood

There isn't much of a differential in a history like Rex's. If he had spent his time watching paid performers on a stage, we wouldn't think a thing about it (neither would the judge). Although he had acted repeatedly on his urges, the only distress he felt was at the prospect of being punished. His complete diagnosis would be as follows:

Axis I	302.82	Voyeurism
Axis II	V71.09	No diagnosis
Axis III		None
Axis IV		Arrest
Axis V	GAF = 61	(current)

302.9 Paraphilia Not Otherwise Specified

A variety of other paraphilic behaviors have been described. Most of these are less common, or less well studied, or both, than the foregoing disorders. Coded as Paraphilia Not Otherwise Specified, they include the following:

Partialism. This is similar to Fetishism, except that it does not involve inanimate objects: The patients are preoccupied with a portion of the body (nose, feet, breasts, buttocks). Some writers consider this a type of Fetishism. There are reports of men who, in a form of negative partialism, are attracted to women with body parts missing (such as a woman with only one leg).

Telephone Scatologia. As the name implies, this is a preoccupation with "talking dirty" on the phone.

Zoophilia. This paraphilia is a preoccupation with having sex with various mammals and other animals.

Necrophilia. Sex with corpses was said to the be only release undertakers had in ancient Egypt. Sex with contemporary cadavers almost demands another Axis I or Axis II diagnosis (perhaps both).

Klismaphilia. In this paraphilia, somewhat allied to Sexual Masochism, some people achieve sexual pleasure by giving themselves enemas. In some such individuals, this behavior is linked with cross-dressing. This behavior has been little studied in the professional literature, though it may be fairly common.

Coprophilia. This is masturbating with one's own feces; it has been rarely reported.

Urophilia. some people become sexually excited by playing or masturbating with urine. This must be distinguished from the form of Sexual Masochism in which the person desires to be urinated upon ("golden showers"). Collectively, preoccupations with enemas and urine are termed "water sports" by those who enjoy them.

Infantilism. In this paraphilia, the patient derives sexual satisfaction from being treated like a baby. This includes wearing diapers and drinking from a bottle.

GENDER IDENTITY DISORDER AND OTHER SEXUAL DISORDERS

302.x Gender Identity Disorder

Patients with Gender Identity Disorder (GID) feel intensely uncomfortable with their own biological sex. Some actually detest their own genitalia. They wish to live as members of the opposite sex, and many of them do take on dress and mannerisms of the opposite sex. Cross-dressing (though not for sexual stimulation) is a common first step toward a complete gender change. Next, they may request to take hormones to suppress menstruation, enlarge their breasts, or otherwise change their body appearance or functioning.

A few persons with GID feel so uncomfortable with their nominal, assigned sex that they request sex reassignment surgery. Although many patients who have such surgery are reportedly satisfied and live contentedly in their new gender, some ultimately request to be changed back. A few males retain their genitals but have their breasts augmented chemically or through surgery.

GID, popularly known as transsexualism, is one of the more recently described disorders in DSM-IV. Until the 1950s, clinicians did not even recognize that people existed who were so intensely uncomfortable with their biological sex. It was only the widespread publicity that occurred in 1952 when Christine Jorgensen received sex reassignment surgery in Denmark and emerged as a woman that this disorder became generally acknowledged.

GID is rare (3 of every 100,000 males, 1 of every 100,000 females). It begins in childhood and appears to be chronic. Many male patients have low sex drive; if they have sex at all, most prefer other men. Nearly all affected women are sexually attracted to women.

It should be noted that it is far more common for boys with gender disturbance to grow up to become homosexual than to develop GID; a minority become normally heterosexual, and only a tiny fraction have GID as adults. Ultimate diagnosis in children or adolescents may required prolonged evaluation.

Criteria for Gender Identity Disorder

- The patient strongly and persistently identifies with the other sex. This is not simply a desire for a perceived cultural advantage of being a member of the other sex. In adolescents and adults, this desire may be manifested by any of the following:

✓ Stated wish to be the other sex
✓ Often passing as the other sex
✓ Wish to live or be treated as the other sex
✓ Belief that the patient's feelings and reactions are typical of the other sex
- There is strong discomfort with the patient's own sex or a feeling that the gender role of that sex is inappropriate for the patient. This is shown by any symptoms such as these:
  ✓ Preoccupation with hormones, surgery, or other physical means to change one's sex characteristics
  ✓ Patient's belief in having been born the wrong sex
- The patient does not have a physical intersex condition.
- These symptoms cause clinically important distress or impair work, social, or personal functioning.

Coding Notes

Assign code number according to current age:

302.85 Gender Identity Disorder in Adolescents or Adults

302.6 Gender Identity Disorder in Children

For patients who are sexually mature, specify whether:

Sexually Attracted to Males

Sexually Attracted to Females

Sexually Attracted to Both Males and Females

Sexually Attracted to Neither Males nor Females

Children who are younger than adolescent age must have four or more of the following signs of identity with the other sex:
  ✓ The child reiterates a desire to be, or insistence in being, the other sex.
  ✓ A boy prefers cross-dressing or simulating female garb; a girl insists on wearing only male clothing.
  ✓ The child persistently and strongly prefers cross-sex roles in fantasy play or repeatedly fantasizes about being the other sex.
  ✓ The child badly wants to participate in games and pastimes of the other sex.
  ✓ The child strongly prefers to play with children of the other sex.

A boy's discomfort with his assigned sex may be shown by any of these:
  ✓ Disgust with his genitals

✓ Assertion that his genitals will disappear or that it would be preferable not to have a penis

✓ Rejection of rough-and-tumble play and male activities, games, and toys

A girl's discomfort with her assigned sex may be shown by any of these:

✓ Rejection of urinating in a seated position

✓ Desire not to develop breasts or menstruate

✓ Claims that she will have a penis

✓ Pronounced dislike for usual female clothing

Billie Worth

"I just want to get rid of it. All of it." Billie Worth was explaining his feelings for the third time that day. He wasn't depressed or melodramatic. Very patiently, he quietly stated the facts.

One of his earliest memories was of watching an actress on TV. When she walked, she brushed her hand against her skirt, causing it to dance. He tried to imitate that walk, to the delight and applause of his mother. His father was in the penitentiary for forgery.

When he was six, Billie discovered that playing with cap pistols and spaceships like the other boys gave him a violent headache. He preferred a Barbie doll that some child had discarded in a dumpster, and he chose his playmates, insofar as he was able, from neighborhood girls who were his age.

When he was a baby, his six-year-old sister, Marsha, had died of meningitis. Billie's mother had kept Marsha's room just as it had been when she died. Some of his happiest childhood afternoons were spent donning one of Marsha's dresses and sitting on her bed with Barbie. Sometimes he pretended to be Marsha. He continued to wedge his feet into her black patent leather shoes until long after he had outgrown them.

When Billie was 13 or 14, about the age that adolescents begin to think seriously about themselves, he realized that he was in fact a girl. "It suddenly struck me that the only masculine thing about me was these revolting things between my legs." Claiming to have chronic asthma, he persuaded a physician to excuse him from gym class throughout his four years of high school. Although he was a good swimmer, his abhorrence of the locker room prevented him from trying out for the team. He took shorthand and home economics (four semesters of each). He did join the science club, which was about as asexual a club as he could find. One year he entered a project in the science fair on the use of various yeasts in baking bread.

When Billie was 16, he bought his first bra and panties with money he had earned babysitting. When he put them on for the first time, he could feel some of the tension drain out of him. Although he sometimes wore his lingerie to school, he did not begin cross-dressing in earnest until he went to college. Because he lived off campus, he had the privacy in which to experiment with skirts, blouses, and makeup. An understanding physician provided him with estrogens, and in his junior year he changed the spelling of his name and began to live as a woman.

Two years out of college, Billie applied for sex reassignment surgery. He had had several male lovers, but they had been unsatisfying because he did not consider himself to be homosexual. "I'm not a gay man; I feel like I'm a straight woman." By now, thanks to hormones, he had small though well-developed breasts; his penis and testicles "just get in the way." He wanted to be rid of them, and told the examining clinician that if necessary he would go to Mexico to have the job done.

Evaluation of Billie Worth

Billie's early realization that he somehow didn't fit in with the other boys is typical of GID patients. He showed this by several sorts of behavior, which constitute the principal criteria for this diagnosis when it is made in children: (1) He preferred wearing his sister's dress and shoes; (2) he preferred dolls to male-oriented play; (3) he fantasized about being a girl; and (4) he preferred playing with girls. Although as a child he apparently didn't articulate the desire to be a girl, he found his penis revolting. These attitudes are far in excess of what DSM-IV calls **nonconformity to stereotypical sex role behavior**.

Billie's realization that he had been born the wrong sex didn't come until adolescence. At about that time, he began a progression—first dressing as a female, then living as a female and taking hormones—culminating in the request for sex reassignment surgery. Although the vignette does not specify that no intersex condition was present, neither does it contain any information that would suggest such a condition. Some of these are described under Gender Identity Disorder Not Otherwise Specified (see below).

The differential diagnosis of GID includes **Schizophrenia**, in which the patient may occasionally have delusions of being the opposite sex. Billie showed no evidence of either delusions or hallucinations, or of any other symptoms typical of Schizophrenia. The absence of sexual excitement as a reaction to cross-dressing would rule out **Transvestic Fetishism**, though some GID patients initially have this paraphilia.

Many (perhaps most) GID patients also have an associated personality disorder such as **Borderline** or **Narcissistic Personality Disorder**. (This may be less often true in female-to-male GID patients.) No evidence of any personality disorder is presented in the vignette. However, Billie's clinician should search diligently for Axis II pathology, which can strongly influence the management and outcome of this condition. As you might expect, **anxiety** and **mood**

disorders are also common associated features. **Substances** (alcohol and/or street drugs) may also be used, especially by female-to-male patients. Billie's full diagnosis would read as follows:

Axis I	302.85	Gender Identity Disorder in Adult, Sexually Attracted to Males
Axis II	799.9	Diagnosis Deferred
Axis III		None
Axis IV		None
Axis V	GAF = 71	(current)

302.6 Gender Identity Disorder Not Otherwise Specified

Several gender identity problems may be coded as Gender Identity Disorder Not Otherwise Specified. There are quite a few of what DSM-IV calls intersex conditions; details can be found in a standard text on endocrinology. Some of these are as follows:

Virilizing adrenal hyperplasia. Excessive androgens *in utero* cause an XX (female) fetus to develop fused labia, enlarged clitoris, and hirsuitism. The most common of the intersex conditions, this one occurs in about 1 per 5,000 live births. These children may be mistaken for males as babies.

Turner's syndrome. These patients are missing one chromosome (X0). They look like females, but they are sterile.

Klinefelter's syndrome. These patients look like males, but have an extra chromosome (XXY). A Klinefelter's male has a small penis.

Androgen insensitivity. This is a rare, X-linked condition in which an XY (male) baby looks like a female. In extreme form, this is called testicular feminization. Evaluation for amenorrhea may first bring this condition to medical attention during adolescence. In less extreme forms, these patients may have a penis and scrotum but a female body shape. Then they resemble Klinefelter's patients.

Other unspecified disorders of gender identity include stress-related, transient cross-dressing and preoccupation with castration without a desire to be the other sex.

302.9 Sexual Disorder Not Otherwise Specified

Sexual problems that don't meet the general qualifications for either a sexual dysfunction or a paraphilia should be coded here. DSM-IV includes several specific examples:

Inadequate sexual performance. Some patients have profound feelings about sexuality or being insufficiently masculine or feminine.

Use of lovers. Some patients are distressed because they regard successive lovers only as objects to be used.

Other sexual orientation problems. This subcategory is for any patient who is significantly distressed about sexual orientation.

Eating Disorders

Quick Guide to the Eating Disorders

As usual, the page number following each item indicates where a more detailed discussion begins.

Primary Eating Disorders

Each of the primary eating disorders is defined by abnormal eating behaviors, and they have a number of other features in common. Patients in both groups may binge and purge with laxatives. Both conditions are encountered mainly in girls and young women; onset is usually during the patient's teens. Anorexia Nervosa is less common than is Bulimia Nervosa, but the overall prevalence of both may be increasing.

Anorexia Nervosa. Despite the fact that they are severely underweight, these patients see themselves as fat (p. 388).

Bulimia Nervosa. These patients eat in binges, then prevent weight gain by self-induced vomiting, purging, and exercise. Although appearance is important to their self-evaluations, these patients do not have the body image distortion characteristic of Anorexia Nervosa (p. 391).

Eating Disorder Not Otherwise Specified. Use this category for disorders of eating that do not meet the criteria for either Anorexia Nervosa or Bulimia Nervosa (p. 394).

Other Causes of Abnormal Weight and Appetite

Mood Disorders. Patients with depression can experience either anorexia with weight loss or increased appetite with weight gain (p. 191).

Schizophrenia and Other Psychotic Disorders. Bizarre eating habits are occasionally encountered in psychotic patients (p. 137).

Somatization Disorder. Complaints of marked weight fluctuation and appetite disturbance may be encountered in these patients (p. 294).

Simple Obesity. This is not a DSM-IV diagnosis (no one knows that it is associated with any defined mental pathology). But emotional problems that contribute to the development or maintenance of obesity can be coded as a Psychological Factor Affecting Medical Condition (p. 533).

Introduction

Eating too little and eating too much have probably been problems as long as there have been people. Nearly everyone has pursued one of these behaviors at one time or another. But like so many behaviors, when they are carried to extremes they can be dangerous. In the case of the eating disorders, they can sometimes be deadly.

As recently as DSM-III-R, the eating disorders were included with other disorders of feeding (Pica, Rumination Disorder) that arise during childhood. Because it is now generally acknowledged that there is no connection between the feeding disorders of children and the eating disorders of adults, Anorexia Nervosa and Bulimia Nervosa have their own section in DSM-IV. Criteria for the childhood feeding disorders are given in Chapter 16 (see p. 522).

307.1 Anorexia Nervosa

Severe loss of weight (body weight reduction of 15% or more), refusal to gain weight, and a distorted body image (patients view themselves as fat, even though they may be dangerously underweight) characterize Anorexia Nervosa. The patient typically fears gaining weight and takes extreme measures to prevent it. When the disorder occurs in a woman, which is the case 95% of the time, her menstrual periods stop.

Recognized for nearly 200 years, this condition can have serious consequences for health. Although it remits spontaneously in most patients, about 5% die of complications from this disease. (When patients are followed over the long term, an even higher mortality rate may be the case.) Anorexia Nervosa may be on the rise, but it still affects less than 1% of the female population. It is more common among adolescent and young adult women.

Criteria for Anorexia Nervosa

- The patient will not maintain a minimum body weight (e.g., 85% of expected weight for height and age).
- Despite being underweight, the patient intensely fears weight gain or obesity.
- Self-perception of the body is abnormal, as shown by at least one of these:
  ✓ Unduly emphasizes weight or shape in self-evaluation
  ✓ Denies seriousness of low weight
  ✓ Has a distorted perception of own body shape or weight
- Due to weight loss, a female patient has missed at least three consecutive menstrual periods (or periods occur only when she is given hormones).

Coding Notes

Specify whether:

Binge-Eating/Purging Type. During an anorectic episode, the patient often purges (vomits, uses laxatives or diuretics) or eats in binges.

Restricting Type. No bingeing and purging during an anorectic episode. This is the more usual type.

Don't adhere too strictly to the 85% figure (see first bullet); it is only a rough guide. For children who are still growing, the criterion is that they fail to *attain* weight gain to 85% of normal weight for height and age.

Marlene Richmond

A statuesque blonde (five feet seven inches tall), Marlene Richmond weighed just over 80 pounds on the day she was admitted to the hospital. Dressed in a jogging suit and leg warmers, she spent part of the initial interview doing deep knee bends. Information for her history was also provided by her older sister, who accompanied her to the hospital.

Marlene grew up in a small town in southern Illinois. Her father, who drilled wells for a living, had a drinking problem. Her mother, severely overweight, started numerous fad diets and never had much success with any of them. One of Marlene's earliest memories was her own resolve that she would not grow up to be like either of her parents.

But the concerns of her 10th grade social circle revolved around appearance, clothing, and diet. That year alone, Marlene dropped 15 pounds from her highest weight ever, which was 125 pounds; even then she complained to her friends that she was too fat. Throughout her high school career, she remained fascinated by food. She took both introductory and advanced home economics. She spent much of her time in computer science class devising a data base that would count the calories in any recipe.

Whenever she was allowed to do so, Marlene ate in her room while watching television. If forced to eat with the family, she spent much of the meal rearranging her food on her plate or mashing it with a fork and taking the smallest bites that would not fall through the tines.

"It's not as if I'm not hungry," she said during her admission interview. "I think about food most of the time. But I look so bloated and disgusting—I can't stand to see myself in the mirror. If I eat even a little bit too much, I feel so stuffed and guilty that I have to bring it back up."

Two years earlier, Marlene had started vomiting whenever she thought she had overeaten. At first she would stick her finger or the end of a pencil down her throat; once she tried some ipecac she found in the medicine cabinet at a friend's house. She quickly learned simply to vomit at will, without any chemical or mechanical aids. She also reduced her weight with diuretics and laxatives. The diuretics helped her shave off a pound or two, but they left her so thirsty that she would soon gain it back. Once or twice a week, she would binge on high-carbohydrate food (she preferred corn chips and cola), then vomit up what she had eaten.

Other than her remarkable thinness and pallor, which was subsequently attributed to anemia, Marlene's appearance at admission was normal. She stopped exercising when the clinician requested it, but she asked whether the hospital had a stair-step exerciser she could use later. Her mood was cheerful and her flow of thought logical. She had no delusions or hallucinations, though she admitted that she was terrified of gaining weight. However, she denied having any other phobias, obsessions, or compulsions; she had never had a panic attack. Most of her spontaneous comments concerned menu planning and cooking; she volunteered that she might like to become a dietitian. She appeared bright and attentive, and made a perfect score on the Mini-Mental State Exam.

Marlene's only health concern was that she hadn't had a menstrual period for five or six months. She knew she wasn't pregnant because she hadn't even had a date for a year. "I think I'd be more attractive if I could just lose another couple of pounds," she said.

Evaluation of Marlene Richmond

Despite the fact that she was at least 15% underweight for her height, Marlene continued to express inappropriate concerns about being overweight. Her disgust at her own image in the mirror is typical of Anorexia Nervosa patients. Her loss of weight was profound enough that she had not had a menstrual period for several months.

Loss of appetite and weight are commonly found in a variety of **general**

medical conditions (liver disease, severe infections, and cancer, to name but a few); these must be ruled out by appropriate medical history and tests. Because the symptoms of Anorexia Nervosa are so distinctive, it is rarely confused with other mental disorders.

Loss of weight and anorexia can be encountered in **Somatization Disorder**, but to receive this diagnosis a patient must have the typical history of multiple somatic complaints. Patients with **Schizophrenia** will sometimes have peculiar eating habits, but unless they become dangerously underweight and have the typical distortion of self-image, both diagnoses should not be made. **Hunger strikes** are usually brief and occur in the context of trying to influence the behavior of others for personal or political benefit. Patients with **Bulimia Nervosa** usually maintain body weight at an acceptable level. Despite the fact that Marlene binged and purged, Bulimia Nervosa should not usually be diagnosed in a patient who also qualifies for Anorexia Nervosa. However, some patients are initially anorectic and later become bulimic. Bulimia Nervosa may also be diagnosed if there is a history of binge–purge cycles that occur during times the patient does not meet criteria for Anorexia Nervosa.

Several mental disorders are often associated with Anorexia Nervosa. **Major Depressive Disorder** could be diagnosed if Marlene had had symptoms of mood disorder. **Panic Disorder**, **Agoraphobia**, **Obsessive–Compulsive Disorder**, and **substance use** may also complicate diagnosis and treatment. Anorexia Nervosa patients may also fear eating in public, in which case a diagnosis of **Social Phobia** should be considered (however, it should not be made if the symptoms are strictly limited to eating behaviors). Specific **personality disorders** have not been identified, but Anorexia Nervosa patients are reported to be somewhat rigid and perfectionistic.

Marlene's history of binge–purge cycles would fit the definition of Binge-Eating/Purging Type; one or the other qualifier must be added in coding. Her full diagnosis would be as follows:

Axis I	307.1	Anorexia Nervosa, Binge-Eating/Purging Type
Axis II	V71.09	No diagnosis
Axis III	263.0	Malnutrition, moderate
Axis IV		None
Axis V	GAF = 45	(current)

307.51 Bulimia Nervosa

In Bulimia Nervosa, there are periods of binge-eating during which enormous amounts of food (usually starches and sweets) may be consumed. To prevent body weight and shape from ballooning, the person compensates by vomiting, exercising, or using laxatives or diuretics. Although bulimic patients are concerned about their weight and appearance, they do not have the distorted self-image typical of Anorexia Nervosa. Bulimia is not limited to underweight people; in fact, it is probably more common in people of normal weight.

Despite the fact that Bulimia Nervosa is a relatively new diagnosis, introduced by DSM-III in 1980, it is more common than Anorexia Nervosa. It affects 1–2% of adult women; there is evidence that the prevalence is probably increasing, but no one is sure why. (There is a lot of dispute about the true prevalence of both Anorexia Nervosa and Bulimia Nervosa, which are diagnosed more commonly by clinicians in North America.)

Criteria for Bulimia Nervosa

- The patient repeatedly eats in binges. In a binge episode, *both* of these are true:
  - The patient consumes much more food than most people would in similar circumstances and in a similar period of time.
  - The patient feels that the eating is out of control.
- The patient repeatedly controls weight gain by inappropriate means, such as fasting, self-induced vomiting, excessive exercise, or abuse of laxatives, diuretics, or other drugs.
- On average, both of the behaviors above (binge eating and inappropriate weight control) have occurred at least twice a month for at least three consecutive months.
- Weight and body shape unduly affect the patient's self-evaluation.
- These symptoms do not occur solely during episodes of Anorexia Nervosa.

Coding Note

Specify whether:

Purging Type: The patient often induces vomiting or misuses diuretics or laxatives. This is the more common type.

Nonpurging type: The patient fasts or exercises excessively, but does not often induce vomiting or misuse diuretics or laxatives.

Bernadine Hawley

"I eat when I'm depressed, and I'm depressed when I eat. I'm totally out of control." As she told her story, Bernadine Hawley frequently dabbed at her eyes with the wad of tissues she had brought with her. She was single and 32; she taught second grade. She had never before sought mental health care.

During her first two years in college, Bernadine had been moderately anorectic. Convinced that she was too fat, she starved and purged herself down to 98 pounds strung out along her five-foot-five-inch frame. In those years she was always hungry and would often go on food binges, during which she would "clean out the refrigerator—mine or anyone else's." She later admitted, "I must have looked pretty sparse." By the time she finished college, her weight had returned to a steady 120 pounds, controlled by self-induced vomiting.

During the intervening 10 years, Bernadine had followed a binge-and-purge pattern. On the average, twice a week she would come home from work, prepare a meal for three, and consume it. She preferred sweets and starches—at a sitting she might consume two lasagna TV dinners, a quart of frozen yogurt, and a dozen sugar donuts, none of which required much effort to prepare. Between courses she vomited up nearly all she took in. If she didn't feel like "cooking," she went out for fast food, wolfing down as many as four Big Macs in half an hour. What she craved seemed to be not the taste but the act of consumption. One evening she ate a stick of butter dipped in confectioner's sugar. In a fit of remorse, she once calculated that during a single evening's binge, she had consumed and regurgitated over 10,000 calories.

She also frequently purged herself with laxatives. The laxatives were effective, but expensive enough that Bernadine felt constrained to steal them. To minimize the chances of detection, she was careful to shoplift only one package at a time. She managed always to keep at least a three-month supply on the shelf at the back of her closet.

Bernadine was the only child of a Midwestern couple she described as "solidly dysfunctional." Because her parents never celebrated the date of their anniversary, she assumed that her own conception had precipitated the marriage. Her mother was cold and controlling; her father, a barber, drank. In the resulting marital strife, Bernadine was alternately censured and ignored. She'd had friends as a child and as an adult, though some of her girlfriends complained that she was overly concerned with her weight and figure. From the few times she had tried sex in college, she'd discovered that she had a healthy sexual appetite. But feelings of shame and embarrassment about her bulimia had kept her from forming any long-lasting relationships with men. She was often lonely and sad, though these feelings never lasted longer than a few days.

Although Bernadine recognized that her weight was currently normal, she was very concerned about it. She clipped low-fat recipes and belonged to a health club. She had often told herself she would give everything she owned to get rid of her bingeing. Recently she had offered a dentist $2,000 to wire her jaws shut. He had pointed out the obvious difficulty that she might then starve, and referred her to the mental health clinic.

Evaluation of Bernadine Hawley

As is true for many bulimic patients, Bernadine's disorder began with behavior typical of mild **Anorexia Nervosa**. She currently would not qualify for that diagnosis (her weight was normal and she did not have a distorted self-image);

in college she might have been diagnosed as having an **Eating Disorder Not Otherwise Specified** (see below). During her recent binge–purge episodes, she lost control and ate far more than normal. She also vomited and used laxatives. Friends had pointed out that she focused excessively on her figure and weight. Her difficulties had lasted far longer than the three-month minimum.

Shoplifting is not a criterion for Bulimia Nervosa, but the two occur together in about one-third of patients. Any history of stealing should raise the possibility of **Antisocial** or **Borderline Personality Disorder**. No evidence for either is given in the vignette.

Rarely, **neurological disorders** (some epilepsies, Kleine–Levin syndrome) can present with overeating. Excessive appetite can also occur in **Major Depressive Disorder With Atypical Features**. Bernadine showed no evidence of either of these conditions. Although she sometimes felt depressed, she had neither the chronicity required for **Dysthymic Disorder** nor enough symptoms for **Major Depressive Disorder**. She did not misuse **alcohol or drugs**, though many Bulimia Nervosa patients do.

> **TIP** All patients with Anorexia Nervosa and Bulimia Nervosa should be closely questioned about concomitant mood disorder. Also, sexual abuse has been reported by about one-quarter of Bulimia Nervosa patients.

Bernadine's complete diagnosis would be as follows:

Axis I	307.51	Bulimia Nervosa, Purging Type
Axis II	V71.09	No diagnosis
Axis III		None
Axis IV		None
Axis V	GAF = 61	(current)

307.50 Eating Disorder Not Otherwise Specified

Use Eating Disorder Not Otherwise Specified for patients who have problems related to appetite, eating, and weight, but who do not meet criteria for Anorexia Nervosa or Bulimia Nervosa. (It is critically important to be sure that these patients also do not have another, more definitive Axis I condition, such as a mood disorder, Schizophrenia, a somatoform disorder, or a disorder due to a general medical condition.) Some patients meet many of the criteria for either Anorexia Nervosa or Bulimia Nervosa. Here are some examples:

Anorexia, normal menses. Although a patient fears becoming fat and has low weight and distorted self-image, she continues to have regular menstrual periods.

Anorexia, normal weight. Some patients lose considerable weight, fear becoming fat, and believe they look fat, yet their weight remains within the normal range.

Bulimia, infrequent binges. A patient meets all the criteria for Bulimia Nervosa but binges less than twice a week.

Bulimia without swallowing. Some patients frequently chew large quantities of food but spit it out without swallowing.

Inappropriate weight control, normal weight. These patients repeatedly vomit or engage in other inappropriate weight control behavior after eating small amounts of food, but their weight remains normal.

Binge-eating disorder. These patients are similar to Bulimia Nervosa in that they eat in binges; however, they do not try to compensate by vomiting, exercising, or using laxatives. This is a new category that has not yet been formally accepted; DSM-IV lists suggested criteria beginning on page 729.

CHAPTER 12

Sleep Disorders

Quick Guide to the Sleep Disorders

DSM-IV has adopted a classification of sleep disorders that is similar to that used by the American Sleep Disorders Association. It currently recognizes two major categories: (1) In the *dyssomnias*, the problem is with the amount or quality of sleep or with its timing. (2) In the *parasomnias*, something abnormal occurs during sleep.

In this Quick Guide, I have arranged the disorders rather differently from DSM-IV, in order to emphasize what I consider to be the most prevalent underlying diagnoses. (As always, the page number following each item indicates where a more detailed discussion begins.) In the bulk of the chapter, however, I have followed DSM-IV's arrangement.

Dyssomnias

A patient with a dyssomnia sleeps too little, too much, or at the wrong time. But the sleep itself is pretty normal.

Sleeping Too Little (Insomnia)

Insomnia is often a symptom; sometimes it is a presenting complaint. Only rarely is it a diagnosis independent of an Axis I or II disorder or a general medical condition (see "Tip," p. 399).

It is impossible to overstate how important it is to evaluate *first* whether another mental disorder or a general medical condition could be the cause of insomnia.

Related to Another Mental Disorder. In a mental health clinic or ward, insomnia is most often encountered in patients suffering from Major Depressive Episodes (p. 191), Manic Episodes (p. 195), or anxiety disorders (p. 245). Criteria are given beginning on page 425.

Due to a General Medical Condition. Many general medical conditions can cause insomnia; the more important of these are detailed beginning on page 431.

Substance-Induced. Most psychoactive substances commonly misused, as well as a variety of prescription medicines, can interfere with sleep (p. 434).

Breathing-Related. Although most patients with breathing problems such as sleep apnea complain of hypersomnia, some instead have insomnia (p. 408).

Primary. Some patients simply sleep too little, and there is no discernible cause (p. 399).

TIP *Primary* (as in *Primary Insomnia*) is one of those funny words that have taken on a clinical meaning different from what is understood by most speakers of English. In the clinical world, *primary* means an illness or symptom for which no cause can be found. Of course, that doesn't mean that there isn't a cause—only that no one knows what it is. It doesn't mean that one condition is more important than another, or that one begins before another one.

If you think this is confusing, consider some of the other words that mean "I haven't the faintest idea what the cause is": *essential*, as in *essential hypertension*; *idiopathic*, as in *idiopathic thrombocytopenic purpura*; *functional*, as in a *functional psychosis*; *cryptogenic*, (literally, "hidden cause"). No wonder clinicians in training have bad dreams.

Sleeping Too Much (Hypersomnia)

You might think that the term *hypersomnia* means that a patient simply sleeps too much. Often, however, it indicates drowsiness at a time when the patient should be alert.

Related to Another Mental Disorder. Excessive drowsiness or sleepiness is not a frequent complaint among patients with other Axis I or Axis II disorders. However, hypersomnia is part of the definition of Major Depressive Episode or Dysthymic Disorder With Atypical Features, and is symptomatic of a few other disorders (p. 428).

Due to a General Medical Condition. Some medical illnesses can result in excessive drowsiness (p. 431).

Substance-Induced. The use of a substance is less likely to produce hypersomnia than insomnia, but it can happen (p. 434).

Breathing Related. Sleep apnea commonly results in excessive daytime sleepiness (p. 408).

Primary. Some patients are simply excessively sleepy for no apparent cause (p. 402).

Sleeping at the Wrong Times

In the following two sleep disorders, the sleep itself is pretty normal, but it occurs during times when the patient should be wakeful.

Narcolepsy. Sleep intrudes into wakefulness, causing patients to fall asleep almost instantly. In extreme cases, this may happen even when they are standing up. Their sleep is brief but refreshing. They may also have sleep paralysis, sudden loss of strength (cataplexy), and hallucinations as they fall asleep or awaken (p. 405).

Circadian Rhythm Sleep Disorder. Three types of mismatches between someone's environment and biological clock have been described: Shift Work, Jet Lag, and Delayed Sleep Phase Types (p. 411).

Other Dyssomnias

Not Otherwise Specified. This category is for dyssomnias that cannot be fitted into any of the categories above (p. 414).

Parasomnias

In the parasomnias, the quality, quantity, and timing of sleep are essentially normal. But something abnormal happens during sleep itself, or during the times when the patient is falling asleep or waking up.

Nightmare Disorder. Bad dreams trouble some people more than others (p. 415).

Sleep Terror Disorder. These patients cry out in apparent fear during the first part of the night. Often they don't really wake up at all. This disorder is not considered pathological in children, but it is in adults (p. 418).

Sleepwalking Disorder. Persistent sleepwalking usually occurs early in the night (p. 421).

Not Otherwise Specified. This category is for parasomnias that cannot be fitted into one of the categories above (p. 424).

Introduction

Keep in mind these several points about the normal sleep of humans:

1. Normality takes in a wide range. This refers to the amount of sleep, how long it takes to fall asleep and to awaken, and what happens in between.

2. Sleep changes throughout the life cycle. Everyone knows that babies sleep most of the time. As people age, the time they take to fall asleep increases, they require less sleep, and they awaken more often throughout the night.

3. Sleep is not uniform; it varies in depth and quality throughout the night. The two principal phases of sleep are rapid-eye-movement (REM) sleep, during which most dreaming takes place, and non-REM sleep. Various disorders can be related to these phases of sleep.

4. Many people sleep less soundly or more briefly than they think they should, but do not have a real disorder of sleep.

As in other areas of DSM-IV, sleep disorder criteria are based solely upon clinical findings. EEG and other studies that might be obtained in a sleep laboratory may be confirmatory, but are not usually required for diagnosis of the conditions described here.

DYSSOMNIAS

307.42 Primary Insomnia

TIP Nobody knows how common it is for a patient who has no other disorder (a general medical condition or an Axis I or II disorder) to complain of insomnia. These patients are probably a tiny minority of those a mental health professional encounters. Perhaps they are more likely to seek help from a primary medical care provider. Although texts say that persistent Primary Insomnia is fairly common, of over 15,000 mental health patients I have treated, exactly *one* had what I considered Primary Insomnia.

Primary Insomnia is what most people understand by insomnia: sleeping too little or unrestfully, without apparent cause. Anxiety, emotional problems, and long-standing tension may lead to Primary Insomnia. Some people may not realize just how tense they are. Some cases may start as insomnia secondary to a general medical condition, such as pain from a broken hip. Even after the hip has healed, the patient may worry about being able to sleep and become conditioned to the idea of being unable to sleep at night. In other words, this insomnia may be learned behavior.

Other people with Primary Insomnia may use their beds for activities other than sleeping or having sex—eating or watching TV, for example. These associations condition them not to sleep when they are in bed. Their sleep may improve during weekends, holidays, and vacations, when they can escape their usual habits and habitats. Whatever the cause, Primary Insomnia can persist forever if it is not addressed. Primary Insomnia is found especially in older patients and in women.

Many people complain of unrefreshing sleep or of being awake when their bed partners say they have slept all night. For this reason, the statement above that insomnia is "sleeping too little" isn't quite right; rather, insomnia is the *complaint* of sleeping too little. But these people do have problems that should not be belittled. Giving them time to state what is on their minds is important in seeking the etiology of their difficulties.

Criteria for Primary Insomnia

- For at least a month, the patient's main complaint has been trouble going to sleep, trouble staying asleep, or feeling unrested.
- The insomnia (or the resulting daytime fatigue) causes clinically important distress or impairs work, social, or personal functioning.
- It does not occur solely in the course of Breathing-Related Sleep Disorder, Circadian Rhythm Sleep Disorder, Narcolepsy, or a parasomnia.
- It does not occur solely in the course of another mental disorder (such as a delirium, Generalized Anxiety Disorder, or Major Depressive Disorder).
- These symptoms are not directly caused by a general medical condition or by the use of substances, including medications.

Curtis Usher

"It's almost spooky. It doesn't seem to make any difference what time I go to bed—9:30, 10:00, 10:30. Whatever, my eyes click open at 2:00 in the morning, and that's it for the rest of the night."

Curtis Usher had had this problem off and on for years. Recently, it was more often on. "Actually, I guess it's usually the worst during the week. Whenever I lie there, I'm worrying about work."

Curtis was a project manager at an advertising agency. It was a wonderful job when times were flush, which they hadn't been for several years. Curtis's boss was a bit of a tyrant who enjoyed saying that he didn't have headaches; he caused them. Curtis didn't have headaches, but he didn't have much sleep, either.

At age 53, Curtis was a healthy man of regular habits. He had lived alone since his wife divorced him three years earlier, claiming he was dull. Occasionally his current girlfriend stayed overnight in his studio apartment, but most evenings he spent lying on his bed watching public television until he couldn't stay awake any longer. He never drank or used drugs, and his mood was good; neither he nor anyone else in his family had ever had any mental health problems.

"I don't take naps during the day," Curtis summed up, "but I might as well. I'm sure not getting much done at work."

Evaluation of Curtis Usher

Curtis clearly had insomnia that had lasted far longer than a month and was causing him distress. The challenge here would be ruling out all of the possible confounding factors. The vignette does not contain enough information to cover every possibility; however, some of the major points have been touched upon.

Curtis probably did not have another Axis I disorder. His mood had been too good for a **Major Depressive Episode**. Although he worried about work, we have no information to suggest that he had an anxiety disorder such as **Generalized Anxiety Disorder**. He certainly did not have **Schizophrenia**. The vignette clearly states that his sleep disorder could not have been **substance-induced**. We have only his own word on his good health to confirm that he did not have a **general medical condition**; his clinician should refer him for a medical evaluation. There is also no information to exclude an Axis II disorder, though these are probably infrequent as a sole cause of a sleep disorder.

What about other sleep disorders? Curtis said that he did not nap, which would seem to rule out **Narcolepsy**. A **Breathing-Related Sleep Disorder** would be more likely to interrupt his sleep throughout the night (*interval sleep disturbance*) than to awaken him once at a set time (*terminal sleep disturbance*). Also, his wife complained of his dullness, not his snoring; the latter would suggest **sleep apnea**. **Circadian Rhythm Sleep Disorder, Delayed Sleep Phase Type**, would result in awakening late rather than early. The vignette contains no information that would support a parasomnia diagnosis, such as **Nightmare Disorder**, **Sleep Terror Disorder**, or **Sleepwalking Disorder**.

Two mechanisms could account for Curtis's insomnia. His work-related anxiety would be one (his boss was demanding, and times were hard in his industry). The other would be that he often lay upon his bed while watching TV. The association of this waking-related activity with bed could be conditioning him to stay awake.

Pending the outcome of a medical evaluation, Curtis's five-axis diagnosis would be as follows:

Axis I	307.42	Primary Insomnia
Axis II	V71.09	No diagnosis
Axis III		None
Axis IV		None
Axis V	GAF = 65	(current)

TIP Generalized Anxiety Disorder is important in this differential diagnosis. Like those with GAD, patients with Primary Insomnia also lie awake worrying. (The difference is that their anxieties are focused on their inability to sleep as well as think they should.) Also watch for "masked depression": Inquire carefully about other vegetative symptoms (appetite, weight loss) of a Major Depressive Episode when evaluating patients who appear to have Primary Insomnia.

307.44 Primary Hypersomnia

Primary Hypersomnia is probably a rare condition; it is certainly less common than Primary Insomnia. These people usually fall asleep easily and rapidly (often in five minutes or less) and may sleep late the next day. They also complain of being chronically tired and sleepy during the day, and they may return to bed for a nap during the day. Total sleep time is greater than nine hours a day, and often much more than that. These naps can occur at any time of the day, even after normal nighttime sleep. If they occur while driving, accidents can result. Although a few days of hypersomnia is not too uncommon, for it to go on and on is decidedly rare.

The causes of Primary Hypersomnia are varied. Some patients have difficulty coping with stress. Others may be trying to fill a void created by a sense of something lacking in their lives. In any event, the response is total sleep time that can be far above normal. Often these people take medications such as central nervous system stimulants or tranquilizers, which only make matters worse.

Criteria for Primary Hypersomnia

- For at least a month (or less, if it is recurrent), the patient's main complaint has been excessive sleepiness. This has been shown by either of these:
  ✓ Prolonged sleep
  ✓ Sleeping during the day, almost daily

- This sleepiness causes clinically important distress or impairs work, social, or personal functioning.
- Neither insomnia nor an inadequate amount of sleep explains the problem better.
- It doesn't occur solely during another sleep disorder (such as Breathing-Related Sleep Disorder, Circadian Rhythm Sleep Disorder, Narcolepsy, or a parasomnia).
- Another mental disorder doesn't explain it better.
- These symptoms are not directly caused by a general medical condition or by the use of substances, including medications.

Coding Note

Specify if: Recurrent. For at least two years, periods of hypersomnia lasting three days or more have occurred several times a year.

Colin Rodebaugh

From the time he was 15, Colin Rodebaugh had dreamed of becoming an architect. He had read biographies of Christopher Wren and Frank Lloyd Wright; in the summers, he worked around construction projects to learn how materials went together. Now he was 23 and in his second year of architectural school, and he couldn't stay awake during class.

"I might as well have weights tied to my eyelids," he said. "For the last six months, two or three times a day, I just have to take a nap. It could be in class, any time. It even happened once when I was making love to my girlfriend—not after, but during!"

Colin complained that he was tired all the time, but his health appeared to be excellent. His father, a family practitioner in Arizona, had insisted that he have a complete physical exam. Colin had been specifically questioned about any history of sudden weakness, loss of consciousness, or seizure disorder, none of which he had had. His mother practiced clinical psychology in Oregon, and she was ready to vouch for his mental health.

"I get plenty of sleep at night—at least nine hours. That's not the problem. It's that I hardly ever feel rested, no matter how much sleep I've had. If I do take a nap, I wake up feeling almost as groggy as when I nodded off."

Even apart from Colin's sleep disorder, school was a frustration. Although he was technically proficient, he'd discovered that he didn't have the eye for design of some of his classmates. During the past semester, he had realized that what talent he had lay in drafting, not design. His advisor hadn't argued with him when they had discussed a possible career change.

Evaluation of Colin Rodebaugh

As with insomnia, the first task in evaluating hypersomnia is to rule out the many conditions that could be causing it. Although the vignette does not contain all the information Colin's clinician would need to make that determination, it does provide an outline.

General medical conditions are probably the most important conditions to rule out in this differential diagnosis. Colin had had a recent workup and physical exam, and was reported to be in good health. Furthermore, there had been no history of sudden weakness or lapses of consciousness that might indicate **psychomotor epilepsy**.

We have no information about **substance use**; Colin's clinician would have to evaluate that. At least his mother, who was a mental health professional, felt that there was no indication of another mental disorder. (**Major Depressive Episode With Atypical Features** would be the most likely Axis I disorder.)

Narcolepsy is another sleep disorder that causes daytime sleepiness. But individuals with Narcolepsy are typically refreshed by their brief naps, whereas Colin felt groggy. **Insufficient nighttime sleep** seems so obvious a possibility that it is sometimes overlooked; suspect it in patients who sleep less than seven hours a night. Colin felt that he got plenty of sleep. At nine hours a night or more, he was not sleep-deprived. His clinician could ask Colin's girlfriend whether he snored or had other symptoms suggestive of a **Breathing-Related Sleep Disorder**.

If we assume that further evaluation would not turn up any other **substance-induced** or **Axis I** or **Axis II disorder**, Colin's difficulty could be one of those rare conditions in which life's disappointments result in lethargy and taking to bed. The condition may cause secondary depression.

As far as we can tell from the vignette, Colin had had only one episode of his sleep disorder, lasting (at the time of his evaluation) about six months. A single episode is the rule, but some patients have multiple episodes, lasting up to several weeks and recurring periodically over the years. To their diagnosis would be added the specifier Recurrent.

Axis I	307.44	Primary Hypersomnia
Axis II	V71.09	No diagnosis
Axis III		None
Axis IV		Inadequate school performance
Axis V	GAF = 65	(current)

TIP Kleine–Levin syndrome is a rare form of recurrent Primary Hypersomnia in which excessive sleep (sometimes as much as 20 hours a day) is associated with compulsive overeating, weight gain, irritability, and inappropriate sexual behavior that includes open masturbation. EEGs are abnormal in this disorder.

347 Narcolepsy

During normal REM sleep, general paralysis of the body muscles occurs. We don't notice this because we are safely asleep. Most of the dreams that we can recall also occur during REM sleep, which occurs throughout the night, usually beginning about 90 minutes after the onset of sleep.

Narcolepsy is a syndrome of excessive sleepiness that has been recognized since about 1880. The classic picture of Narcolepsy includes four symptoms: sleep attacks, cataplexy, hallucinations, and sleep paralysis. However, most patients do not have all of these symptoms.

- In Narcolepsy, REM periods begin within a few minutes of the onset of sleep. Often they will even intrude upon the normal waking state, resulting in the *irresistible urge to sleep*. These sleep attacks last from a few minutes to over an hour, and are particularly notable for being refreshing (in contrast to the grogginess experienced in Primary Hypersomnia). Upon awakening, there is a refractory period of at least one hour, during which the patient will remain completely awake. Sleep attacks can be triggered by stress or by emotion (e.g., laughter or anger).
- The most dramatic symptom is *cataplexy*—sudden, brief episodes of paralysis that can affect nearly all voluntary muscles or just specific muscle groups (such as the jaw or the knees). When it is the former, the patient may collapse completely. When fewer muscle groups are affected or the attack is brief, cataplexy may go almost unnoticed. Cataplexy attacks may occur with the sleep attacks or separately, when there is no loss of consciousness. Often they are precipitated by intense emotion, such as laughter or crying.
- *Hallucinations* may be the first symptom of Narcolepsy; they are predominately visual. They hint that REM sleep is suddenly intruding upon the waking state, because hallucinations occur when the patient is going to sleep or awakening.
- *Sleep paralysis* can be frightening: The patient has the sensation of being awake but unable to move, speak, or even breathe adequately. Sleep paralysis is associated with anxiety and fear of dying; it usually lasts less than 10 minutes and can be accompanied by visual or auditory hallucinations.

A typical history that includes three or four of the classic symptoms is good presumptive evidence for Narcolepsy. But this is a chronic disorder that is difficult to manage and implies lifelong treatment. It is therefore important to confirm diagnosis by appropriate sleep lab studies.

Narcolepsy is strongly hereditary and affects males and females about equally. It is uncommon, though far from rare, affecting less than 1 in 1,000 adults. Onset is usually in puberty, but always by the age of 30. Once it begins, there is usually a slow and steady development. It can lead to depression, impotence, trouble at work, and even accidents on the street or on the job.

TIP Both words derive from Greek, but note the difference between *cataplexy* and *catalepsy*. *Cataplexy* means (approximately) "to strike down"; it is a symptom of Narcolepsy. *Catalepsy* ("to hold down") is a symptom of immobility that occurs in catatonia.

Hypnagogic and *hypnopompic* (see the criteria, below) are two terms widely used to describe events that happen when one is going to sleep or waking up, respectively. (From Greek: *hypn* = "sleep," *agogue* = "leader," *pomp* = "sending away"). Note the different spellings, *hypna-* and *hypno-*.

Criteria for Narcolepsy

• Each day for three months or more, the patient has had irresistible attacks of refreshing sleep.
• The patient experiences either or both of these:
   ✓ Cataplexy (sudden, brief loss of muscle tone bilaterally, usually associated with intense emotion)
   ✓ Intrusions of REM sleep into transitions between waking and sleeping, as shown by *either* of these:
      ✓ Hypnagogic or hypnopompic hallucinations, *or*
      ✓ Sleep paralysis at the beginning or end of sleep
• These symptoms are not directly caused by a general medical condition or by the use of substances, including medications.

Emma Flowers

"It's been happening like this for several years. Only now it's worse," said Eric Flowers, Emma's husband. He had brought her to the clinic because she no longer felt she could drive safely.

Emma herself was slumped in the interview chair next to him. Her chin rested on her chest, and her left arm hung down at her side. She had been soundly asleep for several minutes. "If she hadn't been sitting down, she'd have fallen down," said Eric. "I've had to catch her half a dozen times."

As a teenager, Emma had had vivid, sometimes frightening dreams that occurred as she was going to sleep, even if it was only a brief afternoon nap. By the time she married Eric, she was having occasional "sleep attacks," when she would find the urge to lie down and take a brief nap irresistible. Over the next several years, these naps occurred with increasing frequency. Now, at age 28, Emma found herself napping for 10 minutes or so every three or four hours during the day. Her nighttime sleep seemed entirely normal.

It was the falling attacks that had prompted this evaluation. At first Emma noticed only a sort of weakness in her neck muscles when she felt sleepy. Over the course of a year the weakness had increased, until now it affected every voluntary muscle in her body. It could happen at any time, but usually it was associated with the onset of sudden sleepiness. At these times she seemed to lose all of her strength, sometimes so suddenly that she didn't even have time to sit down. Then she would collapse, right where she had been standing. Today it had happened while she was sitting down. Once it had happened while she was trying to park her car. She had seen a neurologist the month before, but an EEG had revealed no evidence of a seizure disorder, and an MRI was normal.

Emma stirred, yawned, and opened her eyes. "I did it again, didn't I?"

"Feeling better?" asked her husband.

"I always do, don't I?"

Evaluation of Emma Flowers

This vignette illustrates most of the symptoms of Narcolepsy: attacks of irresistible sleep during the day, which the patient experiences as refreshing; cataplexy (though it does not always cause the patient to fall); and vivid dreams that occur during the onset of sleep. Emma did not complain of sleep paralysis, which also occurs unnoticed during normal REM sleep.

Differential diagnosis should include all other possible causes of excessive somnolence: **Substance-Induced Sleep Disorders**; **Major Depressive Episode With Atypical Features**, various **cognitive disorders** (especially delirium); and a panoply of **general medical conditions**, such as hypothyroidism, epilepsy, hypoglycemia, myasthenia gravis, and multiple sclerosis. Emma should, of course, be evaluated for each of these. **Other sleep disorders** associated with daytime sleepiness would also have to be considered. But Emma's history was so typical that Narcolepsy would almost certainly turn out to be her eventual diagnosis.

Many Narcolepsy patients have an associated Axis I diagnosis, most often **Dysthymic Disorder** or **Major Depressive Disorder**, some **substance-related disorder**, or **Generalized Anxiety Disorder**.

Pending the results of a full evaluation, Emma's complete diagnosis would be as follows:

Axis I	347	Narcolepsy
Axis II	V71.09	No diagnosis
Axis III		None
Axis IV		None
Axis V	GAF = 60	(current)

780.59 Breathing-Related Sleep Disorder

There are two main forms of Breathing-Related Sleep Disorder. (Excessive daytime sleepiness is the usual presenting complaint, though some patients may instead complain of insomnia.)

The first form is called *alveolar hypoventilation syndrome*. In this syndrome, respirations do not stop any more often than normal, but blood oxygenation is decreased due to shallow breathing. These patients have shallow breathing when awake, but it worsens during sleep. It is most common in patients who are severely overweight, though it has also been noted in people who have other causes of shallow breathing (e.g., myotonic dystrophy, poliomyelitis, and lesions of the spinal cord or central nervous system). It may be related to sudden infant death as well.

The second major form of Breathing-Related Sleep Disorder is called *sleep apnea*. This is a complete cessation of air exchange during sleep; it is potentially lethal. There are two main subtypes: *obstructive* and *central*.

In the *obstructive* type, airflow through the upper respiratory passages is blocked. During sleep (never while awake), these patients have periods lasting 10 seconds to a minute or longer when they stop breathing completely. The chest continues to heave as the sleeper tries to inhale, but tissues in the mouth and pharynx prevent the normal flow of air. In extreme cases, the struggle continues as long as two minutes. The episode culminates in an extraordinarily loud snore. Most patients have far more than 30 of these episodes per night of sleep. This is the most common form of Breathing-Related Sleep Disorder.

In the *central* type of sleep apnea, the patient (who may be obese) simply stops making any effort to breathe—the diaphragm just stops working. Snoring can be present but is usually not prominent. Males may complain especially of hypersomnia; females may complain of insomnia. (Yet another type begins as an episode of central apnea, then becomes obstructive.)

Regardless of the cause of sleep apnea, the blood becomes depleted of oxygen until breathing starts again. Often, patients are not aware of these events at all, though sometimes they may awaken partly or completely. Besides snoring and daytime sleepiness, there are often problems with hypertension and cardiac arrhythmias; patients may also complain of morning headaches and impotence. During the night, some patients become markedly restless, kicking at bedclothes (or bed partners), standing up, or even walking. Other effects include irritability and cognitive impairment (distractibility, problems with memory or perception, or confusion). Patients may also experience night or morning headaches, heavy sweating, hallucinations when going to sleep, sleep talking, or sleep terrors. *Nocturia* (getting up at night to urinate) is often associated with sleep apnea; *enuresis* (bedwetting) is also occasionally a symptom.

Sleep apnea is relatively common; the incidence increases with advancing age. The onset is usually in middle age; obesity is often a predisposing factor, though some patients are not obese. It is more common in males, though after menopause females are about equally affected.

Because sleep apnea is potentially lethal, it should always be considered in the differential diagnosis of both hypersomnia and insomnia, and appropriate steps should be taken to rule it out. Rapid detection and management can be life-saving. An observant bed partner can provide almost definitive evidence of sleep apnea. But sleep lab evaluation is important in this disorder, to obtain EEG confirmation and to measure how low the blood oxygen saturation goes during the apneic period.

TIP *Ondine's curse* is a term that clinicians and researchers have applied to failure of the brain to stimulate breathing. It is a rare form of alveolar hypoventilation syndrome. The name is taken from a 1939 play by the Frenchman Jean Giraudoux. A knight had been unfaithful to a sea nymph, Ondine (or Undine), who felled him with the curse that unless he focused his attention on breathing, he would forget to breathe and die. Of course, this was exactly what happened when he could no longer remain awake.

Criteria for Breathing-Related Sleep Disorder

- The patient experiences disruption of sleep that causes insomnia or hypersomnia.
- The clinician judges this disruption to be caused by a breathing problem related to sleep, such as central or obstructive sleep apnea or central alveolar hypoventilation syndrome.
- Another mental disorder does not better explain this behavior.
- The symptoms are not directly caused by a general medical condition or by the use of substances, including medications.

Coding Note

On Axis III, also code a sleep-related breathing disorder—for example, 780.57 (obstructive sleep apnea).

Roy Dardis

"I guess it's been going on 30 years and more," said Lily Dardis. It was her husband's snoring she was talking about. "I used to sleep soundly myself, so it didn't bother me. Lately, I've had arthritis that's kept me awake. Roy rattles the windows."

Lying awake nights waiting for the painkiller to take effect, Lily had had the opportunity to study her husband's sleeping habits minutely. As someone who had always slept on his back, Roy had always been a noisy breather at night. But every five minutes or so, his respirations seemed to drop off to nothing. After 20 or 30 seconds, during which his chest would heave, he'd finally break through with an enormous snort. This would be rapidly followed by several additional louder-than-usual snores. "It's a wonder the neighbors don't complain," Lily said.

Roy Dardis was a tall man of enormous bulk, a testament to Lily's country cooking. He guessed he'd always snored some—his brother, with whom he had shared a room as a child, used to tease him about it. Of course, as he jokingly pointed out, the racket didn't bother him because he slept right through it. His complaint was that he just didn't feel rested. He tended to nod off, whether he was at work or watching TV, but that just left him grumpy.

Mornings, Roy often awakened with a headache that seemed localized to the front of his head. Two cups of strong coffee usually took care of the headache.

Evaluation of Roy Dardis

Roy's wife presented strong evidence for Breathing-Related Sleep Disorder: She actually observed that Roy had many periods when he would stop breathing, then resume with an extra-loud snore. From her description of his heaving chest during the apneic periods, this would appear to be an obstructive type of sleep apnea. Roy's bulk, morning headaches, and complaints about dropping off to sleep during the day are also typical of sleep apnea. A clinician should ask any patient like Roy about hallucinations when going to sleep, changes in personality (irritability, aggression, anxiety, depression), loss of sex interest, impotence, night terrors, and sleepwalking; all of these are encountered with varying frequency in sleep apnea.

Other causes of hypersomnia should be considered, though they would not seem likely in Roy's case. Daytime sleepiness and hypnagogic hallucinations occur in **Narcolepsy**, but Roy had no cataplexy and his daytime naps were not refreshing. Of course, many otherwise normal people snore, and this should be considered in the differential diagnosis of any patient whose chief complaint is snoring.

Despite Roy's typical history, sleep lab studies should be pursued, if for no other reason than to evaluate his blood oxygen saturation during an attack of apnea. Other Axis I disorders (especially **mood and anxiety disorders**) and **substance-related disorders** should be evaluated. Some of these—notably **Major Depressive Disorder**, **Panic Disorder**, and **dementia**—may be found as associated diagnoses.

Roy's full diagnosis at this time would be as follows:

Axis I	780.59	Breathing-Related Sleep Disorder
Axis II	V71.09	No diagnosis
Axis III	278.0	Obesity
	780.57	Obstructive sleep apnea
Axis IV		None
Axis V	GAF = 60	(current)

307.45 Circadian Rhythm Sleep Disorder

Circadian is a word that comes from Latin meaning "about one day" (*circa* = "approximately," *dia* = "day"). It refers to the fact that body cycles of sleep, temperature, and hormone production are generated from within the brain. When there are no external time cues (natural phenomena such as daylight or human-made stimuli such as clocks), the free-running human cycle is actually about 25 hours long.

The normal circadian sleep–wake cycle is not constant throughout life. It tends to lengthen during adolescence; that's one reason teenagers tend to stay up late and sleep late. It shortens again in old age, causing older people to fall asleep in their chairs while reading or watching television in the evening. This factor makes both shift work and jet lag more difficult for older people.

There are three main types of Circadian Rhythm Sleep Disorder (which until recently was called Sleep–Wake Schedule Disorder): the Jet Lag and Shift Work Types, which are usually transient and self-correcting, and the Delayed Sleep Phase Type, which is usually chronic.

Jet Lag Type. In this type, individuals feel attacks of intense sleepiness and fatigue after air travel across several time zones; some may complain of nausea or other flu-like symptoms. Adjustment to the new time zone begins by the second day, and is usually completed within one week. (Most people find that time adjustment is faster and easier after flying westward than after flying eastward; this is probably because the body's natural cycle is about 25 hours long, not 24, as noted above. Studies have shown that adjustment to westward flights occurs at the rate of about one and a half hours per day, whereas adjustment to eastward flights is only about one hour per day. This is true whether the traveler lives in the East or in the West.)

Shift Work Type. This type occurs when workers must change from one shift to another, especially when they must be active during their former sleep time. Performance declines and sleepiness ensues. Sleep during the new sleep time is often disrupted and decreased in duration. The symptoms are worst during adjustment to night work, and people vary considerably in the time required for this adjustment. Symptoms may last three weeks or longer, especially if workers try to resume their former sleeping schedules on weekends or holidays.

Delayed Sleep Phase Type. This type differs from the other two in that it is not imposed by external circumstances such as travel or work. These people go to sleep progressively later and awaken late in the day. If they can sleep as late as they wish, they feel fine. But if they must arise to go to work (or supper), they feel sleepy and may even appear "sleep-drunk." Irregular sleep habits and the use of caffeine or other stimulants make it worse. (Note that this disorder type must be distinguished from the life style of some people who *prefer* to go to bed late and sleep late the next day. These people don't try very hard to change and feel quite comfortable with their eccentric schedules. People with Delayed Sleep Phase Type do try to change, and complain of hypersomnolence as a result.)

Criteria for Circadian Rhythm Sleep Disorder

- There is a persisting or repeating mismatch between a patient's sleep–wake pattern and the sleep–wake demands of that patient's environment.
- The mismatch leads to insomnia or hypersomnia.
- This problem causes clinically important distress or impairs work, social, or personal functioning.
- It doesn't occur solely during another mental disorder or sleep disorder.
- It is not directly caused by a general medical condition or by the use of substances, including medications.

Coding Note

Specify:

Delayed Sleep Phase Type. The patient repeatedly has trouble getting to sleep and trouble awakening on time.

Jet Lag Type. Alertness and sleepiness occur at inconvenient times of day after travel across more than one time zone.

Shift Work Type. Because of night shift work or frequently changing job shifts, the patient experiences hypersomnia during the major period of wakefulness or insomnia during the major sleep period.

Unspecified Type.

Marcelle Klinger

Marcelle was a 60-year-old registered nurse, one of seven employed by her small community hospital in the northern California hills. The entire facility had only 32 beds, and although there were nurses' aides and licensed practical nurses to assist, state law required a registered nurse always to be present in the facility. When the nurse who had worked the graveyard shift (11 P.M. to 7:30 A.M.) finally retired, the hospital administrator asked for a volunteer to fill that position.

"Nobody did," said Marcelle, "so some genius decided that it was only fair for everyone to take turns."

The results were four-week shifts. In the course of a year, each nurse would work six of these shifts on days, four on evenings, and two on graveyard. Everyone grumbled, but Marcelle hated it the most. The switch from days to evenings wasn't too bad; she lived close to the hospital, and could be home and in bed by midnight. But the graveyard shift was a disaster.

"I'm the only registered nurse there, and I'm supposed to be awake and alert the whole time. Patients depend on me. But my eyes keep squeezing themselves shut, and my brain seems to hum, as if it's going to sleep. Part of the time I feel sick to my stomach. One time I did fall asleep at work, just for 10 minutes or so. When the phone rang, I woke up feeling hung over."

Marcelle's physical and mental health was excellent. She'd always been a light sleeper, so she found daytime sleeping nearly impossible. Heavy drapes could keep out most of the light, but traffic noises and the sounds from passers-by on the sidewalk outside her bedroom frequently awakened her.

Moreover, the coffee Marcelle drank to keep awake at work prevented her from going to sleep as soon as she went to bed. It also got her up to the bathroom at least once or twice. By the time her husband came home in the afternoon from teaching school, she had seldom logged more than three or four hours of uninterrupted sleep. On weekends, she tried to resume a normal schedule so that she could be with her family, but that only made things worse. "I flew to Paris once and felt jet-lagged for a week. Now I'm sick that way for a whole month."

Evaluation of Marcelle Klinger

Several features of Marcelle's condition could have contributed to her discomfort: (1) Like many people who must work shifts, she tried to re-readjust her sleep–wake schedule on the weekends. (2) Cues from outside her window served to arouse her when she tried to sleep. (3) She was 60; because of the physiology of their sleep, older people are often less able to make these adjustments than are younger people. (4) She drank coffee to stay awake; the dual effects of the caffeine-induced stimulation and her need to get up to urinate interfered further with what sleep she could get.

From her history, we learn that Marcelle had no **general medical condition**, **substance use**, or **other Axis I disorder**. (Although patients with a psychosis such as **Schizophrenia** are sometimes kept up progressively later at night by their hallucinations, **mood** and **anxiety disorders** generally produce only insomnia or hypersomnia.) The vignette provides no evidence for another sleep disorder: When Marcelle napped, it was not refreshing (this would militate against **Narcolepsy**). She had always been a light sleeper anyway, but light sleep per se is not considered a sleep disorder.

The subtype is obvious:

Axis I	307.45	Circadian Rhythm Sleep Disorder, Shift Work Type
Axis II	V71.09	No diagnosis
Axis III		None
Axis IV		Stressful work schedule
Axis V	GAF = 65	(current)

307.47 Dyssomnia Not Otherwise Specified

Problems that have not yet been accorded the status of a better-defined dyssomnia are coded as Dyssomnia Not Otherwise Specified. DSM-IV gives some specific examples:

Nocturnal myoclonus. These are periodic, sustained contractions of the legs that can be associated with brief awakenings. They are not usually clinically important, and are commonly found in the general population. Patients may complain of insomnia or daytime sleepiness. Compare to the restless legs syndrome (see below).

Restless legs syndrome. This condition of unknown etiology produces an almost indescribable discomfort deep within the legs between ankles and knees. Because the discomfort is relieved by movement, patients have an irresistible urge to move their legs. This common disorder often begins before a patient goes to bed, and can delay onset of sleep or awaken the patient during the night. Compare to nocturnal myoclonus.

Other. Use this category for any other hypersomnia, insomnia, or circadian rhythm disorder when you can't decide whether it is primary or caused by substance use or a general medical condition.

PARASOMNIAS

The *parasomnias*, as noted earlier, are problems that intrude upon sleep but don't necessarily cause insomnia or hypersomnia. Motor, cognitive, or autonomic nervous system processes become active during sleep or during the transitions between sleep and wakefulness. Consider the example of nightmares versus sleep apnea. Both occur during sleep, but nightmares are usually problematic because they are scary, not because they interfere with sleeping or cause wakefulness the next day.

307.47 Nightmare Disorder

Most nightmares quickly bring us completely awake; usually we can recall them vividly. They are usually about something that threatens either our safety or our self-esteem. When someone repeatedly has long, terrifying dreams like these, or suffers from daytime sleepiness, irritability, or loss of concentration, the diagnosis of Nightmare Disorder may be warranted.

Nightmares occur during REM sleep, most of which occurs toward the end of the night. They can be increased by withdrawal from REM-suppressing substances; these include antidepressants, barbiturates, and alcohol. Although some degree of rapid heartbeat is common, people with nightmares generally have fewer symptoms of sympathetic nervous system arousal (perspiration, rapid heartbeat, increased blood pressure) than do those who have night terrors.

Nightmares that occur in childhood (especially in young children) have no pathological significance. About half of all adults report nightmares at some time or other. The number who have enough nightmares to be considered pathological is unknown, though perhaps 5% of adults claim to have frequent nightmares. They may be more common in women than in men. To some extent, the tendency to have them may be inherited.

Although adults with frequent nightmares probably have a tendency to psychopathology, there is no consensus among sleep experts as to what that might be. (When it is sorted out, it may turn out to be that the pathology has more to do with who *complains* than with the actual experience of having nightmares.) Vivid nightmares sometimes precede the onset of a psychosis. However, most nightmares may be an expected (hence, normal) reaction to stress; some clinicians believe that they help people to work through traumatic experiences.

> **TIP** At least half the population has had a nightmare at one time or another. So do all these people have a sleep disorder? As with so many other conditions, making this decision is a matter of quantity (number of nightmare episodes) and of the reaction a patient has to the episodes. These factors must be filtered through the judgment of the clinician. Good luck.

Criteria for Nightmare Disorder

- The patient repeatedly awakens with detailed recall of long, frightening dreams. These usually occur in the second half of the sleep or nap period and concern threats to security, self-esteem, or survival.
- The patient quickly becomes alert and oriented upon awakening.
- These experiences (or the resulting sleep disturbance) cause clinically important distress or impair work, social, or personal functioning.
- They don't occur solely during another mental disorder (such as Posttraumatic Stress Disorder or a delirium).
- The symptoms are not directly caused by a general medical condition or by the use of substances, including medications.

Keith Redding

"I wouldn't have come at all, but the other guys made me." Keith Redding twisted his garrison cap in his fingers and looked embarrassed. "Two of them are waiting out in the hallway, in case they're needed for information. I think they really stayed to make sure I kept the appointment."

After six months in the Army, Keith had just been promoted to private first class. He had enlisted right out of high school, thinking that he'd become a mechanic and learn a good trade. But his tests showed he was gifted, so they plunked him into the medics and sent him to school after boot camp. Now he'd been at his new duty station in Texas for two weeks, living in comparative luxury in a barracks room with three roommates.

Having any roommates at all was a problem, because of his sleeping habits. "I have these nightmares," Keith explained. They didn't occur every night, but he did have them several nights a week. He usually awakened an hour or two before reveille, whimpering loudly enough to awaken the others. He'd been having this problem for several years, so he was more or less used to it. But, of course, his roommates objected. It had been worse in the last few months, with the stress of leaving home, moving around, and working at new jobs.

Although Keith's dreams varied, there were some common threads. In one of them he was in a group of people, buck naked. Recently it had been during inspection. All the other troops were lined up, looking smart in their Class A uniforms. He hadn't a stitch on and kept trying to cover himself, though no one seemed to notice. In another, he was the driver of an old "cracker-box" ambulance. For some reason, he had picked up a wounded gorilla. Maddened with pain, the gorilla was pulling itself forward and stretching out a hairy arm to wrap around him.

"Unfortunately, I have terrific recall. I come instantly awake, and every detail of the nightmare is just as sharp as if I'd seen it on TV. Then I'm awake for an hour or more, and so is everyone else."

The balance of Keith's history was unremarkable. He didn't use drugs and didn't drink; his health had been good, and he hadn't been especially depressed or anxious. He had never had blackouts or seizures, and he hadn't been taking medications. He loved his job in the dispensary and believed that his commanding officer found him to be alert and conscientious. He certainly wasn't falling asleep on the job.

"I've met some older guys who've had nightmares after being in combat," Keith said. "I can understand that. But about the worst thing that's ever happened to me since I enlisted has been a flat tire."

Evaluation of Keith Redding

Keith's nightmares didn't bother him much; he had grown used to them. It was his discomfort in regard to his roommates that would qualify his nightmares as sufficiently severe to warrant diagnosis.

Three aspects of Keith's experience are typical of most nightmares: They occurred during the latter part of the night, he came instantly awake, and he clearly recalled their content. (The content of Keith's bad dreams was also typical: threats to his safety or self-respect.) Each of these features serves to differentiate nightmare Disorder from **Sleep Terror Disorder**: Sleep terrors occur early during non-REM sleep, they are poorly remembered, and the patient wakens only partially (if at all). Finally, although there may be some vocalization (in Keith's case, a suppressed whine) when the patient is about to wake up, the paralysis of muscles that normally occurs during REM sleep prevents the loud scream and physical movements that are typical of Sleep Terror Disorder.

If the patient's complaint is of daytime sleepiness, other causes should be considered, such as **Breathing-Related Sleep Disorder**. Keith did not have daytime sleep attacks, though nightmares can be a feature of **Narcolepsy**. Also consider the variety of other Axis I and II disorders in which nightmares can occur: **mood disorders, Schizophrenia, anxiety disorders, somatoform disorders, Adjustment Disorder**, and **personality disorders**.

The fact that Keith had been taking no medications is also important to the differential diagnosis, because withdrawal from **REM-suppressing substances** such as tricyclic antidepressants, alcohol, or barbiturates can sometimes increase the tendency to nightmares. **Seizure disorders** (such as partial complex seizures) can occasionally present with bad dreams; abnormal movements noted by a bed partner during the time of the apparent nightmare could be an indication for EEG studies. As Keith himself noted, nightmares about a traumatic event are frequently encountered in patients who have **Posttraumatic Stress Disorder** (these may occur in non-REM sleep, which is why PTSD patients are more likely to scream).

Keith's full diagnosis would read as follows:

Axis I	307.47	Nightmare Disorder
Axis II	V71.09	No diagnosis
Axis III		None
Axis IV		None
Axis V	GAF = 75	(current)

307.46 Sleep Terror Disorder

Sleep terrors (also known as night terrors) usually affect children. They typically begin between the ages of 4 and 12. When they begin in adulthood, the onset is usually in the 20s or 30s—hardly ever after the age of 40. As is true of nightmares versus Nightmare Disorder (see above), only sleep terrors that are recurrent and produce distress or impairment qualify for a diagnosis of Sleep Terror Disorder.

A sleep terror attack begins with a loud cry or scream during a period of non-REM sleep. (Non-REM is deep or slow-wave sleep, most common early during the night. That is why most sleep terror episodes occur not long after the patient goes to bed.) The person sits up, appears terrified, and seems to be awake but does not respond to attempts at soothing. There will be signs of sympathetic nervous system arousal, such as rapid breathing and heartbeat, sweating, and *piloerection* (hairs standing up on the skin). An attack usually lasts from 5 to 15 minutes and culminates in the person's going back to sleep. Most patients have no memory of the incident the following morning, though some adults may have fragmentary recall.

In Sleep Terror Disorder, there is usually an interval of days to weeks between attacks; stress and fatigue may increase the frequency of attacks. The disorder is equally common in adult males and females.

In children, sleep terrors are not considered pathological. A child almost invariably grows out of them and suffers from no medical or psychological pathology later in life. In adults they are rare and usually associated with some other Axis I disorder (such as an anxiety disorder) or with a personality disorder.

Criteria for Sleep Terror Disorder

- On numerous occasions, the patient awakens abruptly, usually during the first third of sleep and usually beginning with a scream of panic.
- During each episode the patient shows evidence of marked fear and autonomic arousal, such as rapid breathing, rapid heartbeat, and sweating.
- During the episode, the patient responds poorly to the efforts of others to provide comfort.
- The patient cannot recall any dream in detail at the time and cannot recall the whole episode later.
- These symptoms cause clinically important distress or impair work, social, or personal functioning.
- These symptoms are not directly caused by a general medical condition or by the use of substances, including medications.

Bud Stanhope

Bud Stanhope and his wife, Harriette, had just begun marital counseling. They agreed on one thing, which was that many of their problems could be traced to Bud's excessive need for support. They had married on the rebound, soon after Bud's first wife divorced him. "I felt so uncomfortable being alone," said Bud.

His chronically low self-esteem meant that Bud couldn't so much as start a building project around the house without consulting Harriette. Once, when Harriette was out of town at a convention, he even called up his ex-wife for advice. And because he was afraid to disagree with Harriette, they never got anything resolved. "I don't even feel I can tell him how much it bugs me when he wakes me up with those night frights," she said.

"Night frights?" said Bud. "I thought those stopped months ago."

As Harriette described them, Bud's "frights" were always the same. An hour or so after they went to sleep, she'd awaken to his blood-curdling scream. Bud would be sitting bolt upright in bed, a look of stark terror on his face. His eyes wide open, he would be staring off into a corner or toward a wall. She was never sure if he was seeing something, because he never said much that was intelligible—only babble or the occasional random word. He would seem agitated, pluck at his bedclothes, and sometimes start to get out of bed.

"The hairs on his arms will be standing straight up. He's usually breathing fast and perspiring, even if it's cold in the room. Once when I put my hand on his chest, his heart seemed to be beating as fast as a rabbit's."

It would always take Harriette 10 or 15 minutes to soothe Bud. He never fully awakened, but would eventually lie down. Then he would almost instantly fall fast asleep again, while she sometimes lay awake for hours. Bud would have one of these attacks every two or three weeks. Only once did it happen two nights running, and that was during one particularly bad period when he felt sure he was about to lose his job.

Evaluation of Bud Stanhope

Several features of Bud's attacks are distinctive for Sleep Terror Disorder: the degree of autonomic arousal (rapid heartbeat, sweating), the occurrence during the first few hours of sleep, Harriette's inability to console him, his lack of full awakening, and his lack of recall the next day. Taken as a whole, this story is virtually diagnostic. Note that each of these features helps to differentiate this disorder from **Nightmare Disorder**.

Although this did not happen to Bud, **sleepwalking** (sometimes sleep running) occurs in many night terror patients. In adults, you may have to distinguish night terrors from **psychomotor epilepsy**, which can also produce sleepwalking. **Panic Attacks** sometimes occur at night, but these patients awaken completely, without the disorientation and disorganized behavior typical of Sleep Terror Disorder.

Bud also had significant personality problems. As noted in the vignette, he required a great deal of consultation and support (he even went to the extreme of consulting with his ex-wife when Harriette was out of town), and he had trouble disagreeing with others. His discomfort at being alone, low self-confidence, and rush into another marriage when the first one ended would seem to confirm an Axis II diagnosis of **Dependent Personality Disorder**. Other patients may have **Borderline Personality Disorder**. Bud's GAF score was based more on the personality disorder than on the Sleep Terror Disorder. Associated conditions in other patients can include **Posttraumatic Stress Disorder** and **Generalized Anxiety Disorder**.

Axis I	V61.1	Partner Relational Problem
	307.46	Sleep Terror Disorder
Axis II	301.6	Dependent Personality Disorder
Axis III		None
Axis IV		None
Axis V	GAF = 61	(current)

TIP Note that Sleepwalking Disorder (next page) and Sleep Terror Disorder have been given the same code number. This is not a mistake (at least, it isn't *my* mistake). It was that way in DSM-III-R as well. A lot of these issues are decided by international agreement, which isn't necessarily the surest way to do things right.

307.46 Sleepwalking Disorder

Sleepwalking behavior tends to follow a fairly set pattern, usually occurring during the first third of the night (when non-REM sleep is more prevalent). Sleepwalkers first sit up and make some sort of perseverative movement (such as picking at the bedclothes). Then there may be purposeful behavior, such as dressing, eating, or using the toilet. The facial expression is usually blank and staring. If these individuals talk at all, it is usually garbled; speaking sentences is rare. Their movements are usually poorly coordinated. They may put themselves into considerable danger. They usually have amnesia for the episode, although this is variable.

An individual episode usually lasts anywhere from a few seconds to 30 minutes. The person will often be hard to awaken, though spontaneous awakening may occur. If so, there is usually a brief period of disorientation. Some people simply return to bed without awakening. Occasionally, a person who goes to sleep elsewhere will express surprise upon awakening in the wrong location.

Sleepwalking may occur nightly, though usually it is less frequent. As is true of Nightmare Disorder and Sleep Terror Disorder, a diagnosis of Sleepwalking Disorder is not made unless sleepwalking episodes are recurrent and cause impairment or distress. As with so many other sleep disorders, sleepwalking episodes are more likely when a person has been under stress or is tired. The condition appears to have familial and genetic components; some claim that it is a mild form of Sleep Terror Disorder.

Sleepwalking affects 1–5% of all children, in whom it is not considered pathological. It usually begins between the ages of 6 and 12 and lasts for several years, with most children outgrowing it by the age of 15. It affects under 1% of adults, with a typical age of onset between 10 and 15, and tends to be chronic. Men and women are equally susceptible, but it does not usually last past the fourth decade of life. Although adults with Sleepwalking Disorder may have a personality disorder, sleepwalking in children has no prognostic significance.

TIP Sleepwalking has been recognized for hundreds of years, and an extensive, if inaccurate, mythology has been built up about it. Also known as *somnambulism* (which means "sleepwalking"), it has been a reliable device for playwrights (remember Lady Macbeth). One popular myth is that it is dangerous to awaken a sleepwalker. Perhaps this grew out of the observation that it is *difficult* to do so; in any event, I know of no evidence that it is true.

Criteria for Sleepwalking Disorder

- On numerous occasions, the patient arises and walks about, usually during the first third of sleep.
- During sleepwalking, the patient stares blankly, can be awakened only with difficulty, and responds poorly to others' attempts at communication.
- Although there may be a brief period of confusion upon first awakening from the episode, within a few minutes the patient's behavior and mental activity are unimpaired.
- After the episode or the next morning, the patient has no memory for the episode.
- These symptoms cause clinically important distress or impair work, social, or personal functioning.
- The symptoms are not directly caused by a general medical condition or by the use of substances, including medications.

Ross Josephson

"I brought along a video. I thought it might help to explain my problem." Ross Josephson plugged in the portable VCR and small television set. Ross was a college freshman who lived in a dormitory with two roommates; they had provided the videotape.

Ross walked in his sleep. He supposed it had started when he was quite young, though he hadn't fully realized it until he was 12, when he had awakened in his pajamas curled up on the porch swing one hot July dawn. When he told his mother, she remarked that she and her two brothers had all walked in their sleep when they were young. She guessed that Ross would grow out of it, too.

Only he hadn't. A freshman in college now, Ross continued his nocturnal strolls once or twice a month. At first his roommates had been amused; the videotape had been a hit at an impromptu party they had gotten up with some of the girls who lived downstairs. They had lain awake several nights until they caught the complete sequence. Ross had taken the joke well. In fact, he had been fascinated to see how he appeared when sleepwalking.

But last week his roommates had become alarmed when they caught him stepping through an open window onto the third-floor roof of their dormitory building. Other than a low rim around the edge, there was nothing to prevent a nasty 30-foot fall into the grape ivy below. Although they had succeeded in getting him back inside, it had not been without a struggle; Ross clearly had not wanted to be restrained.

After an interview and physical exam by one of the consultants in the student health service, Ross had been pronounced healthy and referred to mental health.

Ross switched on the VCR. The image was grainy, and the camera danced around a good deal, as if the person holding it was trying to contain laughter. It showed a pajama-clad Ross sitting up in bed. Although his eyes were open, he didn't appear to be focused on anything. His face registered no emotion. At first he only pulled—aimlessly, it seemed—at the sheet and blanket. Suddenly he swung his feet to the floor and stood up. He slipped off his pajama top and let it fall onto the bed. Then he walked out through the door into the hallway.

For two or three minutes the camera followed him. He walked up and down the hall several times and finally disappeared into the bathroom, where the camera did not follow. When he emerged, another young man ("That's Ted, one of my roommates," Ross explained) appeared on screen and tried to engage him in conversation. Ross responded with a few syllables, none of which was a recognizable word. Finally, he allowed Ted to guide him gently back to his bed. Almost as soon as he had lain down, he appeared to be asleep. The entire film lasted perhaps 10 minutes.

"When they showed me this the next morning, I was amazed. I hadn't the slightest idea I'd done anything but sleep that night. I never do."

Evaluation of Ross Josephson

Although sleepwalking is not considered pathological in children, adults with Sleepwalking Disorder may have a **personality disorder** or other serious psychopathology. They should be carefully investigated with a full interview. However, occasional sleepwalking may be nonpathological.

The differential diagnosis also includes **psychomotor epilepsy**, which can begin during sleep and present with sleepwalking. The dissociative condition known as **Dissociative Fugue** may sometimes be confused with sleepwalking, but fugues last longer and involve complex behaviors, such as speaking complete sentences. **Sleep drunkenness** is a rare abnormality of awakening in which the patient feels confused for a prolonged period while awakening. It can involve irrational, even violent behavior. Nighttime wandering can also be found in **sleep apnea**. In Ross, there was no evidence for **substance use**.

Other nightime disturbances and sleep disorders can be associated with sleepwalking; these include nocturnal **Enuresis**, **Nightmare Disorder**, and **Sleep Terror Disorder**. **Generalized Anxiety Disorder, Posttraumatic Stress Disorder,** and **mood disorders** can also occur. However, none of these conditions is suggested in the vignette. Ross's complete diagnosis would thus be as follows:

Axis I	307.46	Sleepwalking Disorder
Axis II	V71.09	No diagnosis
Axis III		None
Axis IV		None
Axis V	GAF = 75	(current)

307.47 Parasomnia Not Otherwise Specified

You can use the Parasomnia Not Otherwise Specified category to code parasomnias that don't meet the criteria for Nightmare, Sleep Terror, or Sleepwalking Disorders.

> **REM sleep behavior disorder.** This consists of sometimes violent sudden movements that occur during REM sleep. Upon awakening (which happens readily), the patient reports vivid dreams that correspond to the behavior.

> **Sleep paralysis.** Occurring either at onset of sleep or upon awakening, these episodes can cause profound anxiety, even the fear that the patient is about to die. It is a common component of Narcolepsy, but the two should not both be coded in such cases.

Each of the following conditions, and many other medical conditions that occur during sleep, should be coded on Axis III. They are mentioned for the sake of help with differential diagnosis.

> **Bruxism.** Tooth grinding, which can occur 25 times per night or more, can be loud enough to awaken a bed partner. It usually begins when the patient is a teenager and increases with stress. It is apparently common.

> **Sleep-related cluster headaches.** Patients experience this type of headache as severe pain around the eyes, with tearing and nasal engorgement. Triggered by sleep, it may occur nightly for several weeks, then may be absent for months.

SLEEP DISORDERS RELATED TO ANOTHER MENTAL DISORDER

To a considerable extent, it's a matter of taste whether to diagnosis a sleep disorder that occurs secondary to another Axis I or an Axis II condition. The DSM-IV criteria state that this is appropriate when the problem with sleep is serious enough to justify an evaluation in its own right. If the patient's presenting complaint is the sleep problem, this should be considered evidence of clinical importance. However, the situation is often unclear and usually requires judgment. In the example of a mood disorder, any problem with sleep is almost certainly a *symptom* that will resolve once the depression has been adequately treated. Therefore, no one could be faulted for diagnosing only the mood disorder. In any event, the mood disorder should be listed first, because it is by far the more important.

307.42 Insomnia Related to Another Mental Disorder

As noted earlier in the chapter, sleep disturbance is primarily a symptom; insomnia is symptomatic of many mental disorders. It is often directly proportional to the severity of the mental disorder. Logically, sleep improves once the underlying condition has resolved. Many Axis I and II conditions and disorders often present as sleep problems, for which patients may abuse hypnotic and other medications:

Depression. Insomnia is probably most often a symptom of a mood disorder. In fact, sleep disturbance may be one of the earliest symptoms of depression. Elderly depressed patients are especially likely to have insomnia. In severe depression, terminal insomnia (awakening early in the morning and being unable to get back to sleep) is characteristic.

Anxiety disorders. The criteria for Generalized Anxiety Disorder and for Posttraumatic Stress Disorder specifically mention sleep disturbance as a symptom, but Panic Attacks may also occur during sleep.

Adjustment Disorder. Patients who have developed anxiety or depression in response to a specific stressor may lie awake worrying about their particular stressor or the day's events.

Somatization Disorder. Many somatizing patients will complain of problems with sleep, especially initial and interval insomnia.

Cognitive disorders. Most demented patients have some degree of sleep disturbance, typically interval awakening. They wander at night and suffer from reduced alertness during the day.

Manic and Hypomanic Episodes. In a 24-four hour period, manic and hypomanic patients typically sleep less than they do when they are euthymic. However, they do not complain of insomnia. They feel rested and ready for more activity; their families and friends are the ones who become concerned. If they (or their relatives) do complain, it is usually of lengthened *sleep onset latency* (the time it takes to fall asleep).

Schizophrenia. When they are becoming ill, delusions, hallucinations, or anxiety may keep schizophrenic patients preoccupied later and later into the night. Total sleep time may remain constant, but they arise progressively later, until most of their sleeping occurs during the day. DSM-IV does not provide a way to code a circadian rhythm disorder related to an Axis I disorder; Insomnia Related to Schizophrenia is about the best we can do.

Obsessive–Compulsive Personality Disorder. This personality disorder is commonly cited as an Axis II disorder associated with insomnia.

> **TIP** Anxiety or mania may mask an insomnia that occurs in the course of an Axis I disorder. Patients may not recognize a sleep deficit until they fall asleep at the wheel or suffer an industrial accident. On the other hand, clinicians sometimes focus on the problem with sleep and underdiagnose the underlying mental problem.

Criteria for Insomnia Related to Another Mental Disorder

- For at least a month, the patient's main complaint has been trouble going to sleep, trouble staying asleep, or feeling unrested.
- The insomnia causes daytime fatigue or impairs daytime functioning.
- The insomnia (or its daytime results) causes clinically important distress or impairs work, social, or personal functioning.
- Although it is serious enough to warrant clinical attention, the clinician believes that another Axis I or II disorder (such as Generalized Anxiety Disorder, Major Depressive Disorder, or Adjustment Disorder) causes it.
- Another sleep disorder (such as a parasomnia, Narcolepsy, or Breathing-Related Sleep Disorder) does not explain the symptoms better.
- The insomnia is not directly caused by a general medical condition or by the use of substances, including medications.

Coding Note

Use the name of the actual related mental disorder in the Axis I sleep disorder diagnosis. Also, code the mental disorder itself on Axis I or II, as appropriate.

Sal Camozzi

"I'm just not getting enough sleep to play." Sal Camozzi was a third-year student who attended a small liberal arts college in southern California on a football scholarship. Now it was early November, midway through the season, and he didn't think he could keep up the effort. He had always kept regular hours and "eaten healthy," but for over a month he had been awakening at 2:30 every morning.

"I might as well be setting an alarm," he said. "My eyes click open and there I am, worrying about the next game, or passing chemistry, or whatever. I'm only getting five hours at night, and I've always needed eight. I'm getting desperate."

For a while Sal had tried over-the-counter sleep medications. They helped a little, but mainly they made him feel groggy the next day. He gave them up; he had always avoided alcohol and drugs, and hated the feeling of chemicals in his body.

Sal had had something of the same problem the previous fall, and the one before that. Then he had had the same difficulty with sleep; his appetite had fallen off, too. Neither time had things been as severe as now, however. (This year he had already lost 10 pounds; as a linebacker, he needed to keep his weight up.) Sal also complained that he just didn't seem to enjoy life in general the way he usually did. Although his interest in football and his concentration on the field had diminished, it hadn't been as bad last year, and he had finished the season with respectable statistics.

One summer during high school, Sal had felt listless and slept too much. He'd been tested for infectious mononucleosis and found to be physically well. He was his normal self by the time school started that fall.

Last spring and the one before had been a different matter. When Sal went out for baseball, he seemed to explode with energy, batted .400, and played every game. He didn't sleep much then, either, when he came to think of it, though five hours a night had seemed plenty. "I had loads of energy and never felt happier in my life. I felt like another Babe Ruth."

The coach had noted that Sal had been "terrific during baseball season, all hustle, but he talked too much. Why doesn't he put the same effort into football?"

Evaluation of Sal Camozzi

From Sal's history, he did not have a **Substance-Induced Sleep Disorder** or one related to a **general medical condition**. There was similarly no evidence for **another sleep disorder**.

Sal's sleep difficulty was actually only the tip of his depressive iceberg. The first thing to look for would be other symptoms of a Major Depressive Episode. Although he didn't complain in so many words of feeling depressed, he did report a general loss of zest for life. Besides that and the insomnia, Sal had also lost his appetite, interest, and concentration. Together, his symptoms would barely meet criteria for a **Major Depressive Episode**. The history did not touch on death wishes or suicidal ideas; it should have.

Besides depression, the obvious episodes of high mood would need to be considered in the diagnosis. Sal had had several periods when he felt unusually happy, his energy level increased, he talked a great deal, and his need for sleep decreased. Especially in contrast to his present mood, his self-esteem was markedly increased (he noted that he felt like Babe Ruth). This change in his mood was pronounced enough that others noticed and commented on it, but it did not compromise his functioning or require hospitalization (it would have then instead been diagnosed as a **Manic Episode**). These symptoms would fulfill criteria for a **Hypomanic Episode**.

All of this would add up to a diagnosis of **Bipolar II Disorder** (see p. 219); Sal's current episode would be designated Depressed. He would qualify for none of the episode specifiers, though he would nearly meet the criteria for With Melancholic Features. However, his history of repeated depressions beginning in the same season of the year (fall, in this instance) and consistently either resolving or switching to hypomania during another season (spring) would be typical for the course specifier **With Seasonal Pattern**. Although Sal may have had one episode of depression when he was in high school that did not fit this pattern, most of the episodes did. And the last two years fit the mold exactly.

Sal's sleeplessness would have been clinically significant even without the Bipolar II Disorder, and this would meet the DSM-IV criteria for coding it. As always, however, the diagnosis most in need of clinical intervention would be listed first:

Axis I	296.89	Bipolar II Disorder, Depressed, With Full Interepisode Recovery, With Seasonal Pattern
	307.42	Insomnia Related to Bipolar II Disorder
Axis II	V71.09	No diagnosis
Axis III		None
Axis IV		None
Axis V	GAF = 55	(current)

307.44 Hypersomnia Related to Another Mental Disorder

Hypersomnia is less likely than insomnia to be found with another mental disorder, and fewer mental disorders have been associated with it. Of course, any mental disorder that produces insomnia may lead to daytime sleepiness. However, hypersomnia is a criterion of one important mental disorder subtype and is occasionally associated with several others.

In the With Atypical Features subtype of either Major Depressive Episode or Dysthymic Disorder, the patient complains not of insomnia but of hypersomnia.

Usually relatively young (around college age), these patients complain of feeling unrefreshed from a night's sleep; they may sleep longer than usual in the morning and take naps. The hypersomnia is associated with other symptoms that are somewhat atypical for depression, including increased appetite (rather than decreased), weight gain (not loss), and feeling worse in the evening (instead of in the morning, which is the case for the With Melancholic Features subtype).

In other Axis I disorders, if the patient complains of hypersomnia, it is usually due to daytime drowsiness rather than sleeping excessively at night. This is the case with the somatoform disorders (Hypochondriasis, Somatization Disorder, Conversion Disorder), the dissociative disorders, the personality disorders, and Posttraumatic Stress Disorder. As noted earlier, Schizophrenia patients may suffer from drowsiness resembling that seen in the Delayed Sleep Phase Type of Circadian Rhythm Sleep Disorder.

Criteria for Hypersomnia Related to Another Mental Disorder

- For at least a month, the patient's main complaint has been excessive sleepiness. This has occurred almost daily and has been shown by either or both of these:
  - ✓ Prolonged sleep *or*
  - ✓ Sleeping during the day, almost daily
- This sleepiness causes clinically important distress or impairs work, social, or personal functioning.
- Although it is serious enough to warrant clinical attention, the clinician believes that another Axis I or II disorder (such as Dysthymic Disorder or Major Depressive Disorder) causes it.
- Neither inadequate sleep nor another sleep disorder (such as a parasomnia, Narcolepsy, or Breathing-Related Sleep Disorder) explains the symptoms better.
- The hypersomnia is not directly caused by a general medical condition or by the use of substances, including medications.

Coding Note

Use the name of the actual related mental disorder in the Axis I sleep disorder diagnosis. Also, code the mental disorder itself on Axis I or II, as appropriate.

Adelaide Turner

"I'm going to get fired if I can't get this under control," Adelaide Turner complained. She had appeared 20 minutes late for her appointment. "I was taking a nap," she explained with an embarrassed smile. For weeks she had been nodding off at work. Even when her eyes would stay open, they felt scratchy and frequently filled with tears, and that kept her from seeing her work properly.

Adelaide was 38 and single. She worked in a small shop that assembled computers in Silicon Valley. She liked her job, but she knew that her employer operated on a small profit margin and depended upon her for production.

"What I've produced the most these days has been naps," she said. Her company had a small employees' lounge. For at least a month, Adelaide had felt so tired that she had lain down a few minutes several times a day. These naps were short and dreamless, and left her feeling no better than before.

Adelaide was a single mother, and she thought that this might have something to do with it. Her father had been diagnosed as manic-depressive. After the death of her parents, she had been reared in an orphanage. She had always promised herself she'd do better by her own child.

"He's a good kid, but he's 15, and lately I feel so cross I yell at him for everything. Everything he does—well, everything *everyone* does—seems to annoy me." With questioning, Adelaide realized that she had been feeling depressed most of the time, though the "just angry" had been the most obvious part.

Adelaide didn't use drugs or alcohol. Until this episode, both her physical and mental health had been excellent. She had never before had problems with her mood—or her sleep, for that matter.

Five or six weeks before this appointment, she'd first noticed she was having problems. She had given up her night school class in accounting because she just couldn't keep her mind on the homework. ("And I always loved math in high school.") Without the class, she felt bored and useless, as if she were reaching the end of her life.

Perhaps to compensate, Adelaide ate. She had never been skinny, and now she had put on an additional 25 pounds. About the only bright spot in her life was her relationship with her boyfriend, Jules. "I always feel better when he comes around," she remarked. "For over a year we've talked about getting married, but I've been burned before. Now it's beginning to seem more attractive. Then I could quit work and sleep forever."

Evaluation of Adelaide Turner

Adelaide was a typical example of a patient whose chief complaint is one thing and whose illness is another. Although she complained of excessive sleepiness, which she perceived was about to get her fired, it quickly became apparent that her underlying problem was a depressive disorder. Fortunately, her clinician was alert enough to pick this up. The first task was to identify the mood disorder.

Adelaide admitted to the following symptoms for **Major Depressive Episode**: depressed mood, weight gain, hypersomnia, fatigue, a sense of worthlessness, and trouble concentrating (on her night school homework). All in all, she had been feeling quite different from her usual self for over a month. (She could not have **Dysthymic Disorder**, because she had been depressed far less than two years.) Her health had been good; there was no evidence that her problem was due to a **general medical condition** or to **substance use**.

Adelaide had never had a previous episode of mood disorder, so her diagnosis could not be a **Bipolar I or II Disorder**. This would thus be **Major Depressive Disorder, Single Episode** (see p. 203). According to the severity criteria, she would probably fall between Mild and Severe. She qualified for only one of the episode specifiers, **With Atypical Features**: mood reactivity (she brightened up when she was with Jules, her boyfriend); weight gain and increased appetite; and hypersomnia.

Her clinician decided that Adelaide's sleep disorder warranted a separate diagnosis because drowsiness at work was her presenting complaint. Her complete diagnosis would be as follows:

Axis I	296.22	Major Depressive Disorder, Single Episode, Moderate, With Atypical Features
	307.44	Hypersomnia Related to Major Depressive Disorder
Axis II	V71.09	No diagnosis
Axis III		None
Axis IV		Single mother
Axis V	GAF = 55	(current)

OTHER SLEEP DISORDERS

As with most other groups of disorders in DSM-IV, there are specific codes to use when diagnosing a sleep disorder that you believe is caused by a physical illness or by the use of a substance. Here they are.

780.5x Sleep Disorder Due to a General Medical Condition

Many general medical conditions can result in sleep problems (mostly insomnia). The usual complaints are restlessness, increased sleep onset latency, and frequent awakenings during the night. It should be obvious that such problems occur, especially with medical conditions that can produce discomfort day or night. These include the following:

Fever resulting from a variety of infections.

Pain caused by headache (especially some migraines), rheumatoid arthritis, cancer, painful nocturnal penile erections, or angina.

Itching caused by a variety of systemic and skin disorders.

Breathing problems resulting from asthma or chronic obstructive pulmonary disease (COPD); restricted lung capacity (due to obesity, pregnancy, or spinal deformities); or cystic fibrosis

Endocrine and metabolic diseases, including hyperthyroidism, liver failure, and kidney disease.

Enforced sleeping in one position (e.g., because of wearing a cast)

Neuromuscular disorders, such as muscular dystrophy and poliomyelitis.

Movement and other neurological disorders, such as Huntington's disease, torsion dystonia, Parkinson's disease, and some seizure disorders.

Criteria for Sleep Disorder Due to a General Medical Condition

- The patient has a sleep problem serious enough to warrant clinical attention.
- History, physical exam, or laboratory findings suggest a general medical condition that seems likely to have directly caused this problem.
- The sleep problem causes clinically important distress or impairs work, social, or personal functioning.
- It isn't better explained by another mental disorder (such as Adjustment Disorder, with a serious medical condition as the stressor).
- The problem does not meet criteria for Narcolepsy or a Breathing-Related Sleep Disorder.
- It doesn't occur solely during a delirium.

Coding Notes

Based on predominant symptoms, specify:

780.52	Insomnia Type
780.54	Hypersomnia Type
780.59	Parasomnia Type
780.59	Mixed Type (there is more than one type and none predominates)

Use the name of the actual general medical condition in the Axis I name. Code the general medical condition itself on Axis III.

Hoyle Garner

Hoyle Garner was 58 when he sought treatment for his insomnia. His wife, Edith, accompanied him to the appointment. Together, they ran a "mom and pop" grocery store.

Several years earlier, Hoyle had learned that he had emphysema. A series of pulmonary function tests had prompted his doctor to ask him to quit smoking. After three weeks he had gained 10 pounds and couldn't concentrate well enough to add up the receipts from the store each night. "I was depressed and uptight, and I couldn't sleep two hours without waking up, wanting a cigarette," said Hoyle.

"I begged him to start smoking again," said Edith. "When he did, it was a relief for both of us."

Hoyle quit seeing the doctor, and his sleep returned to normal. Within the past few months, however, he'd begun awakening several times during the course of the night. Some nights this happened as often as every hour. He felt restless and uncomfortable, with some of the same anxiety that he had experienced the time he tried to quit smoking. A few times he tried sitting on the edge of the bed to have a cigarette, but it didn't seem to help. And anyway, Edith complained about the smell of smoke in the night. They still ran their grocery, and Hoyle was having no trouble at all with his columns of figures. He never drank more than a single beer, usually in the afternoon.

"Waking up doesn't bother him much," Edith complained. "He usually goes right back to sleep again. He doesn't even feel sleepy the next day. But it leaves me wide awake, wondering how soon he'll wake up again."

Edith's hours awake had given her plenty of opportunity to observe her husband. After he slept quietly for half an hour or so, his breathing seemed to become rapid and shallow. It never stopped for longer than a few seconds, and he never snored. They had tried having him sleep with extra pillows (it had helped her Uncle Will with his heart failure), but it hadn't eased Hoyle's sleeping any, and it "kinda hurt his neck."

"I hope we can get to the bottom of this," Edith concluded. "It doesn't seem to bother him very much, but I've got to get some sleep."

TIP How do you decide that one event has caused another? Of course, in clinical diagnosis, you can hardly ever be positive. But several features can help you decide with a reasonable degree of certainty that *A* has caused *B*. Some of these are set down in Chapter 18.

Evaluation of Hoyle Garner

Hoyle's sleep problem was less than earth-shaking, but it did cause difficulties for his wife. Typically, a patient with insomnia due to COPD does not complain of daytime drowsiness.

The features of Hoyle's insomnia would *not* suggest a severe **mood disorder**, which might be expected to produce early morning awakening. A mild mood disorder (or **Adjustment Disorder With Depressed Mood**) is typically associated with trouble falling asleep. Based on Edith's observations of his sleep, Hoyle did not have **sleep apnea**. (Do check for sleep apnea in any patient with Sleep Disorder Due to a General Medical Condition; a small number will have two disorders.) There was absolutely no evidence for **Narcolepsy**. He was taking no medications at the time, but many patients with general medical conditions will be doing so; in such cases, **Substance-Induced Sleep Disorder** will have to be ruled out. The type of sleep disturbance determines the last digit of the code number. In Hoyle's case, it was insomnia.

Hoyle could also be diagnosed as having Nicotine Dependence (it was probably responsible for the emphysema in the first place). When he was trying to quit smoking, he clearly experienced Nicotine Withdrawal, and he continued to smoke despite his COPD. His complete diagnosis would thus be as follows:

Axis I	780.52	Sleep Disorder Due to Chronic Obstructive Pulmonary Disease, Insomnia Type
	305.10	Nicotine Dependence
Axis II	V71.09	No diagnosis
Axis III	492.8	Pulmonary emphysema
Axis IV		None
Axis V	GAF = 61	(current)

Substance-Induced Sleep Disorder

As you might expect, substances of abuse can also produce a variety of sleep disorders, most of which will be either insomnia or hypersomnia. The specific problem with sleep can occur during either intoxication or withdrawal.

Alcohol. Heavy alcohol use can produce unrefreshing sleep with strong REM suppression and reduced total sleep time. Patients may experience terminal insomnia, and sometimes hypersomnia. They may continue to have sleep problems that persist for years. Alcohol Withdrawal markedly increases sleep onset latency and produces restless sleep with frequent awakenings. Patients may experience delirium with (especially visual) hallucinations; this was formerly known as delirium tremens.

Sedatives, hypnotics, and anxiolytics. These include barbiturates, over-the-counter antihistamines, bromides, short-acting benzodiazepines, and high doses of long-acting benzodiazepines. Any of these substances may be used in the attempt to remedy insomnia of another origin. They can lead to sleep disorder during either tolerance or withdrawal.

Central nervous system stimulants. Amphetamines and other stimulants typically cause increased sleep onset latency, decreased REM sleep, and more awakenings. Once the drug is discontinued, hypersomnia with restlessness and REM rebound dreams may ensue.

Caffeine. This popular drug produces insomnia with intoxication and hypersomnia upon withdrawal. (No surprises here.)

Other drugs. These include tricyclic antidepressants, neuroleptics, ACTH, anticonvulsants, thyroid medications, marijuana, cocaine, LSD, opioids, PCP, and methyldopa.

Criteria for Substance-Induced Sleep Disorder

- The patient has a sleep problem serious enough to warrant clinical attention.
- History, physical exam, or laboratory data substantiate that *either*
  - ✓ These symptoms have developed within a month of Substance Intoxication or Withdrawal, *or*
  - ✓ Medication use has caused the symptoms.
- No other sleep disorder better accounts for these symptoms.
- The symptoms don't occur solely during a delirium.
- The symptoms cause clinically important distress or impair work, social, or personal functioning.

Coding Notes

Assign a code number based on the specific substance:

291.8	Alcohol
292.89	Amphetamine (or Amphetamine-Like Substance); Caffeine; Cocaine; Opioid; Sedative, Hypnotic, or Anxiolytic; Other [or Unknown] Substance

Depending on the dominant symptomatology, specify:

Insomnia Type
Hypersomnia Type
Parasomnia Type
Mixed Type (there is more than one type and none predominates)

If criteria are met for Substance Intoxication or Withdrawal for the particular substance *and* symptoms develop during that phase, specify:

With Onset During Intoxication

With Onset During Withdrawal

No other sleep disorder must better account for the symptoms than does substance use. Historical information could suggest that this is the case:

Sleep disorder symptoms precede the onset of substance use.

There have been previous episodes of a sleep disorder not related to substance use.

The symptoms are much worse than you would expect for the amount and duration of the substance use.

Sleep disorder symptoms continue long (at least a month) after Substance Intoxication or Withdrawal stops.

The diagnosis of a Substance-Induced Sleep Disorder should be made only when the symptoms considerably exceed what would be expected from an ordinary case of Substance Intoxication or Withdrawal for that specific substance.

Dave Kincaid

Dave Kincaid was a free-lance writer. As Dave explained it, "free-lance" was the industry's way of saying that you were unemployed. He'd actually done reasonably well for himself, specializing in interviews with unimportant (but very interesting) people. Most of his work was published in small magazines and specialized reviews. His two books, a novel and a volume of travel essays, had received good reviews and disappointing sales; they were remaindered early.

When he had to, Dave supported his writing by working. To gather material for his writing, he tried to make his jobs as varied as possible. He had driven a taxi, been a bouncer at a bar, sold real estate, and (in his younger days) been a guide on the Jungle River Cruise at Disneyland. Now 35, he had been supporting his third book, a murder mystery, by working in a coffee roastery north of San Francisco for the last several months. The job didn't pay much over minimum wage, but neither did it demand very much of him. Except for the busy two or three hours around noon, it left him with plenty of time for blocking out the section of his book that he planned to write that night.

It also left Dave time to drink coffee. Besides grinding beans or selling them whole, the roastery served coffee by the cup. Employees could drink what they wanted. Dave was a coffee drinker, but he had always limited himself to three or four cups a day. "It sure isn't enough to explain the way I'm feeling now."

How he was feeling was, in a word, nervous. It was worst at night. "I have this uncomfortable, 'up' sort of feeling, and I want to write. But sometimes I just can't sit still at the word processor. I get that 'live flesh' sensation when your muscles twitch. And my heart beats fast and my gut seems to pour out water, so I have to spend a lot of time in the bathroom."

Dave seldom got to sleep before 2 A.M., sometimes after much tossing and turning. On Sundays he slept until noon, but Monday through Saturday he awakened to his alarm feeling hung over and in desperate need of a cup of coffee.

Dave's health had been excellent. Although he had seldom been in a job where he had a health plan, he had never needed one. Other than the mornings, his mood was good. He had tried marijuana in the past, but didn't like it. He confined his drinking to coffee, but "only three or four cups a day," he said again. He also denied drinking tea, cocoa, or cola beverages. As an afterthought, he added, "Of course, there are the coffee beans."

When things were slow in the afternoon and Dave was thinking about his novel, he would dip into the supply of candy-coated coffee beans the roastery also sold ($4.95 the half-pound). They came coated in white or dark chocolate; he preferred the dark. They also had decaffeinated beans, but these were dipped in yogurt, which he didn't care for at all.

"I don't keep track," said Dave, "but all in all, every afternoon I probably have a few handsful or so."

Evaluation of Dave Kincaid

Dave's symptoms of caffeinism included restlessness, nervousness, muscle twitching, intestinal upset, rapid heartbeat, and above all else, sleeplessness. He needed only five symptoms to fulfill the criteria for **Caffeine Intoxication**.

Although Dave drank fairly modest amounts of coffee, it was very strong and by itself probably contained more than the 250 mg or so usually required for Caffeine Intoxication. He also ate coffee beans; it takes about 35 beans to make a strong cup of brewed coffee, and he consumed several handsful. He may have eaten the equivalent of several additional cups of coffee per day. No wonder he felt nervous.

Associated with his caffeine use, Dave noted increased latency of sleep onset. He felt tired when it was time to get up, and he had to use coffee to get going. Therefore, the basic criteria for a Substance-Induced Sleep Disorder were all met: Use of a substance caused a problem with sleep serious enough to require clinical attention.

Of course, all manner of other sleep disorders could theoretically be responsible (including **Primary Insomnia** and **Sleep Disorder Due to a General Medical Condition, Insomnia Type**), but the rational course is to eliminate (gradually) the caffeine use, then reassess the patient's sleep. This was what Dave's clinician did. In some cases, there can be confusion as to the etiological contributions of the general medical condition and the medications that are used to treat it. At times, two diagnoses may be warranted.

The diagnosis of a Substance-Induced *anything* rests on the clinician's determination that the symptoms are more serious than would be expected from ordinary Substance Intoxication or Withdrawal. This is a judgment call. In the case of Dave Kincaid, the symptoms were sufficiently prominent to bring him for evaluation. With the subtype specifiers required in the criteria, his full diagnosis would be as follows:

Axis I	305.90	Caffeine Intoxication
	292.89	Caffeine-Induced Sleep Disorder, Insomnia Type, With Onset During Intoxication
Axis II	V71.09	No diagnosis
Axis III		None
Axis IV		None
Axis V	GAF = 65	(current)

Impulse-Control Disorders Not Elsewhere Classified

Quick Guide to Impulsive Behavior

As usual, the page number following each item indicates where a more detailed discussion begins.

Impulse-Control Disorders

Intermittent Explosive Disorder. With no other demonstrable pathology (psychological or general medical), these patients have episodes during which they act out aggressively. As a result, they physically harm others or destroy property (p. 441).

Kleptomania. An irresistible impulse to steal objects they don't need causes these patients to do so repeatedly. The phrase "tension and release" characterizes this behavior (p. 443).

Pyromania. Fire setters feel "tension and release" in regard to the behavior of starting fires (p. 445).

Pathological Gambling. These patients repeatedly gamble, often until they lose money, jobs, and friends (p. 448).

Trichotillomania. Pulling hair from various parts of the body is accompanied by feelings of "tension and release" (p. 451).

Impulse-Control Disorder Not Otherwise Specified. Use this category for problems with impulse control that do not meet the criteria either for the disorders above or for any others in DSM-IV (p. 453).

Other Causes of Impulsive Behavior

Paraphilias. Some people (nearly always males) have recurrent sexual urges involving a variety of behaviors that are objectionable to others. They may act upon these urges in order to obtain pleasure (p. 360).

Substance-Related Disorders. "Tension and release" can characterize the impulsive behaviors connected with substance misuse (p. 62).

Bipolar I Disorder. Bipolar I patients may steal, gamble, act out violently, and engage in other socially undesirable behaviors, though this happens only during an acute Manic Episode (p. 195).

Schizophrenia. In response to hallucinations or delusions, schizophrenic patients may impulsively engage in a variety of illegal or otherwise ill-advised behaviors (p. 143).

Antisocial Personality Disorder. Marked impulsivity characterizes antisocial patients, who often act out violently or illegally. They do not experience the "tension and release" typical of some impulse-control disorders (p. 474).

Introduction

The section of DSM-IV covered in this chapter contains a number of leftovers—problems that have characteristics in common with the substance-related disorders and paraphilias, but for obvious reasons are not classified with those disorders. The behaviors described here are violence, stealing, hair pulling, gambling, and fire setting. This is not as uniform a classification as we might wish, but there is a certain cohesiveness to the behaviors it includes. In all cases, the act is *ego-syntonic* (i.e., it takes place in accord with the patient's conscious wishes).

These patients cannot or do not resist impulses, urges, or temptations to do something that harms themselves or others. The behavior in question may occur on the spur of the moment, or it may be planned; it may be (but need not be) accompanied by an attempt to resist it. "Tension and release" is a phrase that describes three of these five conditions. It expresses the typical buildup of anxiety or tension, sometimes for a day or more, until the impulse to act becomes overwhelming. Once the action has been taken, the person experiences a sense of release that may be perceived as relief or pleasure, although remorse or regret may be experienced later.

Two of these disorders do not entail "tension and release" in connection with performing a harmful act. Intermittent Explosive Disorder specifies only that episodes of violent behavior must occur; the criteria for Pathological Gambling are quite similar to those for Substance Dependence. Nonetheless, all of these disorders involve violent, illegal, or harmful acts that can cause unwanted (and often disastrous) consequences for patients and those around them.

> **TIP** There are a number of "-manias" in this chapter. Here, the term is not used by itself in the sense of having a Manic Episode. Instead, as a suffix, it means having a passion or enthusiasm for something.

312.34 Intermittent Explosive Disorder

Intermittent Explosive Disorder is a controversial category. Despite criteria and a few studies, some clinicians still hold that it only exists as a symptom of all the disorders mentioned as exclusions in the diagnostic criteria. What's important about this is that you should vigorously attempt to rule out all other possible causes of explosive episodes before diagnosing this disorder.

A patient's aggressive episodes generally begin suddenly ("hair-trigger temper"). Often they end just as suddenly, with the patient expressing genuine regret for the destructive behavior. Most of these patients are young men. Many have had frequent traffic accidents and moving violations; sexual impulsiveness is another feature sometimes encountered in these patients.

In the past, Intermittent Explosive Disorder has been called *episodic dyscontrol syndrome* and *explosive personality*. By all estimates, it is very rare.

> **TIP** Some of these patients are exquisitely sensitive to alcohol. The condition in which any person has marked loss of behavioral control after just a drink or two used to be called *pathological intoxication*. Although this diagnosis no longer appears in DSM-IV, the concept may have some clinical relevance.

Criteria for Intermittent Explosive Disorder

- On several occasions the patient has lost control of aggressive impulses, leading to serious assault or property destruction.
- The aggression is markedly out of proportion to the seriousness of any social or psychological stressors.

- No other mental disorder or personality disorder better explains the symptoms.
- These symptoms are not directly caused by a general medical condition or by the use of substances, including medications.

Coding Note

DSM-IV specifically mentions Antisocial Personality Disorder, Borderline Personality Disorder, Attention-Deficit/Hyperactivity Disorder, Conduct Disorder, Manic Episode, and psychotic disorders as diagnoses that must be ruled out.

Liam O'Brian

From the time he was a teenager, Liam O'Brian had had a flash-point temper. He had been suspended from 10th grade for using a pair of scissors to assault a classmate who had teased him about wearing the wrong colors on "Clash Day." The following year the police had visited him for breaking a headlamp on the car belonging to the baseball coach, who had called him "out" in a close play at home plate. After he paid for the headlamp, charges were dropped; the coach noted that Liam was "basically a good kid with too much red hair." That year a neurologist reported that his physical exam, EEG and MRI were all normal.

During his first few years of school, Liam had had difficulty sitting still in class and concentrating on his school work. By the time he entered junior high, these behaviors were no longer a problem. In fact, he earned mostly B's and A's, and in the two- to four-month intervals between explosive episodes he was "no more trouble than the average kid," as Liam himself reported to the interviewer.

Following Liam's graduation from high school, his pattern of periodic temper flareups continued pretty much unchanged. After he was fired from two successive jobs for fighting with coworkers, he joined the Army. Within six weeks he had received a bad-conduct discharge for assaulting his first sergeant with a bayonet. Each of these incidents had been triggered by a trivial disagreement or an exchange of words that could hardly be called provocation. Liam said afterwards that he felt bad about his behavior; even the targets of his attacks usually agreed that he "wasn't mean, only touchy."

Liam was now 25, and his most recent evaluation had been ordered by a judge. Liam had been arrested by an off-duty policewoman in a supermarket. He had pushed her after she dumped 15 cans of tuna onto the carousel in the express checkout line. The usual examinations, X-rays, and EEG (this time with esophageal leads and sleep recordings) revealed no pathology. He denied ever having delusions or hallucinations. His father, he said, used to rough up his mother when he was drinking, so Liam had always been afraid to try alcohol or drugs himself.

Liam denied ever having extreme swings of mood, but he did express regret for his unpredictable, explosive behavior. "I just want to get a handle on it," he said. "I'm afraid I just might kill someone, and I'm not mad at anyone."

Evaluation of Liam O'Brian

Liam had a history of many episodes of dyscontrol over a period of at least 10 years. The fact of his behavior would not be the issue here. Rather, a clinician evaluating Liam should carefully search for evidence of exclusions that might indicate a less controversial diagnosis (and perhaps a more readily treatable one).

Liam's mood showed no evidence of either mania or depression, effectively ruling out temper flareups that could be associated with **mood disorder**. At wide intervals he had had two neurological evaluations, neither of which found evidence for **seizures**. He never touched **drugs or alcohol**, and he denied symptoms of **psychosis**. The presence of any such underlying medical disorder would suggest a diagnosis of **Personality Change Due to a General Medical Condition, Aggressive Type**, but there was no evidence of this either.

Patients with **Antisocial Personality Disorder** will often act out violently and unpredictably, but, unlike Liam, they do not feel remorse afterwards. Neither did he have the pervasive history of disregard for the rights of others that is required by DSM-IV for this diagnosis. Patients with **Borderline Personality Disorder** will sometimes have temper outbursts and engage in fights, but Liam did not show other typical traits, such as identity disturbance and affective instability. His five-axis diagnosis would thus read as follows:

Axis I	312.34	Intermittent Explosive Disorder
Axis II	V71.09	No diagnosis
Axis III		None
Axis IV		None
Axis V	GAF = 51	(current)

312.32 Kleptomania

The stealing that occurs in Kleptomania is not a result of need, or even necessarily of desire. These patients characteristically do not need the objects they steal; when caught, they typically have enough money with them to pay for whatever they have taken. Once they have left the scene undetected, they may give away or discard their loot. These patients recognize that their behavior is wrong, but they cannot resist.

Kleptomania is one of the oldest diagnoses in DSM-IV; it dates back over 200 years. It is also probably a highly overused diagnosis—fewer than 1 out of

20 shoplifters can be diagnosed with this disorder. However, when caught, many try to avoid prosecution by claiming that they were driven by an irresistible impulse. Despite its antiquity, Kleptomania remains poorly understood and poorly defined. Once it begins (often in childhood), it tends to be chronic.

Criteria for Kleptomania

- The patient repeatedly yields to the impulse to steal objects that are needed neither for personal use nor for their monetary worth.
- Just before the theft, the patient experiences increasing tension.
- At the time of theft, the patient feels gratification, pleasure, or relief.
- These thefts are committed neither out of anger or revenge nor in response to delusions or hallucinations.
- The thefts are not better explained by Antisocial Personality Disorder, Conduct Disorder, or a Manic Episode.

Roseanne Straub

"Fifteen years!" It was how long Roseanne Straub had been shoplifting, but from the expression on her tear-streaked face, it might have been the length of her sentence.

Roseanne was 27, and this was her second arrest, if you didn't count the one time as a juvenile. Three years earlier, she had been arrested, booked, and released on her own recognizance for walking out of a boutique with a silk blouse worth $150. Fortunately for her, two weeks later the shop fell victim to the recession; the owner, otherwise preoccupied, did not follow through with prosecution. Badly frightened, she had resisted the temptation to shoplift for several months afterwards.

Roseanne was married and had a four-year-old daughter. Her husband worked as a paralegal assistant. After her previous arrest, he had threatened to divorce her and obtain custody of their child if she did it again. She worked as a research assistant for a civilian contractor to the military. A conviction would also doom her security clearance and her job.

"I don't know why I do it. I've asked myself that question a thousand times." Aside from the stealing, Roseanne considered herself a pretty normal person. She had lots of friends and no enemies; most of the time she was quite happy. In every other respect she was law-abiding; she wouldn't even let her husband cheat when he prepared their taxes.

The first time Roseanne had ever stolen from a store was when she was six or seven, but that was on a dare from two school friends. When her mother found the candy she had taken from the convenience store, she had gone with Roseanne and made her return it to the store manager. It was years before she was tempted to steal again.

In junior high, she noticed that periodically a certain tension would build up inside her. It felt as if something deep within her pelvis itched and she couldn't scratch it. For several days she would feel increasingly restless, but with an excited sense of anticipation. Finally she would dart into whatever store she happened to be passing, whisk some article under her coat or into her handbag, and walk out, flooded with relief. For a time it seemed to be associated with her menstrual periods, but by the time she was 17 these episodes had become completely random events.

"I don't know why I do it," Roseanne said again. "Of course, I don't like being caught. But I deserved to be. I've ruined my life and the lives of my family. It's not as if I needed another compact—I must have 15 of them at home."

Evaluation of Roseanne Straub

Ordinary shoplifters plan their thefts and profit from them; they do not have the buildup of tension (with subsequent release) that characterized Roseanne's shoplifting episodes. Patients with **Antisocial Personality Disorder** may steal impulsively, but they will also have histories of committing many other antisocial acts. When criminals falsely claim to have symptoms of Kleptomania, **Malingering** may be diagnosed instead. Patients with **Schizophrenia** will sometimes have hallucinations that order them to steal things. Patients with a **Manic Episode** of **Bipolar I Disorder** may, too.

Anxiety, guilt, and depression are often found in patients with this disorder. Therefore, watch for diagnoses such as **Generalized Anxiety Disorder**, **Dysthymic Disorder**, and **Major Depressive Disorder**. Kleptomania may also be associated with the eating disorders, especially **Bulimia Nervosa**. Patients with **Substance Abuse** or **Dependence** may steal in order to support a drug habit. Many patients with Kleptomania have a concomitant **personality disorder**. None of these, however, applied to Roseanne, so her complete diagnosis would be as follows:

Axis I	312.32	Kleptomania
Axis II	V71.09	No diagnosis
Axis III		None
Axis IV		None
Axis V	GAF = 65	(current)

312.33 Pyromania

As is true of the relationship of Kleptomania to shoplifting, Pyromania accounts for only a small minority of fire setters. Only when there is a typical history of yielding with relief to an irresistible impulse can a diagnosis of Pyromania be sustained.

We have little concrete information about this rare condition. Ninety percent or more of these patients are male; often the behavior begins in childhood. These people may be interested in various aspects of fires, and will turn in false alarms, appear as spectators at fires, and show an interest in the apparatus used by firefighters. They may serve as volunteer firefighters.

Although Pyromania is called an impulse-control disorder, these patients may make advance preparations, such as searching out a site and collecting combustibles. They may also leave clues, almost as if they want to be discovered and apprehended. Fire setters may have low self-esteem and reportedly often have problems getting along with peers.

Criteria for Pyromania

- More than once, the patient has deliberately and purposefully set fires.
- Before the fire setting, the patient experiences tension or excited mood.
- The patient is interested in or attracted to fire and its circumstances and associations (such as firefighting apparatus, uses of fire, or aftermath of fire).
- The patient feels gratification, pleasure, or relief when setting fires or experiencing their consequences.
- These fires are *not* set for any of these reasons:
  - For profit
  - To express a political agenda
  - To conceal crimes
  - To express anger or revenge
  - To improve the patient's living circumstances
  - In response to a hallucination or delusion
  - As a result of impaired judgment (see Coding Note)
- The fire setting is not better explained by Antisocial Personality Disorder, Conduct Disorder, or a Manic Episode.

Coding Note

Of course, setting any fire at all would usually be interpreted as evidence of impaired judgment. What the "impaired judgment" exclusion refers to is the faulty judgment usually associated with other Axis I disorders, such as dementia, Mental Retardation, and Substance Intoxication.

Elwood Telfer

Elwood Telfer's earliest childhood memory was of a candle burning on the kitchen table. He would kneel on a chair as his mother sat in the dark and waited for his father to come home. His father drank, so they often waited a very long time. Periodically, she would put a strand of her own hair into the flame, sending a curl of acrid smoke spiraling toward the ceiling.

"Maybe it's why I've always been fascinated by fire," Elwood told a forensic examiner when he was 27. "I even have a big collection of firefighting memorabilia—old helmets, a badge from an 1896 fire brigade, and so on. I get them at antique shows."

Elwood had set his first fire when he was only seven. He had found an old Zippo lighter that still had enough flint, and he used it on an oily rag that was lying in a hay field. About a quarter-acre burned in the 20 exhilarating minutes before the fire trucks arrived to put it out. He always remembered the day's excitement as being well worth the beating his father administered after sobering up.

Most of Elwood's fires were set in fields or vacant lots. Once or twice he had torched an abandoned house, after first making sure that no one, not even a transient, could be inside. "I never wanted to hurt anyone," he told the examiner. "It's the warmth and the color of the flame and the excitement I like. I'm not mad at anybody."

Elwood had hardly ever had friends. When he entered high school, he was overjoyed to learn that there was a club called the Fire Squad. When he inquired about joining, two upperclassmen laughed and told him that it was an honorary group you could only belong to if you had lettered in football. Elwood felt almost sick with disappointment. That evening he started a small brush fire that consumed a neighbor's tool shed. This was the first time he noticed the healing effect of fire.

Months might go by when he was inactive and calm. Then he would spot a field or empty building that seemed right, and the tension would begin to mount. He might deliberately let it build over several days, to enhance the feeling of release that was almost orgasmic. But he indignantly denied that he ever masturbated at a fire scene. "I'm no pervert," he said.

After he graduated from high school, Elwood took enough accountancy courses to obtain a job as bookkeeper for a security alarm company. He had worked steadily at that job until the present time. He had never married or even dated, and he had no close friends. In fact, he actually felt uncomfortable around other people. The forensic clinician noted no abnormalities of mood, cognition, or the content of thought.

Elwood's only arrest ever, which was the reason for the forensic evaluation, came about because of a change in the weather. It was summertime, and all week the wind had been blowing steadily off the ocean. Elwood had located a promising field of dry grass and manzanita. On Saturday morning he was off work, and the wind still held. With almost uncontrollable excitement, he used a tin of gasoline to start the fire. He reacted with horror and panic when the wind suddenly began to blow toward the ocean; the fire jumped the small service road he had driven in on, and gobbled up his car and several beach dwellings. Firefighters and police found him sitting on the stony beach, crying quietly.

When they searched his apartment, they found a huge videotape collection depicting newscasts of wildfires.

Evaluation of Elwood Telfer

The phenomenon of "tension and release" required for diagnosis of Pyromania is well detailed in the vignette. The clinician's task would be to sort through the differential diagnosis, which is not unlike that for Kleptomania. **Antisocial Personality Disorder** patients will sometimes set fires for either profit or revenge. But Elwood had worked at one job for a decade, and his legal difficulties were restricted to fire setting. **Schizophrenia** patients occasionally set fires in response to hallucinations or delusions; patients with **cognitive disorders** will sometimes set their clothing or kitchens ablaze through inattention. Patients with a **Manic Episode** of **Bipolar I Disorder** may also set fires. However, Elwood had symptoms of none of these conditions.

Patients with Schizophrenia, a Manic Episode, or other severe mental conditions may sometimes set fires to communicate their desires (e.g., to be released from jail, to be returned to a former place of residence). This behavior has been termed **communicative arson**. Another item to consider in the differential diagnosis is **arson with a purpose**: fires set as a matter of political protest or sabotage, or fires set for profit. Persons who set fires for a material purpose will often have a severe **personality disorder**, but will not have the tension and release required for a diagnosis of Pyromania.

Although Elwood had a great deal of difficulty relating to other people, there are insufficient criteria described in this vignette to support a diagnosis of **Avoidant Personality Disorder**. This is not to say that it might not be warranted, only that more information would be needed. The very low GAF was given because of Elwood's potential for harming others with his behavior.

Axis I	312.33	Pyromania
Axis II	V71.09	No diagnosis; avoidant personality features
Axis III		None
Axis IV		None
Axis V	GAF = 20	(current)

312.31 Pathological Gambling

Gambling is extremely common behavior that only becomes a disorder when it is carried to excess. The nascent gambler may be exposed to gambling activities in the home during adolescence. There is a striking similarity between the development of Pathological Gambling and that of Substance Dependence. During an episode, most gamblers report feeling high or aroused, and it is usually several years before the behavior becomes pathological. Initially, success leads to increased gambling; at some point, "the big win" of an amount that may exceed the gambler's yearly earnings produces overconfidence and risk taking. From here on, because all games of chance are weighted toward the house, it is an easy (if painful) spiral into crushing loss, desperate attempts to get even, broken ties of family and friendship, and eventual ruin.

Pathological Gambling is relatively common, affecting about 2% of the adult population. Prevalence estimates range from one to three million individuals in the United States; males outnumber females about two to one. Because it is so common, much more is known about Pathological Gambling than about any other impulse-control disorder.

Criteria for Pathological Gambling

- Persistent, maladaptive gambling is expressed by five or more of the following. The patient:
  ✓ Is preoccupied with gambling (relives past experiences, plans new ventures, or devises ways to obtain seed money)
  ✓ Needs to put increasing amounts of money into play to get the wished-for excitement
  ✓ Has repeatedly tried (and failed) to control or stop gambling
  ✓ Feels restless or irritable when trying to control gambling
  ✓ Uses gambling to escape from problems or to cope with dysphoric mood (such as anxiety, depression, guilt, helplessness)
  ✓ Often tries to recoup losses ("chasing losses")
  ✓ Lies to cover up the extent of gambling
  ✓ Has stolen (embezzlement, forgery, fraud, theft) to finance gambling
  ✓ Has jeopardized a job, important relationship, or opportunity for career or education by gambling
  ✓ Has had to rely on others for money to relieve the consequences of gambling
- A Manic Episode doesn't better explain this behavior.

Randy Porter

The Christmas he was 12, Randy Porter's parents gave him a roulette wheel. It had inlaid numbers and was handmade from shiny ebony. The layout was printed on woven felt, and the ball was ivory. "Best quality you'll find outside of Monte Carlo," his father bragged when Randy opened it up. Throughout high school, Randy loved operating a casino for his friends. Once or twice some adults drifted in from his parents' bingo night; then they played for real money.

Now Randy was 25, divorced, and broke. He'd had a good job managing a restaurant near the Strip in Las Vegas. He couldn't honestly say he had taken his job to be near the action, but after he'd flunked out of college because of too many all-night bridge sessions (penny a point), it had seemed a godsend. It was an easy five-minute walk to two of the most glittering casinos in town—a walk that Randy frequently took on his lunch hour. "I knew everybody there," he reported. "I used to have accounts all over town. But nobody's let me run a tab for years."

Randy's early encounters with a real roulette table had been harmless enough. On his lunch hour he would stroll over to watch the action and place an occasional bet. He won a few dollars and lost a few more. All in all, he found that he could take it or leave it, mostly take it—he loved the surge of adrenaline he felt when he had money in play. He could afford modest losses; by then, he was married and his wife was making good money dealing black-jack at another casino. Then one Saturday afternoon when his wife had to work, black came up seven times in a row, and he walked away from the table with over $55,000 in his pocket. He said, "It was maybe the unluckiest day of my entire life."

In subsequent weeks, Randy lost himself (not to mention the $55,000) in gambling fever. His lunch hour soon stretched to two as he returned to the table again and again in an effort to recoup his losses. After he was caught "borrowing" from his employer, he tried Gamblers Anonymous; he quit be-cause he "didn't believe in a higher power." Over the next two years he became "totally obsessed," as his wife put it on more than one occasion, with the idea of scoring another big win so that he could quit ahead. When she finally left him, it was because she was tired of being ignored and lied to about their finances.

"She said she might as well be married to a one-armed bandit," Randy remarked sadly.

Randy was attentive and pleasant, and sat quietly throughout his inter-view. Though he expressed remorse for the difficulties he had caused himself and others, he described his mood as neither depressed nor ecstatic, but "in the middle." His speech was clear and goal-directed. His cognition and reasoning were excellent.

Before his wife left, Randy had pleaded with her to stay. He promised that he would reform. "I wouldn't bet on it," she had told him.

Evaluation of Randy Porter

In the course of a few years, Randy became thoroughly preoccupied with gam-bling, unsuccessfully tried to control it, chased his losses with more gambling, lied, stole, and eventually lost his wife and his job. He would therefore fully meet the criteria for Pathological Gambling—provided that his behavior was not better accounted for by a **Manic Episode**. Because he had no symptoms of mania, had not been depressed, and there was no evidence of periodicity in his gambling behavior, we can safely rule out **Bipolar I Disorder** as the cause. **Social gamblers** set limits on their losses and gamble in the company of friends; **professional gamblers** respect the odds and maintain strict self-discipline.

The real challenge in evaluating any patient with Pathological Gambling is to determine whether there is an associated mental disorder. Commonly associated Axis I conditions include **mood disorders**, **Panic Disorder**, **Obsessive–Compulsive Disorder**, and **Agoraphobia**. Also look for problems with **substance use** (which may precede or accompany gambling behavior) and **suicide attempts** (which may result from it).

Pathological gamblers are sometimes described as energetic people who are easily bored and big spenders. Of course, people with **Antisocial Personality Disorder** can become heavily involved in gambling, but Randy did not have any of the other behaviors that would be diagnostic of that personality disorder. His full diagnosis would be as follows:

Axis I	312.31	Pathological Gambling
Axis II	V71.09	No diagnosis
Axis III		None
Axis IV		Divorce
Axis V	GAF = 51	(current)

312.39 Trichotillomania

Trichotillomania comes from the Greek meaning "passion for pulling hair." As in Pyromania and Kleptomania, these patients experience mounting tension until they succumb to the urge. When they pull out hair, they experience release. Usually beginning in childhood, these people repeatedly pull out their own hair, beards, eyebrows, or eyelashes. Less often, they will pull hair from armpits, the pubic area, or other body locations. They usually don't report pain associated with the hair pulling, although a tingling sensation may be noted. They may swallow the hair or put it into their mouths. When the onset is in adulthood, it is often associated with psychosis.

These patients are often referred to mental health professionals by dermatologists, who note patchy hair loss. The condition tends to wax and wane, but is usually chronic.

Although Trichotillomania is rarely reported, it is unclear just how common it is. Some reports suggest that it may be found in up to 3% of the adult population, with an overrepresentation among women. It is more common in females than in males, and is especially common in patients who have Mental Retardation.

Criteria for Trichotillomania

- Repeated extraction of the patient's own hair causes noticeable hair loss.
- The patient feels increased tension just before hair pulling or when trying to resist it.
- The patient feels gratification, pleasure, or relief during the hair pulling.
- These symptoms cause clinically important distress or impair work, social, or personal functioning.
- The behavior is not better explained by another mental disorder and is not caused by a general medical condition.

Rosalind Brewer

"I don't know *why* I do it, I just do it." Rosalind Brewer had been referred to the mental health clinic by her dermatologist. "I get to feeling sort of up-tight, and if I just pop one little strand loose, somehow it relieves the tension." She selected a single strand of her long blonde hair, twined it neatly twice around her forefinger, and tweaked it out. She gazed at it a moment before dropping it onto the freshly vacuumed carpet.

Rosalind had been pulling out her hair for nearly half of her 30 years. She thought it had started during her sophomore or junior year in high school, when she was studying for final exams. Perhaps the tingling sensation on her scalp had helped her stay awake, but she didn't know. "Now it's a habit. I've always only pulled the hairs from the very top of my head."

The top of Rosalind's head bore a small, almost-bald spot about the size and shape of a silver dollar. Only a few broken hairs and a sparse growth of new hair sprouted there. It looked like a tonsure.

"It used to make my mom really angry. She said I'd end up looking like Dad. She'd order me to stop, but you know kids. I used to think I had *her* by the short hairs." She laughed bitterly. "Now that I want to stop, I can't."

Rosalind had sucked her thumb until the age of eight, but otherwise her childhood hadn't been remarkable. Her physical health was good; she had no other compulsive behaviors or obsessive thinking. She denied using drugs or alcohol. Although she had no significant symptoms of depression, she admitted that her hair pulling was a serious problem for her. She could wear a hairpiece to hide her bald spot, but the knowledge that it was there had kept her from forming any close relationships with men.

"It's bad enough looking like a monk," Rosalind said. "But this thing has got me living like one, too."

Evaluation of Rosalind Brewer

Rosalind's symptoms included the classic "tension and release" required for a diagnosis of Trichotillomania. She had no evidence of a **dermatological disor-**

der or other **general medical condition** that might explain the condition (she was referred by a dermatologist). The sorts of mental disorders that might be confused with Trichotillomania would include **Obsessive–Compulsive Disorder**, in which compulsive behavior is also found. However, the compulsions of OCD are performed not as an end to themselves, but as a means of preventing anxiety. **Factitious Disorder,** another possibility, would be ruled out because Rosalind gave no indication that she wanted to be a patient. She had no **psychosis** or other evident mental disorder. Thus, her complete diagnosis would be as follows:

Axis I	312.39	Trichotillomania
Axis II	V71.09	No diagnosis
Axis III		None
Axis IV		None
Axis V	GAF = 70	(current)

312.30 Impulse-Control Disorder Not Otherwise Specified

Any problems with the control of impulses that do not meet the criteria for the disorders described above or in other places in DSM-IV can be coded as Impulse-Control Disorder Not Otherwise Specified.

Adjustment Disorder

Introduction

Use the diagnosis of Adjustment Disorder when an identifiable stressor leads to impaired relationships in the patient's work or social life, or when the symptoms seem excessive for the degree of stress that is present. Obviously, in such a definition there is a great deal of room for interpretation (and argument).

Adjustment Disorder patients may be responding to one stress or to many; the stress may happen once or often. It can even be chronic, as when a child or young person is living with parents who fight continually. In clinical situations, the stress has usually affected only one person, but it can affect many (as in a flood or great fire). Almost any relatively commonplace event can be a stressor for someone—getting married or divorced, going away to school, or having to get a job. Whatever the nature of the stressor, the patient feels overwhelmed by the demands of the environment. More severe stresses are more likely to produce an Adjustment Disorder. Personality disorder or cognitive disorder may make a person more vulnerable to stress, and hence to Adjustment Disorder.

The criteria (see below) describes the course, which is usually relatively brief. Symptoms begin soon after the onset of stress, but always within three months. Once the stressor (or its consequences) ends, the symptoms must not persist longer than an additional six months. Of course, if the stressor is one that will be ongoing (such as chronic illness), it may take a very long time for the patient to adjust.

This diagnosis accounts for up to 10% of consultations in a general hospital setting. It may be more justifiable in adults than in adolescents, who often have symptoms that don't add up to much at first but later evolve into a more definitive Axis I diagnosis.

TIP Although some data support the utility of this diagnosis, which has been used clinically for decades, Adjustment Disorder should be reserved as a diagnosis of "almost last resort." It is probably too often used when the clinician simply has no better idea of what is going on. For most patients, another Axis I or an Axis II diagnosis can often be found. When it cannot, consider using the Axis I code 799.9 (Diagnosis Deferred). This has the advantage of preventing premature closure about the patient's problem.

Criteria for Adjustment Disorder

- Within three months of a stressor and in response to it, the patient develops emotional or behavioral symptoms.
- *Either* of the following demonstrates the clinical importance of these symptoms:
  ✓ Distress that markedly exceeds what would normally be expected from such a stressor, *or*
  ✓ Materially impaired job, academic, or social functioning
- These symptoms neither fulfill criteria for an Axis I disorder nor merely represent the worsening of a preexisting Axis I or Axis II disorder.
- The symptoms are not caused by Bereavement.
- They don't last longer than six months after the end of the stressor (or its consequences).

Coding Notes

Depending on the predominant symptoms, code:

309.0	With Depressed Mood. The patient is tearful, sad, hopeless.
309.24	With Anxiety. The patient is nervous, fearful, worried.
309.28	With Mixed Anxiety and Depressed Mood. Combination of the preceding.
309.3	With Disturbance of Conduct. The patient violates rules or rights of others.
309.4	With Mixed Disturbance of Emotions and Conduct. Combinations.
309.9	Unspecified. Examples: job problems, physical complaints, social withdrawal.

Specify whether:

Acute. The symptoms have lasted less than six months.

Chronic. The symptoms have lasted six months or more (use when stressor is chronic or has lasting effects).

Code the specific stressor on Axis IV (for choices, see the Introduction to this book, p. 6).

Clarissa Wetherby

"I know it's temporary and I know I'm overreacting. I sure don't want to, but I just feel upset!"

Clarissa Wetherby was speaking of her husband's new work schedule. Arthur Wetherby was foreman on a road-paving crew whose current job was to widen and resurface a portion of the interstate highway that ran within a few miles of the couple's house. The section the crew was working on now involved an interchange with another major highway. Therefore, the current work had to be done at night.

For the past two months, Arthur had slept days and gone to work at 8:00 P.M. Clarissa worked days as cashier in a restaurant. Except on weekends, when he tried to revert to a normal sleep schedule so he could be with her, they hardly ever saw each other. "I feel like I've been abandoned," she said.

The Wetherbys had been married only three years, and they had no children. Both had been married once before; both were 35. Neither drank or used drugs. Clarissa's only previous encounter with the mental health system had occurred seven years earlier, when her first husband had left her for another man. "I respected his right not to continue living a lie," she said, "but I felt terribly alone and humiliated."

Clarissa's symptoms now were much as they had been then. Most of the time when she was at work, she felt "about normal" and maintained good interest in what she was doing. But when she was alone at home in the evenings, she would be visited by waves of depression. These left her virtually immobilized, unable even to turn on the television set for company. She often cried to herself and felt guilty for giving in to her emotions. "It's not as if someone had died, after all." Although she had some difficulty getting to sleep at night, she slept soundly in the morning. Her weight was constant, her appetite was good, and she had no suicidal ideas or death wishes. She did not report any problems with her concentration. She denied ever having had symptoms of mania.

That other time, she had remained depressed and upset until a few weeks after the divorce was final. Then she seemed suddenly able to put it behind her and begin dating once again.

"I know I'll feel better, once Arthur gets off that schedule," she said. "I guess it just makes me feel worthless, playing second fiddle to an overpass."

Evaluation of Clarissa Wetherby

Clarissa's reaction to the stress of her husband's work schedule might be considered extreme by some observers. That is one of the important points of this diagnosis: The patient's distress often seems out of proportion to the apparent degree of the stress that has caused it. Her history provides a clue as to why she might have reacted as she did: She was reminded of the much more traumatic time her previous husband abandoned her—for good, and under circumstances that she considered humiliating. It is important, however, always to consider carefully whether a patient's reaction may be **nonpathological**.

The time course was right for Adjustment Disorder: Clarissa's symptoms developed shortly after she learned about Arthur's new work schedule. Although we have no way of knowing how long this episode might last, her previous such episode ended after a few months, when the aftermath of her divorce had lessened. Clarissa was not recently **bereaved**, thereby fulfilling another of the criteria.

The differential diagnosis of Adjustment Disorder comprises all the other conditions listed in DSM-IV. For Clarissa, the symptoms of mood disorder were the most prominent. She had never been manic, so could not qualify for a **Bipolar I Disorder**. In fact, her depression was not consistent with **Major Depressive Episode** (even the **With Atypical Features** subtype). She had low mood, but only when alone in the evenings (not most of the day). She maintained interest in her work (rather than experiencing loss of interest in nearly all activities). Without one or both of these symptoms, there could not be a DSM-IV diagnosis of Major Depressive Episode, regardless of her guilt feelings, low energy, and trouble getting to sleep at night. Of course, her symptoms had lasted far less than two years, so she would also fail to meet the criteria for **Dysthymic Disorder**.

The question of **Posttraumatic Stress Disorder** (and **Acute Stress Disorder**) often comes up in the differential diagnosis of Adjustment Disorder. Both of those anxiety diagnoses require that the stressor be of life-threatening proportions and that the patient respond intensely with fear, helplessness, or horror. Another category to consider is that of the **personality disorders**, which may worsen (and hence become more apparent) with stress. Clarissa did not fulfill criteria for any of these.

Each patient will be coded on the basis of the predominant symptoms and whether these are Acute or Chronic. Clarissa's mainly depressive symptoms would be coded as Acute, because she had been symptomatic for less than six months:

Axis I	309.0	Adjustment Disorder, With Depressed Mood, Acute
Axis II	V71.09	No diagnosis
Axis III		None
Axis IV		None
Axis V	GAF = 61	(current)

Personality Disorders

Quick Guide to the Personality Disorders

DSM-IV lists 10 specific personality disorders, one fewer than DSM-III-R (Passive–Aggressive Personality Disorder has been relegated to an appendix to await further study). Five of the 10 have been studied reasonably well and therefore have greater validity than the rest: antisocial, borderline, obsessive–compulsive, schizoid, schizotypal.

The 10 disorders are divided into three clusters, A, B, and C. These clusters have been used since DSM-III to group the personality disorders, but their validity has been heavily criticized. They are perhaps most useful as a device to help you remember the personality disorders.

Cluster A

People with the Cluster A personality disorders can be described as withdrawn, cold, suspicious, or irrational. (Here and throughout the Quick Guide, as usual, the page number following each item indicates where a more detailed discussion begins.)

Paranoid. These people are suspicious and quick to take offense. They often have few confidants and may read hidden meaning into innocent remarks (p. 463).

Schizoid. These people care little for social relationships, have a restricted emotional range, and seem indifferent to criticism or praise. Tending to be solitary, they avoid close (including sexual) relationships (p. 466).

Schizotypal. Interpersonal relationships are so difficult for these people that they appear peculiar or strange to others. They lack close friends and are uncomfortable in social situations. They may show suspiciousness, unusual perceptions or thinking, eccentric speech, and inappropriate affect (p. 470).

Cluster B

People with the Cluster B disorders tend to be dramatic, emotional, and attention-seeking; their moods are labile and often shallow. They often have intense interpersonal conflicts.

Antisocial. The irresponsible, often criminal behavior of these people begins in childhood or early adolescence with truancy, running away, cruelty, fighting, destructiveness, lying, and theft. In addition to criminal behavior, as adults they may default on debts, or otherwise show irresponsibility; act recklessly or impulsively; and show no remorse for their behavior (p. 474).

Borderline. These impulsive people make recurrent suicide threats or attempts. Affectively unstable, they often show intense, inappropriate anger. They feel empty or bored, and they frantically try to avoid abandonment. They are uncertain about who they are, and lack the ability to maintain stable interpersonal relationships (p. 478).

Histrionic. Overly emotional, vague, and attention-seeking, histrionic people need constant reassurance about their attractiveness. They may be self-centered and sexually seductive (p. 482).

Narcissistic. These people are self-important and often preoccupied with envy, fantasies of success, or ruminations about the uniqueness of their own problems. Their sense of entitlement and lack of empathy may cause them to take advantage of others. They vigorously reject criticism, and need constant attention and admiration (p. 485).

Cluster C

People with the Cluster C disorders tend to be anxious and tense, and are often overcontrolled.

Avoidant. These timid people are so easily wounded by criticism that they hesitate to become involved with others. They may fear the embarrassment of showing emotion or of saying things that seem foolish. They may have no close friends, and they exaggerate the risks of undertaking pursuits outside their usual routines (p. 487).

Dependent. These people need the approval of others so much that they have trouble making independent decisions or starting projects; they may even agree with others whom they know to be wrong. They fear abandonment, feel helpless when they are alone, and are miserable when relationships end. They are easily hurt by criticism and will even volunteer for unpleasant tasks to gain the favor of others (p. 490).

Obsessive–Compulsive. Perfectionism and rigidity characterize these people. They are often workaholics, and they tend to be indecisive, excessively scrupulous, and preoccupied with detail. They insist that others do things their way. They have trouble expressing affection, tend to lack generosity, and may even resist throwing away worthless objects they no longer need (p. 493).

Other Personality Disorders

Personality Disorder Not Otherwise Specified. Use this category for personality disturbances that do not meet the criteria for any of the disorders above, or for personality disorders that have not achieved official status (p. 495).

Other Causes of Long-Standing Character Disturbance

Personality Change Due to a General Medical Condition. A medical condition can affect a patient's personality for the worse. This does not qualify as a personality disorder, because it may be less pervasive and not present from an early age (p. 57).

Axis I Disorders. When they persist for a long time (usually years), a variety of Axis I conditions can distort the way a person behaves and relates to others. This can give the appearance of a personality disorder. Such effects are especially likely in the mood disorders (Dysthymic Disorder, Major Depressive Disorder), psychotic disorders (Schizophrenia), and cognitive disorders (dementias). Some studies find that mood disorder patients are more likely to show personality traits or disorders when they are clinically depressed; this may be especially true of Cluster A and Cluster C traits. Depressed patients should be re-evaluated for Axis II disorders once the depression has remitted.

Introduction

All humans (and numerous other species as well) have *personality traits*. These are well-ingrained ways in which individuals experience, interact with, and think about everything that goes on around them. *Personality disorders* are collections of traits that have become rigid and work to individuals' disadvantage, to the point that they impair functioning or cause distress. DSM-IV personality disorders are all patterns of behavior and thinking that have been present since early adult life and have been recognizable in the patient for a long time.

Personality disorders are probably *dimensional*, not *categorical*; this means that their components (traits) are present in normal people, but are accentuated in those with the disorders in question.

As defined in DSM-IV, all personality disorders have in common the following characteristics:

Generic Criteria for Personality Disorders

- A lasting pattern of behavior and inner experience that markedly deviates from norms of the patient's culture. The pattern is manifested in at least two of these areas:
  - ✓ Affect (appropriateness, intensity, lability, and range of emotions)
  - ✓ Cognition (how the patient perceives and interprets self, others, and events)
  - ✓ Impulse control
  - ✓ Interpersonal functioning
- This pattern is fixed and affects many personal and social situations.
- The pattern causes clinically important distress or impairs work, social, or personal functioning.
- This stable pattern has lasted a long time, with roots in adolescence or young adulthood.
- The pattern isn't better explained by another mental disorder.
- It isn't directly caused by a general medical condition or by the use of substances, including medications.

Coding Notes

If there is an Axis I diagnosis but a personality disorder is the main reason the patient has come for evaluation, (Principal Diagnosis) should be appended to the Axis II diagnosis. For example:

Axis I	302.81	Fetishism
Axis II	301.0	Paranoid Personality Disorder (Principal Diagnosis)

A frequently used defense mechanism can be indicated on the Axis II line:

Axis II	301.0	Paranoid Personality Disorder; frequent use of projection

If your patient's personality disorder preceded a psychotic disorder (most often Schizophrenia), the diagnosis might read:

Axis I	295.10	Schizophrenia, Disorganized Type, Continuous, With Prominent Negative Symptoms
Axis II	301.22	Schizoid Personality Disorder (Premorbid)

TIP These generic criteria are new in DSM-IV. It is puzzling that, after the general introduction to the personality disorders, they are never referred to in the criteria sets for the 10 specific disorders in Clusters A, B, and C. But these general criteria are extremely important. They spell out these vital points, central to the diagnosis of any personality disorder: It is lifelong, affects many areas of the patient's life, causes problems, and isn't the product of another illness. Whenever you consider the diagnosis of a personality disorder, keep these basic criteria carefully in mind.

Personality disorders are coded on Axis II, and they often coexist with Axis I disorders. The information they contain gives the clinician a better understanding of the behavior of patients; it can also augment our understanding of the management of many patients.

As you read these criteria and the accompanying vignettes, keep in mind the twin hallmarks of the personality disorders: *early onset* (usually by late teens) and *pervasive nature*, such that a disorder's features affect nearly all aspects of work and social life.

Diagnosing Personality Disorders

The diagnosis of personality disorders presents a variety of problems. These Axis II disorders are often overlooked; on the other hand, sometimes they are overdiagnosed (Borderline Personality Disorder is a notorious example). Some (Antisocial Personality Disorder) carry a poor prognosis; most, if not all, are hard to treat. Their relatively weak validity suggests that no personality disorder should be the sole diagnosis when an Axis I disorder can explain the signs and symptoms that make up the clinical picture. For all of these reasons, it is a good idea to have in mind an outline for making the diagnosis of a personality disorder.

1. Verify the duration of the symptoms. Make sure that your patient's symptoms have been present at least since early adulthood (since age 15 for Antisocial Personality Disorder). Interviewing informants (family, friends, coworkers) will probably give you the most valid material.

2. Verify that the symptoms affect many areas—DSM-IV calls them "contexts"—of the patient's life. Specifically, are work, home life, personal life, sexual life affected?

3. Check that criteria are fully met for the particular diagnosis in question. This means counting symptoms and consulting the 10 sets of diagnostic criteria. Sometimes this will involve a judgment call. Try to be as objective as possible. As with Axis I disorders, you can force a patient into a variety of diagnoses if you are strongly enough motivated to do so.

4. Rule out Axis I pathology, because Axis I disorders are usually more acute and have greater potential for doing harm; they are also easier to treat. Here is where the generic criteria (p.461) can be helpful. They list the specific

areas that must be covered: general medical conditions, substance-related disorders, other mental disorders.

5. This is also a good time to review the generic criteria for any other requirements you may have missed. Note that each patient must have two or more types of lasting problems with behavior, thoughts, or emotions from a list of four: cognitive, affective, interpersonal, and impulsive. (This helps ensure that the patient's problems truly do affect more than one life area.)

6. Search for other Axis II diagnoses. Evaluate the entire history to learn whether any additional personality disorder is present. Many patients fulfill criteria for more than one Axis II disorder; in such cases, diagnose them all. Perhaps more often, you will find too few symptoms to make any diagnosis. Then you have two options:

a. If a patient has elements of one personality disorder (e.g., Avoidant), but too few to meet the diagnostic criteria, you can assign the Axis II code V71.09 No diagnosis; avoidant personality features.

b. If there are elements of two or more disorders, you can assign the Axis II code 301.9 Personality Disorder Not Otherwise Specified. (This category has other uses; see p. 495.)

7. Record all Axis I and Axis II diagnoses. Some examples of how this is done are shown in the Coding Notes for the generic criteria and in the vignettes that follow.

TIP Although you can learn the rudiments of each of these personality disorders from the material I present here, it is important to note that these abbreviated descriptions only begin to tap their rich psychopathology. If you want to make a study of the Axis II disorders, I strongly recommend that you consult standard texts.

CLUSTER A PERSONALITY DISORDERS

301.0 Paranoid Personality Disorder

The central characteristic of patients with Paranoid Personality Disorder is their unjustified distrust and suspicion of others. Because they fear exploitation, they will not confide in others whose behavior should have earned their trust. They read unintended meaning into benign comments and actions. They will interpret untoward occurrences as the result of deliberate intent and will harbor resentment for a long time, perhaps forever.

These people are rigid, often litigious, and have an especially urgent need to be self-sufficient. To others, they appear to be cold, calculating, guarded people who avoid both blame and intimacy. On interview, they may appear tense and have trouble relaxing. This disorder is especially likely to create occupational difficulties: These patients are so aware of rank and power that they frequently have trouble dealing with superiors and coworkers.

Although it is apparently far from rare (it may affect 1% of the general population), Paranoid Personality Disorder rarely comes to clinical attention. When it does, it is usually diagnosed in men. Its relationship (if any) to the development of Schizophrenia, Paranoid Type, remains unclear.

Criteria for Paranoid Personality Disorder

- Beginning by early adult life, the patient is distrustful and suspicious of others, whose motives are seen as malevolent. These attitudes are present in a variety of situations and shown by at least four of the following:
    - ✓ Unfounded suspicion that other are deceiving, exploiting, or harming the patient
    - ✓ Preoccupation with unjustified doubts as to the loyalty or trustworthiness of associates or friends
    - ✓ Reluctance to confide in others, due to unwarranted fears that information will be maliciously used against the patient
    - ✓ Perception of hidden, demeaning, or threatening content in ordinary events or comments
    - ✓ Persistent bearing of grudges
    - ✓ Perception of personal attacks on own reputation or character, not perceived by others; the patient responds quickly with anger or counterattacks
    - ✓ Unjustified, recurring suspicions about the fidelity of spouse or sexual partner
- These symptoms do not occur solely in the course of a psychotic disorder (such as Schizophrenia) or a mood disorder with psychotic features.
- They aren't directly caused by a general medical condition.

Coding Note

If the criteria above are fulfilled prior to the onset of Schizophrenia, (Premorbid) should be added as a qualifier.

TIP For Paranoid Personality Disorder, as for all the personality disorders, the checkmarked criteria are printed in descending order of their frequency (whenever this is known).

Schatzky

A professor of dermatology at University Hospital, Dr. Schatzky had never consulted a mental health professional. But he was well known to the staff at the medical center and notorious among his colleagues. One of them, Dr. Cohen, provided most of the information for this vignette.

Schatzky had been around for several years. He was known as a solid researcher and an excellent clinician. A hard worker, he supervised fellows working on two grants and did more than his share of the teaching.

One of the trainees working in his lab was a physician by the name of Masters. He was a bright, capable young man whose career in academic dermatology seemed destined to soar. When Dr. Masters got an offer from Boston of an assistant professorship and his own lab space, he told Schatzky that he was sorry, but he would leave at the end of the semester. Furthermore, he wanted to use some of their data.

Schatzky was more than upset. He responded by telling Dr. Cohen that the data belonged to the lab and must stay in the lab. He wouldn't allow anyone to "rip him off," and he told Dr. Masters that he would be blackballed if he tried to publish papers based on their findings. Furthermore, Schatzky told him to keep away from the students until he left. This outraged the other dermatologists. Dr. Masters was one of the most popular young teachers in the department, and the notion that he shouldn't have any contact with the students seemed punitive and little short of an assault on academic freedom.

The other dermatologists discussed the situation in a department meeting when Schatzky was out of town. One of the older professors had volunteered to try to persuade him to let Dr. Masters teach anyway. Schatzky refused with the response, "What have I done to you?" He seemed to think the other professor had it in for him.

This professor told Dr. Cohen that he wasn't really surprised. He'd known Schatzky since college, and he'd always been a suspicious type. "He won't confide in anyone without a signed loyalty oath," was how the other professor put it. Schatzky seemed to think that if he said anything nice, it would somehow be turned against him. The only person he seemed to trust completely was his wife, a rabbity little creature who had probably never disagreed with him in her life.

At the meeting, someone else suggested that the department chairman should talk to him and try to "jolly him along a bit." But Schatzky had little sense of humor and "the longest memory for a grudge of anyone on the face of the planet."

In the collective memories of all the staff, Schatzky had never had mood swings or psychosis. "Never out of touch with reality, only nasty," said Dr. Cohen. And at department dinners, he never drank.

Evaluation of Dr. Schatzky

From the information available in this vignette, Dr. Schatzky had never been interviewed by a mental health professional. Any conclusions must therefore be tentative. Clinicians simply have no right to make definitive diagnoses on patients (or just plain people) on whom they have not gathered adequate information.

Dr. Schatzky's symptoms had apparently been quite constant and present throughout his entire adult life (since college). He had had problems with both cognition and interpersonal functioning, which led to problems with his work and personal life.

What symptoms of Paranoid Personality Disorder did Dr. Schatzky have? (1) Without cause, he suspected young Dr. Masters of planning to "rip off" his data. (2) His colleagues noted his long-standing concerns about the loyalty of associates. (3) He would never confide in others. (4) He refused to let Dr. Masters teach, which sounds like grudge holding. (Apparently, however, he had never questioned the loyalty of his wife, which would be another common symptom of this personality disorder.)

Could an Axis I diagnosis explain Dr. Schatsky's behavior as described? Although the information is incomplete, **drug** or **alcohol use** would not appear likely. (It seems unlikely that anyone of middle age could have been taking a medication long enough to produce character disturbance that had lasted his entire adult life.) The vignette provides no evidence of a **general medical condition**. According to the information provided, Dr. Schatzky had never had frank psychosis, such as **Delusional Disorder** or **Schizophrenia, Paranoid Type**, and he had no **mood disorder**. According to the generic criteria for personality disorders, this would seem to cover all the exclusions.

Were there any other personality disorders that Dr. Schatzky might have instead? **Schizoid** patients are cold and aloof, and as a result may appear distrustful, but they do not have the prominent suspiciousness characteristic of paranoid patients. **Schizotypal** patients may have paranoid ideation, but they also appear peculiar or odd, which is not the case for paranoid patients. And Dr. Schatzky did not appear to prefer solitude. Those with **Antisocial Personality Disorder** are often cold and unfeeling, may be suspicious, and have trouble forming interpersonal relationships. However, they rarely have the perseverance to complete professional school, and Dr. Schatzky had no history of criminal behavior or reckless disregard for the safety of others.

Dr. Schatsky's *tentative* five-axis diagnosis would be as follows:

Axis I	V71.09	No diagnosis
Axis II	301.0	Paranoid Personality Disorder
Axis III		None
Axis IV		Loss of colleague
Axis V	GAF = 70	(current)

301.20 Schizoid Personality Disorder

Patients with Schizoid Personality Disorder are indifferent to the society of other people, sometimes profoundly so. Typically, they are lifelong loners who show a restricted emotional range; they appear unsociable, cold, and seclusive.

They may succeed at solitary jobs others find difficult to tolerate. These patients may daydream excessively, become attached to animals, and often do not marry or even form long-lasting romantic relationships. They do retain contact with reality, unless they develop Schizophrenia. However, their relatives are not at increased risk for that disease.

Although it is uncommonly diagnosed, this disorder is relatively common, affecting perhaps a few percent of the general population. Men may be at greater risk than women. The following patient was the younger brother of Lyonel Childs, whose history has been presented in connection with Schizophrenia, Paranoid Type (see p. 145).

Criteria for Schizoid Personality Disorder

- Beginning by early adult life, the patient is isolated from social relationships and shows a restricted emotional range in interpersonal settings. These attitudes are present in a variety of situations and shown by at least four of the following:
  ✓ Neither wants nor likes close relationships, including those within a family
  ✓ Nearly always prefers solitary activities
  ✓ Has little interest in sexual activity with another person
  ✓ Enjoys few activities, if any
  ✓ Other than close relatives, has no close friends or confidants
  ✓ Does not appear affected by criticism or praise
  ✓ Is emotionally cold, detached, or bland
- These symptoms do not occur solely in the course of a psychotic disorder (such as Schizophrenia), a mood disorder with psychotic features, or a pervasive developmental disorder.
- They aren't directly caused by a general medical condition.

Coding Note

If the criteria above are fulfilled prior to the onset of Schizophrenia, (Premorbid) should be added as a qualifier.

Lester Childs

"We brought him in because of what happened to Lyonel. They seemed so much alike, and we were worried." Lester's mother sat primly on the office sofa. "After Lyonel was arrested, that's when we decided I should bring Lester in to see you."

At 20, Lester Childs was in many ways a carbon copy of his older brother. Born several weeks prematurely, he had spent the first several weeks of life in an incubator. But he gained weight rapidly and within a few months was well within the norms for his age.

He walked, talked, and was toilet-trained at the usual ages. Perhaps because they both worked so hard on the farm, perhaps because there were no other young children for Lester and his siblings to play with, his parents noticed nothing wrong until Lester entered first grade. Within a few weeks, his teacher had telephoned to set up a conference.

Lester seemed bright enough, they were told; his school work wasn't in question. But his sociability was next to nil. At recess, when the other children played dodge ball or pom-pom-pullaway, he remained in the classroom to color. He seldom participated in group discussions, and he always sat a few inches back from the others in the reading circle. When his turn for show and tell came, he stood silently in front of the class for a few moments, then pulled a length of kite string from his pocket and dropped it onto the floor. Then he sat down.

Most of this behavior was quite a lot like Lyonel's, so the parents hadn't been too worried. Even so, they took him to see their family doctor, who agreed that it was probably normal for their family and that he would "grow out of it." But Lester never did; he only grew up. He would never even do things with the family. At Christmas, he would open a present, take it over to a corner, and play with it by himself. Even Lyonel never did that.

When Lester entered the room, it was clear that he didn't regard the appointment as much of an occasion. He wore jeans with one knee missing, tattered sneakers, and a T-shirt that at one time surely had had sleeves. Through much of the interview, he continued to leaf through a magazine devoted to astronomy and math. After waiting more than a minute for Lester to say something, the interviewer began. "How are you today?"

"I'm okay." Lester kept on reading.

"Your mom and dad asked you to come in to see me today. Can you tell me why?"

"Not really."

"Do you have any ideas about it?"

"No."

Most of the interview went that way. Lester willingly gave information when he was directly asked, but he seemed completely uninterested in volunteering anything. Sitting quietly, nose in his magazine, he showed no other abnormalities or eccentricities of behavior. His flow of speech (what there was of it) was logical and sequential. He was fully oriented, and on his Mini-Mental State Exam he scored a perfect 30. His mood was "okay"—neither too happy nor too sad. He had never used alcohol or drugs of any kind. He calmly but emphatically denied ever hearing voices, seeing visions, or having beliefs that he was being watched, followed, talked about, or otherwise interfered with. "I'm not like my brother," he said in his longest spontaneous speech up to that point.

When asked what he was like, Lester said it was Greta Garbo—who also wanted to be left alone. He claimed he didn't need friends, and he could also do without his family. Neither did he need sex. He had checked out the sex magazines and anatomy books. Females or males, it was boring. His idea of a good way to spend his life was to live alone on an island, like Robinson Crusoe. "But no Friday."

Tucking his magazine under his arm, Lester walked out of the office, never to return.

Evaluation of Lester Childs

Any diagnosis of personality disorder requires that the difficulties be both pervasive and enduring. Although he was only 20 years old, Lester's problems had certainly been enduring: They were noticeable when he was six. And as far as we can tell, his rejection of interpersonal contact extended into every facet of his life—family, social, and school.

Lester rejected close relationships, even with his family; he preferred solitary activities; he rejected the notion of having a sexual relationship with anyone (although this could conceivably change with maturity and opportunity); he had always lacked close friends; his affect seemed quite flat and detached (although, this could have been an artifact of a first interview with a reluctant interviewee). In any event, Lester met at least four and possibly five of the criteria for Schizoid Personality Disorder. These symptoms would satisfy three of the areas (cognition, affect and interpersonal functioning) required by the generic criteria for personality disorders. His interest in mathematics and astronomy would not be unusual in persons with this disorder, who typically thrive on work that others might find too lonely to enjoy.

Could any Axis I disorder explain his clinical picture? Patients with **depressive disorders** are often withdrawn and unsociable, but these are seldom present on a lifelong basis. Besides, Lester specifically denied feeling depressed or lonely; any doubts on the point could be settled by asking about vegetative symptoms of depression (changes in appetite or sleep). He also denied having symptoms that would suggest **Schizophrenia** (delusions and hallucinations), and this was supported by collateral information from his mother. There were no stereotypies or symptoms of impaired communication, as would be expected for **Autistic Disorder**, or disturbance of consciousness of memory, as would be required for a **cognitive disorder**. From the information we have, he was physically healthy and did not use drugs, alcohol, or medications.

What other Axis II disorders should be considered? Patients with **Schizotypal Personality Disorder** can have constricted affect and unusual appearance. Lester's clothing was out of keeping for most visits to a professional office but would probably be quite usual for a disaffected 20-year-old, and he denied having any beliefs that might seem odd. He did not voice any ideas that seemed especially suspicious or distrusting, such as might be encountered in someone with **Paranoid Personality Disorder**. Patients with **Avoidant Personality Disorder** are also isolated from other people; unlike schizoid patients, however, they do not choose this isolation and they suffer for it.

If Lester later developed Schizophrenia, the qualifier (Premorbid) would be added at that time to the Axis II diagnosis. He would not receive an Axis IV code at the current evaluation, because his thinking and behavior only distressed his parents, not him. For similar reasons, it would be difficult to place him squarely on the GAF Scale. The score given below is to some extent a matter of taste, and arguable.

Axis I	V71.09	No diagnosis
Axis II	301.20	Schizoid Personality Disorder
Axis III		None
Axis IV		None
Axis V	GAF = 65	(highest level past year)

301.22 Schizotypal Personality Disorder

From an early age, patients with Schizotypal Personality Disorder have lasting interpersonal deficiencies that severely reduce their capacity for closeness with others. They also have distorted or eccentric thinking, perceptions, and behaviors that can make them seem odd. They often feel anxious when with strangers, and they have almost no close friends. They may be suspicious and superstitious; their peculiarities of thought include magical thinking and belief in telepathy or other unusual modes of communication. Such patients may talk about sensing a "force" or "presence," or have speech characterized by vagueness, digressions, excessive abstractions, impoverished vocabulary, or unusual use of words.

Schizotypal patients may eventually develop Schizophrenia. Many of them are depressed when they first come to clinical attention. Their eccentric ideas and style of thinking also place them at risk for becoming involved with cults. They get along poorly with others and under stress may become briefly psychotic, but many marry and work despite their odd behavior. This disorder occurs about as often as Schizoid Personality Disorder.

Criteria for Schizotypal Personality Disorder

• Beginning by early adult life, these patients experience isolation and discomfort with social relationships, as well as perceptual or cognitive distortions and peculiar behavior. These qualities are present in a variety of situations and shown by at least five of the following:

✓ Ideas of reference (not delusional)
✓ Behavior influenced by odd beliefs or by magical thinking inconsistent with cultural norms (including marked superstitions, belief in telepathy)
✓ Unusual perceptions or bodily illusions
✓ Odd speech (vague, excessively abstract, impoverished)
✓ Paranoid or suspicious ideas
✓ Affect that is constricted in range or inappropriate to the topic
✓ Odd behavior or appearance
✓ Other than close relatives, no close friends or confidants
✓ In social situations, marked anxiety that is not reduced by familiarity; this is associated with paranoid fears rather than negative self-judgments

- This syndrome does not occur only in the course of Schizophrenia or another psychotic disorder, a mood disorder with psychotic features, or a pervasive developmental disorder.

Coding Notes

If the criteria above are fulfilled before the onset of Schizophrenia, (Premorbid) should be added as a qualifier.

In children, odd beliefs (see second checkmarked item) may be bizarre fantasies or preoccupations.

Timothy Oldham

"But it's *my* baby! I don't care what he had to do with it!" Pregnant and miserable, Charlotte Grenville sat in the interviewer's office and wept with frustration. She was there at the request of the presiding judge in a battle over visitation rights with her yet-unborn child.

The identity of the father was never in doubt. The week after her second missed period, Charlotte had visited a gynecologist and then called Timothy Oldham with the news. She had considered threatening to sue him for child support, but that hadn't been necessary. He made good money installing carpets and had no dependents. He offered her $200 a month, beginning immediately. But he wanted to help rear their child. Charlotte had rejected that idea out of hand and then filed suit. With a crowded court docket, the case had dragged on nearly as long as Charlotte's pregnancy.

"I mean, he's really weird!"

"What do you mean, 'weird?' Give me some examples."

"Well, I've known him for the longest time—several years, anyway. He had a sister who died; he talks about her like she's still alive. And he does *weird* things. Like, when we were making love? Right in the middle he started this babble about 'holy love' and dedicating his seed. It put me right off. I told him to stop and get off, but it was too late. I mean, would you want your kid growing up with that for a father?"

"If he's so peculiar, how did you get involved with him?"

She looked abashed. "Well, we only did it once. And I might have been a little bit drunk at the time."

Compared to Charlotte, Tim was sedate. He sat quietly in the interview chair, a gangly blonde whose hair swept across his forehead nearly to his eyebrows. He told his story in a dull monotone that didn't reveal the slightest trace of emotion.

Timothy Oldham and his twin sister, Miranda, had been orphaned when they were four years old. He had no memory of his parents, other than a vague impression that they might have made their living from a marijuana farm in northern California. The two children had been taken in by an aunt and uncle, Southern Baptists who, he said, made the farm couple in Grant Woods' *American Gothic* look cheerful by comparison. "That painting, it's really them. I have a copy of it in my bedroom. Sometimes I can almost see my uncle moving the pitchfork back and forth to signal me."

"Is it really your uncle, and does the pitchfork really move?" the interviewer wanted to know.

"Well, it's more of a feeling I get ... not really ... a sign of my Christian endeavor ..." Timothy's voice trailed off, but he kept gazing straight ahead.

The "Christian endeavor," he explained, meant that everyone was put on earth for some special purpose. His uncle always used to say that. He thought his purpose might be to help raise the baby growing inside Charlotte. He knew there had to be more to life than laying carpets all day.

Timothy had only a few friends, none of them close. Charlotte herself had spent no more than a few hours in his company. In response to a question, he talked about his sister. Miranda and he had been understandably close; she was the only real friend he had ever had. She died of a brain tumor when they were 16, and Timothy was devastated. "We were webbed together when we were born. I swore at her graveside it would never be undone."

With still no inflection in his voice, Timothy explained that being "webbed together" was something you were born with. He and Miranda still were webbed. It was a Christian endeavor, and she was directing him from beyond the grave to have a baby girl. He said that it would be having Miranda back again. He knew that the baby wouldn't actually *be* Miranda, but said he knew it would be a girl. "It's just one of those feelings. But I know I'm right."

Timothy responded negatively to the usual questions about hallucinations, delusions, abnormal moods, substance use, and medical problems such as head injury and seizure disorders. Then he arose from his seat and left the room without a word.

That evening Charlotte Grenville gave birth—to a healthy baby boy.

Evaluation of Timothy Oldham

Charlotte's testimony would suggest that Timothy's peculiarities had been present for years. Although we don't know much about his school career or work, his symptoms would seem likely to affect most areas of his life. This point should be more fully explored.

Timothy's symptoms of Schizotypal Personality Disorder included odd beliefs (his conviction that the baby would be his sister returned to earth—there is no evidence that he came from a subculture where this sort of thinking was the norm), illusions (the farmer in the picture waving his pitchfork), peculiar speech (he spoke of being "webbed" to his twin sister), constricted affect, and absence of close friends. Unexplored by the interviewer were the presence of ideas of reference, paranoid ideas, odd behavior, and excessive social anxiety. Cognitive, affective, and interpersonal symptoms were represented here, however (see the generic criteria for personality disorders).

This evaluation turned up no indications of an Axis I disorder. Timothy had some peculiarities of speech, but he specifically denied the actual psychotic symptoms necessary to support a diagnosis of **Delusional Disorder** or **Schizophrenia**. Other Axis I disorders that could produce psychotic symptoms include **mood disorder** and **cognitive disorders**, but this interview also produced evidence against both of these.

Other personality diagnoses to consider would include **Schizoid** and **Paranoid Personality Disorder**. Both of these imply some degree of social isolation, but not the eccentric thinking of Schizotypal Personality Disorder. Patients with any of these three Cluster A disorders can decompensate into brief psychoses—a trait in common with **Borderline Personality Disorder**. Some patients may qualify for two diagnoses simultaneously: Borderline and a Cluster A disorder. **Avoidant Personality Disorder** patients are socially isolated, but they suffer from it and lack odd behavior and thinking. Of course, a **Personality Change Due to a General Medical Condition** must be considered in those who have a severe or chronic illness; Timothy didn't.

As of this evaluation, Tim had not developed Schizophrenia, so the qualifier (Premorbid) would not be used:

Axis I	V71.09	No diagnosis
Axis II	301.22	Schizotypal Personality Disorder
Axis III		None
Axis IV		Litigation regarding child visitation
Axis V	GAF = 75	(current)

CLUSTER B PERSONALITY DISORDERS

301.7 Antisocial Personality Disorder

Patients with Antisocial Personality Disorder chronically disregard and violate the rights of other people; they cannot or will not conform to the norms of society. This said, there are a number of ways in which people can be antisocial. Some are engaging con artists; others may be graceless thugs. Women with the disorder are often involved in prostitution. The more traditional aspects of antisociality in others may be obscured by the heavy use (and, generally, purveyance) of illicit drugs.

Although these people often seem superficially charming, many are aggressive and irritable. Their irresponsible behavior affects nearly every life area. Besides substance use, there may be fighting, lying, and criminal behavior of every conceivable sort: theft, violence, confidence schemes, and child and spouse abuse. These people may claim to have guilt feelings, but they do not appear to feel genuine remorse for their behavior. Although they may complain of multiple somatic problems and will occasionally make suicide attempts, their manipulative interactions with others make it difficult to decide whether or not their complaints are genuine.

DSM-IV criteria for Antisocial Personality Disorder specify that the patient must have (1) a history of three or more Conduct Disorder symptoms as a juvenile, and (2) at least four antisocial symptoms as an adult. For convenience, the juvenile symptoms are listed in their entirety in the accompanying criteria.

About 3% of men, but only about 1% of women, have this disorder; it accounts for about three-quarters of penitentiary prisoners. It is more common among lower-class populations and runs in families; it probably has both a genetic and an environmental basis. Male relatives have Antisocial Personality Disorder and substance-related disorders; female relatives have Somatization Disorder and substance-related disorders. Attention-Deficit/Hyperactivity Disorder in childhood is a common precursor.

Although treatment seems to make little difference to antisocial patients, there is some evidence that the disorder decreases with advancing age. Many such people mellow out after the age of 30 or more, to become "only" substance users. Death by suicide or homicide is the lot of others.

> TIP   Generally, the diagnosis of Antisocial Personality Disorder will not be warranted if antisocial behavior occurs only in the context of substance abuse. Individuals who misuse substances sometimes engage in

criminal behavior, but only when in pursuit of drugs. It is crucial to learn whether patients with possible Antisocial Personality Disorder have engaged in illicit acts when *not* using substances.

Although these patients often have a childhood marked by incorrigibility, delinquency, and school problems such as truancy, fewer than half the children with such a background eventually develop the full adult syndrome. Therefore, this diagnosis should never be made before age 18.

Finally, this is a serious disorder, with no known effective treatment. It is therefore a diagnosis of last resort. Before making it, redouble efforts to rule out other Axis I and II disorders.

Criteria for Antisocial Personality Disorder

- *Before* age 15, for 12 months or more the patient repeatedly violated rules, age-appropriate societal norms, or the rights of others (Conduct Disorder; see p. 520). This was shown by at least three of these:

Aggression against people or animals

✓ Engaged in frequent bullying or threatening
✓ Often started fights
✓ Used a weapon that could cause serious injury (gun, knife, club, broken glass)
✓ Showed physical cruelty to people
✓ Showed physical cruelty to animals
✓ Engaged in theft with confrontation (armed robbery, extortion, mugging, purse snatching)
✓ Forced sex upon someone

Property destruction

✓ Deliberately set fires to cause serious damage
✓ Deliberately destroyed the property of others (except for fire setting)

Lying or theft

✓ Broke into building, car, or house belonging to someone else
✓ Frequently lied or broke promises for gain or to avoid obligations ("conning")
✓ Stole valuables without confrontation (burglary, forgery, shoplifting)

Serious rule violation

✓ Beginning before age 13, frequently stayed out at night against parents' wishes

✓ Ran away from parents overnight twice or more (once if for an extended period)

✓ Beginning before age 13, engaged in frequent truancy

- *Since* age 15, the patient has shown disregard for the rights of others in a variety of situations. This is demonstrated by at least three of these:

✓ Engages in repeated behaviors that are grounds for arrest, whether arrested or not

✓ Lies, uses aliases, or cons others for gain or gratification

✓ Is impulsive or does not plan ahead

✓ Shows irritability and aggression through recurrent physical fights or assaults

✓ Recklessly disregards safety of self or others

✓ Shows irresponsibility through repeated failure to sustain employment or honor financial obligations

✓ Lacks remorse for own injurious behavior (shows indifference or rationalizes)

- The patient is currently at least 18 years old.
- The antisocial behavior does not occur solely during a Manic Episode or Schizophrenia.

TIP The criteria suggest some sort of behavioral change at age 15. Actually, juvenile and adult misbehaviors exist on two continuums (chronology and severity), the one flowing into the other. The point is that these patients begin to misbehave when they are very young and continue to do so, at least through their early adult years.

Milo Tark

Milo Tark was 23, good-looking, and smart. When he worked, he was well paid as a heating and air conditioning installer. He had broken into that trade when he left high school, which happened somewhere in the middle of his 10th-grade year. Since then, he had had at least 15 different jobs; the longest of them had lasted six months.

Milo was referred for evaluation after he was caught trying to con money from elderly patrons at an automatic teller machine (ATM). The machine was one of two that served the branch bank where his mother worked as assistant manager.

"The little devil!" his father exclaimed during the initial interview. "He was always a difficult one to raise, even when he was a kid. Kinda reminded me of me, sometimes. Only I pulled out of it."

Milo picked a lot of fights when he was a boy. He had bloodied his first nose when he was only five, and the world-class spanking his father had given him had taught him nothing about keeping his fists to himself. Later he was suspended from the seventh grade for extorting $3 and change from an eight-year-old. When the suspension was finally lifted, he responded by ditching class for 47 straight days. Then began a string of encounters with the police, beginning with shoplifting (condoms) and progressing through breaking and entering (four counts) to grand theft auto when he was 15. For stealing the Toyota, he was sent for half a year to a camp run by the state youth authority. "It was the only six months his mother and I ever knew where he was at night," his father observed.

Milo's time in detention seemed to have done him some good, at least initially. Although he never returned to school, for the next two years he avoided arrest and intermittently applied himself to learning his trade. Then he celebrated his 19th birthday by getting drunk and joining the Army. Within a few months he was out on the street again, with a bad-conduct discharge for sharing cocaine in his barracks and assaulting two corporals, his first sergeant, and a second lieutenant. For the next several years, he worked when he needed cash and couldn't get it any other way. Not long before this evaluation, he had gotten a 16-year-old girl pregnant.

"She was just a ditsy broad." Milo lounged back, one leg over the arm of the interview chair. He had managed to grow a scraggly beard, and he rolled a toothpick around in the corner of his mouth. The letters H-A-T-E and L-O-V-E were clumsily tattooed across the knuckles of either hand. "She didn't object when she was gettin' laid."

Milo's mood was good now, and he had never had anything that resembled mania. There had never been symptoms of psychosis, except for the time he was coming off speed. He "felt a little paranoid" then, but it didn't last.

The ATM job was a scam thought up by a friend. The friend had read something like it in the newspaper and decided it would be a good way to obtain fast cash. They had never thought they might be caught, and Milo hadn't considered the effect it would have on his mother. He merely yawned and said, "She can always get another job."

Evaluation of Milo Tark

Milo's behavior persistently affected all aspects of his life: school, work, family, and interpersonal relations. By the time he was 15, he easily met criteria for **Conduct Disorder** (see the "Before age 15" criteria list above). After that, he moved into full-blown adult criminality that persisted through his early 20s: repeated illegal acts, assaults (on Army personnel), poor work record, impulsivity (no planning about breaking into the ATM), and lack of remorse (toward his mother and the girl he impregnated). His symptoms touched on the areas of cognition, affect, interpersonal functioning, and impulse control (see the generic criteria for personality disorders).

Patients with a **Manic Episode** or **Schizophrenia** will sometimes engage in criminal activity, but it is episodic and accompanied by other manic or psychotic symptoms. Milo steadfastly denied any behavior suggesting either a mood or a psychotic disorder. **Mentally retarded** patients may break the law, either because they do not realize that it is wrong or because they have been influenced by others. Although Milo did not do especially well in school, there is no indication that he was held back in school or had specific learning disabilities.

Substance-related disorders are important in the differential diagnosis, because many addicted patients will do nearly anything to obtain money for their substance of choice. Milo had used cocaine and amphetamines, but (according to him) only briefly. Most of his antisocial behaviors were not associated with drug use. Patients with **impulse-control disorders** will engage in illegal activities, but this is confined to the context of **Pathological Gambling**, **Kleptomania**, or **Pyromania**. Patients with the eating disorder **Bulimia Nervosa** sometimes shoplift, but Milo had no evidence of bulimic episodes. Of course, many of these disorders (as well as **anxiety disorders**) can be encountered as associated diagnoses in antisocial patients.

Career criminals whose antisocial behavior is confined to their "professional lives" may not fulfill all of the criteria for Antisocial Personality Disorder. They may instead be diagnosed as having **Adult Antisocial Behavior**, which is recorded as a V code (V71.01) on Axis I. It constitutes part of the differential diagnosis of the personality disorder.

Milo's complete diagnosis would be as follows:

Axis I	V71.09	No diagnosis
Axis II	301.7	Antisocial Personality Disorder
Axis III		None
Axis IV		Arrest for ATM fraud
Axis V	GAF = 35	(current)

301.83 Borderline Personality Disorder

Patients with Borderline Personality Disorder sustain a pattern of instability throughout their adult lives. They often appear to be in a crisis of mood, behavior, or interpersonal relationships. Many feel empty and bored; they attach themselves strongly to others, then become intensely angry or hostile when they believe that they are being ignored or mistreated by those they depend on. They may impulsively try to harm or mutilate themselves; these actions are expressions of anger, cries for help, or attempts to numb themselves to their emotional pain. Although borderline patients may experience brief psychotic episodes, these episodes resolve so quickly that they are seldom confused with psychoses like Schizophrenia. Intense and rapid mood swings, impulsivity, and unstable interpersonal relationships make it difficult for borderline patients to achieve their full potential socially, at work, or in school

Borderline Personality Disorder runs in families. These people are truly miserable and in some cases (up to 10%) complete suicide.

TIP The concept of Borderline Personality Disorder was devised about the middle of the 20th century. These patients were originally (and sometimes still are) said to be on the borderline between neurosis and psychosis. The existence of this borderline is disputed by many clinicians. As the concept has evolved into a personality disorder, it has achieved remarkable popularity, perhaps because so many patients can be shoehorned into its capacious definition.

Although 1–2% of the general population may legitimately qualify for the diagnosis of Borderline Personality Disorder, it is probably applied to a far greater proportion of the patients who seek mental health care. It may still be the most overdiagnosed condition in DSM-IV. Many of these patients have Axis I disorders that are more readily treatable; these include Major Depressive Disorder, Somatization Disorder, and substance-related disorders.

Criteria for Borderline Personality Disorder

• Beginning by early adult life, the patient has unstable impulse control, interpersonal relationships, moods, and self-image. These persistent or recurrent qualities are present in a variety of situations and shown by at least five of the following:
  ✓ Frantic attempts to prevent abandonment, whether this is real or imagined (don't include self-injurious or suicidal behaviors, covered below)
  ✓ Unstable relationships that alternate between idealization and devaluation
  ✓ Identity disturbance (severely unstable self-image or sense of self)
  ✓ Potentially self-damaging impulsiveness in at least two areas, such as binge eating, reckless driving, sex, spending, substance use (don't include suicidal or self-mutilating behaviors)
  ✓ Self-mutilation or suicide thoughts, threats, or other behavior
  ✓ Severe reactivity of mood leading to marked instability (mood swings of intense anxiety, depression, or irritability, lasting a few hours to a few days)

✓ Chronic feelings of emptiness
✓ Anger that is out of control or inappropriate and intense (demonstrated by frequent temper displays, repeated physical fights, or feeling constantly angry)
✓ Brief paranoid ideas or severe dissociative symptoms related to stress

Josephine Armitage

"I'm cutting myself!" The voice on the telephone was high-pitched and quavering. "I'm cutting myself right now! Ow! There, I've started." The voice howled with pain and rage.

Twenty minutes later, the clinician had Josephine's address and her promise that she would come in to the emergency room right away. Two hours later, her left forearm swathed in bandages, Josephine Armitage was sitting in an office in the mental health department. Criss-crossing scars furrowed her right arm from wrist to elbow. She was 33, a bit overweight, and chewing gum.

"I feel a lot better," she said with a smile. "I really think you saved my life."

The clinician glanced at her nonswathed arm. "This isn't the first time, is it?"

"I should think that would be pretty obvious. Are you going to be terminally dense, just like my last shrink?" She scowled and turned 90 degrees to look at the wall. "Sheesh!"

Her previous therapist had seen Josephine for a reduced fee, but had been unable to give her more time when she requested it. She had responded by letting the air out of all four tires of the therapist's new BMW.

Her current trouble was with her boyfriend. One of her girlfriends had been "pretty sure" James had been out with another woman two nights ago. Yesterday morning, Josephine had called in sick to work and staked out James's workplace so she could confront him. He hadn't appeared, so last evening she had banged on the door of his apartment until neighbors threatened to call the police. Before leaving, she'd kicked a hole in the wall beside James's door. Then she got drunk and drove up and down the main drag, trying to pick up a date.

"Sounds dangerous," observed the clinician.

"I was looking for Mr. Goodbar, but no one turned up. I decided I'd have to cut myself again. It always seems to help." Josephine's anger had once again evaporated, and she had turned away from the wall. "Life's a bitch, and then you die."

"When you cut yourself, do you ever really intend to kill yourself?"

"Well, let's see." She chewed her gum thoughtfully. "I get so angry and depressed, I just don't care what happens. My last shrink said all my life I've felt like a shell of a person, and I guess that's right. It feels like there's no one living inside, so I might just as well pour out the blood and finish the job."

Evaluation of Josephine Armitage

The first thing this clinician would have to do would be to determine whether the behaviors reported (and observed) had been present since Josephine's late teen years. From her report of the comment made by her "last shrink," this would seem to be the case, but it would have to be verified. These behaviors were pervasive: Her work was affected (calling in sick on a whim is problematic behavior), and her relations with her boyfriend and her previous therapist were certainly affected.

Josephine had an abundance of symptoms. The entire episode of staking out James's apartment would seem to be a frantic effort to avoid abandonment. Even her initial moments with the present clinician revealed some swings between idealization and devaluation. She showed evidence of dangerous impulsivity (driving while under the influence of alcohol, trying to pick up a stranger), and she had made repeated suicide attempts. Her mood, even within the confines of this vignette, would seem markedly unstable and reactive to what she perceived to be the clinician's reaction toward her, and her anger was sudden, inappropriate, and intense. She agreed with a description of herself as an "empty shell." Although patients with Borderline Personality Disorder are often described as having identity disturbance and occasional, brief psychotic lapses, the vignette gives no evidence of either of these in Josephine. Even so, she had six or seven symptoms, whereas only five are required.

A long list of Axis I disorders can be confused with Borderline Personality Disorder; each must be considered before settling on this disorder as a sole (or principal) diagnosis. Many borderline patients also have a **Major Depressive Disorder** or **Dysthymic Disorder**. You must establish that suicidal behaviors, anger, and feelings of emptiness are not experienced only during episodes of depression. Similarly, you must establish that affective instability is not due to **Cyclothymic Disorder**.

Borderline patients can have **psychotic episodes**, but these are brief, are stress-related, and resolve quickly and spontaneously, so they should not be confused with **Schizophrenia**. The misuse of various substances can lead to suicide behavior, instability of mood, and reduced impulse control. **Substance-related disorders** are also often found as a concomitant with Borderline Personality Disorder, and should always be asked about carefully. **Somatization Disorder** patients are often quite dramatic and may misuse substances and make suicide attempts. Although this vignette contains no evidence for these disorders (other than getting drunk—was this an isolated event?), the evaluating clinician would need to consider carefully the list just given.

Multiple Axis II personality disorders are not infrequent in borderline patients. Josephine's presentation was dramatic, suggesting **Histrionic Personality Disorder**. With further interviewing and observation, she might qualify for both of these diagnoses. Borderline patients can also show features of other personality disorders. **Narcissistic** patients are also self-centered, though without Josephine's impulsivity. **Antisocial** patients are impulsive and do not control their anger; although some of Josephine's behaviors were destructive, she did not engage in overtly criminal activity. Assuming the verification of her history, her diagnosis would be as given below.

If you want to alert others to the severity of a patient's disorder (as indicated by the number of symptoms and by persistent self-endangerment), the severity code Severe can be used, as discussed in the Introduction to this book (p. 5). Let us assume that this would be done in Josephine's case:

Axis I	V71.09	No diagnosis
Axis II	301.83	Borderline Personality Disorder, Severe
Axis III	881.00	Lacerations of forearm
Axis IV		None
Axis V	GAF = 51	(current)

301.50 Histrionic Personality Disorder

Patients with Histrionic Personality Disorder have a long-standing pattern of excessive emotionality and attention-seeking that seeps into all areas of their lives. These people satisfy their need to be at center stage in two main ways: (1) Their interests and topics of conversation focus on their own desires and activities; and (2) their behavior, including speech, continually calls attention to themselves. They are overly concerned with physical attractiveness (of themselves and of others, as it relates to them), and they will express themselves so extravagantly that it seems almost a parody of normal emotionality. Their need for approval can cause them to be seductive, often inappropriately (even flamboyantly) so. Many lead normal sex lives, but some may be promiscuous, and still others may have difficulty with frigidity or impotence.

These people are often so insecure that they constantly need the approval of others. Dependence on the favor of others may cause their moods to seem shallow or excessively reactive to their surroundings. Low tolerance for frustration may spawn temper tantrums. They usually like to talk with mental health professionals (it is another chance to be the center of attention), but because their speech is often vague and full of exaggerations, they can prove frustrating to interview.

Quick to form new friendships, histrionic people are also quick to become demanding. Because they are trusting and easily influenced, their behavior may appear inconsistent. They don't think very analytically, so they may have difficulty with tasks that require logical thinking, such as doing mental arithmetic. However, they may succeed in jobs that set a premium on creativity and imagination. Their craving for novelty sometimes leads to legal problems as they seek sensation or stimulation. Some have a remarkable tendency to forget affect-laden material.

This disorder has not been especially well studied, but it is reportedly quite common. It may run in families. The classical patient is female, though the disorder can occur in men.

Criteria For Histrionic Personality Disorder

- Beginning by early adult life, emotional excess and attention-seeking behaviors are present in a variety of situations and shown by at least five of these:
  ✓ Discomfort with situations in which the patient is not the center of attention
  ✓ Relationships that are frequently fraught with inappropriately seductive or sexually provocative behavior
  ✓ Expression of emotion that is shallow and rapidly shifting
  ✓ Frequent focusing of attention on self through use of physical appearance
  ✓ Speech that is vague and lacks detail
  ✓ Overly dramatic expression of emotion
  ✓ Easy suggestibility (patient is readily influenced by opinions of other people or by circumstances)
  ✓ Belief that relationships are more intimate than they really are

Angela Black

Angela Black and her husband, Donald, had come for marriage counseling; as usual, they were fighting.

"He never listens to me. I might as well be talking to the dog!" Tears and mascara dripped onto the front of Angela's low-cut silk dress.

"What's there to listen to?" Donald retorted. "I know I irritate her, because she complains so much. But when I ask how she'd like me to change, she can never put her finger on it."

Angela and Donald were both 37 years old, and they had been married nearly 10 years. Already they had been separated twice. Donald made excellent money as a corporate lawyer; Angela had been a fashion model. She didn't work often any more, but her husband made enough to keep her well dressed and shod. "I don't think she's ever worn the same dress twice," Donald grumbled.

"Yes, I have," she snapped back.

"When? Name one time."

"I do it all the time. Especially recently." For several sentences Angela defended herself, without ever making a concrete statement of fact.

"*Res ipsa loquitur*," said Donald with satisfaction.

"Oh, God, Latin!" She nearly howled. "When he puts in his superior, gratuitous Latin, it makes me want to cut my wrists!"

The Blacks agreed on one thing: For them, this was a typical conversation.

He worked late most nights and weekends, which upset her. She spent far too much money on jewelry and clothing. She relished the fact that she could still attract men. "I wouldn't do it if you paid more attention to me," she said, pouting.

"You wouldn't do it if you didn't listen to Marilyn," he retorted.

Marilyn and Angela had been best friends since their cheerleading days in high school. Marilyn was wealthy and independent; she didn't care what people thought, and behaved accordingly. Usually, Angela followed right along.

"Like the pool party last summer," put in Donald, "when you took off your suits to 'practice cheers' for the races. Or was that your idea?"

"What would you know about it? You were working late. Besides, it was only the tops."

Evaluation of Angela Black

Angela's personality style had a profound effect on her marriage, though the vignette hints that her other social relationships (e.g., men at the party) were affected as well. More information would be needed to establish that she had been this way throughout her adult life. However, it would seem unlikely that this personality style had developed recently.

Angela's symptoms included a strong need to be the center of attention and sexual provocation (inferred from her dancing topless); overconcern with physical appearance; dramatic emotional expression; suggestibility (following the lead of her friend Marilyn); and vague speech (commented on by her husband). In all, she had five or six symptoms of Histrionic Personality Disorder.

Her clinician should gather information adequate to determine that Angela did *not* have any of the Axis I disorders that commonly accompany Histrionic Personality Disorder. These include **Somatization Disorder** (had she been in good physical health?) and **substance-related disorders**.

Would Angela qualify for other Axis II diagnoses? She was centrally concerned with herself, and she liked to be admired. However, she lacked the sense of grandiose accomplishment that characterizes patients with **Narcissistic Personality Disorder**. Patients with **Borderline Personality Disorder** often also have histrionic features. In fact, DSM-III (1980) included suicidal behaviors as a criterion for both of these disorders. Angela's mood was somewhat labile, but she did not report interpersonal instability, identity disturbance, transient paranoid ideation, or other symptoms that characterize borderline patients. Her easy suggestibility might suggest **Dependent Personality Disorder**, but she was so far from leaning on her husband for support that she actively fought with him. Her full diagnosis would thus be as follows:

Axis I	V71.09	No diagnosis
Axis II	301.50	Histrionic Personality Disorder
Axis III		None
Axis IV		Partner Relational Problem
Axis V	GAF = 65	(current)

301.81 Narcissistic Personality Disorder

People with Narcissistic Personality Disorder have a lifelong pattern of grandiosity (in behavior and in fantasy), thirst for admiration, and lack of empathy. These attitudes permeate most aspects of their lives. They feel that they are unusually special; they are self-important individuals who commonly exaggerate their accomplishments to make themselves seem bigger than life. (It should be noted from the outset, however, that these traits constitute a personality disorder only in adults. Children and teenagers are naturally self-centered; in this age range, narcissistic traits don't necessarily imply ultimate personality disorder.)

Despite their grandiose attitudes, narcissistic individuals have fragile self-esteem and often feel unworthy; even at times of great personal success, they may feel fraudulent or undeserving. They remain overly sensitive to what others think about them, and feel compelled to extract compliments. When criticized, they may cover their distress with a façade of icy indifference. As sensitive as they are about their own feelings, they have little apparent understanding of the feelings and needs of others and may feign empathy, just as they may lie to cover their own faults.

Narcissistic people often fantasize about wild success and envy those who have achieved it. They may choose friends they think can help them get what they want. Their job performance can suffer (due to interpersonal problems) or can be enhanced (due to their eternal drive for success). Because they tend to be concerned with grooming and value their youthful looks, they may become increasingly depressed as they age.

This disorder has been very poorly studied. It is probably uncommon; reportedly, most patients are men. There is no information about family history, environmental antecedents, or other background material that might help us to understand these difficult personalities.

Criteria for Narcissistic Personality Disorder

- Beginning by early adult life, grandiosity (fantasized or actual), lack of empathy, and need for admiration are present in a variety of situations and shown by at least five of these:
    - ✓ A grandiose sense of self-importance (patient exaggerates own abilities and accomplishments)
    - ✓ Preoccupation with fantasies of beauty, brilliance, ideal love, power, or limitless success
    - ✓ Belief that personal uniqueness renders the patient fit only for association with (or understanding by) people or institutions of rarefied status
    - ✓ Need for excessive admiration
    - ✓ A sense of entitlement (patient unreasonably expects favorable treatment or automatic granting of own wishes)

✓ Exploitation of others to achieve personal goals
✓ Lack of empathy (patient does not recognize or identify with the feelings and needs of others)
✓ Frequent envy of others or belief that others envy patient
✓ Arrogance or haughtiness in attitude or behavior

Berna Whitlow

"Dr. Whitlow, you're my backup for emergency clinic this afternoon. I've got to have some help from you!" Eleanor Bondurak, a social worker at the mental health clinic, was red-faced with anger and frustration. It wasn't the first time she had had difficulty working with this psychologist.

At the age of 50, Berna Whitlow had worked at nearly every mental health clinic in the metropolitan area. She was well trained and highly intelligent, and she read voraciously in her specialty. Those were the qualities that over the years had landed her job after job. The qualities that kept her moving from one job to another were known better to those who worked with her than to those who hired her. She was famous among coworkers for being pompous and self-centered.

"She said she wasn't going to take orders from me. And her attitude said for her, 'You're nothing but a social worker.'" Eleanor was now reliving the moment in a heated discussion with the clinical director. "She said she'd talk to my boss or to you. I pointed out that neither of you was in the building at the time, and that the patient had brought in a gun in his briefcase. So then she said I should 'write it up and submit it,' and she would 'decide what action to take.' That's when I had you paged."

With the crisis over (the gun had been unloaded, the patient not dangerous), the clinical director had dropped in to chat with Dr. Whitlow. "Look, Berna, it's true that ordinarily the social worker usually sees the patient and does a writeup before the psychologist steps in. But this wasn't exactly an ordinary case! Especially in emergencies, the whole team has to act together."

Berna Whitlow was tall, with a straight nose and jutting chin that seemed to radiate authority. Her long hair was thick and blond. She raised her chin a bit higher. "You hardly need to lecture me on the team approach. I've been a leader in nearly every clinic in town. I'm a superb team leader. You can ask anyone." As she spoke, she rubbed the gold rings that encircled nearly every finger.

"But being a team leader involves more than just giving orders. It's also about gathering information, building consensus, caring about the feelings of oth— "

"Listen," she interrupted, "it's her job to work on my team. It's my job to provide the leadership and make the decisions."

Evaluation of Berna Whitlow

From the material we have (again, the conclusions drawn must be tentative), Dr. Whitlow's personality traits would seem to have caused difficulties for many years. They affected her broadly, interfering with work (many jobs) and interpersonal relationships. Of course, a full assessment would inquire about her personality as it affected her home and social life.

Her symptoms suggestive of narcissism included haughty attitude, exaggerating her own accomplishments ("I'm a superb team leader"), insisting that she only receive orders or requests from persons of high rank, expecting obedience, and lacking empathy with fellow workers. Affective, cognitive, and interpersonal features were present here (see the generic criteria for personality disorders).

Although **Dysthymic Disorder** and **Major Depressive Disorder** frequently accompany this personality disorder, there is no evidence in the vignette to support either of those diagnoses. An interviewing clinician could ask about sensitive issues such as mood and character disorder.

Several other personality disorders can either accompany or be confused with Narcissistic Personality Disorder. **Histrionic** patients are also extremely self-centered, but Dr. Whitlow was not as theatrical (although she did wear ostentatious rings). As is the case in **Borderline Personality Disorder** (and most others), narcissistic patients have a great deal of trouble relating to other people. But they (including Dr. Whitlow) are not especially prone to unstable moods, suicidal behavior, or brief psychoses under stress. Although there is a hint of the deceitful in narcissistic exaggerations, these people lack the pervasive criminality and disregard for the rights of others that are typical of **Antisocial Personality Disorder**.

Dr. Whitlow's *tentative* five-axis diagnosis would be as follows:

Axis I	V71.09	No diagnosis
Axis II	301.81	Narcissistic Personality Disorder
Axis III		None
Axis IV		None
Axis V	GAF = 61	(current)

CLUSTER C PERSONALITY DISORDERS

301.82 Avoidant Personality Disorder

People with Avoidant Personality Disorder feel inadequate and are socially inhibited and overly sensitive to criticism. These characteristics are present throughout adult life, and affect most aspects of daily life. (Like narcissistic traits, avoidant traits are common in children and do not necessarily imply eventual personality disorder.)

Their sensitivity to criticism and disapproval makes these people self-ef-facing and eager to please others, but it can also lead to marked social isola-tion. They may misinterpret innocent comments as critical; often they refuse to begin a relationship unless they are sure they will be accepted. They will hang back in social situations for fear of saying something foolish, and will avoid occupations that involve social demands. Other than their parents, siblings, or children, they tend to have few close friends. Comfortable with routine, they may go to great lengths to avoid departing from their set ways. In an interview they may appear tense and anxious; they may misinterpret even benign state-ments as criticism.

This category was new in DSM-III, and the research to support it has been sparse. It is uncommon as personality disorders go, and there is almost no in-formation about sex distribution and family pattern. Many such patients marry and work, although they may become depressed or anxious if they lose their support systems. This disorder may be associated with a disfiguring illness or condition. Avoidant Personality Disorder is not often seen clinically; these pa-tients tend to come for evaluation only when another illness supervenes.

Criteria for Avoidant Personality Disorder

- Beginning by early adult life, social inhibition, hypersensitivity to criticism, and feelings of inadequacy are present in a variety of situations and shown by at least four of these:
  ✓ Fears criticism, disapproval, or rejection to the extent of avoiding ma-terial interpersonal contact in an occupation
  ✓ Will only become involved with others if certain of being liked
  ✓ Is restrained in intimate relationships for fear of ridicule or shame
  ✓ In social situations, is preoccupied with concerns of being criticized or rejected
  ✓ Experiences inhibitions in new relationships, stemming from feelings of inadequacy
  ✓ Is convinced of being inferior, unappealing, or inept
  ✓ For fear of embarrassment, avoids personal risk or new activities

Jack Weiblich

Jack Weiblich was feeling worse when he ought to be feeling better. At least, that's what his new acquaintances in Alcoholics Anonymous had told him. One had reminded him that 30 days sobriety was "time enough to detox every last cell" in his body. Another thought he was having a dry drunk.

"Whatever a dry drunk is," Jack observed later. "All I know is that af-ter five weeks without alcohol, I'm feeling every bit as bad as I did 15 years ago, before I'd ever had a drop. I've enjoyed hangovers more than this!"

By age 32 Jack had a lot of hangovers to choose from. He'd had his first drink when he was only a senior in high school. He had been a strange, lonely sort of kid who'd had a great deal of difficulty meeting other people. While he was still in high school, he had begun to lose his hair; now, with the exception of his eyebrows and eyelashes, he was totally bald. He was also afflicted with a slight, persistent nodding of his head. "Titubation," the neurologist had said; "don't worry about it." The sight of his balding, nodding head in the mirror every morning looked grotesque, even to Jack. As a teenager he found it almost impossible to form relationships; he was positive that no one could like someone as peculiar as he was.

Then one evening Jack found alcohol. "Right from the first drink, I knew I'd discovered something important. With two beers on board, I forgot all about my head. I even asked a girl out. She turned me down, but it didn't seem to matter that much. I had found a *life*." But the following morning, he found that he still had his old personality. He experimented for months before he learned when and how much he could drink and maintain a glow sufficiently rosy to help him feel well, but not too rosy for him to function. During a three-week period in his senior year at law school when he sobered up completely, he discovered that without alcohol, he still had the same old feelings of isolation and rejection.

"When I'm not drinking, I don't feel sad or anxious," Jack observed. "But I'm lonely and uncomfortable with myself, and I feel that other people will feel the same about me. I guess that's why I just don't make friends."

After law school, Jack went to work for a small firm that specialized in corporate law. They called him "The Mole," because he spent nearly all of every work day in the law library doing research. "I just didn't feel comfortable meeting the clients—I never get along well with new people."

The only exception to this life style was Jack's membership in the stamp club. From his grandfather, he had inherited a large collection of commemorative plate blocks. When he took these to the Philatelic Society, he thought they'd welcome him with open arms, and they did. He continued to build upon his grandfather's collection and attended meetings once a month. "I guess I feel okay there because I don't have to worry whether they'll like me. I've got a great stamp collection for them to admire."

Evaluation of Jack Weiblich

Jack's symptoms were pervasive enough (profoundly affecting his work and social life) and had been present long enough (since he was a teenager) for a personality disorder. They included the following typical criteria for Avoidant Personality Disorder: He avoided interpersonal contact (e.g., with clients at the law firm); he felt that he was unappealing; although he joined the stamp club, he was pretty sure that his collection would be accepted; he worried a lot about being rejected. Cognitive and interpersonal areas are involved (see the generic criteria for personality disorders).

Depression and anxiety are both common in avoidant patients. Therefore, it is important to search for evidence of **mood disorders** and **anxiety disorders** (especially **Social Phobia, Generalized**) in patients who avoid contact with others. Jack stated explicitly that he felt neither sad nor anxious, but he admitted that he had severely misused alcohol. The **substance-related disorders** are other Axis I disorders that commonly bring a patient with Avoidant Personality Disorder to the attention of mental health care providers.

In both Avoidant and **Schizoid Personality Disorder**, patients spend most of their time alone. The difference, of course, is that avoidant patients are unhappy with their condition, whereas schizoid people prefer it that way. A somewhat more difficult differential diagnosis may be that between Avoidant and **Dependent Personality Disorder**. (Dependent patients, like Jack, avoid positions of responsibility.) Note that Jack's avoidant life style may have had its genesis in his twin physical peculiarities, baldness and nodding head.

Although Jack was alcohol-dependent, his clinician felt that it was causing him little current difficulty and that the personality disorder was the fundamental problem needing treatment (other clinicians might argue with this decision). It was therefore listed as his principal diagnosis:

Axis I	303.90	Alcohol Dependence
Axis II	301.82	Avoidant Personality Disorder (Principal Diagnosis)
Axis III	704.09	Alopecia totalis
	781.0	Nodding of head
Axis IV		None
Axis V	GAF = 61	(current)

301.6 Dependent Personality Disorder

Much more so than most, patients with Dependent Personality Disorder feel the need to be taken care of. Because they desperately fear separation, their behavior becomes so submissive and clinging that it may result in others' taking advantage of them or rejecting them. They may feel anxious if they are thrust into a position of leadership, and they feel helpless and uncomfortable when they are alone. Because they typically need much reassurance, they may have trouble making decisions. Such patients have trouble initiating projects and sticking to a job on their own, though they may do well under the careful direction of someone else. They tend to belittle themselves and to agree with people who they know are wrong. They may also tolerate considerable abuse (even battering).

Though it may occur commonly, this condition has not been well studied. Some writers believe that it is difficult to distinguish it from Avoidant Personality Disorder. It has been found more often among women than men. Bud Stanhope, a patient with Sleep Terror Disorder, also had Dependent Personality Disorder; his history is given on page 419.

Criteria for Dependent Personality Disorder

- Beginning by early adult life, a need to be taken care of leads to clinging, submissive behavior and fears of separation that are present in a variety of situations and shown by at least five of these:
  ✓ Need for excessive advice and reassurance to make everyday decisions
  ✓ Need for others to be responsible for most major life areas
  ✓ Feared loss of approval or support, leading to difficulty with expressing disagreement (don't count fears of retaliation that are realistic)
  ✓ Trouble with starting projects or carrying them out independently (this must be due to low self-confidence, not due to low motivation or energy)
  ✓ To gain nurture and support, willingness to go to excessive lengths (even to volunteer for unpleasant tasks)
  ✓ When alone, exaggerated fears of incapacity for self-care, leading to feelings of discomfort or helplessness
  ✓ If one close relationship is lost, urgent seeking of another to provide care and support
  ✓ Preoccupation with unrealistic fears of being abandoned to provide own care

Janet Greenspan

A secretary in a large Silicon Valley company, Janet Greenspan was one of the best workers there. She was never sick or absent, and she could do anything— she'd even had some bookkeeping experience. Her supervisor noted that she was polite on the phone, typed like a demon, and would volunteer for anything. When the building maintenance crew went out on strike, Janet came in early every day for a week to clean the toilets and sinks. But somehow, she just wasn't working out.

Her supervisor's complaint was that Janet needed too much direction, even for simple things—such as what sort of paper to type form letters on. When she was asked what she thought the answer should be, her judgment was good, but she always wanted guidance anyway. Her constant need for reassurance took an inordinate amount of her supervisor's time. That was why she had been referred to the company mental health consultant for an evaluation.

At 28, Janet was slender, attractive, and very carefully dressed. Her chestnut hair already showed streaks of gray. She appeared at the doorway of the office and asked, "Where would you like me to sit?" Once she started talking, she spoke readily about her life and her work.

She had always felt timid and unsure of herself. She and her two sisters had grown up with a father who was affectionate but dictatorial; their mouse of a mother seemed to accept his loving tyranny gladly. At her mother's knee, Janet had learned obedience well.

When Janet was 18, her father suddenly died; within a few months her mother remarried and moved to another state. Janet felt bereft and panic-stricken. Instead of beginning college, she took a job as a teller in a bank; soon afterward, she married one of her customers. He was a 30-year-old bachelor, set in his ways, and he soon let it be known that he preferred to make all of the couple's decisions himself. For the first time in a year, Janet relaxed.

But even security bred its own anxieties. "Sometimes at night I wake up, wondering what I'd do if I lost him," Janet told the interviewer. "It makes my heart beat so fast I think it might stop from exhaustion. I just don't think I could manage on my own."

Evaluation of Janet Greenspan

Janet had the following symptoms of Dependent Personality Disorder: She needed considerable advice to make everyday decisions; she wanted her husband to make their decisions; panic-stricken when her father died and her mother left town, she fled into an early marriage; she feared being left to fend for herself, even though she had had no indication that this was likely. She even volunteered to clean the office toilet, probably to secure the favor of the rest of the staff. We have no evidence that she was reluctant to disagree with others, but otherwise she would seem to fit the criteria well. Janet reported that she had been this way since childhood; from the history, her character traits would seem to have affected both work and social life. Fortunately, she married someone who wanted to be in charge and who didn't seem to object to her dependency. Cognitive, affective, and interpersonal areas were involved (see the generic criteria for personality disorders).

Dependent behavior is found in several Axis I conditions and disorders that Janet did not appear to have, including **Somatization Disorder** and **Agoraphobia**. The person with the secondary psychosis in **Shared Psychotic Disorder** often has a dependent personality. **Major Depressive Disorder** and **Dysthymic Disorder** are important in the differential diagnosis; either of these may become prominent when patients lose those upon whom they depend. Even if Janet had all the required physiological symptoms for **Generalized Anxiety Disorder**, she would not be given this diagnosis, because her worries were evidently limited to fears of abandonment.

Patients with Dependent Personality Disorder must be differentiated from those with **Histrionic Personality Disorder**, who are impressionable and easily influenced by others (but Janet did not seem to be especially attention-seeking). Other personality disorders usually included in the differential diagnosis are **Borderline** and **Avoidant**.

Janet's full diagnosis would read as follows:

Axis I	V71.09	No diagnosis
Axis II	301.6	Dependent Personality Disorder
Axis III		None
Axis IV		None
Axis V	GAF = 70	(current)

301.4 Obsessive–Compulsive Personality Disorder

People with Obsessive–Compulsive Personality Disorder are perfectionistic and preoccupied with orderliness; they need to exert interpersonal and mental control. These traits exist on a lifelong basis, at the expense of efficiency, flexibility, and candor. Obsessive–Compulsive Personality Disorder is not just Axis I Obsessive–Compulsive Disorder (OCD) writ small. Many patients with the personality disorder have no actual obsessions or compulsions at all, though some eventually develop OCD.

The rigid perfectionism of these patients often results in indecisiveness, preoccupation with detail, scrupulosity, and insistence that others do things their way. These behaviors can interfere with their effectiveness in work or social situations. They may have trouble expressing affection; often they seem quite depressed, and this depression may wax and wane, sometimes to the point that it drives them into treatment. Sometimes these people are stingy; they may be savers, refusing to throw away even worthless objects they no longer need.

These people are list makers who allocate their own time poorly, workaholics who must meticulously plan even their own pleasure. Once a vacation is planned, they may only postpone it. They resist the authority of others, but insist on their own. They may be perceived as stilted, stiff, or moralistic.

This condition is probably fairly common. It is diagnosed more often in males than in females, and it probably runs in families.

Criteria for Obsessive–Compulsive Personality Disorder

• Beginning by early adult life, a preoccupation with control, orderliness, and perfection overshadow qualities of efficiency, flexibility, and candor. These behaviors are present in a variety of situations and shown by at least four of the following:

✓ Is absorbed with details, lists, order, organization, rules, or schedules to such an extent that the purpose of the activity is lost ("can't see the forest for the trees")
✓ Is perfectionistic to a degree that interferes with completing the task
✓ Is a workaholic (works to exclusion of leisure activities)
✓ To a degree out of keeping with cultural or religious influence, is overly conscientious, inflexible, or scrupulous about ethics, morals, or values
✓ Saves worthless items of no real or sentimental value
✓ Won't cooperate or delegate tasks unless others agree to do things the patient's way
✓ Is stingy toward self and others; hoards money against future need
✓ Is rigid and stubborn

Robin Chatterjee

"I admit it—I'm over the top in neatness." Robin Chatterjee straightened a fold in her traditional Indian sari. Robin was a graduate student in biology, born in Bombay and educated in London. Now she spent part of her time as a teaching assistant in biology, and the rest struggling through her own course work at a major U.S. university. She gazed steadily at the interviewer

According to her preceptor, a slightly dour Scot named Dr. MacLeish who had asked her to come for the interview, the problem wasn't neatness. It was completing the work. Every paper she turned in was wonderful—every fact was there, every conclusion correct, not even a misspelling. He had asked her why she couldn't learn to let go of them a little sooner, "before the rats die of old age?" She had thought it funny at the time, but it made her think.

Robin had always been orderly. Her mother had made her keep neat little lists of her chores, and the habit stuck. Robin admitted that she became so "lost in lists" that sometimes she hardly had time to finish the work. Her students seemed fond of her, but several had said they wished she'd give them more responsibility. One had told Dr. MacLeish that Robin seemed afraid even to let them do their own dissections—their methods weren't as compulsively correct as hers were, so she tried to do them herself. Finally, she also admitted that nearly every night, her work habits kept her in the lab until late. It had been weeks since she'd had a date—or any social life at all. This realization was what spurred her to follow Dr. MacLeish's advice and come in for a mental health evaluation.

Evaluation of Robin Chatterjee

Robin would barely meet the criteria for Obsessive–Compulsive Personality Disorder. She was workaholic and perfectionistic, to the point that it interfered with the learning of her students. She had a great deal of difficulty delegating work—even the students' own dissections! And she concentrated so on her lists of tasks that she sometimes didn't accomplish the tasks themselves. She had had these tendencies throughout her young adult life. Interpersonal and cognitive areas were involved (see the generic criteria).

Depressed mood is common in these patients. The common Axis I disorders that should be looked for in a patient with Obsessive–Compulsive Personality Disorder include **OCD**, **Major Depressive Disorder**, and **Dysthymic Disorder**. Robin was not depressed and, unlike so many patients with Obsessive–Compulsive Personality Disorder, seemed to have no other disorder. Because she barely met the criteria and was functioning well overall, the extent of her personality disorder would be judged to be Mild:

Axis I	V71.09	No diagnosis
Axis II	301.4	Obsessive–Compulsive Personality Disorder, Mild
Axis III		None
Axis IV		None
Axis V	GAF = 70	(current)

OTHER PERSONALITY DISORDERS

301.9 Personality Disorder Not Otherwise Specified

The Personality Disorder Not Otherwise Specified category can be used for patients who have insufficient features for any better-defined personality disorder, but who appear to have long-standing personality traits that have caused difficulties in many life areas. It can also be used for other personality disorders that have not yet received official DSM sanction, such as Depressive Personality Disorder (or have recently lost it, such as Passive–Aggressive Personality Disorder). Such a case would be coded on Axis II as, for example, Personality Disorder Not Otherwise Specified (passive–aggressive). In DSM-IV, see page 732 for suggested research criteria for Depressive Personality Disorder, and page 733 for those for Passive–Aggressive Personality Disorder.

CHAPTER 16

Disorders Usually First Diagnosed in Infancy, Childhood, or Adolescence

Quick Guide to Disorders Beginning in Infancy, Childhood, or Adolescence

Of course, many of the disorders considered earlier in this book can be first encountered in children (or at least young adolescents); Anorexia Nervosa and Schizophrenia are but two examples that come quickly to mind. Conversely, many of the disorders discussed in this chapter can continue to cause problems during adulthood. But only a few commonly constitute a focus of attention for clinicians who evaluate and treat adults. These are considered in detail in this chapter, and are marked in the Quick Guide by an asterisk (*). For the remainder of the disorders DSM-IV includes in the section of the manual corresponding to this chapter, I provide the diagnostic criteria only. (Also mentioned below are some conditions arising in early life that are assigned V-codes in DSM-IV and covered in the section of the manual titled "Other Conditions That May Be a Focus of Clinical Attention"; I discuss these conditions briefly in Chapter 17.) As always in the Quick Guide, the page number following each item refers to the point at which a discussion of it begins.

Limitations of Intellectual Functioning

*Mental Retardation. Beginning before the age of 18, these people have low intelligence that causes them to need special help in coping with life. Note that Mental Retardation is coded on Axis II of DSM-IV and is assigned a code number according to its severity: Mild, Moderate, Severe, Profound, or Unspecified. It is described in detail beginning on page 501.

Borderline Intellectual Functioning. This V-code is used for persons in the IQ range of 71 –84, without the problems in coping with life associated with Mental Retardation (p.540).

Learning Disorders

As the label suggests, people with learning disorders have far more difficulty than normal in learning specific academic skills. Although they will be suspected on the basis of classroom reports, each of these diagnoses must be made on the basis of a standardized, individualized test. In DSM-III-R these were called academic skills disorders and were coded on Axis II; in DSM-IV they are coded on Axis I.

Reading Disorder. The patient's reading skills develop far more slowly than those of peers (p.506).

Mathematics Disorder. Math skills are markedly less than expected for the patient's age (p.507).

Disorder of Written Expression. Writing skills are slow to develop (p.507).

Learning Disorder Not Otherwise Specified. Use this category for learning disorders, such as spelling, that do not meet the criteria for any of the disorders above (p.508).

Academic Problem. This V-code is used when scholastic problems are the focus of treatment (p.541).

Motor Skills Disorder

Developmental Coordination Disorder. The patient is slow to develop motor coordination and is *not* necessarily mentally retarded (p.508). This category was coded on Axis II in DSM-III-R, but is coded on Axis I of DSM-IV.

Communication Disorders

Communication disorders, like the disorders in the preceding two groups, have been moved from Axis II in DSM-III-R to Axis I in DSM-IV.

Expressive Language Disorder. Patients may have small vocabularies or trouble producing grammatically correct sentences (p.509).

Mixed Receptive–Expressive Language Disorder. A patient has the problems noted above, plus problems understanding words or sentences (p.509).

Phonological Disorder. Speech develops slowly for the patient's age or dialect (p.510).

Stuttering. There is frequent disruption in the normal fluency of speech (p.510).

Pervasive Developmental Disorders

In the pervasive developmental disorders (which, again, DSM-III-R placed on Axis II, but DSM-IV places on Axis I) children fail to develop normally in a number of areas; these include the ability to interact socially, to communicate verbally and nonverbally, and to use their imaginations. Of course, once such a child grows up these conditions will continue to affect adult life, but they will hardly ever be the focus of an initial evaluation of an adult.

Autistic Disorder. The child has impaired social interactions and communications, and develops stereotyped behaviors and interests (p.511).

Rett's Disorder. After six months of apparently normal development, the child has abnormal development as shown by slow head growth, delayed language, poorly coordinated gait, and loss of purposeful hand movements and of social engagement (p.512).

Childhood Disintegrative Disorder. Following two years of normal development, the child loses acquired skills (p.513).

Asperger's Disorder. This condition is similar to Autistic Disorder, except that children with Asperger's Disorder do not have delayed or impaired language (p.514).

Pervasive Developmental Disorder Not Otherwise Specified. This category is used for such conditions as atypical autism (p.514).

Attention-Deficit and Disruptive Behavior Disorders

Attention-Deficit/Hyperactivity Disorder. In this common condition, abbreviated as ADHD, patients are hyperactive, impulsive, or inattentive, and often all three (p.515).

Attention-Deficit/Hyperactivity Disorder Not Otherwise Specified. Use this category for symptoms of hyperactivity, impulsivity, or inattention that do not meet the criteria for ADHD (p.520).

Conduct Disorder. The patient violates rules or the rights of others (p.520). It is a common precursor to Antisocial Personality Disorder, for which it forms a portion of the criteria (p.474).

Oppositional Defiant Disorder. Multiple examples of negativistic behavior persist for at least six months (p.521).

Child or Adolescent Antisocial Behavior. This V-code can be used in instances where antisocial behavior cannot be ascribed to a mental disorder such as Oppositional Defiant Disorder, Conduct Disorder, or ADHD (p.540).

Disruptive Behavior Disorder Not Otherwise Specified. Use this category for disturbances of conduct or oppositional behaviors that do not meet the criteria for Conduct Disorder or Oppositional Defiant Disorder (p.522).

Feeding and Eating Disorders of Infancy or Early Childhood

Pica. The patient eats material that is not food (p.522).

Rumination Disorder. There is persistent regurgitation and chewing of food already eaten (p.523).

Feeding Disorder of Infancy or Early Childhood. A child's failure to eat enough leads to weight loss or a failure to gain weight (p.523).

Tic Disorders

*Tourette's Disorder. Multiple vocal and motor tics occur frequently throughout the day in these patients (p.523).

Chronic Motor or Vocal Tic Disorder. A patient has either motor or vocal tics, but not both (p.526).

Transient Tic Disorder. Tics occur for no longer than one year in these patients (p.527).

Tic Disorder Not Otherwise Specified. Use this category for tics that do not meet the criteria for any of the preceding (p.527).

Elimination Disorders

Encopresis. At the age of four years or later, the patient repeatedly passes feces into clothing or onto the floor (p.528).

Enuresis. At the age of five years or later, there is repeated voiding of urine (it can be voluntary or involuntary) into bedding or clothing (p.528).

Other Disorders of Infancy, Childhood, or Adolescence

Separation Anxiety Disorder. The patient becomes anxious when separated from parent or home (p.529).

Selective Mutism. The patient elects not to talk (p.530).

Reactive Attachment Disorder of Infancy or Early Childhood. Beginning before age five, a child doesn't relate appropriately to others (p.530).

Stereotypic Movement Disorder. Patients repeatedly rock, bang their heads, bite themselves, or pick at their own skin or body orifices (p.531).

Parent–Child Relational Problem. This V-code is used when there is no mental disorder, but a child and parent have problems getting along (e.g., overprotection or inconsistent discipline) (p.537).

Sibling Relational Problem. This V-code is used for difficulties between siblings (p.537).

Problems Related to Abuse or Neglect. A single V-code number is used to cover the categories of difficulties that arise from neglect or from physical or sexual abuse of children (p.538).

Disorder of Infancy, Childhood, or Adolescence Not Otherwise Specified. This is a catch-all category for mental disorders beginning in early life that do not meet the criteria for *any* disorder described above (p.532).

Introduction

The title of this chapter means exactly what it says: The onset of these Disorders is usually sometime during childhood. It does not mean that these disorders occur only during the early years of a person's life, nor does it mean that a child cannot have a disorder listed elsewhere in DSM-IV.

The principal aim of this book is to provide information about the diagnosis of mental health disorders that affect adults. But a few of the childhood disorders listed in this chapter persist long enough to become a focus for evaluation or treatment in adult life. For convenience, I give criteria for all the disorders that begin in infancy, childhood, or adolescence. But I provide descriptions and vignettes only for those you are likely to encounter in adults who come for evaluation.

MENTAL RETARDATION

Mental Retardation

Mental Retardation is a behavioral syndrome related to low intelligence. By definition, it begins before the age of 18. Of course, in most instances the onset is far earlier—usually in infancy, or even before birth. If the onset of the behavior occurs at age 18 or after, it is called a dementia. These two diagnoses can coexist.

Besides age of onset, there are two other basic criteria for this diagnosis:

1. The patient's intelligence level, as determined by a standard individual test (not a group test, which is less accurate), must be markedly below average. In practical terms, this means an IQ of less than 70.

2. At this IQ level, most people need special help to cope with life. This need defines the other important criterion for diagnosis: The patient's ability to adapt to the demands of normal life must be impaired in some important way. How well this adaptation succeeds depends on the patient's education, job training, motivation, personality, and support from significant others. Of course, adaptation also varies inversely with the severity of retardation.

The second criterion is important for two reasons, each of which suggests the value of flexibility when interpreting a low IQ score. Some people with unusually low IQs are able to get along without assistance, whereas others who score higher than 70 need help in coping. Also, cultural differences, illness, and mental set can all affect the accuracy of IQ testing.

A variety of behavioral problems commonly associated with Mental Retardation do not constitute criteria for diagnosis. Among them are aggression, dependency, impulsivity, passivity, self-injury, stubbornness, low self-esteem, and poor frustration tolerance. Many of these people also suffer from mood disorders (which are often underdiagnosed), psychotic disorders, poor attention span, and hyperactivity. However, many others are quite placid, loving, and pleasant people whom others find enjoyable to live and associate with.

Although many mentally retarded people are physically normal, others have abnormalities that make them conspicuous, even to the untrained eye. These include short stature, seizures, hemangioma, and malformations of the eyes, ears, and other parts of the face. A diagnosis of mental retardation is likely to be made earlier when there are associated physical abnormalities (e.g., those seen in Down's syndrome).

The many causes of Mental Retardation include genetic abnormalities, chemical effects, structural brain damage, inborn errors of metabolism, and childhood disease. An individual may have biological or social causes, or both. Some of these (with the approximate percentage of all cases of Mental Retardation they represent) are given below:

Genetic Causes (About 5%). Chromosomal abnormalities, Tay–Sachs, tuberous sclerosis.

Early Pregnancy Factors (about 30%). Trisomy 21 (Down's syndrome), substance use by mother, infections.

Later Pregnancy and Perinatal Factors (about 10%). Prematurity, anoxia, birth trauma, fetal malnutrition.

Acquired Childhood Physical Conditions (about 5%). Lead poisoning, infections, trauma.

Environmental Influences and Mental Disorders (about 20%). Cultural deprivation, early-onset Schizophrenia.

Unknown Factors (about 30%). No identifiable cause.

As defined above, about 1% of the general population has Mental Retardation. Males outnumber females about three to two. The vast majority of these people (85%) have Mild Mental Retardation (IQ of 50 to 70); these people are usually considered "educable." They can be expected to attain roughly sixth-grade academic skills by the time they are grown, and with support can often live in the community. Individuals with Moderate Mental Retardation (IQ level from the high 30s to low 50s) constitute about 10% of all mentally retarded persons. They usually learn to communicate while still young, and can learn social and occupational skills. They may be able to work in sheltered workshops, but will probably never live independently. Those with Severe Mental Retardation (IQ level from the low 20s to high 30s) constitute under 5%. They may learn to communicate when they are in school, and, under supervision, may learn to perform simple jobs. They may even learn to read a few words. Persons with Profound Mental Retardation (IQ in the low 20s or below) constitute only 1–2%; usually a serious neurological disorder has caused their retardation.

TIP Even individually administered IQ tests will have a few points of error. That is why some patients with measured IQs as high as 75 can sometimes be diagnosed as having Mental Retardation—they have problems with adaptive functioning that help define the condition. On the other hand, an occasional person with an IQ of less than 70 may function quite well, and therefore not qualify for this diagnosis.

Interpretation of IQ scores also must consider the possibility of *scatter* (better performance on verbal tests than on performance tests, or vice versa), as well as physical, cultural, and emotional disabilities. This is not an easy area in which to make interpretations, and the help of a skilled psychometrist may be needed in many instances.

Finally, like the personality disorders, Mental Retardation is a lifelong condition that is coded on Axis II.

Criteria for Mental Retardation

- The patient's intellectual functioning is markedly below average (IQ of 70 or less on a standard, individually administered test).
- In two or more of the following areas, the patient has more trouble functioning than would be expected for age and cultural group:
  ✓ Communicating
  ✓ Caring for self
  ✓ Living at home
  ✓ Relating to others
  ✓ Using community resources
  ✓ Directing self
  ✓ Academic functioning
  ✓ Working
  ✓ Using free time
  ✓ Health
  ✓ Safety
- The condition begins before age 18.

Coding Notes

Code based on approximate IQ range:

317	Mild Mental Retardation (IQ 50–55 to 70)
318.0	Moderate Mental Retardation (IQ 35–40 to 50–55)
318.1	Severe Mental Retardation (IQ 20–25 to 35–40)

| 318.2 | Profound Mental Retardation (IQ less than 20–25) |
| 319 | Mental Retardation, Severity Unspecified (the patient cannot be tested, but retardation seems highly likely) |

Mental Retardation is coded on Axis II. On Axis I, code any associated mental disorders; on Axis III, code any general medical condition that has caused the Mental Retardation.

For infants, the clinician must make a subjective judgment of intellectual functioning.

Grover Peary

When Grover Peary was born, his mother was only 15. She was an obese, unpopular girl who hadn't even realized she was pregnant until her sixth month. Then she hadn't bothered to seek prenatal care. Born after a hard 30-hour labor, Grover hadn't breathed right away. After the delivery, his mother had lost interest in him; he had been reared alternately by his grandmother and aunt. Grover was now 28 years old.

Grover had walked at 20 months and spoken his first words when he was two and a half.

After a pediatrician diagnosed him as being "somewhat slow," his grandmother enrolled him in an infant school for the developmentally disabled. At the age of seven, he had done well enough to be "mainstreamed" in his local elementary school. Throughout the remainder of his school career, he worked with a special education teacher for two hours each day and attended regular class for the rest of the day. Testing when he was in the 4th and 10th grades placed his IQ at 70 and 72, respectively.

Despite his handicap, Grover loved school. He had learned to read by the time he was eight, and he spent much of his free time poring over books on geography and natural science. (He had a great deal of free time, especially at recess and lunch hour. He was clumsy and physically undersized, and the other children routinely excluded him from their games.) He talked at one time of becoming a geologist, but was steered toward a general curriculum. Because he lived in a county that provided special education and training for the mentally handicapped, he learned to navigate the complicated public transportation. A job coach helped him to find work washing dishes at a restaurant in a downtown hotel, and to learn the skills necessary to maintain the job. The restaurant manager got him a room in the hotel basement.

The waitresses at the restaurant often gave Grover a few quarters out of their tips. Living at the hotel, he didn't need much money—his room and food were taken care of, and in the tiny dish room where he worked, he didn't need much of a wardrobe. He spent most of his money on his CD collection and going to the baseball games. His aunt, who saw him every week, helped him with grooming and reminded him to shave. She and her husband also took him to ballgames; otherwise, he would have spent nearly all of his free time in his room, listening to his stereo and reading magazines.

When an earthquake hit the city where Grover lived, the hotel was so badly damaged that it closed with no notice at all. Thrown out of work, all of Grover's fellow employees were too busy taking care of their own families to think about Grover. His aunt was out of town on vacation, so he had nowhere to turn. It was summertime, so he placed the few possessions he had rescued in a heavy-duty lawn and leaf bag and walked the streets until he grew tired; he then rolled out some blankets in the park. He slept this way for nearly two weeks, eating what he could scrounge from other campers. Although federal emergency relief workers had been sent to help those hit by the earthquake, Grover did not request relief. Finally, a park ranger recognized his plight and referred him to the clinic.

During that first interview, Grover's shaggy hair and thin face gave him the appearance of someone older than 28. Dressed in a soiled shirt and a baggy pair of pants (they appeared to be someone's castoffs), he sat still in his chair and gave poor eye contact. He spoke hesitantly at first, but he was clear and coherent, and could eventually communicate well with the interviewer. (Much of the information given above, however, was obtained from old school records and from his aunt upon her return from vacation.)

Grover's mood was surprisingly good, about medium in quality. He smiled when he talked about his aunt, but looked serious when he was asked where he was going to stay. He had no delusions, hallucinations, obsessions, compulsions, or phobias. He denied having any Panic Attacks, though he admitted he felt "sorta worried" when he had to sleep in the park.

Grover scored 25 out of 30 on the Mini-Mental State Exam. He was oriented except to day and month; he spent a great deal of effort subtracting sevens, and finally got two correct. He was able to recall three objects after five minutes, and managed a perfect score on the language section. He recognized that he had a problem with where to live, but, aside from asking his aunt when she returned, he didn't have the slightest idea how to go about solving the problem.

Evaluation of Grover Peary

Had Grover been evaluated before the hotel closed, he might not have fulfilled the criteria for Mental Retardation. At that time he had a place to live, food to eat, and activities to occupy him. However, his aunt had to remind him about shaving and staying presentable. Despite low scores on at least two IQ tests, he was functioning pretty well in a highly, if informally, structured environment.

But once this support system collapsed (quite literally), Grover could not cope with change. He did not make use of the resources available to others who had lost their homes. He was unable to find work. Through the generosity of others, he managed to eat. Therefore, despite the fact that his IQ had hovered in the low 70s, he was judged impaired enough to warrant a diagnosis of Mild Mental Retardation.

The differential diagnosis of Mental Retardation includes a variety of **learn-**

ing disorders and communication disorders, the criteria for which are given later in this chapter. Dementia would have been diagnosed if Grover's problem with cognition had represented a marked decline from his previous level of functioning. (The two diagnoses can coexist, though they can be difficult to discriminate.) Even at his IQ level, Grover might have been diagnosed as having Borderline Intellectual Functioning if he had not had such obvious difficulties in coping with life.

Mentally retarded youngsters and adults often have associated Axis I disorders, which include Attention-Deficit/Hyperactivity Disorder and pervasive developmental disorders. Mood disorders are often present, though clinicians may not recognize them without adequate collateral information. Personality traits such as stubbornness are also sometimes concomitant. Down's syndrome patients are at high risk for developing Dementia of the Alzheimer's Type as they approach their 40s. Grover's five-Axis diagnosis would be as follows:

Axis I	V71.09	No diagnosis
Axis II	317	Mild Mental Retardation
Axis III		None
Axis IV		Homeless
		Unemployed
Axis V	GAF = 45	(current)

> TIP Note that the term *developmental disability* as it is used in law is not restricted to people with Mental Retardation. This term applies to anyone who by age 22 has permanent problems functioning in at least three areas because of mental or physical impairment.

LEARNING DISORDERS

315.00 Reading Disorder

Criteria for Reading Disorder

- As measured by a standardized test that is given individually, the patient's ability to read (accuracy or comprehension) is substantially less than would be expected from the patient's age, intelligence, and education.

- This deficiency materially impedes academic achievement or daily living.
- If there is also a sensory defect, the reading deficiency is worse than would be expected from it.

Coding Note

On Axis III, code any sensory deficit or general medical condition (such as a neurological disorder).

315.1 Mathematics Disorder

Criteria for Mathematics Disorder

- As measured by a standardized test that is given individually, the patient's mathematical ability is substantially less than would be expected from the patient's age, intelligence, and education.
- This deficiency materially impedes academic achievement or daily living.
- If there is also a sensory defect, the mathematics deficiency is worse than would be expected from it.

Coding Note

On Axis III, code any sensory deficit or general medical condition (such as a neurological disorder).

315.2 Disorder of Written Expression

Criteria for Disorder of Written Expression

- As measured by functional assessment or by a standardized test that is given individually, the patient's writing ability is substantially less than would be expected from the patient's age, intelligence, and education.
- The difficulty with writing grammatically correct sentences and organized paragraphs materially impedes academic achievement or daily living.
- If there is also a sensory defect, the writing deficiency is worse than would be expected from it.

Coding Note

On Axis III, code any sensory deficit or general medical condition (such as a neurological disorder).

315.9 Learning Disorder Not Otherwise Specified

Problems of learning that don't meet criteria for any more specific disorder can be coded as Learning Disorder Not Otherwise Specified. DSM-IV gives the example of reading, mathematical, and writing problems that only together impede academic ability.

MOTOR SKILLS DISORDER

315.4 Developmental Coordination Disorder

Criteria for Developmental Coordination Disorder

- Motor coordination in daily activities is substantially less than would be expected from the patient's age and intelligence. This may be shown by dropping things, general clumsiness, poor handwriting, or poor sports ability, or by pronounced delays in developmental motor milestones (such as sitting, crawling, or walking.)
- This incoordination materially impedes academic achievement or daily living.
- It is not due to a general medical condition, such as cerebral palsy or muscular dystrophy.
- Criteria for a pervasive developmental disorder are not fulfilled.
- If there is Mental Retardation, the incoordination is worse than would be expected from it.

Coding Note

On Axis III, code any sensory deficit or general medical condition (such as a neurological disorder).

COMMUNICATION DISORDERS

315.31 Expressive Language Disorder

Criteria for Expressive Language Disorder

- As measured by standardized tests that are given individually, the patient's scores for expressive language development are materially lower than those for *both* nonverbal intellectual capacity and receptive language development. Clinically, the patient may have severely limited vocabulary, make errors of tense, recall words poorly, or produce sentences that are shorter or less complex than is developmentally appropriate.
- This disorder interferes with educational or occupational achievement or with social communication.
- It does not fulfill criteria for a Mixed Receptive–Expressive Language Disorder or a pervasive developmental disorder.
- If the patient also has Mental Retardation, environmental deprivation, or a speech–motor or sensory deficit, the problems with language are worse than would be expected from these problems.

Coding Note

On Axis III, code any neurological condition or a speech–motor or sensory deficit.

315.31 Mixed Receptive–Expressive Language Disorder

Criteria for Mixed Receptive–Expressive Language Disorder

- As measured by standardized tests that are given individually, the patient's receptive *and* expressive language development scores are materially lower than those for nonverbal intellectual capacity. Clinically, the patient may have the same problems as with Expressive Language Disorder, as well as problems understanding sentences, words, or specific classes of words (such as spatial terms).

- This disorder interferes with educational or occupational achievement or with social communication.
- It does not fulfill criteria for a pervasive developmental disorder.
- If the patient also has Mental Retardation, environmental deprivation or a speech–motor or sensory deficit, the problems with language are worse than would be expected from these problems.

Coding Note

On Axis III, code any neurological condition or a speech–motor or sensory deficit.

315.39 Phonological Disorder

Criteria for Phonological Disorder

- The patient doesn't use speech sounds that are expected for age and dialect. Examples: substituting consonant sounds for one another, omitting final consonants.
- This problem interferes with educational or occupational achievement or with social communication.
- If the patient also has Mental Retardation, environmental deprivation or a speech–motor or sensory deficit, the problems with language are worse than would be expected from these problems.

Coding Note

On Axis III, code any neurological condition or a speech–motor or sensory deficit.

307.0 Stuttering

Criteria for Stuttering

- The patient lacks normal fluency and time patterning of speech that are appropriate for age. This is characterized by frequent occurrences of at least one of the following:
  ✓ Repetitions of sounds and syllables

✓ Sound prolongations
✓ Interjections
✓ Broken words (pauses within words)
✓ Blocking that is audible or silent
✓ Circumlocutions (substitutions to avoid words that are hard to pronounce)
✓ Words spoken with excessive physical tension
✓ Repetitions of monosyllabic whole words (such as "A-a-a-a-a dog bit me")
• These problems interfere with educational or occupational achievement or with social communication.
• If the patient also has a sensory or speech-motor deficit, the problems with language are worse than would be expected from these problems.

Coding Note

On Axis III, code any neurological condition or a sensory or speech–motor deficit.

307.9 Communication Disorder Not Otherwise Specified

Use Communication Disorder Not Otherwise Specified for patients whose problems of communication don't fit the criteria for any more specific disorder. DSM-IV gives examples of abnormalities in the pitch, loudness, quality, tone, or resonance of the voice.

PERVASIVE DEVELOPMENTAL DISORDERS

299.00 Autistic Disorder

Criteria for Autistic Disorder

• The patient fulfills a total of at least six criteria from the following three lists, distributed as indicated:

- Impaired social interaction (at least two):
  - ✓ Markedly deficient regulation of social interaction through multiple nonverbal behaviors, such as eye contact, facial expression, body posture, and gestures
  - ✓ Lack of peer relationships that are appropriate to developmental level
  - ✓ Absence of seeking to share achievements, interests, or pleasure with others
  - ✓ Absence of social or emotional reciprocity
- Impaired communication (at least one):
  - ✓ Delayed or absent development of spoken language, for which the patient *doesn't* try to compensate with gestures
  - ✓ In patients who can speak, notable deficiency in ability to begin or sustain a conversation
  - ✓ Language that is repetitive, stereotyped, or idiosyncratic
  - ✓ Appropriate to developmental stage, absence of social imitative play or spontaneous, make-believe play
- Activities, behaviors, and interests that are repetitive, restricted, and stereotyped (at least one):
  - ✓ Abnormal (in focus or intensity) preoccupation with interests that are restricted and stereotyped (such as spinning things)
  - ✓ Rigid performance of routines or rituals that don't appear to have a function
  - ✓ Repetitive, stereotyped motor mannerisms (such as hand flapping)
  - ✓ Persistent absorption with parts of objects
- Before age three, the patient shows delayed or abnormal functioning in one or more of these areas:
  - ✓ Social interaction
  - ✓ Language used in social communication
  - ✓ Imaginative or symbolic play
- These symptoms are not better explained by Childhood Disintegrative Disorder or Rett's Disorder.

299.80 Rett's Disorder

Criteria for Rett's Disorder

- *All* of the following suggest normal early development:
  - Prenatal and perinatal development

- Psychomotor development, at least until age 5 months
- Head circumference at birth
- After this apparently normal beginning, *all* of these occur:
  - Head growth slows abnormally between 5 and 48 months.
  - Between 5 and 30 months, the child loses already acquired purposeful hand movements and develops stereotyped hand movements, such as hand washing or hand wringing.
  - Early in the course, the child loses interest in the social environment. (However, social interaction often develops later.)
  - Gait or movements of trunk are poorly coordinated.
  - Severe psychomotor retardation and impairment of expressive and receptive language.

299.10 Childhood Disintegrative Disorder

Criteria for Childhood Disintegrative Disorder

- At least until age two, the child develops normally, as shown by age-appropriate adaptive behavior, play, social relationships, and both nonverbal and verbal communication.
- Before age 10, the child experiences clinically important loss of previously learned skills in the following areas (two or more required):
  - ✓ Language (expressive or receptive)
  - ✓ Adaptive behavior or social skills
  - ✓ Bladder or bowel control
  - ✓ Play
  - ✓ Motor skills
- The child functions abnormally in two or more of the following ways:
  - ✓ Social interaction is characterized by impaired nonverbal behaviors, peer relationships, or emotional or social reciprocity.
  - ✓ Communication is characterized by delayed or absent spoken language, inability to converse, language use that is repetitive or stereotyped, or absence of varied make-believe play.
  - ✓ Activities, behavior, and interests are repetitive, restricted, and stereotyped; this includes motor mannerisms and stereotypies.
- These symptoms are not better explained by Schizophrenia or by another specific pervasive developmental disorder.

299.80 Asperger's Disorder

Criteria for Asperger's Disorder

- At least two demonstrations of impaired social interaction:
  - ✓ Markedly deficient regulation of social interaction through multiple non-verbal behaviors, such as eye contact, facial expression, body posture, and gestures.
  - ✓ Lack of peer relationships that are appropriate to developmental level
  - ✓ Absence of seeking to share achievements, interests, or pleasure with others
  - ✓ Absence of social or emotional reciprocity
- At least one demonstration of activities, behavior, and interests that are repetitive, restricted, and stereotyped:
  - ✓ Abnormal (in focus or intensity) preoccupation with interests that are restricted and stereotyped (such as spinning things)
  - ✓ Rigid performance of routines or rituals that don't appear to have a function
  - ✓ Repetitive, stereotyped motor mannerisms (such as hand flapping)
  - ✓ Persistent absorption with parts of objects
- The symptoms cause clinically important impairment in social, occupational, or personal functioning.
- There is *no* clinically important general language delay (the child can speak words by age two, phrases by age three).
- There is *no* clinically important delay in developing cognition, age-appropriate self-help skills, adaptive behavior (except social interaction), and normal curiosity about the environment.
- The patient doesn't fulfill criteria for Schizophrenia or for another specific pervasive developmental disorder.

299.80 Pervasive Developmental Disorder Not Otherwise Specified

Use Pervasive Developmental Disorder Not Otherwise Specified for severe, pervasive developmental disturbances that do not meet criteria for one of the specific disorders described above or for Schizophrenia, Schizotypal Personality Disorder, or Avoidant Personality Disorder. DSM-IV particularly mentions atypical autism, which is a label used for disturbances that don't meet criteria for Autistic Disorder because of late age of onset, too few symptoms, or atypical symptoms.

ATTENTION-DEFICIT AND DISRUPTIVE BEHAVIOR DISORDERS

314.xx Attention-Deficit/Hyperactivity Disorder

Attention-Deficit/Hyperactivity Disorder (ADHD), which has had a long string of names since it was first described in 1902, is one of the most common behavioral disorders of childhood. But only in the last few years have clinicians widely acknowledged that symptoms of ADHD can persist into adult life.

Although this disorder is usually not diagnosed until the age of nine, symptoms typically begin before the child goes to school. (DSM-IV criteria require some symptoms before age seven.) Mothers sometimes report that their ADHD children cried more than their other babies, that they were colicky or irritable, or that they slept less. Some even swear that these children kicked more before they were born.

Developmental milestones may occur early; these children may be described as never walking, but running. They are "motorically driven" and have trouble sitting quietly. They may also be clumsy and have problems with their coordination. At least one study has found that they require more emergency care than do non-ADHD children for injuries and accidental poisonings. They often cannot focus on schoolwork; therefore, though IQ is usually normal, they may perform poorly in school. They tend to be impulsive, to say things that hurt the feelings of others, and to be unpopular. They may be so unhappy that they also fulfill criteria for Dysthymic Disorder.

All of these behaviors usually decrease with adolescence, when many ADHD patients settle down and become normally active and capable students. But some use substances or develop other forms of delinquent behavior. Adults may continue to have interpersonal problems, alcohol or drug use, or personality disorders. Adults may also complain of trouble concentrating, disorganization, impulsivity, mood lability, overactivity, quick temper, and intolerance of stress.

ADHD affects about 2% of boys and a much smaller percentage of girls (the ratio ranges between four to one and seven to one). No one knows how many adults are still affected by remnants of this disorder. The condition tends to run in families: Parents and siblings are more likely than average to be affected. Alcoholism and divorce, as well as other causes of family disruption, are common in the family backgrounds of these people. There may be a genetic association with Antisocial Personality Disorder and Somatization Disorder. Also associated with ADHD are various learning disabilities, especially problems with reading.

Criteria for Attention-deficit/Hyperactivity Disorder

- The patient has *either* **inattention** or **hyperactivity–impulsivity** (or both), persisting for at least six months to a degree that is maladaptive and immature, as shown by the following:
    - ✓ **Inattention.** At least six of the following *often* apply:
        - ✓ Fails to pay close attention to details or makes careless errors in schoolwork, work, or other activities
        - ✓ Has trouble keeping attention on tasks or play
        - ✓ Doesn't appear to listen when being told something
        - ✓ Neither follows through on instructions nor completes chores, schoolwork, or jobs (*not* because of oppositional behavior or failure to understand)
        - ✓ Has trouble organizing activities and tasks
        - ✓ Dislikes or avoids tasks that involve sustained mental effort (homework, schoolwork)
        - ✓ Loses materials needed for activities (assignments, books, pencils, tools, toys)
        - ✓ Is easily distracted by external stimuli
        - ✓ Is forgetful

    - ✓ **Hyperactivity–impulsivity.** At least six of the following *often* apply:

    Hyperactivity

    - ✓ Squirms in seat or fidgets
    - ✓ Inappropriately leaves seat
    - ✓ Inappropriately runs or climbs (in adolescents or adults, this may be only a subjective feeling of restlessness)
    - ✓ Has trouble quietly playing or engaging in leisure activity
    - ✓ Appears driven or "on the go"
    - ✓ Talks excessively

    Impulsivity

    - ✓ Answers questions before they have been completely asked
    - ✓ Has trouble awaiting turn
    - ✓ Interrupts or intrudes on others
- Some of the symptoms above began before age seven.
- Symptoms are present in at least two types of situations, such as school, work, home.
- The disorder impairs school, social, or occupational functioning.
- The symptoms do not occur solely during a pervasive developmental disorder or any psychotic disorder, including Schizophrenia.
- The symptoms are not explained better by a mood, anxiety, dissociative, or personality disorder.

Coding Notes

Code is based on the symptoms during the past six months:

3 I 4.00	Attention-Deficit/Hyperactivity Disorder, Predominantly Inattentive Type. The patient has recently met the criteria for inattention but not for hyperactivity–impulsivity.
3 I 4.0 I	Attention-deficit/Hyperactivity Disorder, Predominantly Hyperactive–Impulsive Type. The patient has recently met the criteria for hyperactivity–impulsivity but not for inattention.
3 I 4.0 I	Attention-Deficit/Hyperactivity Disorder, Combined Type. The patient has recently met the criteria for both inattention *and* hyperactivity–impulsivity. (Most ADHD children have symptoms of the Combined Type.)

Specify "In Partial Remission" for patients (especially adults or adolescents) whose *current* symptoms do not fulfill the criteria.

Denis Tourney

"I think I've got what my son has."

Denis Tourney was a 37-year-old married man who worked as a research chemist.

Throughout his life, he had had trouble focusing his attention on any task at hand. Because he was very bright and personable, he had been able to overcome his handicap and succeed at his job for a major pharmaceutical manufacturer.

At home one evening the week before this appointment, Denis had been working on plans for a new chemical synthesis. His wife and children were in bed and it was quiet, but he had been having an unusually hard time keeping his mind on his work. Everything seemed to distract him—the ticking of the clock, the cat jumping up onto the table. Besides, his head was beginning to pound, so he grabbed what he thought were two aspirin tablets and washed them down with a glass of milk.

"What happened next seemed like magic," he said. "It was as if somebody had put my brain waves through a funnel and squirted them onto the paper I was working on. Within half an hour I had shut out everything but my work. In two hours I accomplished what would ordinarily take a day or more to get done. Then I got suspicious and looked at the pill bottle. I had taken two of the tablets that were prescribed last month for Randy."

Denis's son was eight, and until a month ago he had been considered the terror of the second grade. But in the four weeks that he had been taking Ritalin, he had seemed less driven; his grades had improved; and he had become "almost a pleasure to live with."

For years, Denis had suspected that he himself might have been hyperactive as a child. Like Randy, during the first few grades of elementary school he had been unable to sit still in his seat—bouncing up to use the pencil sharpener or to watch a passing ambulance. His teacher had once written a note home complaining that he talked constantly and that he "squirmed like a bug on a griddle." It was part of the family mythology that he had "crawled at eight months, run at ten." On questioning, Denis admitted that as a kid he was always on the go and could hardly tolerate waiting his turn for anything ("I felt like I was going to climb right out of my skin").

He was almost stupifyingly forgetful. "Still am. I really can't recall much else about my attention span when I was a kid—it was too long ago," he said. "But I have the general impression that I didn't listen very well, just like I am today. Except when I took those two pills by mistake."

Denis had been born in Ceylon, where his parents were both stationed as career diplomats with the foreign service. His father drank himself into an early grave, but not before divorcing his mother when their only child was seven or eight. Denis vividly remembered their last major argument, because it was about him. His mother had pleaded to have Denis's problems evaluated, but his father had banged his fist and sworn that no kid of his was "going to see some damn shrink." Not long afterwards, his parents had split up.

Denis felt he had learned a lot from his father's example—he didn't drink, had never tried drugs, didn't argue with his wife, and had readily agreed when she suggested having Randy evaluated. "You always dream that your kids will have what you never did," he said. "In this case, it's Ritalin."

The remainder of Denis's evaluation was unremarkable. His physical health was excellent, and he had had no other mental health problems. Apart from a certain tendency to fidget in his chair, his appearance was unremarkable. His speech and affect were both completely normal, and he earned a perfect score on the Mini-Mental State Exam.

Evaluation of Denis Tourney

As a child, Denis undoubtedly had a number of symptoms of ADHD. It was easiest for him to remember the problems relating to his activity level. Those included the childhood symptoms of squirming, inability to remain seated or wait his turn, always being on the go, excessive running, and excessive talking. He also thought that he had had problems with his attention span, though he was less clear about the exact symptoms. But even at a remove of three decades, he remembered enough hyperactivity–impulsivity symptoms to justify the diagnosis.

As an adult, Denis continued to have severe problems concentrating. Just as he had done as a child, he was able to overcome them on the strength of raw intelligence. As a result, until he compared his normal concentration to the kind of work he could do with medication, he never realized just how handicapped he had been.

In children, a number of other conditions make up the differential diagnosis. (Note that in a clinician's office, many ADHD children are able to sit still and focus attention well; the diagnosis is best made on the basis of historical information.) Those with **Mental Retardation** learn slowly and may be overly active and impulsive, but ADHD patients, once their attention is captured, are able to learn normally. Unlike children with **Autistic Disorder**, ADHD patients communicate normally. **Depressed** patients may be agitated or have a poor attention span, but the duration is not usually lifelong. Many patients with **Tourette's Disorder** are also hyperactive, but those who only have ADHD will not show motor and vocal tics.

Children reared in a **chaotic social environment** may also have difficulty with hyperactivity and inattention; ADHD should only be diagnosed in a child who lives in a stable social environment. Other **behavior disorders** (oppositional, conduct) may involve behavior that runs afoul of adults or peers, but the behaviors appear purposeful and are not accompanied by the feelings of remorse typical of ADHD behavior. However, many children with ADHD also have **Conduct Disorder** or **Oppositional Defiant Disorder**, as well as Tourette's Disorder.

The differential diagnosis in adults includes **Antisocial Personality Disorder** and **mood disorders** (mood disorder patients can have problems with concentration). The diagnosis should not be made if the symptoms are better explained by **Schizophrenia**, an **anxiety disorder**, or a **personality disorder**.

Because Denis had had elements of inattention and hyperactivity as a child, he was given the type diagnosis of Combined Type, even though as an adult he could not recall enough symptoms to fulfill the criteria. This was a judgment call by his clinician.

Axis I	314.01	Attention-Deficit/Hyperactivity Disorder, Combined Type, In Partial Remission
Axis II	V71.09	No diagnosis
Axis III		None
Axis IV		None
Axis V	GAF = 70	(current)

> **TIP** ADHD is a diagnosis that is probably severely underdiagnosed in adults. Although some clinicians have expressed skepticism about its validity, the evidence of the legitimacy of this disorder is increasing.

314.9 Attention-Deficit/Hyperactivity Disorder Not Otherwise Specified

Use the Attention-Deficit/Hyperactivity Disorder Not Otherwise Specified category for patients with prominent symptoms that have never met the criteria for ADHD proper.

312.8 Conduct Disorder

Criteria for Conduct Disorder

- For 12 months or more, the patient has repeatedly violated rules, age-appropriate societal norms, or the rights of others. This is shown by three or more of the following, at least one of which has occurred in the previous six months:

Aggression against people or animals

✓ Engages in frequent bullying or threatening
✓ Often starts fights
✓ Has used a weapon that could cause serious injury (gun, knife, club, broken glass)
✓ Has shown physical cruelty to people
✓ Has shown physical cruelty to animals
✓ Has engaged in theft with confrontation (armed robbery, extortion, mugging, purse snatching)
✓ Has forced sex upon someone

Property destruction

✓ Has deliberately set fires to cause serious damage
✓ Has deliberately destroyed the property of others (except for fire setting)

Lying or theft

✓ Has broken into building, car or house belonging to someone else
✓ Frequently lies or breaks promises for gain or to avoid obligations ("conning")
✓ Has stolen valuables without confrontation (burglary, forgery, shoplifting)

Serious rule violation

✓ Beginning before age 13, frequently stays out at night against parents' wishes
✓ Has run away from parents overnight twice or more (once if for an extended period)
✓ Beginning before age 13, engages in frequent truancy
• These symptoms cause clinically important job, school, or social impairment.
• If older than age 18, the patient does not meet criteria for Antisocial Personality Disorder.

Coding Notes

Based on age of onset, specify:

Childhood-Onset Type. At least one problem with conduct before age 10.

Adolescent-Onset Type. No problems with conduct before age 10.

Specify severity:

Mild (both are required). There are few problems with conduct beyond those needed to make the diagnosis, *and* all of these problems cause little harm to other people.

Moderate. Number and effect of conduct problems is between Mild and Severe.

Severe (either or both of). Many more conduct symptoms than are needed to make the diagnosis, *or* the conduct symptoms cause other people considerable harm.

313.81 Oppositional Defiant Disorder

Criteria for Oppositional Defiant Disorder

• For at least six months, the patient shows defiant, hostile, negativistic behavior; four or more of the following often apply:
✓ Losing temper
✓ Arguing with adults
✓ Actively defying or refusing to carry out the rules or requests of adults
✓ Deliberately doing things that annoy others
✓ Blaming others for own mistakes or misbehavior
✓ Being touchy or easily annoyed by others

- ✓ Being angry and resentful
- ✓ Being spiteful or vindictive
- The symptoms cause clinically important distress or impair work, school, or social functioning.
- The symptoms do not occur in the course of a mood or psychotic disorder.
- The symptoms do not fulfill criteria for Conduct Disorder.
- If older than age 18, the patient does not meet criteria for Antisocial Personality Disorder.

Coding Note

Only score a criterion as positive if that behavior occurs more often than expected for age and developmental level.

312.9 Disruptive Behavior Disorder Not Otherwise Specified

A patient who has clinically important conduct problems or oppositional behaviors that do not meet the criteria for either Conduct Disorder or Oppositional Defiant Disorder can be coded as having Disruptive Behavior Disorder Not Otherwise Specified.

FEEDING AND EATING DISORDERS OF INFANCY OR EARLY CHILDHOOD

307.52 Pica

Criteria for Pica

- For at least one month, the patient persists in eating dirt or other nonnutritive substances.
- This behavior is not appropriate to the patient's developmental level.
- It is not sanctioned in the patient's culture.
- If this behavior occurs solely in the context of another mental disorder (such as Mental Retardation, a pervasive developmental disorder, or Schizophrenia), it is serious enough to require independent clinical attention.

307.53 Rumination Disorder

Criteria for Rumination Disorder

- After a period of normal functioning, for at least one month the patient repeatedly regurgitates and rechews food.
- This behavior is not caused by a gastrointestinal illness or other general medical condition (such as esophageal reflux).
- The behavior doesn't occur solely during Anorexia Nervosa or Bulimia Nervosa.
- If it occurs solely during Mental Retardation or a pervasive developmental disorder, it is serious enough to require independent clinical attention.

307.59 Feeding Disorder of Infancy or Childhood

Criteria for Feeding Disorder of Infancy or Childhood

- For one month or more, the patient has persistently failed to eat adequately and has either not gained weight or lost weight.
- This behavior is not due to a gastrointestinal illness or other general medical condition (such as esophageal reflux).
- Neither another mental disorder (such as Rumination Disorder) nor the lack of available food better explains the symptoms.
- The disorder begins before age six.

TIC DISORDERS

307.23 Tourette's Disorder

A *tic* is any stereotyped movement or vocalization that is nonrhythmic, rapid, repeated, stereotyped, and sudden. Although tics are often described as involuntary, many patients can suppress them for a time. Patients who have Tourette's Disorder have many tics that affect various parts of the body. Motor tics of the head are usually present (eye blinking is often the first symptom to appear). Some patients have complex motor tics (e.g., they may do deep knee bends). The location and severity of tics typically change with time.

But the *vocal* tics are what cause this disorder to be so distinctive and bring these patients to the attention of mental health clinicians (rather than neurologists). Vocal tics can include an astonishing variety of barks, clicks, coughs, grunts, and understandable words. A sizable minority (ranging from 10 to 30%) of patients have *coprolalia*, which means that they utter obscenities or other language that renders the condition intolerable by family and acquaintances. Mental coprolalia (intrusive dirty thoughts) can also occur.

This unusual and distressing disorder was named for the French neurologist Gilles de la Tourette, who first wrote about it in 1885. It is a relatively rare condition, affecting about 1 person in 2,000. Males are two to three times more likely than females to be affected. Associated symptoms include self-injury due to banging the head and picking at the skin. It is said that the tendency to develop Tourette's is inherited as an autosomal dominant gene, though not everyone who has the gene develops tics (there is incomplete penetrance). There is often a family history of tics and of Obsessive–Compulsive Disorder (OCD).

On average, onset of this distressing condition occurs at age seven; most patients have become symptomatic by their early teen years. It usually lasts throughout life, though there may be periods of remission. With maturity, it can disappear or be reduced in severity.

Criteria for Tourette's Disorder

- At some time during the illness, though not necessarily at the same time, the patient has had both of these:
  - At least one vocal tic *and*
  - Multiple motor tics
- For longer than one year, these tics have occurred many times each day, nearly every day or at intervals.
- During this time, the patient never goes longer than three months without the tics.
- These symptoms cause marked distress or materially impair work, social, or personal functioning.
- The symptoms begin before age 18.
- The symptoms are not directly caused by the effects of a general medical condition (such as Huntington's disease or a postviral encephalitis) or by the use of a substance (such as a central nervous system stimulant).

Coding Note

In the criteria for this and the other tic disorders, a *tic* is defined as a motor movement or vocalization that is nonrhythmic, rapid, repeated, stereotyped, and sudden.

Gordon Whitmore

Gordon was a 20-year-old college student who came to the clinic with this chief complaint: "I stopped my medicine and my Tourette's is back."

The product of a full-term pregnancy and uncomplicated delivery, Gordon had developed normally until he was eight and a half. That was when his mother noticed his first tic. At the breakfast table, she was looking at him across the top of a box of Post Toasties. As he read what was written on the back, every few seconds he would blink his eyes, squeezing them shut and then opening them wide.

"She asked me what was wrong, said she wondered if I was having a convulsion," Gordon told the mental health clinician. He suddenly interrupted his story to yell, "Shit-fuck! Shit-fuck!" As he bellowed out each exclamation, he twisted his head sharply to the right and shook it so that his teeth actually rattled. "But I never lost consciousness or anything like that. It was only the beginning of my Tourette's."

Undisconcerted at his sudden outburst, Gordon calmly continued his story. Throughout the rest of his childhood, he gradually accumulated an assortment of facial twitches and other abrupt movements of his head and upper body. Each new motor tic earned renewed taunts from his classmates, but these were mild compared with the abuse he suffered once the vocal tics began.

Not long after he turned 13, Gordon noticed that a certain tension would seem to accumulate in the back of his throat. He couldn't describe it—it didn't tickle and it didn't have a taste. It wasn't something he could swallow down. Sometimes a cough would temporarily relieve it, but more often it seemed to require some form of vocalization to ease it. A bark or yelp worked just fine. When it was most intense, only an obscenity would do.

"Shit-fuck! Shit-fuck!" he yelled again. Then, "Cunt!" Gordon shook his head again and hooted twice.

Halfway through his junior year in high school, the vocal tics got so bad that Gordon was placed on "permanent suspension" until he could learn to sit in a classroom without creating pandemonium. The third clinician his parents took him to prescribed haloperidol. This relieved his symptoms completely, except for the tendency to blink when he was under stress.

He had remained on this drug until a month earlier, when he read an article about tardive dyskinesia and began to worry about side effects. Once he stopped taking the medication, the full spectrum of tics rapidly returned. He had recently been evaluated by his general physician, who had pronounced him healthy. He had never abused street drugs or alcohol.

Gordon was a neatly dressed, pleasant-appearing young man who sat quietly for most of the interview. He really seemed quite ordinary, aside from exaggerated blinking, which occurred several times a minute. He sometimes accompanied the blinks by opening his mouth and curling his lips around his teeth. But every few minutes there occurred a small explosion of hoots, grunts, yelps, or barks, along with a variety of tics that involved his face, head, and shoulders. Irregularly but with some frequency, his outbursts would include expletives, as recorded above; these with more volume than conviction. Afterwards, without any apparent embarrassment, he would take up the thread of conversation where it had been left off.

The remainder of Gordon's mental status was not remarkable. When he was not having tics, his speech was clear, coherent, relevant, and spontaneous. He was worried about his symptoms, but denied feeling depressed or especially anxious. He had never had hallucinations, delusions, or suicidal ideas. He also denied having obsessions and compulsions. "You mean like Uncle George," he said. "He does rituals." Gordon scored a perfect 30 on the Mini-Mental State Exam.

Evaluation of Gordon Whitmore

Gordon's symptoms included vocal as well as multiple motor tics, which certainly had occurred frequently enough and long enough to qualify him fully for a diagnosis of Tourette's Disorder. He was otherwise healthy, so that a **general medical condition** (especially neurological disorders such as dystonia) would not appear to be a likely cause of his symptoms. Other Axis I disorders associated with abnormal movements include **Schizophrenia** and **Amphetamine Intoxication**, but Gordon presented no evidence for either of these. The duration and full spectrum of vocal and multiple motor tics distinguished his condition from other tic disorders (**Chronic Motor or Vocal Tic Disorder, Transient Tic Disorder**).

You should also inquire about conditions that may be associated with Tourette's. These include **ADHD** of childhood and **OCD**. (Gordon's uncle may have had OCD. Although there is still controversy, some studies report associations of these conditions.)

Gordon's full diagnosis would be as follows:

Axis I	307.23	Tourette's Disorder
Axis II	V71.09	No diagnosis
Axis III		None
Axis IV		None
Axis V	GAF = 55	(current)

307.22 Chronic Motor or Vocal Tic Disorder

Criteria for Chronic Motor or Vocal Tic Disorders

- At some time, the patient has had either, *but not both*, vocal or motor tics.
- For longer than one year, these tics have occurred many times each day, nearly every day or at intervals.

- During this time, the patient never goes longer than three months without the tics.
- These symptoms cause marked distress or materially impair work, social, or personal functioning.
- The symptoms begin before age 18.
- The symptoms are not directly caused by a general medical condition (such as Huntington's disease or a postviral encephalitis) or by the use of a substance (such as a central nervous system stimulant).
- The patient has never fulfilled criteria for Tourette's Disorder.

307.21 Transient Tic Disorder

Criteria for Transient Tic Disorder

- The patient has vocal or motor tics, or both. They can be single or multiple.
- For at least four weeks but no longer than 12 consecutive months, these tics have occurred many times each day, nearly every day.
- These symptoms cause marked distress or materially impair work, social, or personal functioning.
- The symptoms begin before age 18.
- The symptoms are not directly caused by a general medical condition (such as Huntington's disease or a postviral encephalitis) or by the use of a substance (such as a central nervous system stimulant).
- The patient has never fulfilled criteria for Tourette's Disorder or for Chronic Motor or Vocal Tic Disorder.

Coding Note

Specify whether:

Single Episode

Recurrent

307.20 Tic Disorder Not Otherwise Specified

Use the Tic Disorder Not Otherwise Specified category to code tics that don't fulfill criteria for one of the preceding tic disorders.

ELIMINATION DISORDERS

Encopresis

Criteria for Encopresis

- Accidentally or on purpose, the patient repeatedly passes feces into inappropriate places (clothing, the floor).
- For at least three months, this has happened at least once per month.
- The patient is at least four years old (or the developmental equivalent).
- This behavior is not caused solely by the use of substances (such as laxatives) or by a general medical condition (except through some mechanism that involves constipation).

Coding Notes

Code by specific type:

787.6	Encopresis With Constipation and Overflow Incontinence
307.7	Encopresis Without Constipation and Overflow Incontinence

Mechanisms that involve constipation may include hypothyroidism, side effects of medication, or a febrile illness that causes dehydration.

307.6 Enuresis

Criteria for Enuresis

- Accidentally or on purpose, the patient repeatedly urinates into clothing or the bed.
- The clinical importance of this behavior is shown by *either* of these:
  - ✓ It occurs at least twice a week for at least three consecutive months, *or*
  - ✓ It causes clinically important distress or impairs work (scholastic), social, or personal functioning.

- The patient is at least five years old (or the developmental equivalent).
- This behavior is not directly caused by a general medical condition (such as diabetes, seizures, or spina bifida) or by the use of a substance (such as a diuretic).

Coding Note

Specify type:

Nocturnal Only

Diurnal Only

Nocturnal and Diurnal

OTHER DISORDERS OF INFANCY, CHILDHOOD, OR ADOLESCENCE

309.21 Separation Anxiety Disorder

Criteria for Separation Anxiety Disorder

- The patient has excessive, developmentally inappropriate anxiety about being separated from home or from those to whom the patient is attached. Of the following symptoms, three or more persist or recur:
  ✓ Excessive distress when anticipating or experiencing separation from home or parents
  ✓ Excessive worry about loss of or harm to parents
  ✓ Excessive worry about being separated from a parent by a serious event (such as being kidnapped or becoming lost)
  ✓ Refusal or reluctance to go somewhere (such as school) due to separation fears
  ✓ Excessive fears of being alone or without parents at home, or without important adults elsewhere
  ✓ Refusal or reluctance to sleep away from home or to go to sleep without being near a parent
  ✓ Recurrent nightmares about separation

✓ Recurrent physical symptoms (such as abdominal pain, nausea, vomiting, headache) when anticipating or experiencing separation from parents
- These symptoms last four weeks or more.
- They begin before age 18.
- They cause clinically important distress or impair school (work), social, or personal functioning.
- The symptoms do not occur solely during a pervasive developmental disorder or any psychotic disorder, including Schizophrenia.
- In adolescents and adults, the symptoms are not better explained by Panic Disorder With Agoraphobia.

Coding Note

Specify if: Early Onset (begins before age 6).

313.23 Selective Mutism

Criteria for Selective Mutism

- Despite speaking in other situations, the patient consistently does not speak in specific social situations where speech is expected, such as at school.
- This behavior interferes with educational or occupational achievement or with social communication.
- It has lasted at least one month (excluding the first month of school).
- It is not caused by unfamiliarity or discomfort with the spoken language needed in the social situation.
- It is not better explained by a communication disorder (such as Stuttering).
- It does not occur solely during a pervasive developmental disorder or by any psychotic disorder (such as Schizophrenia).

313.89 Reactive Attachment Disorder of Infancy or Early Childhood

Criteria for Reactive Attachment Disorder of Infancy or Early Childhood

- The patient's social relatedness is markedly disturbed and developmentally inappropriate. This begins before age five and occurs in most situations; it is shown by *either* of these:

✓ Inhibitions. In most social situations, the child doesn't interact in a developmentally appropriate way. This is shown by responses that are excessively inhibited, hypervigilant, or ambivalent and contradictory. For example, the child responds to caregivers with frozen watchfulness or mixed approach–avoidance and resistance to comforting.

✓ Disinhibitions. The child's attachments are diffuse, as shown by indiscriminate sociability with inability to form appropriate selective attachments. For example, the child is overly familiar with strangers or lacks selectivity in choosing attachment figures.

- This behavior is not explained solely by a developmental delay (such as Mental Retardation), and it does not fulfill criteria for a pervasive developmental disorder.
- Evidence of persistent pathogenic care is shown by one or more of these:
  ✓ The caregiver neglects the child's basic emotional needs for affection, comfort, and stimulation.
  ✓ The caregiver neglects the child's basic physical needs.
  ✓ Stable attachments cannot form because of repeated changes of primary caregiver (such as frequent changes of foster care).
- It appears that the pathogenic care just described has caused the disturbed behavior; for example, the behavior began after the pathogenic care did.

Coding Note

Specify type, based on predominant clinical presentation:

Inhibited Type. Failure to interact predominates.

Disinhibited Type. Indiscriminate sociability predominates.

307.3 Stereotypic Movement Disorder

Criteria for Stereotypic Movement Disorder

- The patient's motor behavior seems driven, repetitive and nonfunctional. Examples include biting or hitting self, body rocking, hand shaking or waving, head banging, mouthing of objects, and picking at skin or body openings.
- This behavior seriously interferes with normal activities or causes physical injury that requires medical treatment (or would, if the behavior were not interfered with).
- If the patient also has Mental Retardation, the stereotypic behavior is serious enough to be a focus of treatment.
- The behavior is not better explained by a compulsion (as in Obsessive–Com-

pulsive Disorder), a tic (as in a tic disorder), hair pulling (as in Trichotillomania), or a pervasive developmental disorder.
- It is not directly caused by a general medical condition or by the effects of substance use.
- The behavior has persisted for at least four weeks.

Coding Note

Specify if: With Self-Injurious Behavior. The behavior causes bodily injury that requires medical treatment (or would, if the behavior were not interfered with).

313.9 Disorder of Infancy, Childhood, or Adolescence Not Otherwise Specified

Disorder of Infancy, Childhood, or Adolescence Not Otherwise Specified is the ultimate catch-all category for this group of disorders: It is used for *any* other disorder that begins before adulthood that is not better defined above.

Other Factors That May Need Clinical Attention

A variety of other problems or disorders that are not mental disorders them-selves, strictly speaking, can cause someone to need attention. These may or may not be related to a mental disorder. (I indicate below those for which DSM-IV has provided or suggested criteria.) At the end of the chapter, I also provide some codes that are sometimes helpful for administrative purposes.

316 Psychological Factor Affecting Medical Condition

Mental health professionals deal with a number of types of problems that can influence the course or care of a medical condition. For example, proper care of diabetes can be hindered by a patient who refuses to follow the recom-mended dose of insulin; smoking can increase the risk of further heart attacks. The diagnosis of Psychological Factor Affecting Medical Condition, coded on Axis I, can be used to identify such patients. All of the possibilities are men-tioned in the following criteria.

Criteria for Psychological Factor Affecting Medical Condition

- The patient has a general medical condition (coded on Axis III).
- This condition has been affected by at least one psychological factor, as shown in at least one of these ways:
  - ✓ Development of, worsening of, or delay in recovery from the general medical condition closely follows the factor.
  - ✓ The factor interferes with treatment of the general medical condition.

533

✓ The factor worsens the risk to the health of the patient.
✓ Stress from the factor evokes or worsens symptoms of the general medical condition (such as chest pain in a patient with heart disease).

Coding Notes

On Axis III, code the name of the general medical condition.

The exact name used for a psychological factor depends on the type of factor. If more than one psychological factor is present, choose the most prominent one:

Mental Disorder Affecting [General Medical Condition]. For example, a man with Schizophrenia hears voices that tell him to refuse dialysis for his kidney disease. This would be coded as follows:

Axis I	295.30	Schizophrenia, Paranoid Type, Continuous
	316	Mental Disorder Affecting Renal Disease
Axis III	585	Chronic Renal Failure

Psychological Symptoms Affecting [General Medical Condition]. Use this when criteria for a mental disorder are not fulfilled, but symptoms do cause problems—for example, a patient's anxiety worsens her hypertension.

Personality Traits or Coping Style Affecting [General Medical Condition]. For example, a patient with a life-threatening condition that could be corrected by surgery denies the need for an operation.

Maladaptive Health Behaviors Affecting [General Medical Condition]. DSM-IV gives the examples of excessive eating, avoidance of exercise, and risky sex.

Stress-Related Physiological Response Affecting [General Medical Condition]. For example, a patient's ulcers are exacerbated by stress.

Other or Unspecified Psychological Factors Affecting [General Medical Condition].

TIP Of course, you can find at least one psychological factor in nearly any general medical condition. To use this diagnosis effectively, reserve it for situations in which it is clear that the psychological factor is adversely influencing the course of the general medical condition. An example would be refusal to give up high-salt, high-fat junk food in a person who has high blood pressure and heart disease.

MEDICATION-INDUCED MOVEMENT DISORDERS

Medication-induced movement disorders are important in mental health care for two reasons:

- They may be mistaken for Axis I conditions (such as tic disorders, Schizophrenia, or anxiety disorders).
- They can affect the management of patients who are receiving psychotropic medications.

332.1 Neuroleptic-Induced Parkinsonism

Most of the antipsychotic agents that have been developed and used over the past 40 years can induce a frozen face, shuffling gait, and pill-rolling tremor that much resemble naturally occurring Parkinson's disease. Suggested research criteria are given beginning on page 736 of DSM-IV.

333.92 Neuroleptic Malignant Syndrome

In Neuroleptic Malignant Syndrome, the use of a neuroleptic medication leads to muscle rigidity, fever, and other problems (which can include sweating, trouble swallowing, incontinence, and delirium). Suggested research criteria for this uncommon condition are given beginning on page 739 of DSM-IV.

333.7 Neuroleptic-Induced Acute Dystonia

Abruptly contracting muscles of the head, neck, or other portions of the body can produce painful, often frightening spasms. These are due to the use of neuroleptic medications and occur quite commonly. Suggested research criteria are given on page 742 of DSM-IV.

333.99 Neuroleptic-Induced Acute Akathisia

Shortly after beginning or increasing the dose of a neuroleptic drug, some patients become acutely restless and unable to remain seated. Suggested research criteria are given beginning on page 744 of DSM-IV.

333.82 Neuroleptic-Induced Tardive Dyskinesia

After a patient has taken a neuroleptic medication for a few months or longer, involuntary movements of the face, jaw, tongue, or limbs may become noticeable. Once begun, these movements can become permanent, even if the neuroleptic medication responsible is discontinued. Suggested research criteria are given beginning on page 747 of DSM-IV.

333.1 Medication-Induced Postural Tremor

A fine tremor associated with efforts to maintain a posture may develop with the use of medications such as antidepressants, lithium, or valproate. Suggested research criteria are given beginning on page 749 of DSM-IV.

333.90 Medication-Induced Movement Disorder Not Otherwise Specified

DSM-IV suggests that Medication-Induced Movement Disorder Not Otherwise Specified may be useful for tardive dystonia and for nearly all of the syndromes above when they are associated with medications other than neuroleptics.

995.2 Adverse Effects of Medication Not Otherwise Specified

Adverse Effects of Medication Not Otherwise Specified can be used for this category for unwanted effects that are not movement disorders that become an important focus for clinical attention. Examples include severe hypotension caused by neuroleptics or priapism caused by trazodone.

RELATIONAL PROBLEMS

V61.9 Relational Problem Related to a Mental Disorder or General Medical Condition

You should use this somewhat confusingly named category if your patient's main difficulty is due to interaction with a relative or significant other who has a mental disorder or physical disease.

V61.20 Parent–Child Relational Problem

Use Parent–Child Relational Problem when clinically important symptoms or negative effects on functioning are associated with the way a parent and child interact. The problematic interaction pattern may include faulty communication, ineffective discipline, or overprotection.

V61.1 Partner Relational Problem

Use Partner Relational Problem when clinically important symptoms or negative effects on functioning are associated with the way a patient and spouse or partner interact. The problematic interaction pattern may include faulty communication or an absense of communication.

V61.8 Sibling Relational Problem

Use Sibling Relational Problem when clinically important symptoms or negative effects on functioning are associated with the way siblings interact.

V62.81 Relational Problem Not Otherwise Specified

When the need for evaluation centers around relational problems not covered by the above-mentioned categories, use Relational Problem Not Otherwise Specified. DSM-IV suggests the example of problems with coworkers.

PROBLEMS RELATED TO ABUSE OR NEGLECT

The titles of the following V-codes are pretty much self-explanatory.

V61.21 Physical Abuse of Child

Specify 995.5 if clinical attention is focused on the victim.

V61.21 Sexual Abuse of Child

Specify 995.5 if clinical attention is focused on the victim.

V61.21 Neglect of Child

Specify 995.5 if clinical attention is focused on the victim.

V61.1 Physical Abuse of Adult

Physical Abuse of Adult is the category used for elder and spousal abuse. Specify 995.81 if clinical attention is focused on the victim.

V61.1 Sexual Abuse of Adult

Sexual Abuse of Adult is used for problems such as rape. Specify 995.81 if clinical attention is focused on the victim.

OTHER CONDITIONS THAT MAY BE A FOCUS OF CLINICAL ATTENTION

V15.81 Noncompliance With Treatment

Noncompliance With Treatment identifies a patient who requires attention because the patient has ignored or controverted attempts at treatment for a mental disorder or a general medical condition. An example would be a patient with Schizophrenia who requires repeated hospitalization for refusal to take medication.

V65.2 Malingering

Malingering is defined as the intentional production of the signs or symptoms of a physical or mental disorder. The purpose is some sort of gain: obtaining something desirable (money, drugs, insurance settlement) or avoiding something unpleasant (punishment, work, military service, jury duty). Malingering is often confused with Factitious Disorder (in which the motive is not external gain but a wish to occupy the sick role) and the somatoform disorders (in which the symptoms are not intentionally produced at all).

Malingering should be suspected in any of these situations:

- The patient has legal problems or the prospect of financial gain.
- The patient has Antisocial Personality Disorder.
- The patient tells a story that does not accord with informants' accounts or with other known facts.
- The patient does not cooperate with the evaluation.

TIP Malingering is easy to suspect and difficult to prove. In the absence of an observation of definitive behavior (you watch someone place sand into a urine specimen or hold a thermometer over a glowing light bulb), a resolute and clever malingerer can be almost impossible to detect. When Malingering involves symptoms that are strictly mental or emotional, detection may be impossible. Moreover, the consequences of this diagnosis are dire: It provides closure in such a way as to totally alienate the clinician from the patient. I therefore recommend that you make this diagnosis only in the most obvious and imperative of circumstances.

V71.01 Adult Antisocial Behavior

If the reason for clinical attention is antisocial behavior that is not part of a pattern (and hence not attributable to Antisocial Personality Disorder, Conduct Disorder, or a disorder of impulse control), Adult Antisocial Behavior can be coded. Examples would include the activities of career criminals who do not have any of the disorders just mentioned.

V71.02 Childhood or Adolescent Antisocial Behavior

Childhood or Adolescent Antisocial Behavior is the juvenile equivalent of the adult code described above.

V62.89 Borderline Intellectual Functioning

Use Borderline Intellectual Functioning for a patient whose IQ and level of functioning fall within the range of 71 to 84. In the face of other Axis I diagnoses (psychotic or cognitive disorders, for example), the differential diagnosis between Borderline Intellectual Functioning and Mild Mental Retardation can be quite difficult. Code this, like Mental Retardation, on Axis II.

780.9 Age-Related Cognitive Decline

You should only use Age-Related Cognitive Decline once you have determined (probably through neuropsychological testing) that your patient does *not* have a cognitive disorder such as dementia. In other words, the decline in memory must be severe enough to cause the patient distress, but must also be within the limits of normality for the patient's age.

V62.82 Bereavement

When a relative or close friend dies, it is quite natural to grieve. When the symptoms of the grieving process are a reason for receiving clinical attention, DSM-IV allows you to make a diagnosis of Bereavement—provided that the symptoms don't last too long and aren't too severe. The problem is that the sadness of grief can closely resemble the sadness associated with a Major Depressive Episode. DSM-IV points out certain symptoms to help you decide whether, in addition to being bereaved, the patient is suffering from a Major Depressive Episode:

- Guilt feelings (other than about actions that might have prevented the death)
- Death wishes (other than the survivor's wishing to have died with the loved one)
- Slowed-down psychomotor activity
- Severe preoccupation with worthlessness
- Severely impaired functioning for an unusually long time
- Hallucinations (other than of seeing or hearing the deceased)

In addition, people who are "only" bereaved typically regard their moods as normal. A diagnosis of depressive illness is usually withheld in these cases until after the symptoms have lasted longer than two months.

TIP The fact that a patient has a "reason" to be depressed is no reason to ignore the symptoms of a mood disorder. Even when they occur soon after a loved one's death, serious symptoms such as feelings of worthlessness, suicidal ideas, insomnia, and loss of appetite should be carefully evaluated and followed. The consequences of doing otherwise can be dire.

V62.3 Academic Problem

Use Academic Problem for a patient whose problem is related to scholastic endeavors and who does not have a learning disorder or other mental disorder that accounts for the problem. Even if another disorder can account for the problem, the Academic Problem itself may be so severe that it independently justifies clinical attention. For example, see the vignette of Colin Rodebaugh (p. 403).

V62.2 Occupational Problem

Occupational Problem is the work-related equivalent of Academic Problem, just discussed. DSM-IV includes examples of problems in choosing a career and of dissatisfaction with one's job.

313.82 Identity Problem

Identity Problem may be applied to patients who are uncertain about identity-related issues, such as career, friendships, goals, morals, or sexual orientation. (Of course, this is entirely different from disorientation as to person, which is a symptom of several cognitive disorders.)

V62.89 Religious or Spiritual Problem

Patients who require evaluation or treatment for issues pertaining to religious faith (or its lack) may be given the Religious or Spiritual Problem code.

V62.4 Acculturation Problem

Acculturation Problem may be useful for patients whose problems center on a move from one culture to another (e.g., migrants and immigrants).

V62.89 Phase of Life Problem

Phase of Life Problem is a code you can use for a patient whose problem is not due to a mental disorder but to a life change, such as marriage, divorce, new job, or retirement. It must be discriminated from Adjustment Disorder.

ADDITIONAL CODES

Several other codes are useful for administrative purposes. Two of them state that your patient has no diagnosis on one of the first two axes. Others provide you with ways to indicate that you don't know what's wrong, if anything.

300.9 Unspecified Mental Disorder (nonpsychotic)

There are one or two situations in which a diagnosis of Unspecified Mental Disorder may be appropriate:

- The diagnosis you want to give is not contained in DSM-IV.
- You know that a patient has a mental disorder, but you have insufficient information to state what it is, and no Not Otherwise Specified category seems appropriate. Once you have obtained more information, you should be able to change this to a more specific diagnosis.

V71.09 No Diagnosis or Condition on Axis I

No Diagnosis or Condition on Axis I means that the patient does not have a major mental disorder or V-code condition that is the focus of clinical attention. However, the patient may still have an Axis II disorder that is the focus of clinical attention, which becomes the principal diagnosis.

V71.09 No Diagnosis on Axis II

No Diagnosis on Axis II means that the patient does not have a personality disorder or Mental Retardation. However, most patients appearing for mental health evaluation will have an Axis I disorder.

799.9 Diagnosis or Condition Deferred on Axis I

Diagnosis or Condition Deferred on Axis I means that there is not enough information to make any Axis I diagnosis. It is even possible that the patient may eventually prove to have no diagnosis on Axis I.

799.9 Diagnosis Deferred on Axis II

Diagnosis Deferred on Axis II means that there is not enough information to make any Axis II diagnosis. It is even possible that the patient may eventually prove to have no diagnosis on Axis II.

Evaluating the Mental Health Patient

Making a diagnosis is usually not as simple as comparing one list of symptoms to a set of criteria. Patients often have many symptoms; sometimes these can suggest a number of different disorders. In most cases, you will sift through your patient's history and mental status examination to help you decide which diagnoses are most likely.

Principles for Selecting Diagnostic Information

Experienced clinicians use a number of principles to help them arrive at a diagnosis. (They don't always realize they use them, but they are there.) While you are learning, keep these principles in mind. They should help focus your attention on the information crucial to your choice of appropriate diagnosis. You will encounter them again and again in the case histories given later in this chapter, and in your life as a clinician.

1. History is better than cross-sectional observation. This crucial principle recognizes that patients with widely differing diagnoses can have symptoms that appear strikingly similar to an observer. To illustrate, consider the example of a 35-year-old man who hears voices. With no other information, you couldn't make a diagnosis or even judge how serious your patient's illness is. Here's how historical information about your patient could help:

> If he initially became ill 15 years ago and has been that way ever since, you would strongly consider Schizophrenia.

> If he has previously recovered completely from an episode of psychosis with excitable, elevated mood, you would consider Bipolar I Disorder.

> If he has been ill for less than six months, you might diagnose Schizophreniform Disorder.

If he has recently stopped drinking after months of heavy alcohol intake, you should consider Alcohol-Induced Psychotic Disorder, With Hallucinations.

2. Recent history is better than ancient history. This principle reminds us that illnesses develop sequentially. Patients change, and often the evolving symptoms of an illness will help you to evaluate it better. A diagnosis that seemed reasonable 10 years ago may be untenable in the light of more recent symptoms. Here are some examples:

At 17, a graduating high school senior's introspection and moodiness are diagnosed as Adjustment Disorder With Depressed Mood. A year later, the same patient now has inappropriate affect and incoherent speech; Schizophrenia is diagnosed.

A 25-year-old man suffers from depression and is diagnosed as having Major Depressive Disorder, Single Episode. Two years later, when he becomes acutely manic, the diagnosis is changed to Bipolar I Disorder, Most Recent Episode Manic.

A 58-year-old woman complains of anxiety and is diagnosed is having Generalized Anxiety Disorder. Two months later she is found to have a hyperactive thyroid; her diagnosis then becomes Anxiety Disorder Due to Hyperthyroidism.

3. Collateral information augments history from the patient. Informants often have information or a point of view that augments (or sometimes contradicts) what you have obtained from the patient. Consider these examples:

A 19-year-old woman has repressed the fact that she was molested by an uncle when she was five; her sister recalls it.

A college student complains of trouble concentrating when he studies; his roommate confides that the patient stays up late at night having conversations with voices no one else can hear.

A depressed woman knows nothing of her family history; her father reports that a grandparent was diagnosed as having Schizophrenia.

A young attorney complains of Panic Attacks; his wife reveals that he has been smoking crack cocaine.

4. Signs are better than symptoms. *Symptoms* (what your patient complains of) may be distorted by either of two factors: the patient's interpretation and yours. But *signs* (what you observe about your patient's behavior) are subject only to the inaccuracies of your own interpretation. For example:

Although a man complains only of "anxiety," you notice fresh needle tracks on his arm.

A woman denies hearing voices, but during an interview she pauses and seems to be listening to something.

5. Objective assessments are better than subjective judgments. This principle reminds us to be wary of any diagnosis based on intuition (or hunches). Until the last few decades, mental health diagnosis was often unscientific and had little predictive value. One goal of DSM-IV is to encourage diagnosis that can predict the future course of an illness, its probable response to treatment, and the likelihood of its being passed on to the patient's children. Consider this example:

A patient became acutely excited and sold a valuable automobile for $500. A clinician diagnosed Schizophrenia, because "selling a car so cheap seemed like a crazy thing to do." Later rediagnosed as having Bipolar I Disorder, the patient was successfully treated with lithium.

6. Crisis-generated data are suspect. How someone responds to emergencies may yield valuable insights, but may not reveal much about ordinary, day-to-day behavior. But relying too heavily on your observations of behavior under stress could distort your assessment of such patients as these:

The normally cheerful salesman who is depressed just after losing a large account.

The ebullient demeanor of the lottery winner who has temporarily forgotten the misery caused by her recent divorce.

Rules for Formulating a Rational Diagnosis

The list of all diagnoses possible for any given patient is called the *differential diagnosis*. Traditionally, the possibilities are arranged in order of likelihood, with the most probable diagnosis listed first. Such a list is valuable for several reasons. First, it helps you to plan your further diagnostic efforts; second, it tells you what you should consider treating first; third, it should help you organize your thinking about prognosis. At the bottom of the list will appear some diagnoses you consider pretty unlikely. Include them anyway. This is especially true if there is some doubt as to the correct diagnosis; a broad and inclusive list improves your chances for selecting the correct diagnosis. More information on this is contained in my book on interviewing, *The First Interview*.

Several rules can assist you in selecting the most likely diagnosis for the top of your differential diagnostic list. This is the diagnosis that you will want to investigate first or that urgently requires treatment. Here is a set of rules that can help you select a working diagnosis for your patient. The rules are arranged approximately in descending order of importance.

A. Disorders due to general medical conditions, or cognitive disorders, pre-empt all other diagnoses that could produce the same symptoms. Many general medical conditions produce mental symptoms and require urgent evaluation and treatment to prevent serious medical complications. (Some of these conditions are listed in Appendix B.) For example, a patient's depression and lethargy could be due to a mood disorder, but is a hypothyroid condition remotely possible? If so, it should be listed first, because hypothyroidism can progress to coma and death.

B. Try to explain all the symptoms with the fewest diagnoses possible. It is possible for a patient with three symptoms to have three independent diagnoses, but it isn't likely. It is more reasonable to look for a single illness that explains all of the symptoms. This is called the rule of *parsimony*. Of course, it is by no means an absolute requirement. But parsimony is simple and elegant, and it carries the force of logic. "Thinking small" also helps to focus your therapy on what is most important. And it has been a staple of mental health diagnosis for over 100 years.

C. Consider first disorders that have been present longer. Here's another rule that clinicians have used for years. It suggests that if a patient with disorder *A* later develops disorder *B*, perhaps *A* caused *B*. It also suggests the possibility of treating two diseases by attacking one. For instance, suppose that a woman with long-standing Alcohol Dependence becomes depressed. Of course, she could have developed an independent Major Depressive Disorder. A better bet, however, is that she has Alcohol-Induced Mood Disorder With Depressive Features. (This also illustrates parsimony, Rule B.)

D. Use family history as a guide. Mental disorders run in families. Whether the mode of transmission is environmental (e.g., imitation or learning) or hereditary, the presence of a relative with disorder *X* suggests that your patient may also have disorder *X*.

E. If all else fails, use the safest diagnosis. By *safest*, I mean that one diagnosis may have a better outcome (it remits spontaneously or responds well to treatment) than other diagnoses lower on the list. All diagnoses can be ranked on a hierarchy of safety, as I have done in Table 18.1. (As a further aid to diagnosis, I also supply a frequency-based hierarchy in Table 18.2) Clinicians might disagree as to the exact placement of diagnoses in Table 18.1, but most would probably agree that, all other factors being equal, you should choose first the diagnosis that is more treatable and has a better prognosis. Consider these examples:

> A patient who becomes hyperactive and delusional could have either Bipolar I Disorder or Schizophrenia. The safety principle would direct you to place Bipolar I Disorder higher on your list, because it has the better prognosis.

> A patient who suffers memory lapses could have either Dementia of the Alzheimer's Type or Major Depressive Disorder. Unless you are absolutely certain that no other, more treatable illness is more likely, you shouldn't diagnose Alzheimer's.

Table 18.1   Hierarchy of Conservative (Safe) Diagnoses

Most favorable (most treatable, best outcome):

Major Depressive Disorder, Single Episode or Recurrent
Bipolar I Disorder

Middle ground:

Alcohol Dependence
Panic Disorder
Specific or Social Phobia
Obsessive–Compulsive Disorder
Anorexia Nervosa
Substance Dependence (other than Alcohol Dependence)
Borderline Personality Disorder

Least favorable:

Schizophrenia
Antisocial Personality Disorder
Dementia Due to HIV Disease
Dementia of the Alzheimer's Type

Note. Adapted by permission from *Boarding Time* (p. 95) by J. Morrison and R. A. Muñoz, 1991, Washington, DC: American Psychiatric Press. Copyright 1991 by the American Psychiatric Association.

Case Histories

With experience, sorting through the information from a patient's history and mental status exam becomes gradually easier. After you have evaluated 200 patients or so, you will find that the evaluation process has become virtually second nature. In the remainder of this chapter, I present a number of case histories. Here is your opportunity to try your own diagnostic skills on a variety of patients, some with multiple mental disorders. Such patients may be the norm rather than the exception. A recent national survey of adults in the general population found that of those who had a lifetime history of at least one disorder, over 60% had more than one. About 14% of all Americans have three or more lifetime diagnoses.

Due to space requirements, these case histories have been somewhat abridged. Other clinicians might disagree with some of my conclusions; my main purpose in presenting them is to demonstrate a reasoned approach to diagnosis. I refer periodically to the principles (1–6) and rules (A–E) described above. Generally, I have put first the cases that are less complicated.

Table 18.2 Most Valid Diagnoses, in Descending Order
of Frequency Expected in a General Mental Health Population

Common:

    Major Depressive Disorder, Single Episode
    Alcohol Dependence
    Bipolar I Disorder
    Schizophrenia
    Major Depressive Disorder, Recurrent
    Somatization Disorder
    Borderline Personality Disorder

Less common:

    Panic Disorder, With or Without Agoraphobia
    Dementias (including Alzheimer's, Vascular, Due to HIV Disease)
    Antisocial Personality Disorder
    Obsessive–Compulsive Disorder
    Mental Retardation, if specific etiology (e.g., Down's syndrome,
       phenylketonuria)
    Anorexia Nervosa

Rare:

    Learning disorders
    Gender Identity Disorder
    Tourette's Disorder
    Autistic Disorder
    Delusional Disorder

Note. Adapted by permission from *Boarding Time* (p. 92) by J. Morrison, and R. A. Muñoz, 1991, Washington, DC: American Psychiatric Press. Copyright 1991 by the American Psychiatric Association.

Laura Freitas

Laura Freitas, a 32-year-old divorced woman, was admitted to a mental health unit with this chief complaint: "I'm God." She was referred from an outpatient clinic and served as her own chief informant.

    Laura had had her first episode of mental illness at age 19, after her second baby was born. She could remember little about this period, except that it was called a "postpartum psychosis" and she had spent some time in isolation for dancing nude in the hospital day room. She had recovered and remained well until three years ago, when, for reasons she could not remember, she was placed on lithium carbonate. She had taken this medication from then until seven or eight days ago, when she stopped because "I felt so well, so *powerful* that I knew I didn't need it." Over the next several days she became increasingly agitated, slept little, and talked a great deal, until friends finally brought her for treatment.

Laura had been born in Illinois, where her father was an automobile mechanic. She was an only child who often felt that her parents would have been happier with no children at all. They were both alcoholics, and she had run away overnight on at least one occasion when she was 13. She had experimented with marijuana on two occasions when she was a teenager, but she denied using other drugs, including alcohol.

At 18 Laura had been briefly married to a bread salesman, to whom she had borne two children. The daughter, 13, lived with her father. The son, 14, was hyperactive and had at one time been treated with Ritalin. Laura was a fallen-away Catholic who for the past two years had worked at a travel agency. She stated that her health had been "above perfect," meaning that she had had no allergies or medical problems, other than a tonsillectomy when she was six and a tubal ligation after the birth of her daughter.

Family history was positive for alcoholism not only in both parents, but in both grandfathers. A paternal aunt would intermittently "go to pieces," becoming excessively religious and imagining various sins to feel guilty about.

Laura was a somewhat overweight woman who looked about her stated age. She was quite agitated, jumping out of her chair every few moments to pace back and forth to the door. She was given her breakfast during a part of this interview; she intentionally smeared grape jelly onto the trousers of a passing nurse. Subsequently, she lay down on the floor and kicked her legs in the air, apparently in ecstasy.

Laura seemed to be struggling to control her speech; even so, she skipped from one subject to another. However, the rate at which she spoke was approximately normal. Her affect was clearly elevated, and she declared that she had never felt better in her life. She admitted that she might hear voices singing (no music could be heard by the interviewer), and that she enjoyed singing along with what she heard. She stated that she was "The All-Powerful One," and that she now realized that she had no need for medication.

Laura was oriented to person, place, and time. She named five recent presidents, and correctly (and extremely rapidly) subtracted serial sevens into the negative numbers. When she finished, she apologized for taking so long to complete a task working with numbers. "After all," she said, "I created them."

Evaluation of Laura Freitas

Two diagnostic areas stand out in Laura's case—psychosis and mood disturbance. Psychosis can be dealt with summarily: Her delusions were too brief for any of the psychotic diagnoses except **Brief Psychotic Disorder** or a **Sub-**

stance-Induced Psychotic Disorder. However, each of these requires that a mood disorder does not explain the symptoms better. Because Laura had apparently had previous Manic Episodes (see below), she would not qualify for any psychotic disorder.

Laura's current symptoms would strongly suggest a **Manic Episode**. It appears that a previous clinician also thought so: She was successfully treated with lithium (which is specific for the bipolar disorders) until shortly before this admission. Let us work through the steps necessary to diagnose Manic Episode:

1. **Quality of Mood**. Elevated mood was shown in the expansive way Laura expressed herself and in her statement that she had never felt better.

2. **Duration**. Her current symptoms had lasted at least one week. Information from informants (Principle 3) would probably establish that the onset of her present episode was even longer ago, perhaps at the point that she began to feel increasingly "well."

3. **Symptoms**. She had at least four symptoms (three required) of a Manic Episode. She was grandiose, stating that she was God and that her physical health was "above perfect." She also had agitation, excessive speech, and decreased need for sleep.

4. **Impairment**. This was clearly demonstrated by Laura's admission to the hospital, where she smeared jelly on a nurse.

5. **Exclusions**. None were noted, including **substance use** (she had used marijuana only when she was a teenager) and **general medical conditions**. However, hyperthyroidism and other endocrine disorders should be ruled out by routine laboratory testing upon admission.

Laura would therefore fulfill the basic criteria for Manic Episode. No general medical condition or cognitive disorder would seem more likely (Rule A). If any further confirmation was needed, she had an aunt who might have had a recurrent psychosis. This sort of family history (Rule D) would better support a remitting condition such as **Bipolar I Disorder** than a chronic psychosis such as **Schizophrenia**.

The vignette does not indicate whether Laura had ever had an episode of depression; for coding purposes, it doesn't matter. Her most recent (current) episode was Manic, and she had had at least two prior episodes (one 13 years ago, one 3 years ago when she started lithium). Psychosis would qualify her for the fifth-digit severity level of .x4. Her delusion that she was God would be mood-congruent for mania.

Laura would not qualify for any episode specifiers (see Table 5.1), but she had been well after her previous episode, yielding the course specifier of **With Full Interepisode Recovery**. The vignette gives no information suggesting that she also had an Axis II personality disorder. Her physical health (Axis III) was good. There is no evidence that her divorced status or the treatment of her son for hyperactivity would have any effect on the treatment of her mania, so no Axis IV problem should be listed. Her GAF would be scored on the basis that she was currently quite ill, with behavior influenced by delusions, but that she did not seem to be in danger of hurting herself or others. Her five-axis diagnosis would thus be as follows:

Axis I	296.44	Bipolar I Disorder, Most Recent Episode Manic, Severe With Mood-Congruent Psychotic Features, With Full Interepisode Recovery
Axis II	V71.09	No diagnosis
Axis III		None
Axis IV		None
Axis V	GAF = 25	(on admission)

Adrian Branscom

Adrian Branscom was a 49-year-old executive who referred himself to his company's mental health clinician. "I never thought I'd be talking to a shrink," was his first comment upon entering the office.

After serving two years as a junior officer in the Army Ordnance Corps, Adrian had been recruited by a subsidiary of one of the large petroleum companies that specialized in oil field development. He was bright and energetic, and he climbed rapidly through the ranks of middle management. He was in line for a vice-presidency when the recession hit. Although his share of the restructuring turned out to be no vice-presidency and a 10% pay cut, Adrian felt lucky that he still had a job. His wife's view was less sanguine.

Yoshiko was a Japanese war bride. They had married during a whirlwind two-week leave he had spent in Tokyo during Adrian's tour of duty in Vietnam. For the past 20 years, since the birth of their daughter and son, she had stayed home with the children.

"She wishes she had stayed home in Japan," Adrian commented wryly. Almost since their wedding, Yoshiko had accused him of taking her away from her people so he could "dump her." In all the years they had lived together, she had never made friends. She spent most of her free time acquiring a collection of Japanese porcelain artifacts. Now she deeply resented her husband's demotion and their loss of income.

"We hadn't been getting along well for years," said Adrian, "but for the last several years we've hit one new low after another. She says if I were a real man, I'd provide better for her."

On many occasions, Adrian had told Yoshiko he thought they should discuss their problems. Her usual response was "So go ahead and discuss it!" When he tried to state his viewpoint, she would listen for half a sentence; then "She always begins to talk over me. After starting six or eight sentences, I usually give up."

Every suggestion Adrian made that they seek marital counseling provoked a torrent of invective from Yoshiko and the demand for a divorce. When he tried to discuss divorce, she cried and said that he was trying to get rid of her and that they'd all be better off if she committed suicide. These tirades made him feel guilty, and they had worsened in the past month or so.

Although Adrian was usually a "happy-go-lucky sort of fellow," for most of the past six weeks he had been depressed and anxious. His appetite and energy had been unchanged, but he had had trouble sleeping most nights; he had often awakened with a pounding heart and the feeling that he was about to smother. His concentration at work and his self-confidence had both plummeted. Increasingly over the past week, he had been thinking about death and the shotgun he still had somewhere up in his attic. Frightened, he had finally decided to seek help.

Adrian had been born in west central Texas, where his father taught school and did a little farming. He was the youngest of three children, all of whom managed to go to college and succeed in business or the professions. "It wasn't until I was out of college that I realized just how dirt poor my parents were," he said. "I guess we seemed well off because we were all happy."

The family history was negative for substance use or for any other mental disorder. Adrian had never used drugs or alcohol, and had never had moods that were excessively elevated or irritable. He spent most of his time at work and had very few friends; he had never strayed from the marital bed ("or twin beds," as he put it). At home, he enjoyed collecting rocks and hiking with his son.

Adrian was a conservatively dressed, somewhat overweight man who looked his stated age. He sat quietly in the office chair during the interview. Once or twice he reached for a fresh tissue to wipe his eyes. His speech was clear, coherent, relevant, and spontaneous. His mood was appropriate to the content of thought and showed normal lability. He denied having any hallucinations or delusions. He stated that he had always been "a fixer"—that he felt it was his job to make things work for everyone. He earned a perfect score on the Mini-Mental State Exam. His insight and judgment seemed unimpaired. "I think we'd all be better off if we lived apart," he concluded. "This is one thing I don't think I can fix."

Evaluation of Adrian Branscom

A rapid reading of Adrian's history suggests three possible diagnostic areas: mood disorder, anxiety disorder, and problems of adjustment. To consider **Adjustment Disorder** first, it would be easy to suppose that Adrian's difficulties could be laid completely at the doorstep of his marital difficulties. After all, he had no past history of mental disorder, and he did have an extremely troubled marriage. But he had enough symptoms to qualify for a mood disorder (see below), and the criteria for Adjustment Disorder With Depressed Mood quite clearly require that the criteria for no other Axis I disorder be fulfilled. From the information we have, his character structure, though perhaps a bit naïve, revealed none of the sorts of interpersonal difficulties we would expect for an Axis II personality disorder. However, in a later interview, the clinician should obtain information from informants; the vignette gives only Adrian's interpretation of his marital difficulties.

As for the anxiety disorders, Adrian had episodes of awakening from sleep with pounding heart and shortness of breath, and he had felt anxious for much of the previous few weeks. These symptoms did not qualify for a **Panic Attack** (which can occur during sleep); therefore, **Panic Disorder** would not be diagnosed. None of his symptoms would suggest **Specific Phobia**, **Social Phobia**, **Agoraphobia**, or **Obsessive–Compulsive Disorder**. Although he was a war veteran, he was evidently not exposed to extremely traumatic events (as would be the case in **Posttraumatic Stress Disorder**). **Generalized Anxiety Disorder** requires a six-month duration and more symptoms. Although Adrian was overweight, obesity does not have any known relationship to anxiety symptoms; it should be mentioned on Axis III, however.

Finally, Adrian did have some clear-cut mood symptoms; these included feeling depressed most of the time, insomnia, problems with concentration, feelings of guilt, and an increasing preoccupation with suicide. (DSM-IV does not credit low self-confidence and weeping as depressive symptoms.) His symptoms had been constantly present for over a month and were causing him trouble with his job. None of the exclusions would apply (**Bereavement**, **general medical condition**, or **substance use**), so he would fulfill criteria for a **Major Depressive Episode** and for **Major Depressive Disorder, Single Episode**. None of the course or episode specifiers would apply (see Chapter 5, Table 5.1). He fulfilled only the minimum number of symptoms, but one of these (suicidal ideas) was serious; his clinician thought this deserved a severity rating of Moderate.

The coding and recording of Adrian's depression would thus be quite straightforward. But what if he had had just two fewer symptoms of depression? He would then qualify for none of the specific mood disorders. Although he could be diagnosed as having an **Adjustment Disorder with Depressed Mood**, I would prefer to diagnose him as having **Depressive Disorder Not Otherwise Specified**. This would remind me to watch for additional depressive symptoms. The GAF score below was assigned on the basis of having moderate symptoms. Although Adrian had had some thoughts about suicide, he had no plans and did not appear to be at serious immediate risk. His complete diagnosis would be as follows:

Axis I	296.22	Major Depressive Disorder, Single Episode, Moderate
Axis II	V71.09	No diagnosis
Axis III	278.0	Obesity
Axis IV		Marital discord
Axis V	GAF = 60	(current)

James Chatterton

When James Chatterton was 18, he cut his wrist on the glass of a window he had just broken; that earned him his first admission to a mental hospital. James's aunt was the chief informant on this occasion. "He always seemed a little cold. Kind of like his cousin, my Betty," she said.

James had been pretty unconventional, even when he was little. He cared so little what other people thought that in fourth grade, when he called the teacher "Gristle Butt," he didn't even acknowledge the suppressed laughter of the other children. "I don't think he had a single friend in school," said his aunt. "He never cracked a smile, never got angry—not even when he said he thought the other kids were talking about him. He said that quite a lot, as I recall." Even when he was older, he had never showed the slightest interest in girls or curiosity about sex.

When James was 14, his mother died suddenly. His father, working in another state, had no time to care for him, so he was sent to live with his aunt. With no friends to speak of, he had plenty of time to study and did well during his first two or three years in high school. He was fond of science. Well past the time when most boys give up that sort of thing, he continued to play with the chemistry set he had received for Christmas the year he was nine.

One day toward spring of his senior year, when his cousin Betty was home from college with her "sickness," she lifted her skirt and offered to let James touch her. "He came and told me about it immediately," said his aunt. "He said it made him feel nauseated." On the following day, the entire family was relieved when Betty was rehospitalized for Schizophrenia.

For the next several months, James seemed to go into a decline. When his grades fell and his aunt asked why, he only shrugged. He showed no interest either in going to college or in getting a job. He spent most of his free time reading chemistry texts and making notes in the margins. Sometimes when his aunt awakened in the early hours of the morning, she thought she heard him walking around in his room. Several times he seemed to be laughing to himself. He took to sleeping late, often past noon; gradually he stopped going to school at all.

That summer, Betty returned from the hospital, vastly improved on neuroleptic medication. Within a week she confided to her mother that James had warned her not to take the medication. It was part of a plot by Mormons, he had told her, to make her sterile. Several times during the next two months, he lectured her about extraterrestrials.

James had stopped eating much of anything and lost at least 20 pounds. Weight loss and sleep disturbance made him look gaunt and older. It was just before Thanksgiving when he broke the window and cut himself, and was finally admitted to the same hospital where Betty had been a patient.

Apart from his lack of friends and his separation from his parents, James's early life had not been remarkable. He had experimented with marijuana a few times, but had never used other street drugs or alcohol. He smoked about a pack a day of cigarettes. His only medical problem had been an operation for an umbilical hernia when he was five. Besides his cousin, the family history was positive for alcoholism in his paternal grandfather and hyperthyroidism in both his father and an uncle. His mother had been "nervous."

James was thin and sallow and looked several years older than his age. He was dressed in tattered, cut-off blue jean shorts and a T-shirt. His tennis shoes had no laces, so he scuffed slowly into the interview room, head down and eyes to the ground. Though his facial expression was almost always blank, he would occasionally laugh and turn his head to the side as if he had heard something. He initially denied that he was hearing voices, but later in the day admitted to a second interviewer that a woman's voice kept telling him to "jack off." He denied having any delusions, including grandeur or persecution. Asked directly about a Mormon conspiracy to sterilize his cousin, he said that he wasn't at liberty to discuss it.

James claimed not to be depressed or suicidal; he said he had broken the window and lacerated his arm because he was "upset." He scored 28 out of 30 on the Mini-Mental State Exam (he did not know the date within two days or the name of the hospital). Although he agreed that he needed medical attention for his arm, he had no insight about his psychiatric disorder.

Evaluation of James Chatterton

James had symptoms in three principal areas: psychotic thinking, somatic symptoms, and social and personality problems. The somatic symptoms included loss of appetite and weight loss, and a family history of hyperthyroidism should cause his clinician to consider a **general medical condition** as a possible cause of his psychosis (Rule A). Upon admission he would receive a complete physical exam and relevant laboratory testing, which would include thyroid tests. For the purposes of this discussion, let us assume that no evidence of thyroid disease was found.

The discussion of James's psychotic thinking follows the outline of the section in Chapter 4 called "Distinguishing Schizophrenia from Other Psychotic Disorders." First, the *extent of symptoms* must be considered: Did James have enough to meet the "A" criteria for Schizophrenia? His active psychotic symptoms included persecutory delusions (the Mormon plot, extraterrestrials) and the hallucinated woman's voice giving him commands. These two symptoms by themselves would be enough to fulfill the "A" criteria, but he also had the negative symptom of loss of volition (his grades declined and he showed no interest in work or college). Although his behavior suggested otherwise, James at first denied hearing voices. This demonstrates the value of Principle 4, which was confirmed later when he admitted to another interviewer that he was having auditory hallucinations. Laughing to himself (possibly responding to something funny his hallucinated voices said) and having a relative with Schizophrenia would also point strongly to a diagnosis of **Schizophrenia**.

The *course* of a psychotic disorder is extremely important in determining the exact diagnosis. James's disorder began gradually, without precipitating factors, and progressed without remission or recovery. Including the prodromal period when he began to withdraw and to show lack of volition, he had been ill longer than six months (from about April to November). Premorbid personality is discussed below. The *consequences* were also severe enough for a diagnosis of Schizophrenia: They severely interfered with James's social life and his ability to attend school.

The next step in considering psychotic thinking must be to rule out any possible *exclusions* for Schizophrenia. The possibility of a general medical condition has already been discussed (and, for the sake of argument, dismissed). James had tried marijuana a few times, but had not **used substances** enough to account for his remarkable deterioration. He scored two points short of perfect on the Mini-Mental State Exam, well above the range for a **cognitive disorder**. The last exclusion would concern **mood disorder**. Although James had lost weight, slept poorly, and cut his wrist on glass, when he was admitted to the hospital he could not explain why he had cut the wrist. Moreover, he not only denied feeling depressed; his affect was at times inappropriate.

Finally, social and personality problems must be considered. According to his aunt, from the time he was a little boy James had been identified by others as "different." He was emotionally distant, didn't care what others thought, had no close friends, showed few expressions of emotion, and preferred solitary activities—all symptoms of **Schizoid Personality Disorder**. We have only his aunt's perspective on his lack of interest in sex, though he apparently never dated. (However, it does not seem surprising that he would be upset at the frank sexual offering of a disturbed cousin.) He also had some ideas of reference (the other children might be talking about him). This is a symptom of **Schizotypal Personality Disorder**, but his aunt did not report other odd beliefs or peculiar speech or behaviors. James was generally more aloof than peculiar. The absence of other symptoms of suspiciousness would also rule out **Paranoid Personality Disorder**.

The diagnosis of James's Schizophrenia subtype would require some thought. He had both delusions and hallucinations, but would not be diagnosed as having the **Paranoid Type** because his affect was generally flat and often inappropriate (giggling). Yet he also could not be diagnosed as having the **Disorganized Type**, because neither his speech nor behavior was disorganized. Of course, he had no features of the **Catatonic Type** at all. **Undifferentiated Type** would remain as the diagnosis of exclusion. He had not yet been ill with active-phase symptoms for a year, so he would receive no course specifier. I have already noted his Axis II personality disorder, to which the qualifier (**Premorbid**) would be added because it was present long before his Schizophrenia began.

James also had a notable problem with sleep, but should it receive an independent diagnosis? He would meet most of the criteria for **Insomnia Re-**

lated to **Schizophrenia**, but it was neither the predominant complaint nor a major focus for treatment. Persistent insomnia of this sort usually normalizes once the Schizophrenia has been successfully treated. James's full diagnosis would thus be as follows:

Axis I	295.90	Schizophrenia, Undifferentiated Type
Axis II	301.20	Schizoid Personality Disorder (Premorbid)
Axis III	881.02	Laceration of wrist
Axis IV		None
Axis V	GAF = 20	(on admission)

Gail Downey

"Go ahead, cut!" Gail lay flat on her hospital bed, staring at the ceiling. Her hair was carefully washed and combed, but her expression was stiff. "I want a lobotomy. I'll sign the papers. I can't take this any more."

Gail was an attractive 34-year-old divorcee with three children. For five years she had had depressions but no manias or hypomanias. Her treatment had been marked by frequent suicide attempts and hospitalizations. In her current episode, which had lasted nearly five weeks, she had felt severely depressed throughout nearly every day. She complained that she lay awake until the early hours of each night; she had no pep, interest, or appetite. She cried frequently, and she was so distracted by her emotional turmoil that her boss had reluctantly let her go. She had been prescribed at least six antidepressants, often in combination. Most of these seemed to help the depression initially, raising her mood enough that she could at least return home. She also had responded positively to each of several courses of ECT. Within a few months of each new treatment she would relapse and return to the hospital, often with a fresh set of stitches in her wrist. While on a brief pass from the present hospitalization, she had swallowed a nearly fatal overdose of chloral hydrate.

After Gail's parents had divorced when she was nine, she had been reared by her mother. Since the age of 13, Gail had been arrested three or four times for taking small items such as pantyhose or a lipstick from department stores. Each of these incidents had occurred while she was under particular stress, usually because a job or personal relationship was going sour. She always noted increasing tension before taking these items, and felt nearly explosive joy each time she left the store with her trophy in the pocket of her overcoat. As a juvenile, whenever she was caught she had been remanded to the custody of her mother; once she had paid a fine. The most recent episode had occurred just before this hospitalization. This time, the charges had been dropped because of her repeated suicide attempts.

Gail's medical history read like a catalog of symptoms. It included urinary retention, a lump in her throat that seemed about to strangle her, chest pains, severe menstrual cramps, vomiting spells, chronic diarrhea, heart palpitations, migraine headaches (a neurologist said they were "not typical"), and even a brief episode of blindness (from which she had recovered without treatment). At the time of the divorce, Gail's husband had confided that she had been "frigid" and often complained of pain during intercourse. Starting in her teens, she had taken medicine or consulted a physician for more than 30 of these symptoms. The doctors had never found much wrong with her physically; they had either given her tranquilizers or referred her to a succession of psychiatrists.

After several years Gail had been evicted from her apartment, and her husband had obtained custody of their three children. The only nonmedical person she ever talked to was her mother. Now she was demanding an operation that would permanently sever some of the connections within her brain.

Evaluation of Gail Downey

Gail had more than enough mood symptoms (low mood, loss of pleasure, insomnia, anorexia, suicide ideas, loss of energy, trouble thinking) to qualify her current episode as a **Major Depressive Episode**. She did not abuse substances; the exclusions for general medical conditions and substance use are discussed below. Any patient who presents with severe depression should be evaluated for **Major Depressive Disorder**, which is potentially life-threatening and often responds quickly to the appropriate therapy. Gail had had numerous episodes of depression, no manias or hypomanias, and no psychotic symptoms; she had also apparently recovered for at least two months between episodes. She would therefore qualify for a diagnosis of Major Depressive Disorder, Recurrent. The persistent suicide attempts would mark it as **Severe Without Psychotic Features**. The vignette does not give enough information to support an episode specifier. But the fact that Gail's depression had been treated so often and so unsuccessfully would cause one to suspect some other underlying condition.

Since her teens Gail had had a variety of somatic symptoms, at least some of which (like the migraines) were atypical. She had well over eight of the DSM-IV **Somatization Disorder** symptoms, which were distributed appropriately for that diagnosis. Among the medical and neurological disorders to consider would be multiple sclerosis, spinal cord tumors, and diseases of the heart and lungs. The fact that she had been unsuccessfully treated by so many physicians would reduce the likelihood that she instead had a series of **general medical conditions** (Rule A). The vignette provides no evidence that Gail consciously feigned her symptoms for gain (**Malingering**) or for less obvious motives (**Factitious Disorder**).

No additional diagnosis is needed for Gail's **anorexia**; any problem with maintaining body weight was not due to refusal of food, but to her lack of appetite. Her **insomnia** could be given a separate Axis I diagnosis (307.42, Insomnia Related to Somatization Disorder) had it been serious enough to warrant independent clinical evaluation; it wasn't. Similarly, her **sexual dysfunction** would not be independently coded (even if the vignette gave enough specifics as to its exact nature), because it is easily explained as a symptom of Somatization Disorder.

Finally, Gail's history (see Principle 3) revealed a pattern of repeated shoplifting characterized by tension and release. Nothing else in her history would lead us to believe that she had **Antisocial Personality Disorder**, and she had certainly never had had a **Manic Episode**. She would thus qualify for a diagnosis of **Kleptomania**.

> **TIP** Many Somatization Disorder patients also have panic attacks and other symptoms of a variety of **anxiety disorders**. As with depressive disease, there is the danger that clinicians will make an incomplete diagnosis of an anxiety disorder and ignore the underlying Somatization Disorder.

Gail thus had three codable Axis I diagnoses. How should they be listed? Her Major Depressive Disorder was serious enough that it had been the focus of treatment for at least five years; at the beginning of her treatment, that approach was probably sound (it followed the safety rule, Rule E). However, Principle 1 and Rule C would now suggest that Somatization Disorder should become the focus of her care. Although the Somatization Disorder criteria do not specify severity, Gail's clinician, who wanted to indicate how seriously ill she had been, used the generic severity criteria that can be applied to most DSM-IV diagnoses (see the Introduction, p. 5).

The vignette gives little information about her personality; to indicate the need for further exploration, the code for Diagnosis Deferred should be assigned on Axis II. Considering her past history, the Axis III code seems something of an irony.

Axis I	300.81	Somatization Disorder, Severe
	296.33	Major Depressive Disorder, Recurrent, Severe Without Psychotic Features
	312.32	Kleptomania
Axis II	799.9	Diagnosis Deferred
Axis III		None
Axis IV		Unemployment, Loss of child custody, Eviction
Axis V	GAF = 40	(current)

Sara Winkler

Sara Winkler crossed herself three times before she sat down. She and her husband were each 25 and they had been married four years.

"I've known her since we were 16," Loren Winkler said, "and she's always been pretty careful. You know, checking the stove to see that it's turned off or the doors to make sure that they're really locked before we go out. It's only been the last couple of years that it's been so much worse."

Sara was a college graduate who had worked briefly as a paralegal assistant before taking time out to have a family. She was healthy and had no history of alcohol or drug use. When Jonathan, their son, was only six months old, she had had a terrifying dream in which she plunged a paring knife into the chest of a doll as it lay on the kitchen table. She recognized the doll as one she had owned as a child. But as the knife entered the plastic body, its arms and legs began to move, and she saw that it was a real child. On the kitchen wall, the word *KILL* seemed to scroll upward before her eyes, and she awakened screaming. It had taken her several hours to get back to sleep.

The following evening, while slicing carrots for a salad, she suddenly had this thought: "Would I ever harm Jonathan?" Although the idea seemed absurd, it was accompanied by some of the same anxieties she had felt the night before. She took the baby in to her husband while she finished preparing dinner.

After that, thoughts of knives and of stabbing someone smaller and weaker had increasingly wormed their way into Sara's consciousness. Even if her mind was fixed on reading or watching television, she might suddenly visualize the giant block letters *KILL* arising before her.

The idea that she would actually harm Jonathan seemed irrational to her, but the nagging doubts and anxiety tormented her daily. She no longer trusted herself in the kitchen with him. Sometimes she could almost feel the muscles of her forearm begin to contract in the act of reaching for a knife. Although she had never followed through on one of these impulses, the thought that she might do so terrified her constantly. Now she refused even to open the knife drawer. Any cutting had to be done with scissors or the food processor, or else her husband had to do it.

Not long after her dream, Sara began trying to ward off her troubling thoughts and impulses. A fallen-away Catholic, she reverted to some of the practices she had known as a child. When she had one of her frightening thoughts, she initially felt comforted if she crossed herself. If she was carrying packages or Jonathan, she muttered a Hail Mary.

With time, the power of these simple measures seemed to weaken. Then Sara found that if she crossed herself three times or said three Hail Marys (or any combination, in threes), she felt better. Eventually, however, she needed nine of these behaviors before she felt she had adequately protected her son and herself. When she was in public, she could cross herself once and complete the ritual by murmuring Hail Marys under her breath.

Now Jonathan was nearly a year old, and several hours a day were being consumed in Sara's repetitive thoughts and activities. Jonathan was fretful, and her husband was cooking virtually all of their meals. For several weeks she had felt increasingly depressed; she admitted that her mood was bad nearly all the time, though she had not had suicidal ideas or death wishes. Nothing interested her much, and she was always tired. She had lost over 10 pounds and had insomnia; she frequently awakened screaming at night. When her husband found her doing penance 27 times in a row, he insisted they come for help.

"I know it seems crazy," Sara said tearfully, "but I just can't seem to get these stupid ideas out of my head."

Evaluation of Sara Winkler

For longer than two weeks, Sara had been depressed most of the time. Her symptoms included insomnia, fatigue, and loss of interest and weight. She was physically healthy (no **general medical conditions**) and had no history of **substance use** (Rule A). It is hard to be sure whether she was being impaired by the depression or the symptoms of **Obsessive–Compulsive Disorder (OCD)**; it seems reasonable that she would be having problems from both. If so, she would fulfill the criteria for **Major Depressive Episode**. With no prior Major Depressive, **Manic**, or **Hypomanic Episodes**, her diagnosis would be **Major Depressive Disorder, Single Episode**. The severity specifier would be **Moderate** (few symptoms, no suicidal ideas, but considerable distress), and there was very little danger that she would ever actually harm her son.

As for Sara's anxiety—her more obvious area of difficulty—she had neither **Panic Attacks** nor **Generalized Anxiety Disorder**. Rather, Sara had obsessions and compulsions, both of which fulfilled criteria for OCD. (Although she had another Axis I disorder, her obsessions were not confined to guilty ruminations related to her Major Depressive Disorder.) Her OCD symptoms occupied more than an hour a day, and she was severely distressed. Clearly, Sara's concern was not just an exaggeration of a real-life problem, so her focus of concern was pathological. She herself recognized that she was being unreasonable, so the specifier **With Poor Insight** would not apply.

In the reading of Sara's Axis I diagnoses, the depression was listed first to indicate that her clinician regarded it as the aspect that required clinical attention first. (Others might well disagree.) Her GAF score would be justified by the severity of her rituals.

Axis I	296.22	Major Depressive Disorder, Single Episode, Moderate
	300.3	Obsessive–Compulsive Disorder
Axis II	V71.09	No diagnosis
Axis III		None
Axis IV		None
Axis V	GAF = 45	(on admission)

Gemma Livingstone

"I eat, then I throw up." That was how Gemma Livingstone described her problem during her first interview. Beginning when she was 23, this behavior had been almost continual in the intervening four years.

Even as a teenager, Gemma was concerned about the way she looked. With some of the other girls in high school, from time to time she had crash-dieted. But her weight had seldom varied by more than a few pounds from 116. At five feet, six inches tall, she had been svelte but not too thin. Throughout her adolescence and early adulthood, she had the feeling that if she did not tightly control her eating habits, she would rapidly gain weight—"puff up like a toad," as she put it.

Dealing with the aftermath of an unwanted pregnancy and a subsequent abortion, Gemma had had the opportunity to test her theory. Eating what she wanted, she had ballooned from a size 8 to a size 14 in less than half a year. Once she finally regained control, she vowed she would never lose it again. For three years, she had bought nothing larger than a size 4.

When Gemma was a teenager, she and her friends simply didn't eat. When dining in a restaurant or with friends, she would still push her food around on her plate to disguise how little she was actually taking in. But when she was at home she would often eat a full meal, then retire to the bathroom and throw up. At first, this had required touching the back of her throat with the handle of a teaspoon she kept in the bathroom for that purpose. With practice, she had learned to regurgitate just by willing it. "It's as easy as blowing your nose," she said.

Gemma's fear of obesity had become the organizing principle of her life. On her refrigerator door, she kept a picture of herself when she was in her "toad" phase. She said that every time she looked at it, she lost her appetite. Whereas she used to use laxatives for constipation, recently she had begun to use them as another means of purging her system: "If I don't have a bowel movement every day, I feel as if I'll burst. Even my eyes get all puffy." She had also taken some diuretics, but had stopped doing so when her periods stopped. She didn't really believe there was a connection, but recently she had begun to menstruate again. If there was one thing she feared more than getting fat, it was getting pregnant. She had never been very active sexually, but now she and her husband seldom had intercourse more than about once a month. Even then, she insisted on using both a diaphragm and a condom.

Other than her weight, which had fallen to less than 90 pounds, Gemma appeared to be in good health. A review of systems was positive only for abdominal bloating. Although she occasionally had a day or two of low mood and feeling sorry for herself, she laughed it off as "PMS" and added that it certainly wasn't bothering her now. She had never had Manic Episodes, hallucinations, obsessions, compulsions, phobias, panic attacks, or thoughts about suicide.

Gemma had been born in Virginia Beach, Virginia, where her father was stationed when he was in the Navy. Subsequently he owned his own heating and air conditioning company, and the family was reasonably well off. She was an only child. There had been no history of any kind of difficulties with learning or conduct while she was in school. She and her husband were married when she was 21, after she had worked for three years as a bank teller. They had two children, a son who was seven and a daughter aged five.

Gemma's only brush with the law had occurred two years earlier, when she'd forged some prescriptions to obtain amphetamines for dieting. She had copped a plea and been placed on probation for a year; she had not used amphetamines since then. She had tried marijuana once or twice when she was first out of high school, but had never used alcohol or tobacco. Her only surgical procedure had been bilateral breast augmentation, which had been done with autologous fat rather than silicone.

In a separate interview, Gemma's husband stated that he thought his wife felt inadequate and insecure. He said that she usually dressed in revealing, even alluring clothing, which looked less enticing now that she had lost so much weight. When she did not get her way, she would sometimes pout for hours, though he didn't think there was much real feeling behind this expression of her emotion. "She loves to be the center of attention," he said, "but a lot of people don't buy into her act any more. I think it frustrates her."

Gemma was a dark-haired, slightly built woman who had probably been quite pretty before she lost so much weight. She smiled readily and somewhat self-consciously, as if she were trying to make her cheeks dimple. She wore a V-necked blouse and a very short skirt that she did not attempt to pull down when she crossed her legs. She spoke with a good deal of rolling of eyes and varying inflection of her voice, but her answers to the examiner's questions were themselves vague and often discursive. She denied feeling depressed or wishing she were dead; she had never had delusions or hallucinations, but she claimed that she was still "fat as a pig." To illustrate, she pinched between thumb and forefinger a fold of skin that hung loosely from her arm. She scored a perfect 30 on the Mini-Mental State Exam.

Evaluation of Gemma Livingstone

Gemma had a history of disordered eating that dated back to her high school years. She was gaunt and fearful of gaining weight; she perceived herself as being fat. Because she was once again having her periods, she might have been diagnosed as **Eating Disorder Not Otherwise Specified**. DSM-IV specifically mentions that Anorexia Nervosa *with* regular menses is one of the conditions that can be so coded. However, to her clinician it seemed artificial not to give Gemma a full **Anorexia Nervosa** diagnosis. If she had been evaluated several months earlier, she would have qualified; if she were a man, she would qualify now. However, the specifier **In Partial Remission** was used (see page 5). Her current subtype was **Binge-Eating/Purging Type**; as a teenager, she had been of the **Restricting Type**.

Based only on the information she herself provided, Gemma could not have been given a definitive Axis II diagnosis. But from her husband's information (Principle 3) and that of the mental status evaluation, the following criteria for **Histrionic Personality Disorder** were established: needing to be the center of attention, shifting and shallow emotion, drawing attention to herself (wearing revealing clothing and crossing her legs), speaking vaguely, and expressing herself dramatically. **Somatization Disorder** is often associated with this diagnosis, but a review of systems revealed minimal symptoms—far too few to make any sort of somatoform diagnosis.

Would other Axis I or II diagnoses be possible? Forging prescriptions and using drugs were illegal, but Gemma did not continue with either behavior; thus, they would not constitute evidence of diagnosable pathology. Her complete diagnosis would therefore read as follows:

Axis I	307.1	Anorexia Nervosa, Binge-Eating/Purging Type, In Partial Remission
Axis II	301.50	Histrionic Personality Disorder
Axis III		None
Axis IV		None
Axis V	GAF = 61	(current)

Edith Roman

Edith Roman was a 76-year-old woman admitted to the hospital on the complaint of Sylvia, her daughter: "She's been depressed since her stroke."

Beginning about a year earlier, Edith had become forgetful. This first became apparent when for three weeks out of four she neglected to place her Friday night telephone call to Sylvia, who at that time lived several hundred miles away. Each time her daughter called instead, and Edith seemed surprised to get the call.

When she finally took a week off work for a visit, Sylvia discovered that Edith had also been neglecting the marketing and housecleaning: The sink was full and the refrigerator was nearly empty, and dust thickly coated everything. Although Edith's speech and physical appearance hadn't changed, something was clearly wrong. By the end of the week, Sylvia had the answer from a neurologist: early Alzheimer's disease. She took an extra week off work to move her mother across the state and into her own home. A companion was hired to stay with Edith during the day, when Sylvia was away at work.

This arrangement worked well for several months. Edith's deterioration was gradual and minimal, until her stroke left her limping and unable to remember words. Now her memory was worse than ever, and this was when the depression began. When Edith talked at all, she complained to the companion about how useless and lonely she felt. She slept poorly, ate very little, cried often, and said she was a burden.

Edith had been born in St. Louis, where, until she was 12, her parents had run a small dry-cleaning business. Then her father died and her mother soon married Edith's paternal uncle, who came equipped with two teenagers of his own. They all got along quite well, and Edith graduated from high school, got married, and had her only child. Throughout life, she had been a pleasant, spunky woman who had been interested in crafts and many other aspects of homemaking. After her husband died, she continued to be active in her social and bridge clubs. Until a year ago, her physical health had been good; she had never used alcohol or tobacco.

An elderly woman dressed in a cotton nightgown and a quilted wrap, Edith sat upright on the edge of her bed, her left hand lying uselessly in her lap. She made good eye contact with the examiner; though she did not speak spontaneously, she did respond to all questions. Her monosyllabic speech was clear, but she sometimes had difficulty finding the words she wanted. Asked to identify a magazine, she thought for a moment and called it "this papers." She admitted feeling depressed, said that she saw no future for herself, and hoped she could die soon. She denied ever experiencing hallucinations or delusions. On the Mini-Mental State Exam, she scored only 16 out of a possible 30.

Evaluation of Edith Roman

The symptoms of Edith's **dementia** included failing memory and deteriorating ability to care for herself (evidence of loss of executive functioning). These symptoms had begun gradually and were gradually worsening when she had her stroke. At that point, her memory abruptly worsened further and she developed an aphasia (she couldn't think of certain words she wanted to use). She maintained eye contact and appeared to focus her attention on the examiner—evidence against a **delirium**. A neurological exam earlier had not found evidence of other **general medical conditions** that might better explain her symptoms.

For far longer than two weeks, Edith had also had symptoms of depression. These included constantly depressed mood, loss of appetite and sleep, death wishes, and the feeling of being a burden (more or less equivalent to a sense of worthlessness). Her symptoms would seem to qualify for **Major Depressive Episode**, except that she also had a severe cognitive disorder (Rule A).

Edith's dementia had two causes, and each of them had created difficulties for her and her daughter with communication and with everyday functioning. This would fulfill the criteria for **Dementia Due to Multiple Etiologies**, which is not really a diagnosis. Instead, it is a reminder to record on Axis I and on Axis III each cause of dementia. Edith's clinician presumed that her depression was a result of the combined effects of **Dementia of the Alzheimer's Type** and **Vascular Dementia**; her symptoms did not rate the specifier **With Behavioral Disturbance**. However, her depression was coded in the fifth digit of both types of dementia. Her daughter noted that her premorbid personality had been cheerful, so no Axis II diagnosis was given.

Axis I	290.21	Dementia of the Alzheimer's Type, With Late Onset, With Depressed Mood
	290.43	Vascular Dementia, With Depressed Mood
Axis II	V71.09	No diagnosis
Axis III	331.0	Alzheimer's disease
	436	Cerebrovascular accident
Axis IV		None
Axis V	GAF = 31	(on admission)

Reggie Ansnes

When he was 35, Reggie Ansnes was admitted to a mental hospital 3,000 miles from home. The admitting note reported that he was agitated, was somewhat grandiose, and didn't even know what city he was in. Although he talked a lot, nothing he said made much sense. "I have Schizophrenia," was one of his few unambiguous statements.

"It must be his Schizophrenia," said his wife on the telephone to the clinician who admitted him. "He told me he had it once before. We've only been married three years."

Five years earlier, Reggie had been admitted with psychosis to a mental hospital in Boston. His wife thought that he had believed he was the son of Jesus, but she didn't know anything else about his symptoms. A doctor had told him he had Schizophrenia of the Paranoid Type. He had been treated with chlorpromazine; she knew that because he was still taking it when they began dating.

For about two years after that hospitalization, Reggie had been somewhat depressed. He used to complain of trouble concentrating at work, and his wife knew that not long after he was discharged from the hospital he had had suicidal ideas. However, the depression had gradually remitted, leaving him with relatively mild problems with appetite and sleep. Even these had resolved about the time they got married, and he had been well ever since. It had now been several years since he had taken any medication at all.

For several days before Reggie left on his business trip, he had seemed unusually cheerful. He talked a lot, seemed to have more energy than usual, and arose early to get caught up with the work he would miss while he was gone.

Reggie's wife stated that her husband was in good physical health except for a "slight thyroid condition." He took a small dose of a thyroid medication; she thought that he had had it checked the last time he visited his doctor, three months earlier. He didn't drink or use drugs, to her knowledge.

Admission blood testing included a thyroid level and a toxicity screen for drugs and alcohol. During his first day in the hospital, Reggie was extremely hyperactive and did not sleep at all. His mood was markedly elevated, and his rapid speech was often unintelligible. His statements that could be understood included "I am the son of God," and he shared some ideas for improving the operation of the hospital. He paid little attention to whatever task was at hand, so the Mini-Mental State Exam could not be completed.

Evaluation of Reggie Ansnes

Thyroid disease is a general medical condition that can cause mood symptoms; however, Reggie's physician had recently evaluated his thyroid condition, and it had never before produced symptoms that resembled his current condition. Re-evaluation of thyroid function tests would be a reasonable course to follow, in any event (Rule A).

As for substance use, the history from Reggie's wife would militate against **Substance-Induced Psychotic Disorder, With Onset During Withdrawal**. However, the blood toxicity screen should rule out the possibility of such a psychosis **With Onset During Intoxication** (e.g., Phencyclidine Intoxication). With the other history available, this would seem highly unlikely. It is much more usual for patients to use alcohol to attenuate the uncomfortable, driven feeling caused by mania or other psychosis.

A mood disorder would seem a much stronger possibility. Five years earlier, Reggie had had grandiose delusions; afterward, he had been depressed for months or years. After a two-year period of apparent complete normality, he had once again become psychotic, with elevated mood, hyperactivity, insomnia (a decreased need for sleep), and distractibility. Assuming that the tests for thyroid function and toxic screen were normal, he would completely fulfill the criteria for a **Manic Episode**, and thus for **Bipolar I Disorder, Most Recent Episode Manic**.

The previous history of Schizophrenia might appear to provide a ready-made diagnosis for this obviously psychotic patient. If Reggie's earlier illness really had been Schizophrenia (Paranoid or Undifferentiated Type), until the current episode it would have carried the specifier **Single Episode In Full Remission**. In any case this would be highly unusual, and would not be possible at all if mood symptoms had been as prominent then as they were now. Any current Schizophrenia diagnosis would have to be listed as **Provisional** until symptoms had been present for at least six months. An apparent mood disorder now and Schizophrenia years ago would violate the parsimony rule (Rule B), as well as the basic criteria for Schizophrenia.

The fourth- and fifth-digit codes listed below are self-explanatory. Reggie's previous Schizophrenia diagnosis was simply wrong, and should be expunged from his records. The second GAF score was added to emphasize the acute nature of his symptoms.

Axis I	296.44	Bipolar I Disorder, Most Recent Episode Manic, Severe With Mood-Congruent Psychotic Features, With Full Interepisode Recovery
Axis II	V71.09	No diagnosis
Axis III	244.9	Acquired hypothyroidism
Axis IV		None
Axis V	GAF = 30	(on admission)
	GAF = 90	(highest level past year)

Jeremy Dowling

"I feel miserable," was the chief complaint of Jeremy Dowling, a 24-year-old graduate student. Jeremy was a lifelong perfectionist, and a thesis deadline two weeks away wasn't improving matters. He was weeks behind schedule, partly because he needed to perfect every paragraph before he began to write the next. Most of the time since his teen years, he had felt "not good enough" and somewhat depressed. He had never had a Manic Episode. He was socially withdrawn and claimed never to take much pleasure in things. "I'm a pessimist, more or less," he said.

Jeremy described his appetite as being fine, and he had never had suicidal ideas: "Life is too meaningful, and I'm wasting it." His sleep, however, was another matter. With the approaching thesis deadline, he felt that he had to stay up most nights in order to do his work. Therefore, he drank lots of coffee. "If I have to sleep less than eight hours a night, I drink a cup every two or three hours. When I'm up all night, it's four or five cups. *Strong* coffee." Other than coffee, Jeremy denied ever misusing substances such as alcohol or street drugs.

Lately, Jeremy had stayed up all night three nights a week; he always felt tired. He also admitted to chronic feelings of guilt and irritability. He had never had crying spells, but his concentration was "a lifelong major problem." For example, while he was working at the computer other thoughts and worries intruded upon his consciousness, to the point that he had difficulty getting his work done.

Jeremy complained of anxiety. Toward the end of supper, for example, he would begin to worry about the amount of work he had to do. He would feel a knot in his stomach, and the world would seem to be closing in. He felt no better at one time or day or another, but he did improve briefly once he turned in a major assignment such as a term paper. However, he denied ever having problems with shortness of breath, muscle twitching, or palpitations of his heart, unless he had had an extraordinarily large amount of coffee. At those times, he also would notice that he felt nervous and often had an upset stomach, sometimes to the point that he had to stay home from class. He never had a feeling of impending doom or disaster.

Jeremy had always been a list maker, but did not describe any obsessional thinking or compulsive behavior. ("I do sometimes straighten out my sock drawer," he was careful to point out.) He described himself as a person who had always had difficulty making decisions, even to the point that he couldn't discard worthless things that he no longer needed—an Easter basket from when he was 10, for example.

Jeremy was born in Brazil, where his father had been studying insects of the rain forests. The family returned to live in southern California when Jeremy was four. His mother was a professional harpist; she had been in therapy with one counselor or another for 25 years. She had always been somewhat dour and had never gotten much pleasure out of life. When Jeremy was 16, she had obtained a divorce because she had never felt that her husband was committed to their relationship. After the divorce, she had changed to such an extent that she had finally consented to take an antidepressant medication. It had "turned her life around," and now she was happy for the first time in her life. It was partly at her urging that Jeremy was now seeking treatment.

Several maternal relatives had had depression, including a cousin who'd killed himself by drinking antifreeze. Another relative had also committed suicide, but Jeremy did not know the details.

When Jeremy was in high school, he had been "born again"; since then he had attended a strongly fundamentalist church. He strongly condemned his father for living with another woman without marrying her; for over two years, father and son hadn't spoken. Jeremy's only physical problem was that he chewed his nails. He had never had any legal difficulties. He had a serious girlfriend, and they were "trying very hard" to refrain from overcommitting themselves sexually until they got married.

Jeremy was a tall, rather gangling man whose haggard face and baggy eyes made him look over 30. Although he moved normally and smiled readily, prominent worry lines were emerging on his forehead. His speech was clear, coherent, relevant, and spontaneous. When he talked spontaneously, it was largely to discuss his concerns about getting his thesis done; he denied any death wishes or suicidal ideas. He was fully oriented, had an excellent fund of information, and could do calculations quickly. His recent and remote memory were unimpaired; his insight and judgment were excellent.

Evaluation of Jeremy Dowling

In evaluating any mood disorder, the first business at hand is to determine whether either a **Major Depressive** or **Manic Episode** has been present. Jeremy came close to satisfying criteria for the former: He had been "somewhat depressed" for a long time, perhaps most of his adult life. The depression was present most of the time, and he never took much pleasure in things; He felt chronically guilty and had poor concentration and low self-esteem. However, from history and direct observation he had had no problems with appetite or weight, suicidal ideas, or level of psychomotor activity. Although he did complain of fatigue, this symptom appeared related to his coffee drinking. His family history was strongly positive for a mood disorder (his mother had been depressed, and two relatives had committed suicide).

Jeremy had four symptoms (five required) of Major Depressive Episode, and two symptoms (two required) of **Dysthymic Disorder**, which cannot be diagnosed in the presence of a Major Depressive Episode (at least not for the first two years). But is it reasonable to insist that a patient *exactly* fulfill the criteria? After all, Jeremy *nearly* met criteria for Major Depressive Episode, and his family history *was* strongly positive. A diagnosis of **Major Depressive Disorder** would point the way to treatment and alert clinicians to possible worsening symptoms (such as suicidal ideas) later on. But this clinician felt that it was more important to emphasize the prolonged course of Jeremy's symptoms, which seemed almost to shade into his personality disorder (see below). Dysthymic Disorder often sets the stage for later Major Depressive Disorder; the two together are sometimes called *double depression*. Here is an area where two excellent diagnosticians may disagree forever.

Jeremy had never had anxiety attacks, phobias, obsessions, or compulsions. He had had a good deal of anxiety, however, and was worried about a variety of things—school, his personality, the intensity of his relationship with his girlfriend. He complained of fatiguability, troubles with his sleep, and concentration, which would seem (barely) enough to qualify for a diagnosis of **Generalized Anxiety Disorder**. However, it is vital to know that his symptoms did not occur solely during the course of a mood disorder. He definitely had some sort of mood disorder, which had persisted throughout the time he had anxiety symptoms. Therefore, his clinician felt that no concurrent anxiety diagnosis could be made.

As for substance use, although Jeremy had never used alcohol or street drugs, his coffee use had on many occasions produced nervousness, upset stomach, palpitations, muscle twitching, and insomnia. These were sometimes serious enough that he couldn't go to school; the symptoms would qualify for a diagnosis of **Caffeine Intoxication**. An additional diagnosis of **Caffeine Dependence** would hardly ever be warranted.

Finally, self-described as a perfectionistic pessimist who chronically felt he was not good enough, Jeremy was also a list maker and a drawer straightener. He also had trouble making decisions and couldn't discard things. These features, plus his moralistic condemnation of his father, would be diagnostic of **Obsessive–Compulsive Personality Disorder**.

Jeremy's Dysthymic Disorder appeared to have begun years ago, probably when he was still a teenager. He did qualify for **With Atypical Features** (hypersomnia, increased appetite), which is the only episode specifier you can give in Dysthymic Disorder. An Axis IV problem was noted because it could affect management, at least for the next two weeks. His GAF was scored on the basis of his combined Axis I and II disorders.

Axis I	300.4	Dysthymic Disorder, Early Onset
	305.90	Caffeine Intoxication
Axis II	301.4	Obsessive–Compulsive Personality Disorder
Axis III		None
Axis IV		Thesis deadline
Axis V	GAF = 65	(current)

Cookie Coates

Cookie was a 23-year-old single woman who was admitted to a mental health unit with the chief complaint of "seeing spiders."

According to the records, the doctor had been late for Cookie's birth, which a nurse had tried to hold back by pressure on her head. "I don't know if it would have made any difference, anyway," her mother reportedly told a social worker at the time. "I had measles during my pregnancy."

Whatever the cause, Cookie was slow to develop. She walked at 18 months, spoke words at two years, and uttered sentences at three. She was a withdrawn, frightened child who clung so tightly to her mother that she could not even be left with a babysitter. She did not begin school until she was nearly seven. With an IQ that hovered in the low 70s, she attended special classes for her first two years, and was then "mainstreamed" into regular classes.

In her early school years, Cookie developed a reputation for biting and kicking other children. When she was 11, she was disciplined on a number of occasions for stealing (and eating) lunches belonging to other children. At about the same time, she began to pull out her hair. She would generally pull only a few strands at a time from the front of her head, but worked away at it assiduously throughout the day. By the end of the school day, there would be little accumulations of hair all around her desk.

However, it was Cookie's persistent tendency to hurt and mutilate herself that first brought her into mental health care. At nine, she bit her lip until it bled. The following year, she gradually fell into the habit of repeatedly banging her forearms on the edge of a table; this produced chronic swelling and bruising, and eventually a constantly running sore. When she was 13, she cut long troughs in her face with a razor and then rubbed dirt into the wounds, producing a permanent, hypertrophic scar.

Several of these episodes prompted admission to mental health facilities. Most of them were for short stays, but once, when she was 16 and set fire to her pantyhose, she was kept for four months. During this admission it was learned that from the age of seven, Cookie had been sexually molested almost weekly by her father and two older brothers. She was subsequently admitted to the first in a series of group homes for the developmentally disabled.

Cookie's pattern in each of these facilities was to form an immediate, strong relationship with one or more staff members, especially males. Typically, she would call one of them "Daddy." When a staff member disappointed her (as inevitably each of them did), she would say that she hated the staffer. This animosity could last for weeks, during which she would sometimes sulk and say she was depressed, sometimes lose her temper and throw things in her room. At still other times she would accuse her counselors of conspiring to drive her crazy, so they could return her to the hospital. As she became more familiar with a facility, she would request special privileges (extra food at supper, staying up late) and injure herself in some dramatic way when it was not forthcoming.

Cookie was also found to engage in episodes of sexual acting out. During parties or other activities with patients from the men's group home, she would lie with her head in the lap of nearly any male patient or run her hand between his thighs. Repeated cautioning and counseling from her own staff counselors did nothing to eliminate this sort of behavior; it only caused her to become more cautious about where and when she did it. Also in the various group homes, she was noted to be prone to episodes of opportunistic binge eating. She habitually ate large quantities for each meal. But she also ate from the plates of others when they were finished, to the point that she often volunteered to clear away the table, even when it was not her turn. None of the staffers who provided information to the admitting clinician were aware of any self-induced vomiting or use of laxatives. They described her activity level while she was in her most recent group home as "couch potato."

On admission to the unit, Cookie was an obese woman who wore no makeup and was dressed in a sweat shirt and sweat pants. She fiddled with strands of her hair; although she did not pull any out during the interview, there were several patches the size of a half-dollar on her scalp where she was nearly bald. She denied feeling a sense of either tension or relief in regard to her hair pulling. She sat quietly, showing no evidence of abnormal movements, and cooperated with the examiner. She said that she felt "hopeless," and her mood showed a decreased lability and appeared appropriate to these thoughts. She spoke slowly and did not volunteer information, but she always responded to questions. Her thinking was sequential and goal-oriented, with no evidence of loose associations.

Cookie reported occasionally seeing "showers of spiders" falling from the ventilator in the ceiling of her bedroom. For several years she had intermittently heard voices directing her to harm herself. She usually noticed them when she was unhappy. They were quite clearly audible, were not the voices of anyone she knew, and were located within her own head. Upon close questioning, she agreed that they could be her own thoughts. She did not think anyone else could hear them. She talked freely about the sexual abuse she had suffered from her father and brothers, and described it in graphic (and seemingly accurate) detail. However, close questioning failed to reveal evidence of either reliving or repressing these experiences.

Cookie scored 28 out of 30 on the Mini-Mental State Exam (she could remember only two of three objects at five minutes, and missed the correct date by several days). Although she maintained good attention, she could only perform very simple calculations. She recognized that there was something wrong with her, but attributed it to others: her parents and a worker at her previous residence who had "dissed" (disrespected) her by laughing when she said she heard voices. She did not feel she needed to be in the hospital, and said that she would like to get her own apartment and a job as a waitress.

Evaluation of Cookie Coates

Cookie presented with a wide variety of clinical problems and symptoms, potentially encompassing psychotic, mood, anxiety, impulse-control, eating, and personality disorders, as well as mental subnormality.

Let us consider the mental subnormality first. Cookie was slow to develop and consistently had IQ scores that were in the very low 70s. She performed well on the Mini-Mental State Exam and had no problems with attention, so she would not seem to qualify for a cognitive disorder such as a **delirium** or **dementia**. She could be diagnosed as having the V-coded (V62.89) **Borderline Intellectual Functioning**, but her clinician felt that the extent of her deficits (problems with self-care, home living, social/interpersonal skills, self-direction, and safety) warranted a diagnosis of **Mild Mental Retardation**.

Other disorders can now be considered. Cookie reported feeling hopeless and **depressed**, but these symptoms appeared to be transitory, reactive to her circumstances, and to some extent manipulative. Symptoms of **psychosis** (seeing spiders, hearing voices) did not carry the conviction of true hallucinations: They often occurred when she was unhappy, and she noted that the voices could be her own thoughts. She had no loose associations, catatonic behavior, or negative symptoms typical of **Schizophrenia**. In fact, no psychotic diagnosis seemed justified. Although she ate in binges, there was no history of vomiting or use of laxatives or diuretics, and her self-evaluation did not overemphasize her weight or body shape. One clinician felt that her history had some of the features of **Posttraumatic Stress Disorder**, but she had no history of reliving the sexual abuse she had endured as a child.

Cookie's acting-out behaviors included biting, kicking, hair pulling, and stealing, which began when she was about 11. These behaviors did not appear to be part of a larger problem with violating societal norms or the rights of others, ruling out **Conduct Disorder**. The hair pulling was not associated with the tension-and-release phenomenon, so **Trichotillomania** could not be diagnosed. Self-injury can be encountered in **Stereotypic Movement Disorder**, but Cookie's behavior did not appear to be repetitive and stereotypical. Rather, most of her self-destructive behaviors seemed better explained by **Borderline Personality Disorder**. Beginning in her teens and affecting many life areas, the relevant symptoms included self-harm, intense interpersonal relations (those with various staff members), impulsivity (eating, sexual acting out), reactive mood (temper tantrums), and paranoid ideation.

Although Cookie did not have all the symptoms of Borderline Personality Disorder, those she did have were specified as **Severe**. The GAF was scored as a composite of all of her difficulties.

Axis I	317	Mild Mental Retardation
Axis II	301.83	Borderline Personality Disorder, Severe
Axis III	278.0	Obesity
Axis IV		None
Axis V	GAF = 30	(current)

Dean Wannamaker

"I keep hearing voices that I can't turn off," said Dean Wannamaker. They bothered him every day, and he wasn't sure how much longer he could stand it.

Dean was 54, but he had first heard voices when he was only in his early 40s. In fact, he had been hospitalized on three separate occasions, but each time he had been successfully treated with medication. It had now been over six years since he was last hospitalized.

"They're in my head, but they sound just as loud and clear as a radio," Dean said. The voices were mostly men, but there were a few women as well. He didn't recognize any of them. They spoke only phrases, not sentences, but they seemed to be trying to order him around. They would tell him that it was time to go home or that it would be okay to have another drink. "Mostly, they seemed to be looking out for me." He thought that he'd been hearing them for about three weeks this time.

Dean admitted that he was a drinker. He had begun drinking sweet wine when he was only 12. In the military he had had a few fights and was even threatened with court-martial once, but he'd managed to "escape with an honorable discharge." Over the years, he'd been arrested several times for driving while under the influence of alcohol; the most recent time was only two weeks ago.

Dean's usual pattern was to drink heavily for several months, then stop suddenly and stay dry for years. His three previous benders had occurred 3, 5, and 11 years earlier, respectively. The bender 11 years ago was when his wife had walked out on him for good; she was tired of paying his traffic tickets and supporting him when he got fired for missing work. He'd had a girlfriend, Annie—the same one he was with now—so he didn't mind so much about his wife. What he remembered most vividly was the time he'd heard voices for nearly three months. "It was enough to drive a man to drink," he commented, without a trace of irony.

On the present occasion the IRS had "driven him to drink." He made good money at his trade (he was a meat cutter), and, apparently in the throes of his last bender three years before, he had neglected to report some of it. Now he was being dunned for back taxes, penalties and interest, and he didn't even have any records.

"This time I didn't intend to start drinking," he said. "I only meant to take a drink." Now he had been drinking over a quart of bourbon a day for two months. Annie added that he never seemed drunk, and confirmed that he only had these hallucinations after he'd been drinking for a while.

The middle of three children, Dean had been born in Chicago, where his father worked as a meat salesman. His parents had divorced when he was only nine; his mother had remarried twice. In the course of a depression four years earlier, his older brother had shot himself to death. His sister was a nurse who had once been hospitalized for abusing barbiturates.

After the military, Dean had attended two years of junior college, but he didn't think it ever did him much good. "I've never been anything more than a big, dumb city slicker who cuts up dead animals for a living," he said.

Annie reported that Dean had been depressed most of the time for the last month and a half—not quite as long as he'd been drinking. He had cried some and slept poorly, often awakening early in the morning, unable to get back to sleep. His appetite had diminished, and he'd lost about 20 pounds. He seemed chronically tired and his sex interest was diminished, except when he was drunk, which was most of the time.

Dean looked closer to 60 than to 54. He had clearly lost weight. He was over six feet tall, but his outsized clothes seemed to diminish his size. He slumped quietly in his chair and only spoke when spoken to. His voice was a low monotone, but his speech was relevant and coherent. He was fully alert, and he paid close attention to the conversation. There was very little variation in his mood, which he admitted was depressed. He was fully oriented to time, place, and person; he scored 29 of 30 on the Mini-Mental State Exam, failing only to recall a street address after five minutes. He had never had delusions, but neither did he seem to have any insight into the fact that what he heard was not real.

Dean had had some thoughts about dying. They had begun with the depression, and now the voices had jumped on the idea. "They aren't ordering me to do it or anything like that," he said. "They just think I might be a lot better off."

Evaluation of Dean Wannamaker

To begin with, what were Dean's diagnosable drinking behaviors? Of course, he had many of the social symptoms (divorce, arrests) required for a diagnosis of **Alcohol Abuse**. But would he meet the stricter criteria for **Alcohol Depen-**

dence? During the current episode of drinking, he demonstrated tolerance (he didn't appear drunk on a quart per day of hard liquor), continued to drink despite having hallucinations, and used more alcohol than he intended ("I only meant to take a drink"). Even if withdrawal symptoms were not taken into account, he would qualify for a diagnosis of Alcohol Dependence. He had been actively drinking within the past month, so he could have no course specifier.

Dean's somatic complaints included appetite and weight loss, reduced libido, and insomnia. These represent three separate DSM-IV categories (eating, sleep, and sexual disorders), and a differential diagnosis could be constructed for each. However, the resulting burden of independent Axis I diagnoses would be highly unlikely, from either a statistical or a logical viewpoint (Rule B). These somatic complaints can all be found in patients who have depression, psychosis, or alcohol-related disorders. A **Mood Disorder Due to a General Medical Condition** must always be considered, especially in a patient who has been ignoring health needs (Rule A). A physical examination and laboratory tests would be needed to rule out such conditions as hypothyroidism and others listed in Appendix B. However, no information given in the vignette suggests that Dean had any such medical disorder.

Throughout his later adult life, Dan had intermittently heard voices. A principal concern for any psychotic patient is whether **Schizophrenia** is a possibility. But Dean lacked the "A" portion of the basic criteria. He had hallucinations but no other symptoms (though his affect was constricted, this was probably due to the depression). Annie pointed out that he only had hallucinations after he had been drinking. The lack of "A" criteria would also rule out **Schizophreniform** and **Schizoaffective Disorders**. The results of his Mini-Mental State Exam would rule out **delirium** and **dementia**; the history would exclude **Psychotic Disorder Due to a General Medical Condition**. Of course, all other psychotic disorders require that the symptoms not be directly related to the use of a substance. Furthermore, neither **Delusional Disorder** nor **Brief Psychotic Disorder** can be diagnosed if a mood disorder is more likely.

Look at the criteria for **Substance-Induced Psychotic Disorder** in Chapter 4. These require prominent hallucinations or delusions. If hallucinations are present, the patient (like Dean) must not have insight that they are caused by the substance. Inasmuch as Dean always drank before the hallucinations appeared and they never lasted longer than a few weeks after the drinking stopped, he would seem to fulfill the criteria for an **Alcohol-Induced Psychotic Disorder, With Hallucinations**. If this became the working diagnosis, the qualifier **With Onset During Withdrawal** would have to be added.

As for mood disorder, Dean fulfilled the inclusion criteria for **Major Depressive Episode**: six weeks of persistent low mood, fatigue, weight loss, insomnia, and thoughts of suicide. His symptoms represented a change from his usual self and were distressing. They were not the result of **Bereavement**. However, they did occur subsequent to the time he began drinking, and therefore *could* be alcohol-related; if so, this would rule out **Major Depressive Disorder**.

The criteria for **Substance-Induced Mood Disorder** are simple. Dean would appear to fulfill them: He was persistently depressed, he had been intoxicated for several months, and the symptoms caused him distress. He fulfilled none of the several bits of evidence the criteria mention that would support a non-substance-related depression. Although his brother had shot himself during a depression, we do not know whether he was also a drinker; a sister had used drugs.

Major Depressive Disorder is treatable, and it can be lethal. It should be given a high priority for investigation and possible treatment (Rule E). However, it should not be diagnosed automatically in a substance-using patient; many instances of mood disorder will improve with cessation of the substance use.

Therefore, symptoms of substance use, mood disorder, and psychosis must be accounted for in Dean's final diagnosis. It would not appear that cognitive or general medical conditions can explain these symptoms (Rule A). It would be elegant to explain all of them simply, on the basis of one underlying disease mechanism (Rule B). Because substance use was surely the first of these symptom groups to appear (Rule C)—Dean began drinking at age 12 and had some behavioral problems resulting from it when he was a young man in the military—it is reasonable to consider it first.

Now we have two ways of looking at Dean's symptoms: (1) Alcohol Dependence induced a psychosis *and* he had an independent Major Depressive Disorder; (2) Alcohol Dependence induced both a psychosis and a mood disorder. Unhappily, Rule D doesn't help us: Dean's family had both substance use and depression. But the simplicity of the second formulation, plus the desire not to rush in with possibly unnecessary treatment before it is needed, would lead a conservative clinician initially to regard the mood disorder as substance-induced—at least until Dean could be withdrawn completely from alcohol. The clinician's perception that the alcoholism was the underlying problem, and thus the one that should be addressed first, would determine the order of diagnoses on Axis I:

Axis I	303.90	Alcohol Dependence
	291.3	Alcohol-Induced Psychotic Disorder, With Hallucinations, With Onset During Withdrawal
	291.8	Alcohol-Induced Mood Disorder, With Depressive Features, With Onset During Intoxication
Axis II	V71.09	No diagnosis
Axis III		None
Axis IV		None
Axis V	GAF = 40	(current)

TIP While writing up these cases histories, I was struck by the difficulty of getting onto paper the way clinicians think. The problem is that of describing parallel processing. Experienced clinicians tend not to think sequentially but to consider many factors all at once. For example, in interviewing Dean Wannamaker, I considered general medical conditions, substance-induced disorders, primary mood and psychotic disorders almost simultaneously. This is an ability that most clinicians develop with experience—some time after their first 200 interviews. Clearly, you will be needing a lot of patience.

Appendix A. Global Assessment of Functioning (GAF) Scale

Consider psychological, social, and occupational functioning on a hypothetical continuum of mental health–illness. Do not include impairment in functioning due to physical (or environmental) limitations.

Code   (**Note:** Use intermediate numbers when appropriate, e.g., 45, 68, 72.)

100
| **Superior functioning in a wide range of activities, life's problems never seem to get out of hand, is sought by others because of his or her many positive qualities. No symp-**
91   **toms.**

90   Absent or minimal symptoms (e.g., mild anxiety before an exam), **good functioning in all**
| **areas, interested and involved in a wide range of activities, socially effective, generally**
| **satisfied with life, no more than everyday problems or concerns** (e.g., an occasional argu-
81   ment with family members).

80   **If symptoms are present, they are transient and expectable reactions to psychosocial**
| **stressors** (e.g., difficulty concentrating after family argument); **no more than slight impair-**
| **ment in social, occupational, or school functioning** (e.g., temporarily falling behind in
71   schoolwork).

70   Some mild symptoms (e.g., depressed mood and mild insomnia) **OR some difficulty in so-**
| **cial, occupational, or school functioning** (e.g., occasional truancy, or theft within the house-
| hold), **but generally functioning pretty well, has some meaningful interpersonal rela-**
61   **tionships.**

60   Moderate symptoms (e.g., flat affect and circumstantial speech, occasional panic attacks)
| **OR moderate difficulty in social, occupational, or school functioning** (e.g., few friends,
51   conflicts with peers or co-workers).

50   Serious symptoms (e.g., suicidal ideation, severe obsessional rituals, frequent shoplifting)
| **OR any serious impairment in social, occupational, or school functioning** (e.g., no friends,
41   unable to keep a job).

40   **Some impairment in reality testing or communication** (e.g., speech is at times illogical,
| obscure, or irrelevant) **OR major impairment in several areas, such as work or school,**
| **family relations, judgment, thinking, or mood** (e.g., depressed man avoids friends, ne-
| glects family, and is unable to work; child frequently beats up younger children, is defiant at
31   home, and is failing at school).

30   **Behavior is considerably influenced by delusions or hallucinations OR serious impair-**
| **ment in communication or judgment** (e.g., sometimes incoherent, acts grossly inappropri-
| ately, suicidal preoccupation) **OR inability to function in almost all areas** (e.g., stays in bed
21   all day; no job, home, or friends).

20   Some danger of hurting self or others (e.g., suicide attempts without clear expectation of
| death; frequently violent; manic excitement) **OR occasionally fails to maintain minimal**
| **personal hygiene** (e.g., smears feces) **OR gross impairment in communication** (e.g., largely
11   incoherent or mute).

10   **Persistent danger of severely hurting self or others** (e.g., recurrent violence) **OR persis-**
| **tent inability to maintain minimal personal hygiene OR serious suicidal act with clear**
1   **expectation of death.**

0   Inadequate information.

Note. Reprinted by permission from the *Diagnostic and Statistical Manual of Mental Disorders*, 4th ed. (p. 32), by the American Psychiatric Association, 1994, Washington, DC: Author. Copyright 1994 by the American Psychiatric Association.

Appendix B. General Medical Disorders as They Affect Mental Diagnosis

Medical disorder	Anx	Depr	Mania	Psych	Delir	Dem	Cata	Pers Chng	Erect	Ejac	Dyspar	Anorg
Cardiovascular												
Anemia	X											
Angina	X											
Aortic aneurysm									X			
Arrhythmia	X				X							
Arteriovenous malformation							X					
Congestive heart failure	X				X				X			
Hypertension	X				X							
Myocardial infarction	X											
Mitral valve prolapse	X											
Paroxysmal atrial tachycardia	X											
Shock	X				X							
Endocrine												
Addison's	X	X			X				X			
Carcinoid	X											
Cushing's	X	X	X		X			X				
Diabetes	X								X			X
Hyperparathyroidism						X						
Hyperthyroidism	X	X	X		X				X			
Hypoglycemia	X	X			X	X						
Hypoparathyroidism	X	X										
Hypothyroidism	X	X		X		X		X	X			X
Inappropriate ADH					X							
Klinefelter's									X			
Menopause	X										X	
Pancreatic tumor		X										
Pheochromocytoma	X											
Premenstrual syndrome	X											
Hyperprolactinemia												X
Infections												
AIDS	X	X	X			X		X				
Brain abscess					X							
Subacute bacterial endocarditis	X											
Syphilis						X						
Systemic infection	X				X							

Appendix B. *(cont'd)*

Medical disorder	Anx	Depr	Mania	Psych	Delir	Dem	Cata	Pers Chng	Erect	Ejac	Dyspar	Anorg
Urinary tract infection					X							
Vaginitis											X	
Viral infection		X										
Toxicity												
Aminophylline					X							
Anticholinergics	X			X	X							
Anticonvulsants				X								
Antidepressants				X	X				X	X		X
Antihypertensives				X					X	X		X
Antiparkinsonians				X					X	X		
Antipsychotics					X				X	X		X
Aspirin intolerance	X											
Bromide				X								
Cimetidine					X							
Digitalis					X							
Disulfiram				X	X							
Estrogens									X			
Fluorides							X					
Heavy metals	X	X										
Herbicides									X			
L-dopa					X							
Muscle relaxants				X								
Nonsteriodal anti-inflammatory agents				X								
Steroids				X								
Theophylline	X											
Metabolic												
Electrolyte imbalance	X				X							
Hepatic disease		X			X	X			X			
Hypercarbia					X							
Hyperventilation	X											
Hypocalcemia	X											
Hypokalemia	X	X										
Hypoxia					X							
Malnutrition		X			X				X			
Porphyria	X							X				
Renal disease	X				X	X			X			
Neurological												
Alzheimer-Pick						X						
Amyotrophic lateral sclerosis						X			X			
Brain tumor	X				X	X	X	X	X			

Appendix B. *(cont'd)*

Medical disorder	Anx	Depr	Mania	Psych	Delir	Dem	Cata	Pers Chng	Erect	Ejac	Dyspar	Anorg
Cerebellar degeneration						X						
Cerebrovascular accident	X							X				
Encephalitis	X				X	X	X					
Epilepsy, seizures	X	X			X	X		X				
Extradural hematoma					X							
Head trauma	X				X	X	X	X				
Huntington's	X	X				X		X				
Intracerebral hematoma					X							
Jakob-Creutzfeldt						X						
Meniere's	X											
Meningitis					X							
Migraine	X											
Multiple sclerosis	X	X	X			X		X	X			
Multi-infarct						X						
Neurosyphilis			X		X	X		X	X			
Normal-pressure hydrocephalus						X						
Parkinson's						X			X			X
Postanoxia						X						
Progressive supra-nuclear palsy						X						
Spinal cord disease									X			
Subarachnoid hemorrhage					X		X					
Subdural hematoma					X	X	X					
Transient ischemic attack	X				X							
Wilson's	X							X				
Other												
Collagen	X											
Endometriosis											X	
Pelvic disease									X		X	X
Peyronie's disease									X			
Postoperative states					X							
Systemic lupus erythematosis	X	X		X	X			X				
Temporal arteritis	X											
Pulmonary												
Asthma	X											
Chronic obstructive lung disease	X				X				X			
Hyperventilation	X											
Pulmonary embolus	X											

Appendix B. *(cont'd)*

Medical disorder	Anx	Depr	Mania	Psych	Delir	Dem	Cata	Pers Chng	Erect	Ejac	Dyspar	Anorg
Vitamin Deficiency												
B^{12} (pernicious anemia)	X	X				X						
Folic acid						X						
Niacin (nicotinic) pellagra					X	X						
Thiamine (B^1) Wernicke's					X	X						

Note. Key to mental diagnoses: Anx, anxiety; Depr, depression; Mania, mania; Psych, psychosis; Delir, delirium; Dem, dementia; Cata, catatonia; Pers Chng, personality change; Erect, erectile disorder; Ejac, ejaculatory dysfunction; Dyspar, dyspareunia; Anorg, anorgasmia.

Appendix C. Mini-Mental State Exam

Maximum score	Score	
		Orientation
5	( )	What is the (year)(season)(date)(month)?
5	( )	Where are we? (state)(country)(town)(building)(floor)
		Registration
3	( )	Name three objects: Allow 1 second to say each. Then ask the patient all three after you have said them. Give 1 point for each correct answer. Then repeat them until all three are learned. Count trials and record.
		Trials_____
		Attention and Calculations
5	( )	Serial sevens. Give 1 point for each correct answer. Stop after five answers. Alternatively, spell *world* backward.
		Recall
3	( )	Ask for three objects repeated previously. Give 1 point for each correct.
		Language
9	( )	Name a pencil and watch. (2 points) Repeat the following: "No ifs, ands, or buts." (1 point) Follow a three-stage command: "Take a paper in your right hand, fold it in half, and put it on the floor." (3 points) Read and obey the following: "Close your eyes." (1 point) "Write a sentence." (1 point) "Copy a design." (1 point)
__Total score		

Assess level of consciousness: _____

Alert	Drowsy	Stupor	Coma

Index

Entries with **boldfaced** page numbers include DSM-IV diagnostic criteria.
Entries with *italicized* page numbers include a definition.